Dietary Fiber
and
Health

T0320951

Dietary Fiber
and
Health

Edited by
Susan S. Cho • Nelson Almeida

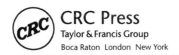
CRC Press
Taylor & Francis Group
Boca Raton London New York

CRC Press is an imprint of the
Taylor & Francis Group, an **informa** business

CRC Press
Taylor & Francis Group
6000 Broken Sound Parkway NW, Suite 300
Boca Raton, FL 33487-2742

First issued in paperback 2017

© 2012 by Taylor & Francis Group, LLC
CRC Press is an imprint of Taylor & Francis Group, an Informa business

No claim to original U.S. Government works

ISBN-13: 978-1-4398-9929-8 (hbk)
ISBN-13: 978-1-138-19979-8 (pbk)

Library of Congress Cataloging-in-Publication Data

Dietary fiber and health / Susan Cho, Nelson Almeida, editors.
    p. ; cm.
    Includes bibliographical references and index.
    ISBN 978-1-4398-9929-8 (hardcover : alk. paper)
    I. Cho, Sungsoo. II. Almeida, Nelson. III. Vahouny Fiber Symposium (9th : 2010 : Bethesda, Maryland)
    [DNLM: 1. Dietary Fiber--therapeutic use. 2. Dietary Fiber--analysis. 3. Nutritional Requirements. WB 427]

615.8'54--dc23   2012013737

Visit the Taylor & Francis Web site at
http://www.taylorandfrancis.com

and the CRC Press Web site at
http://www.crcpress.com

Contents

Preface

Fiber offers a variety of health benefits and is essential in reducing the risk of chronic diseases such as diabetes, obesity, cardiovascular disease, and diverticulitis. According to the Institute of Medicine (IOM), adequate intake (AI) of total fiber should be 14 g/1000 kcal. The IOM recommendation is joined by those from a variety of government public health agencies that promote increased fiber consumption, but a majority of people in developed countries still fall short of recommended values.

On average, Americans consume only half of the required intake, and approximately 90% of the U.S. population fails to meet AI goals. The problem stems largely from the fact that most conventional high-fiber foods are not tasty. Their organoleptic properties lack the kind of sensory attributes that people seek in the foods they eat. This makes it imperative for food companies to formulate tasty foods with high fiber content to improve population-wide consumption. Many have done so with new fiber ingredients that satisfy consumer demands while delivering the health benefits of fiber.

This book discusses findings from the Ninth Vahouny Fiber Symposium, which was held in Bethesda, Maryland, in June 2010. It includes a definition of fiber developed through expert consensus and delves into the many health benefits of fiber, including its prebiotic effects and roles in weight management, glycemic control, cardiovascular health, and intestinal regularity. It also reviews a variety of fiber ingredients that can be used in many appealing foods. The book provides details of claim opportunities for fiber ingredients and fiber-containing foods as well as a list of global suppliers of these ingredients. It is designed for use by food product developers, nutritionists, dietitians, and regulatory agencies.

Contributors

Nelson Almeida
The Kellogg Company
Battle Creek, Michigan

James W. Anderson
Department of Medicine
and
Department of Clinical Nutrition
University of Kentucky
Lexington, Kentucky

Nicolas Auriou
Nestlé Research Centre
Lausanne, Switzerland

David J. Baer
Agricultural Research Service
United States Department of
    Agriculture
Beltsville Human Nutrition Research
    Center
Beltsville, Maryland

Olivier Ballèvre
Nestlé R&D
Beijing, China

Sebastien Baray
Colloïdes Naturels International
Rouen, France

Jacqueline S. Barrett
Gastroenterology Department
Central Clinical School
Alfred Medical Research
    and Education Precinct
Monash University
Melbourne, Victoria, Australia

Victoria A. Betteridge
Tate & Lyle PLC
London, United Kingdom

J.R. Biesiekierski
Gastroenterology Department
Central Clinical School
Alfred Medical Research
    and Education Precinct
Monash University
Melbourne, Victoria, Australia

Anthony R. Bird
CSIRO Food and Nutritional Sciences
Adelaide, South Australia, Australia

Anne M. Birkett
Corn Products International
Westchester, Illinois

Charles T. Bonfield
Vahouny Symposia, Ret.
Delray Beach, Florida

Allan W. Buck
Archer Daniels Midland Company
Decatur, Illinois

Wim Caers
BENEO Group
Tienen, Belgium

Iris L. Case
NutraSource, Inc.
Clarksville, Maryland

Martine Champ
Institut National de la Recherche
    Agronomique
Centre de Recherche en Nutrition
    Humaine
Physiologie des Adaptations
    Nutritionnelles
Nantes, France

Jason A. Charrier
Louisiana State University
    Agricultural Center
Baton Rouge, Louisiana

Yu-Ting Chiu
Department of Human Nutrition,
    Food and Animal Science
University of Hawaii at Manoa
Honolulu, Hawaii

Susan S. Cho
NutraSource, Inc.
Clarksville, Maryland

Anthony E. Civitarese
John S. McIlhenny Laboratory
The Pennington Biomedical
    Research Center
Baton Rouge, Louisiana

and

Department of Metabolic Biology
Arizona State University
Tempe, Arizona

Emilie Combet
Centre for Population and Health
    Sciences
College of Medical, Veterinary and
    Life Sciences
Yorkhill Hospitals
Glasgow University
Glasgow, United Kingdom

Stuart A.S. Craig
Danisco A/S
Tarrytown, New York

Tyler Culpepper
Emerging Pathogens Institute
University of Florida
Gainesville, Florida

Jon DeVries
General Mills
and
ILSI-NA Carbohydrate Committee
    Chair
Minneapolis, Minnesota

Christine A. Edwards
Centre for Population and Health
    Sciences
College of Medical, Veterinary and
    Life Sciences
Yorkhill Hospitals
Glasgow University
Glasgow, United Kingdom

Hans Ulrich Endress
Herbstreith & Fox KG
Neuenbuerg, Germany

Marc Enslen
Nestlé Research Centre
Lausanne, Switzerland

Bassam Faress
Garuda International
Exeter, California

Véronique Ferchaud-Roucher
Centre de Recherche en Nutrition
    Humaine
Nantes, France

Juana Fernández-López
Agro-Food Technology Department
Miguel Hernández University
Alicante, Spain

Jürgen Fischer
Herbafood Ingredients GmbH
Werder, Germany

Laurent Flet
Centre de Recherche en Nutrition
Humaine
Nantes, France

Alice Fu
Shangdong Longlive
Qingdao, China

Evangélica Fuentes-Zaragoza
Agro-Food Technology Department
Miguel Hernández University
Alicante, Spain

Daniel D. Gallaher
Department of Food Science and
Nutrition
University of Minnesota
St. Paul, Minnesota

Ada L. Garcia
School of Medicine
College of Medical, Veterinary and
Life Sciences
Yorkhill Hospitals
Glasgow University
Glasgow, United Kingdom

Peter R. Gibson
Gastroenterology Department
Central Clinical School
Alfred Medical Research
and Education Precinct
Monash University
Melbourne, Victoria, Australia

Jean-Philippe Godin
Nestlé Research Centre
Lausanne, Switzerland

Felicia Goldsmith
Louisiana State University
Agricultural Center
Baton Rouge, Louisiana

Dennis T. Gordon
Matsutani Chemical Industry Co., Ltd.
Itami City, Japan

and

PIC&PC
Cathlamet, Washington

Laetitia Guérin-Deremaux
Roquette
Lestrem, France

Emma P. Halmos
Gastroenterology Department
Central Clinical School
Alfred Medical Research
and Education Precinct
Monash University
Melbourne, Victoria, Australia

Hiroshi Hara
Division of Applied Bioscience
Laboratory of Nutritional
Biochemistry
Graduate School of Agriculture
Hokkaido University
Sapporo, Japan

Robert Hesslink
Imagenetix, Inc.,
San Diego, California

John F. Howlett
Exponent International Limited
Derby, United Kingdom

Dan Inman
J. Rettenmaier USA LP
Schoolcraft, Michigan

Ajmila Islam
Department of Food Science and
Nutrition
University of Minnesota
St. Paul, Minnesota

Marlene Janes
Louisiana State University
    Agricultural Center
Baton Rouge, Louisiana

Manan Jhaveri
Department of Medicine
and
Department of Clinical Nutrition
University of Kentucky
Lexington, Kentucky

Julie Miller Jones
Department of Family
    Consumer and Nutritional Sciences
St. Catherine University
St. Paul, Minnesota

Sumiko Kanahori
Matsutani Chemical Industry Co., Ltd.
Itami City, Japan

Michael J. Keenan
Louisiana State University
    Agricultural Center
Baton Rouge, Louisiana

Kazunari Kitamori
College of Human Life and
    Environment
Kinjo Gakuin University
Nagoya, Japan

Tomoko Koda
Faculty of Human Life and Science
Doshisha Women's College of Liberal
    Arts
Kyōtanabe, Japan

Laura Kotowski
Department of Food Science and
    Nutrition
University of Minnesota
St. Paul, Minnesota

Michel Krempf
Centre de Recherche en Nutrition
    Humaine
Nantes, France

David W. Lafond
The Kellogg Company
Battle Creek, Michigan

Bobbi Langkamp-Henken
Food Science and Human Nutrition
    Department
University of Florida
Gainesville, Florida

Albert W. Lee
NutraSource, Inc.
Clarksville, Maryland

Catherine Lefranc-Millot
Roquette
Lestrem, France

Geoffrey Livesey
Independent Nutrition Logic Ltd.
Wymondham, Norfolk,
    United Kingdom

Joanne R. Lupton
Department of Nutrition and Food
    Science
Texas A&M University
College Station, Texas

Katherine Macé
Nestlé Research Centre
Lausanne, Switzerland

Valérie Macioce
Roquette
Lestrem, France

Volker Mai
Emerging Pathogens Institute
University of Florida
Gainesville, Florida

Kevin C. Maki
Provident Clinical Research
Glen Ellyn, Illinois

Roy J. Martin
Louisiana State University
 Agricultural Center
Baton Rouge, Louisiana

and

USDA Center
University of California-Davis
Davis, California

Ana Martin-Sánchez
Agro-Food Technology Department
Miguel Hernández University
Alicante, Spain

Satomi Maruyama
College of Human Life and
 Environment
Kinjo Gakuin University
Nagoya, Japan

Noriko Matsukawa
Division of Applied Bioscience
Laboratory of Nutritional
 Biochemistry
Graduate School of Agriculture
Hokkaido University
Sapporo, Japan

Megumi Matsumoto
Department of Physical Education
College of Humanities and Science
Nihon University
Tokyo, Japan

Frank Mattes
Herbstreith & Fox KG
Neuenbuerg, Germany

Bruce May
CSIRO Food and Nutritional Sciences
Adelaide, South Australia, Australia

Kathleen L. McCutcheon
Louisiana State University
 Agricultural Center
Baton Rouge, Louisiana

Agnes Meheust
ILSI
Brussels, Belgium

Diederick Meyer
Sensus BV
Roosendaal, the Netherlands

Shaylyn B. Mitchell
Gastroenterology Department
Central Clinical School
Alfred Medical Research
 and Education Precinct
Monash University
Melbourne, Victoria, Australia

Matthew K. Morell
CSIRO Food Futures Flagship
CSIRO Plant Industry
Australian Capital Territory, Australia

Jane G. Muir
Gastroenterology Department
Central Clinical School
Alfred Medical Research
 and Education Precinct
Monash University
Melbourne, Victoria, Australia

Mitsuko Naoi
Department of Food and Health
 Sciences
International College of Arts and
 Sciences
Fukuoka Women's University
Fukuoka, Japan

Casilda Navarro
Agro-Food Technology Department
Miguel Hernández University
Alicante, Spain

Julie-Anne Nazare
Department of Food Science and
    Nutrition
University of Minnesota
St. Paul, Minnesota

Theresa A. Nicklas
Department of Pediatrics
Children's Nutrition Research Center
Baylor College of Medicine
Houston, Texas

Stephanie Nishi
NutraSource, Inc.
Clarksville, Maryland

Mari Noborikawa
Faculty of Human Life Science
Mimasaka University
Okayama, Japan

Sen-ichi Oda
Department of Zoology
Okayama University of Science
Okayama, Japan

Kazuhiro Okuma
Matsutani Chemical Industry Co., Ltd.
Itami City, Japan

Carol E. O'Neil
Louisiana State University
    Agricultural Center
Baton Rouge, Louisiana

Derrick K. Ong
Gastroenterology Department
Central Clinical School
Alfred Medical Research
    and Education Precinct
Monash University
Melbourne, Victoria, Australia

Deirdre E. Ortiz
The Kellogg Company
Battle Creek, Michigan

Morine Paintin
Nestlé Research Centre
Lausanne, Switzerland

Jin-Hee Park
Seoul, Korea

José A. Pérez-Álvarez
Agro-Food Technology Department
Miguel Hernández University
Alicante, Spain

Etienne Pouteau
Nestlé Research Centre
Lausanne, Switzerland

Anne M. Raggio
Louisiana State University
    Agricultural Center
Baton Rouge, Louisiana

Rosemary Rose
Gastroenterology Department
Central Clinical School
Alfred Medical Research
    and Education Precinct
Monash University
Melbourne, Victoria, Australia

Ouriana Rosella
Gastroenterology Department
Central Clinical School
Alfred Medical Research
    and Education Precinct
Monash University
Melbourne, Victoria, Australia

Yolanda Ruiz-Navajas
Agro-Food Technology Department
Miguel Hernández University
Alicante, Spain

Elena Sánchez-Zapata
Agro-Food Technology Department
Miguel Hernández University
Alicante, Spain

Estrella Sayas-Barberá
Agro-Food Technology Department
Miguel Hernández University
Alicante, Spain

Esther Sendra
Agro-Food Technology Department
Miguel Hernández University
Alicante, Spain

Reshani Senevirathne
Louisiana State University
    Agricultural Center
Baton Rouge, Louisiana

Li Shen
Louisiana State University
    Agricultural Center
Baton Rouge, Louisiana

Susan J. Shepherd
Gastroenterology Department
Central Clinical School
Alfred Medical Research
    and Education Precinct
Monash University
Melbourne, Victoria, Australia

Joanne L. Slavin
Department of Food Science and
    Nutrition
University of Minnesota
St. Paul, Minnesota

Maria Stewart
Department of Human Nutrition,
    Food and Animal Science
University of Hawaii at Manoa
Honolulu, Hawaii

Hiroyuki Tagami
Matsutani Chemical Industry Co., Ltd.
Itami City, Japan

Toru Takahashi
Department of Food and Health
    Sciences
International College of Arts and
    Sciences
Fukuoka Women's University
Fukuoka, Japan

Miki Tokunaga
Department of Food and Health
    Sciences
International College of Arts and
    Sciences
Fukuoka Women's University
Fukuoka, Japan

David L. Topping
CSIRO Food and Nutritional Sciences
Adelaide, South Australia, Australia

Paula R. Trumbo
Center for Food Safety and Applied
    Nutrition
United States Food and Drug
    Administration
College Park, Maryland

Richard T. Tulley
Louisiana State University
    Agricultural Center
Baton Rouge, Louisiana

Maria Ukhanova
Emerging Pathogens Institute
University of Florida
Gainesville, Florida

Sylvia Usher
CSIRO Food and Nutritional Sciences
Adelaide, South Australia, Australia

Kirk Vidrine
Louisiana State University
    Agricultural Center
Baton Rouge, Louisiana

Manuel Viuda-Martos
Agro-Food Technology Department
Miguel Hernández University
Alicante, Spain

Cathy Williams
Louisiana State University
    Agricultural Center
Baton Rouge, Louisiana

Chu K. Yao
Gastroenterology Department
Central Clinical School
Alfred Medical Research
    and Education Precinct
Monash University
Melbourne, Victoria, Australia

Jianping Ye
Pennington Biomedical Research
    Center
Baton Rouge, Louisiana

Yassine Zair
Centre de Recherche en Nutrition
    Humaine
Nantes, France

June Zhou
Laboratory of Geriatric
    Endocrinology and Metabolism
Veterans Affairs Medical Center
Washington, District of Columbia

1

Reflections on 30 Years of the Vahouny Fiber Symposia

CHARLES T. BONFIELD

Contents

1.1 Introduction

The Vahouny Fiber Symposium is the preeminent international meeting on dietary fiber research. The meeting attracts leading international scientists who present and discuss the results of their current work in dietary fiber research. These symposia are usually 3 or 3-1/2 day meetings and have been held in Washington, DC, in 1981, 1984, 1988, 1992, 1996, 2000, and 2010. The proceedings of these symposia were published in six books (1981–1996) and a CD (2000 symposium).

A 1 day Vahouny Symposium on Dietary Fiber in Health and Disease was held in conjunction with Nutrition Adelaide 98, a joint meeting of the Australasian Clinical Nutrition Society and the Nutrition Society of Australia. The proceedings of this symposium were published in a special supplement of the *Asia Pacific Journal of Clinical Nutrition*, Vol. 8, 1999.

The Seventh International Vahouny Symposium was held at the Royal College of Physicians in Edinburgh, Scotland, in May 2002. The proceedings of this symposium were published in a special supplement to the *Proceedings of the Nutrition Society*, Vol. 62, No. 1, February 2003.

The (Eighth) Vahouny-ILSI Japan International Symposium on Non-Digestible Carbohydrate was held at the National Olympics Memorial Youth

1

Center in Tokyo, Japan, on September 2004. The proceedings of this symposium were published in the *Foods & Food Ingredients Journal of Japan*, Vol. 210, 2005.

In his foreword to Dietary Fiber: Basic and Clinical Aspects (the Proceedings of the Second Vahouny Fiber Symposium, 1984), Denis Burkitt began with the following comment: "Only 15 years ago a conference on dietary fiber, let alone an international conference, would have been considered extremely unlikely, and in fact an unthinkable event." Yet this "unthinkable event" has continued for 30 years.

Any review of the Vahouny Symposia must start with a memoriam to George Vartkas Vahouny, the originator of these symposia. Dr. Vahouny was professor of biochemistry at the George Washington University School of Medicine in Washington, DC, United States, and was one of the early investigators in the field of dietary fiber research. He conducted research into various aspects of the physiological effects of dietary fiber in the gastrointestinal tract and was published extensively. Most of his research used animal models that he had developed himself—he was also involved in several clinical research studies in humans. Dr. Vahouny's research interest was not limited to dietary fiber; he also conducted research studies and published a number of papers on dietary lipids and cholesterol. Dr. Vahouny was the organizer of the First Washington Dietary Fiber Symposium held in 1981 (later to be called the Vahouny Symposia, beginning in 1988). Dr. Vahouny was also an enthusiastic educator. He taught physiology and nutrition courses at the medical school and was a mentor for a number of doctorial students.

Also, any such review must also recognize the contributions to this field, and to all nutrition science, by David Kritchevsky. Dr. Kritchevsky was the Casper Wistar Scholar at the Wistar Institute in Philadelphia, Pennsylvania. He published extensively on various nutritional subjects, but most extensively on dietary lipids and dietary fiber. He also served on many editorial boards and scientific advisory committees. Dr. Kritchevsky was an adviser to Dr. Vahouny during Vahouny's PhD program, and the relationship between these two scientists grew larger and closer over the years. David Kritchevsky was instrumental in developing the program and selecting speakers for most of the Vahouny Symposia.

1.2 First International Vahouny Fiber Symposium

The First Washington Symposium on Dietary Fiber was organized in 1981 by George Vahouny and David Kritchevsky and was held in Washington, DC. George Vahouny was the spark and energy behind the planning and organization of this meeting. He felt that there should be a fiber conference where scientific researchers could meet in a collegial atmosphere to engage in give-and-take discussions about current research results and to explore future research activities that might provide information to help us understand the chemical, physiological, and health benefits of this very interesting macronutrient.

Highlights of this symposium included presentations from John Cummings on "Consequences of the Metabolism of Fiber in the Human Large Intestine," Martin Eastwood on "Dietary Fiber and Colon Function in a Population Aged 18–80 Years," Michael Hill on "Colonic Bacterial Activity—Effect of

Fiber on Substrate Concentration and on Enzyme Action," Anthony Leeds on "Modification of Intestinal Absorption by Dietary Fiber and Fiber Components," James W. Anderson on "Dietary Fiber and Diabetes," and George V. Vahouny himself on "Dietary Fiber and Intestinal Absorption of Lipids."

The proceedings of this symposium were published in a book entitled Dietary Fiber in Health and Disease, edited by Vahouny and Kritchevsky and published by Plenum Press, 1982.

1.3 Second International Vahouny Fiber Symposium

The Second Washington Symposium on Dietary Fiber was held in Washington, DC, in April 1984, and was organized by George Vahouny, David Kritchevsky, and Charles Bonfield. This meeting, like the one in 1981, was conducted with informality and openness. The conference was honored to have Denis Burkitt as the keynote speaker.

Dr. Burkitt fascinated all attendees with his historical perspective of early observations of the health benefits of a high-fiber diet. He properly acknowledged the first observations of Dr. T.L. Cleave in his pioneering book entitled *The Saccharine Disease* published in 1975. He also cited the major contributions to dietary fiber research by his close colleagues, Hugh Trowell and A.R.P. Walker, who like himself, spent much of their professional careers serving and observing the native populations in undeveloped areas of Africa.

This symposium had many highlights. Leon Prosky, Hans Englyst, and David Southgate presented significant papers on dietary fiber analysis and the relationship between dietary fiber composition and physiological effects. David Jenkins reviewed his work on the glycemic index. Abigail Salyers discussed "Diet and the Colonic Environment." Jon Story gave a paper on "Modification of Steroid Excretion in Response to Dietary Fiber." Barbara Schneeman talked about the "Effects of Fiber on Plasma Lipoprotein Concentration."

This conference also included two satellite symposia. The session on Dietary Fiber and Cancer was sponsored by the U.S. National Cancer Institute and included papers on etiological and nutritional factors associated with dietary fiber and colorectal cancer. The session on Dietary Fiber and Obesity featured papers on the effects of various dietary fibers on insulin and glucose metabolism, high-fiber diets for obese diabetic men, and the treatment of overweight outpatients with high-fiber diets.

Proceedings of the main program and the Fiber and Cancer satellite were published in the book entitled *Dietary Fiber: Basic and Clinical Aspects*, edited by Vahouny and Kritchevsky and published by Plenum Press, 1986. Proceedings of the Dietary Fiber and Obesity satellite were published in the book *Dietary Fiber and Obesity*, edited by Bjoernthorp, Vahouny, and Kritchevsky and published by Alan R. Liss, Inc., 1985.

1.4 Third International Vahouny Fiber Symposium

The Third International Vahouny Fiber Symposium was held in Washington, DC, in April 1988. The symposium series was renamed after George Vahouny, who tragically passed away in 1986. David Kritchevsky, his long-time friend and colleague, penned the following appropriate remembrance for this meeting: "George Vahouny's lamentably short but inordinately productive career can be characterized in the words of Albert Szent-Gyorgy; 'Research is to see what everybody else has seen and to think what nobody else has thought.' George Vahouny was, above all, an innovator whose originality touched every area of biology in which he worked. The field of dietary fiber was one of his later career interests, but with characteristic skill and devotion he became one of its leading practitioners in a very short time."

We were very fortunate, at this conference, to be able to hear papers and talk with Denis Burkitt, Hugh Trowell, and Alec Walker—three pioneers in early dietary fiber research. The organizers of this symposium presented each of these individuals with a framed certificate that recognized their long-time contributions to the dietary fiber field. We believe that this was the last meeting that was attended by all three of these early pioneers in dietary fiber research.

The meeting opened with sessions on the structure and function of dietary fiber and on the effects of fiber on nutrient absorption. The program on the second day included sessions on physiology and microflora, and dietary fiber and obesity. The sessions on the third day were fiber and diseases, and fiber metabolism. The final day was devoted to a satellite symposium on Future Directions in Research on Dietary Fiber and Cancer, sponsored by the U.S. National Cancer Institute.

Proceedings of this meeting were published in the book *Dietary Fiber: Chemistry, Physiology and Health Effects*, edited by David Kritchevsky, Charles Bonfield, and James Anderson and published by Plenum Press, 1990.

1.5 Fourth International Vahouny Fiber Symposium

The Fourth International Vahouny Fiber Symposium opened with a videotaped welcome and message from Denis Burkitt. Dr. Burkitt was unable to travel to the United States, but we were able to hear his talk on the "History of Fiber" via the videotape. On this first day, we also heard some interesting papers by Alec Walker on "Dietary Fiber in Health and Disease: The South African Experience," Edwin R. Morris on "Fiber in Foods," Geoffrey Livesey on "Energy Value of Fiber," and Christine Edwards on "The Physiological Effects of Dietary Fiber."

The program for the first afternoon was devoted to Lipids and Nutrient Metabolism. Barbara Schneeman, Michihiro Sugano, Daniel Gallaher, and Joanne Lupton presented papers on the effects of dietary fiber, particularly viscous fibers, on lipid absorption and metabolism. James Anderson, David Jenkins, and Bjorn Eggum talked about the effects of fiber on fat, carbohydrate, and protein absorption. Sessions were held on Fiber and Cancer and on Fiber's Nutritional Effects. An interesting session was devoted to In Vivo and In Vitro Laboratory Models for Evaluating Fiber's Effects.

Another highlight of this meeting was the introduction of unstructured workshops. Four concurrent workshops were held in two successive one and one-half-hour sessions. The workshops captured George Vahouny's penchant for meetings that encourage free and open discussion by all participants, not just the speaker. The moderators were asked to give a 10–15 min introduction on their subject and then to open the workshop for discussion. Discussions were so intense in some of the workshops that it was difficult to terminate the workshop at the scheduled time.

The Fourth International Vahouny Fiber Symposium was held in Washington, DC, in April 1992. The organizers were Charles Bonfield and David Kritchevsky. The proceedings were published in the book *Dietary Fiber in Health and Disease*, edited by Kritchevsky and Bonfield and published by Eagan Press, 1995.

1.6 Fifth International Vahouny Fiber Symposium

The Fifth International Vahouny Fiber Symposium was held in Washington, DC, in March 1996. This symposium featured four half-day minisymposia on (1) complex carbohydrates, (2) soluble fiber, (3) short-chain fatty acids, and (4) nutrients contributing to the fiber effect. The half-day session on complex carbohydrates was sponsored by the International Life Sciences Institute (ILSI) and included presentations on analysis, classification, product labeling perspectives, U.S. dietary guidelines, and application in the food industry. The half-day session on soluble fiber was sponsored by The Quaker Oats Company and featured presentations on the physiological effects of soluble fiber on blood pressure, body weight, glycemic index, lipid digestion and absorption, cholesterol management, mechanisms of action, and future directions for soluble fiber research. The minisymposium on short-chain fatty acids included presentations on butyrate, intestinal adaptation, gene expression, gut motility, butyrate and colonic neoplasia, calcium absorption, and intestinal growth and function. The session on nutrients contributing to the fiber effect heard presentations on resistant starch, oligosaccharides, fructooligosaccharides, phytosterols, and lignans.

This symposium also continued with the unstructured workshop format with subjects such as (1) clinical study design, (2) fiber and cancer, (3) dietary guidelines, (4) fiber content of food, (5) fiber and heart disease, (6) fiber and body weight management, (7) animal models in fiber research, and (8) soluble fiber analysis.

The Fifth International Vahouny Fiber Symposium was organized by Charles Bonfield and David Kritchevsky. The proceedings were published in the book *Dietary Fiber in Health and Disease*, edited by Kritchevsky and Bonfield and published by Plenum Press, 1997.

1.7 1998 Satellite Symposium in Association with Nutrition Adelaide 98

On December 3, 1998, a 1 day satellite symposium was organized in association with Nutrition Adelaide 98—a joint meeting of the Australasian Clinical Nutrition Society and the Nutrition Society of Australia.

The meeting was held in Adelaide, Australia, and was organized by Charles Bonfield and David Kritchevsky. Papers in the morning session presented research on the effects of carbohydrates in the large intestine. The afternoon session included papers on fiber and cancer.

The proceedings of this symposium were published in a special supplement to the *Asia Pacific Journal of Clinical Nutrition*, Vol. 8, 1999, pp. S1–S60. Supplement editors were Charles Bonfield and David Kritchevsky.

1.8 Sixth International Vahouny Fiber Symposium

The Sixth International Vahouny Fiber Symposium was held in Washington, DC, in March 2000 and featured half-day sessions on (1) fiber and cancer, (2) glycemic index, (3) health effects of whole grains, and (4) nutrients contributing to the fiber effect.

In the fiber and cancer session, Calvert and Klurfeld discussed the results of research on dietary fiber and colon cancer in animal models. J. Lupton presented results of her research on butyrate and colon cancer. E. Giovannucci, J. Marshall, and E. Lanza discussed the results of clinical and epidemiological studies on human colon cancer, and Mike Hill reviewed European Cancer Research.

In the "glycemic index" session, Kendall presented a historical perspective, and Tom Wolever discussed glycemic index measurement. Parks presented information on "The Relationship of Glycemic Index to Lipogenesis," Kohrt on "Aging, Physical Activity and Insulin Action," and Schneeman on "Fiber, CCK and Insulin/Glucose Response."

In the "health effects of whole grains" session, Anderson discussed "Overall Health Benefits," Fulcher talked about "Functional Compartmentalization of Grain Nutrients," Miller about "Grain Antioxidants," Liu on "Intake of Whole Grains, in Relation to Diabetes and Coronary Heart Disease," Jacobs on "Whole Grains and Cancer," and Cleveland on "Whole Grain Intake in the United States." And in the "nutrients contributing to the fiber effect session," Asp, Roberfroid, Shortt, Craig, Jones, Giovannucci, and Erdman presented papers on various oligosaccharides, inulin, polydextrose, phytosterols, folate, and carotenoids.

The following workshops were held: (1) fiber and hypercholesterolemia, (2) fiber and lipids, (3) fiber and cancer, (4) probiotics and prebiotics, (5) fiber and insulin sensitivity/resistance, (6) short-chain fatty acids, and (7) definition of dietary fiber.

Bonfield chaired the closing session, where presentations were made by Sakata on "Influences of Succinic and Lactic Acids on Gut Functions," Story on "Dietary Fiber-Bile Acids Interactions in Atherosclerosis and Colon Cancer Risk," and Asp on "Health Claims and Regulatory Aspects of Dietary Fiber Products."

The Sixth International Vahouny Fiber Symposium was organized by Charles Bonfield and David Kritchevsky, and the proceedings were published on compact disk (CD) by the Vahouny Symposia, Delray Beach, Florida, 2003.

1.9 Seventh International Vahouny Fiber Symposium

The Seventh International Vahouny Symposium was held in Edinburgh, Scotland, in May 2002 and was organized by Charles Bonfield, Martin Eastwood, and David Kritchevsky. This very successful meeting was the first Vahouny Symposium held in Europe and was well attended by scientists from all over the world. There were half-day sessions on (1) general aspects of fiber, (2) whole cereal grains, (3) fiber and human cancer, (4) short-chain fatty acids, (5) health effects of whole grains, (6) nutrients contributing to the fiber effect, (7) physiological aspects of fiber, and (8) open workshops.

We were fortunate to be able to hold this symposium at the Royal College of Physicians facilities in Edinburgh. These facilities are very beautiful and historic, and the library holds many old original medical texts dating from the 1400s including a first edition of Celsus De Medicina dated in 1478.

The General Aspects session included papers by Kritchevsky, McCleary (fiber analysis), Lairon (Suvimax French Study), Edwards (fiber and children), Rimm (fiber and weight loss), Eastwood (fiber and diverticulosis), and DeVries (fiber definition). The session on Whole Grains, Fiber, and Human Cancer featured presentations by La Vecchia (report of Northern Italian Studies), Riboli (The EPIC Study), Mathers (report from the CAPP 1 Study), Rennert (diet and cancer), and Hill (the future for fiber and cancer).

In the session on Short-Chain Fatty Acids, papers were presented by Macfarlane (SCFA regulation), Sakata (influences of pro-biotic bacteria), Bach Knudsen (butyrate metabolism), Pouteau (metabolism of SCFAs), Cherbut (SCFA and GI Motility), Blottiere (intestinal cell proliferation), and Mathers (anti-cancer effects of butyrate).

The Health Effects of Whole Grains Session featured reports on the effects of milling, consumption of whole grains, protective effects of whole grains, protection against cardiovascular disease, protection against diabetes, health claims in the United States, and health claims in Europe.

Papers presented in the Nutrients Contributing to the Fiber Effect session were: Topping on resistant starch Delzenne on oligosaccharides, Ghisolfi on pre-biotics in infant formulas, Nyman on bioactivity of dietary fiber, Hallmanson rye lignans and human health, and Bjorck on fibre and the Glycemic Index.

The Physiological Aspects of Fiber Sessions included papers by Marlett, Phillips, Edwards, Chapin, and Tucker on various aspects on psyllium seed husk or ispaghula and included Strugala and Brownlee on colonic mucin.

The proceedings of this symposium were published in a special supplement to the *Proceedings of the Nutrition Society*, Vol. 62, No. 1, February 2003. Supplement editors were Bonfield, Eastwood, and Kritchevsky.

1.10 Eighth International Vahouny Fiber Symposium (Vahouny-ILSI Japan International Symposium on Non-Digestible Carbohydrate)

The (Eighth) Vahouny-ILSI Japan International Symposium on Non-Digestible Carbohydrate was held at the National Olympics Memorial Youth Center in Tokyo, Japan, in September 2004. This symposium was a conjoint effort of the Vahouny Symposia, ILSI Japan, and ILSI International. The symposium was organized by Takashi Sakata, Hajime Sasaki, and Charles Bonfield.

In the history of dietary fiber Session, Bonfield presented a paper on the history of the Vahouny Symposia and historical overview of dietary fiber (for Dr. Kritchevsky who could not be present). Sugano discussed dietary fiber and lipid metabolism, and Cho presented on dietary fiber and intestinal regularity.

In the physiology and immunology session, Sakata discussed SCFAs and colonic epithelial cells, Ishizuka presented on fiber and immune cells around intestinal crypts, Totsuka discussed the gut immune system, Rauonen talked about colonic fermentation, Takahashi discussed fiber and viscosity and flow behavior, and Yoshimura discussed fibers' influence on enzymatic reaction of soy protein.

In the nutrition session, Ohta presented on fiber and mineral absorption, Mineo discussed fiber effects on calcium absorption, Sakaguchi reviewed protein nutrition from nondigestible carbohydrates, Knudsen reported on rate of SCFA delivery to peripheral tissues, and Prieto discussed soluble fibers in research studies.

In the glycemic index session, Brouns reviewed global aspects of the glycemic index, Delport talked about glycemic response and weight control, Sugiyama discussed glycemic index and Japanese foods, Livesey presented on glycemic control, Daimon reviewed postprandial hyperglycemia, and Komindr presented on the effect of local foods on glucose and protein conservation.

In the pro- and prebiotic session, Ushida discussed colonic microflora effects of pro- and prebiotics, Hojberg presented on the GI microbial system effects on carbohydrate fermentation rate, Matsueda presented on inflammatory bowel disease and dietary fiber, Uchida reviewed efficacy of *P. freudenreichii* ET3, and Umesaki presented on minimum flora for development of intestinal mucosa. The ILSI Japan Research Committee on Sugars organized a special session on a new method for evaluating glucose response—the glucose release rate.

Two workshops were featured. Taiyo Kagaku sponsored a workshop on dietary fiber and intestinal bacterial ecosystem and Matsutani Chemical Industry Co., Ltd. sponsored a workshop on glycemic response—current aspects. The proceedings of this symposium were published in the *Foods & Food Ingredients Journal of Japan*, Vol. 210, Nos. 10–12, 2005.

1.11 Ninth Vahouny International Fiber Symposium

The Ninth International Vahouny Symposium was held in Washington, DC (Bethesda, MD), in June 2010 and was organized by Susan Cho with help from James Anderson, Anne Birkett, Tom Boileau, David Klufeld, Christine Edwards, Georgy Fahey, Brinda Govindarajan, David Jenkins, and Lisa Sanders.

In the fiber and weight management session, Moshfegh, Rimm, Nicklas, Cho, Gallaher, and Wanders presented papers on various aspects of dietary fiber intakes and overweightedness. The fiber and heart disease/cancer session featured papers by Anderson (epidemiological studies), Kendall (portfolio diet and cardiovascular risk reduction), Falk (health effects of whole grains), and Kristensen (hypocaloric diet and whole grains in weight loss and cardiovascular disease).

The fiber and glucose metabolism session included papers by Jenkins (fiber, glycemic index, and diabetes), Vuksan (viscosity determines lipid lowering effects), Maki (measurement techniques for insulin sensitivity), Pouteau (glucose turnover reduced, not insulin resistance, with indigestible carbohydrates), and Takahashi (cellulose decreases diffusion of glucose in the GI lumen). The prebiotic effects of fiber session included papers by Gibson (characteristics and modulation of healthy flora), Guarner (prebiotics and bowel function), and Delzenne (prebiotics and body weight management).

In the session on health benefits of novel fibers, papers were presented by Dahl (overview of fiber, inulin, and digestive health), Abnous (oat bran or wheat bran alters composition of fecal community), Meyer (inulin, gut microbes, and health), Kruger (laxation produced by galactooligosaccharide), and Leach (intake of inulin-type fructans in prehistoric community). The novel fibers and weight management session featured papers by Slavin (dietary fiber and satiety/fiber and weight management), Delzenne (control of energy metabolism by non-digestible oligosaccharides), and Shinoki (improved insulin sensitivity with fructooligosaccharides).

The session on Fibersol-2 included papers by Buck, Hendrich, Livesey, Baer, Mai, and Gordon on characteristics of maltodextrin, Fibersol-2, and low viscous fiber on satiety, glycemia, microbiota, and other properties.

One of the most interesting and controversial sessions was the implementation issues of Codex fiber definition session. Lupton, DeVries, Slavin, Caers, Miller-Jones, and Champ presented the new definition of dietary fiber published by the Codex Alimentarius Commission 2009. The Codex definition starts as follows: "Dietary fiber means carbohydrate polymers with 10 or more monomeric units, which are not hydrolyzed by the endogenous enzymes in the small intestine of humans...," and ended with the following comment: "Decision on whether to include carbohydrates from three to nine monomeric units should be left to national authorities." The sense of many attendees at the Vahouny Symposium was that three to nine manometric units should be included in the definition and that it should be left to national authorities to opt out of including three to nine units if they elected to do so. A petition in this effect was drafted and signed by many attendees.

In the session on galactooligosaccharides: next-generation probiotic, Birlett, Hutkins, Langcamp-Henken, and Gardner presented papers on the properties, clinical immunological effects, and reduction of severity of colitis in rats.

The fiber and gastrointestinal health session included the following research: the role of the colon in the metabolism of potentially bioactive molecules (Edwards), poorly absorbed and fermentable short-chain fatty acids (Muir), characterization of rice dietary fiber from rice bran (Park), sourdough fermentation of wholemeal wheat bread decreases postprandial glucose and insulin in diabetics (Lappi), and sugar beet fiber promotes accumulation of CD8+ intraepithelial lymphocytes (Ishizuka).

On Friday, there were two concurrent sessions. The resistant starch and associated compounds session included papers on the following: resistant starch alters gut fermentation and neuroendocrinology to reduce body fat (Keenan); resistant starch measurement, intakes, and dietary targets (Bird); resistant starch content increases after refrigeration (Stewart); resistant starch is an insulin sensitizer (Robertson); lower food intake associated with resistant starch (Harvey); role of viscosity on satiety and adiposity (Gallaher); and mechanism of flavonoid glycoside absorption by nondigestible saccharide (Matsukawa).

The session on oat and other fibers featured papers on the following: cell wall components of rye, barley, and oats (Lehtinen); oat bran with different viscosities differs in capacities to lower serum LDL cholesterol (Tosh); oat fiber influences gene sets related to inflammation (Ulmius); effects of oat bran of different molecular weights on plasma cholesterol and SCFAs (Immerstrand); viscosity and fermentability of NSP affect digestion and hormone secretion (Hooda); fig fruit as a source of dietary fiber (Sanchez-Zapata); and antioxidant properties of pomegranate peel (Sanchez-Zapata).

The final session on regulatory issues featured a discussion on GRAS notice procedure (Ramos-Valle) and health claims and structure–function claims (Susan Cho).

1.12 Vahouny Medal

In 1992, a vote was taken by attendees of the Fourth International Vahouny Fiber Symposium to conceive and strike a medal that would then be presented to individuals who have made significant contributions to the field of dietary fiber research and dietary fiber knowledge. Since it was intended that this medal would be presented from colleagues in this field, funds were solicited from individual scientists attending the symposium. The medal is named in honor of the late George Vartkes Vahouny. The medal is usually presented during a session at the symposia.

The following individuals have been awarded the Vahouny Medal: David Kritchevsky, Martin Eastwood, David Jenkins, Alec Walker, Nils Asp, Mike Hill, Charles Bonfield, Jim Anderson, Takashi Sakata, Christine Edwards, and Joanne Lupton.

1.13 Conclusion

The Vahouny Symposia in the early 1980s used scientific methodology that included measuring stool weights, chemical analysis of fecal contents, and long discussions on the appropriate laboratory methodology for the analysis of dietary fiber in foods. Today, we consider this type of research to be rather fundamental. And, in truth it was, but this research and these papers laid the groundwork for subsequent investigation into the impact of dietary fiber on human health and disease and provided us with the fundamentals that have been necessary for the research that was discussed in subsequent symposia. Indeed we are making progress in developing methods for the investigation of dietary fiber in health and disease. In his closing remarks at the 1992 symposium, our colleague, Martin Eastwood, challenged the attendees to learn, develop, and employ more sophisticated technology in order to expand knowledge in the science of nondigestible carbohydrates. In recent symposia, we see this challenge is being met.

2

Discussions Relating to the Definition of Dietary Fiber at the Ninth Vahouny Fiber Symposium
Building Scientific Agreement

JOHN F. HOWLETT, VICTORIA A. BETTERIDGE, MARTINE CHAMP,
STUART A.S. CRAIG, AGNES MEHEUST, and JULIE MILLER JONES

Contents

2.1 Introduction

The Ninth Vahouny Symposium on Dietary Fiber, which was held in Bethesda, Maryland, United States, from June 8 to 11, 2010, was attended by more than 150 participants from academia, industry, and regulatory agencies. It was the first Vahouny Symposium to have been held since the adoption of a definition for dietary fiber by the Codex Alimentarius Commission in 2009 and, as such, presented an opportunity for issues surrounding the implementation of the Codex definition to be discussed by a body of scientific and regulatory experts preeminent in the field. Session 10 was jointly sponsored by ILSI North America and ILSI Europe with this objective in mind. The session took the form of a workshop facilitated by Julie Miller Jones, professor of nutrition at St. Catherine University, St. Paul, Minnesota, United States, and Dr. Martine Champ of the Nutritional Physiology Unit of the National Institute for Agronomic Research (INRA), Nantes, France.

The goals of the session were to address critical aspects of the Codex definition of dietary fiber affecting its global implementation in a harmonized fashion and to provide a forum for experts in the field to address these impacts. This session was preceded by a session chaired by Tate & Lyle in which speakers had presented an overview of the Codex definition (Joanne Lupton, Texas A&M University, United States), an account of the methodology available for the analysis of dietary fiber in foods and beverages (Jon DeVries, General Mills, United States), an overview of European and international perspectives regarding the Codex definition (Wim Caers, Beneo-Group, Belgium), and the characterization of physiological benefits of dietary fiber (Joanne Slavin, University of Minnesota, United States).

2.2 Proceedings of the Session

A summary of the implementation issues identified in the previous session was provided by Joanne Lupton to start the discussion. She reviewed the Codex definition for dietary fiber as adopted by the Codex Alimentarius Commission in 2009 [1] and noted that despite the adoption of the definition denoting a significant step forward for a global consensus on the nature and identity of dietary fiber, the following elements of the definition would benefit from further debate:

- Footnote 2 to the definition, which leaves the inclusion of undigestible carbohydrates with degrees of polymerization (DP) in the range 3–9 to the discretion of national authorities
- The absence of a list of beneficial physiological effects and appropriate criteria for their substantiation for the purpose of compliance with the definition
- The analytical methodology by which fiber in food is to be quantified

Various aspects of these issues were the subject of discussion during the remaining part of Session 10.

2.2.1 Exclusion/Inclusion of Carbohydrates with Degrees of Polymerization in the Range 3–9

Debate about the exclusion or inclusion of carbohydrates with DPs in the range 3–9 was focused on two major areas: (1) the lack of scientific support for differences in physiological effects between those oligomers with DP 3–9 and those with higher DP and the absence of readily applicable methods that could clearly distinguish between them, and (2) the fact that the coexistence of regulations allowing two different standards for the same definition undermines the validity of the definition.

All those who spoke regarding physiological aspects argued that there was no basis for distinguishing between carbohydrates with a $DP \geq 10$ and those with $DP \leq 9$ because there were carbohydrates both above and below this cutoff point which exhibited one or more beneficial physiological effect(s) generally associated with fiber. The view was expressed that carbohydrates exhibiting beneficial physiological effects are distributed along a continuous spectrum of chain lengths with no clear differentiation at any particular DP.

Similarly, all those who spoke about methodological aspects were of the view that a universal cutoff point at a DP of 10 and above did not reflect methodological capability. Among those who spoke, there was a view that historically the cutoff point of DP $\geq$ 10* had gained currency in the mistaken belief that it was consistently applicable to all carbohydrates in the frame for consideration as dietary fibers through precipitation in alcohol. In practice, this is not the case, and methodology provides no reliable basis for imposing a distinction between carbohydrates with or without fiber-like properties on the basis of chain length alone.

In addition, many contributors to the debate were of the view that to provide a discretionary approach at the national level to excluding or including carbohydrate fractions within the scope of the definition was undesirable. For nutrition research and assessment, the absence of a common definition creates difficulties for the comparison of fiber intakes across different geographic regions and in the interpretation of studies assessing possible beneficial physiological effects where datasets are drawn from different regions. For consumers and food manufacturers, the application of different interpretations of what constitutes dietary fiber can result in confusing nutrition messages for consumers, demand differences in food labeling of the same food marketed in different countries, and create difficulties for food manufacturers seeking to formulate products for a global market.

Nevertheless, if there had been a necessity for compromise in order to achieve agreement on a definition, then it would have been preferable to default to a position that included carbohydrates with DPs in the range 3–9 within the body of the definition, with discretion included in the footnote for those who disagreed, rather than in the opposite manner as is currently in the Codex definition. If structured in this way, the default form of the definition would have been fully inclusive, more aligned with other existing definitions, and would have more accurately reflected the majority of opinion in the scientific community.

In summary, there was strong consensus among contributors that there is no sound scientific basis for a cutoff point at a DP $\geq$ 10. The difficulty of achieving a reconsideration of this issue within the Codex Alimentarius was acknowledged. It was suggested that the reaffirmation of the existing scientific agreement on the issue would provide better, practical support to national authorities in their implementation.

2.2.2 Agreement on a List of Beneficial Physiological Effects

Initiating the discussion of beneficial physiological effects, Joanne Lupton drew attention to the three categories of dietary fiber differentiated within the Codex definition by their source: those occurring naturally in food as consumed; those

---

* Prior to Codex discussion of a definition for dietary fiber, debate had centered on other cutoff points on the basis that oligomers below the cutoff DPs were soluble in 80% ethanol and those above were not. In practice, no clear cutoff point can be distinguished on the basis of solubility in 80% ethanol because solubility is also determined by the chemical nature of the constituent monosaccharides rather than the number of units alone and, therefore, the relationship between chain length and solubility in ethanol is imprecise.

obtained from food raw material by physical, enzymatic, or chemical means; and those that are synthetic in origin. Of the three categories, the definition requires that the latter two must be shown to have a physiological benefit to health, while for those occurring naturally in food as consumed, no such beneficial effect is required to be demonstrated. At the same time, the definition provides no description of what constitutes a beneficial physiological effect so, to the extent that this remains open to interpretation, it provides no clear indication of the qualifying features of fibers falling within the last two categories.

There is a diverse list of beneficial effects in common use in academia and by institutes, agencies, and authorities worldwide. Until the 2008 session of the Codex Committee on Nutrition and Foods for Special Dietary Uses (CCNFSDU) where the current definition was recommended for adoption, the Codex definition of dietary fiber itself had been presented in conjunction with an illustrative list of relevant beneficial physiological effects and had met with a clear majority of support among participating governments and observer organizations [2]. The list was removed during the 2008 CCNFSDU session to simplify the definition [3], but the list's removal potentially leads to risks of higher levels of confusion as beneficial physiological effects are now open for different interpretations at the national level.

Dr. Lupton suggested that progress might be made by attempting to characterize effects in relation to three levels of agreement on the certainty of their validation:

1. Well-established beneficial effects
2. Probable beneficial effects
3. Possible beneficial effects

In this way, an agreed core list of beneficial effects could be drawn up to provide a working basis for the definition, but at the same time, the list could remain open to additions as emerging science provided sufficient validation.

During discussion, the following physiological effects received support:

- Reduced blood total and/or LDL cholesterol levels
- Attenuation of postprandial glycemia/insulinemia
- Reduced blood pressure
- Increased fecal bulk/laxation
- Decreased transit time
- Increased colonic fermentation/short-chain fatty acid production
- Positive modulation of colonic microflora
- Weight loss/reduction in adiposity
- Increased satiety

Support was not unequivocal in every case. The occurrence of most of the effects was considered to be well established for fibers in general, but the health impact of some effects was the subject of discussion. While in a few cases (reduced blood total cholesterol, reduced blood pressure) there were considered to be clear associations between the endpoints measured and the reduction of disease risk, in other cases (increased colonic fermentability, attenuation of postprandial glycemia/insulinemia, increased satiety), the relevance of the endpoint measured was considered by some to be indeterminate. It was also noted that there is an ongoing discussion about relevant methods and the interpretation of the magnitude of effect, from the perspective of a contribution to health.

Furthermore, it was pointed out that agreement of the substantiation of the beneficial nature of any proposed effects is a case-by-case process.

The view was expressed that in considering beneficial effects in the context of a definition for dietary fiber and resultant nutrient content claims, it is important to keep in mind the consumption of fibers of all types. The total fiber content of the diet contributes several different effects simultaneously, and the overall benefit, however achieved mechanistically, derives primarily from the fact that fiber is not digested in the small intestine and passes to the colon intact. The beneficial outcomes of individual fiber types in individual foods should be seen in terms of their contribution to the overall benefit achieved through their contribution to total dietary fiber intake as reflected in nutrient content claims. This is in contrast to health claims made in relation to individual components where the claim is product specific and requires to be substantiated on a case-by-case basis in relation to the individual food ingredient.

The distinction between these two circumstances is reflected in the nature of the claims made. In the case of fiber content claims, the primary consideration of beneficial effect is in relation to the total fiber content of the diet and the value to consumers of an awareness of the importance of maintaining an adequate intake of dietary fiber from a variety of sources. In the case of health claims, the consideration is entirely product specific with the objective of making an on-pack claim, in a language understood by consumers, for products containing the effective amount of the specific component.

Overall, there was enthusiasm for agreeing on a core list of beneficial physiological effects.

2.2.3 Postsession Survey

At the suggestion of the audience, participants were invited to express by survey their views on whether or not carbohydrates with DPs in the range 3–9 should be included in the definition of dietary fiber and, if a list of beneficial physiological effects were to be compiled, to express their preferences for the effects that should be included. Participants were asked to respond to the statements of the survey presented in Figure 2.1; the results are displayed in Table 2.1.

2.3 Overall Conclusions from the Session and the Survey

There was overwhelming support among the participants during discussion in the session for the inclusion in the definition for dietary fiber of carbohydrate polymers with DPs in the range 3–9, and of the responses to the survey, 86% were in favor of including them and 3% were opposed. For reasons unknown, 11% of

Following the discussion held during the joint ILSI North America–ILSI Europe session at the Ninth Vahouny Fiber Symposium, Thursday, June 10, 2010, do you agree with the following?

The Codex Alimentarius definition of dietary fiber should include carbohydrate polymers of DP 3 and above, which are not hydrolyzed by the endogenous enzymes in the small intestine of humans and showing a physiological effect of benefit to health when pertaining to categories 2 and 3 (as described in the Codex Alimentarius definition of dietary fiber adopted in June 2009) as dietary fibers: Yes/No

In order to qualify as a dietary fiber, the carbohydrate falling into the categories 2 and 3 of the Codex Alimentarius definition (as adopted in June 2009) should demonstrate scientific evidence of at least one of, but not limited to, the following physiological effects listed.

Which of the following physiological effects of benefit to health should be included on the list?
- Reduction in blood total and/or LDL cholesterol levels   Yes/No
- Reduction in postprandial blood glucose and/or insulin levels   Yes/No
- Increased stool bulk and/or decreased gut transit time   Yes/No
- Fermentability by colonic microflora   Yes/No
- Other effect(s)   Yes/No

Figure 2.1 Survey circulated during the ILSI North America–ILSI Europe session.

Table 2.1 Summary of 75 Responses to the Survey Questionnaire

	Positive Answer (%)	Negative Answer (%)	No Answer (%)
Agree with the inclusion of DP 3–9	86.7	2.7	10.6[a]
Agree with physiological response			
Reduction in blood total and/or LDL cholesterol	98.7	1.3	—
Reduction in postprandial blood glucose and/or insulin levels	96	2.7	1.3
Increased stool bulk and/or decreased transit time	98.7	1.3	—
Fermentability by colonic microflora	82.7	6.7	10.6
Proposed other physiological effects	30.7		69.3

[a] Three persons declined to answer the question DP 3–9 on grounds of insufficient information to allow a decision, and five persons left the answer to the question concerning DP 3–9 blank.

respondents did not address the question. Taken together, the discussion during the session and the level of support shown by the survey indicate a convincing level of agreement among experts in the field that the science supports the inclusion of carbohydrate polymers with DPs in the range 3–9 and provides a rationale for science-based decision making by national authorities in their implementation of the Codex definition.

In discussion during the session, there was clear support for the establishment of a list of beneficial physiological effects associated with the consumption of dietary fiber. More than 80% (and, in the case of the first three, more than 95%) of respondents to the survey indicated support for the inclusion of at least the following effects in the list:

- Reduction in blood total and/or LDL cholesterol
- Reduction in postprandial blood glucose and/or insulin levels
- Increased stool bulk and/or decreased transit time
- Fermentability by colonic microflora

Almost a third of respondents to the survey (30%) proposed the inclusion of effects additional to these four. This response would seem to argue strongly for the adoption of an open list of beneficial effects comprising in the first instance the four previously listed functions and leaving open the possibility of the addition of other effects to the list as and when they achieve a similar level of acceptance as a result of developing science.

These results are consistent with several previous consensus documents. An international survey of fiber experts [4] found strong support for inclusion of oligosaccharides that are resistant to hydrolysis by human alimentary enzymes. Also, several recent regional expert opinions or definitions include oligosaccharides and/or a similar list of physiological effects [5–8].

2.4 Conflict of Interest and Funding

John F. Howlett is an employee of Exponent International Limited. John received an honorarium for the drafting of this chapter. Victoria A. Betteridge is an employee of Tate & Lyle PLC and a member of the ILSI Europe Dietary Carbohydrates Task Force. Stuart A.S. Craig is an employee of Danisco A/S and a member of the ILSI North America Technical Committee on Carbohydrates. Agnes Meheust is an employee of ILSI Europe, which is partly funded by the food and related industries. Julie Miller Jones is the scientific advisor of the ILSI North America Technical Committee on Carbohydrates and is a consultant for some not-for-profits and some food companies. The Vahouny symposium session and writing of this chapter was sponsored by both the Dietary Carbohydrates Task Force of the European branch and the Carbohydrates Committee of the North American branch of the International Life Sciences Institute (ILSI). ILSI's programs are supported primarily by its industry membership. Industry members of the Dietary Carbohydrates Task Force of ILSI Europe are AkzoNobel National Starch Food Innovation, Cargill, Coca-Cola Europe, Colloïdes Naturels International, Danisco, Danone, Kellogg Europe, Kraft Foods, Nestlé, Premier Foods, Südzucker/BENEO Group, Syral, and Tate & Lyle. Industry members of the Carbohydrates Committee of ILSI North America are Archer Daniels Midland Company, BENEO Group, Cargill Incorporated, The Coca-Cola Company, Corn Products International, Danisco USA Incorporated, Dr Pepper Snapple Group Incorporated, General Mills, The Hershey Company, Kellogg

Company, Kraft Foods Incorporated, Mars Incorporated, McNeil Nutritionals, Mead Johnson Nutritionals, National Starch Food Innovation, Nestlé USA Incorporated, PepsiCo Incorporated, and Tate & Lyle. The opinions expressed herein are those of the authors or discussion participants and do not necessarily represent the views of ILSI Europe or ILSI North America.

Acknowledgments

John Howlett had primary responsibility for final content; Victoria Betteridge, Martine Champ, and Julie Jones chaired the scientific session discussion and provided substantive input into the paper content; Agnes Meheust and Stuart Craig contributed substantially to writing and editing. All authors read and approved the final manuscript. The authors would like to particularly thank Dr. Jon deVries, Dr. Gunhild Kozianowski, Dr. Lisa Sanders, and Marie Latulippe for their contributions to this paper.

References

1. Codex Alimentarius. 2010. Guidelines on nutrition labeling CAC/GL 2-1985 as last amended 2010. Joint FAO/WHO Food Standards Programme, Secretariat of the Codex Alimentarius Commission, FAO, Rome.
2. Codex Alimentarius. 2007. Report of the 29th session of the Codex Committee on nutrition and foods for special dietary uses, Bad Neuenahr-Ahrweiler, Germany, November 12–16, 2007, ALINORM 08/31/26.
3. Codex Alimentarius. 2008. Report of the 30th session of the Codex Committee on nutrition and foods for special dietary uses, Cape Town, South Africa, November 3–7, 2008, ALINORM 09/32/26.
4. Lee, S.C. and Prosky, L. 1995. International survey on dietary fiber: Definition, analysis and reference materials. *Journal of AOAC International*, 78(1), 22–36.
5. American Association of Cereal Chemists (AACC). 2001. Definition of dietary fiber: Report of the Dietary Fiber Definition Committee to the Board of Directors of the American Association of Cereal Chemists. *Cereal Foods World*, 6(3), 112–126. Accessible at http://www.aaccnet.org/news/pdfs/DFDef.pdf
6. The National Academies of Science, Institute of Medicine (IOM). 2002. *Dietary Reference Intakes for Energy, Carbohydrate, Fiber, Fat, Fatty Acids, Cholesterol, Protein, and Amino Acids*. National Academies Press, Washington, DC, pp. 339–361. Accessible at http://www.nap.edu/openbook.php?record_id=10490&page=339
7. Food Standards Australia New Zealand (FSANZ). Food Standards Australia New Zealand Code Issue 115, Standard 1.2.8 Nutrition Information Requirements. p. 2.
8. EFSA. 2007. Statement of the scientific panel on dietetic products, nutrition and allergies on a request from the commission related to dietary fiber (Request N° EFSA-Q-2007-121). Expressed on July 6, 2007 at its 17th plenary meeting corresponding to item 10.1 of the Agenda.

3

Implementation Issues of the Codex Definition of Dietary Fiber

Degree of Polymerization, Physiological, and Methodological Considerations

VICTORIA A. BETTERIDGE, WIM CAERS, JOANNE R. LUPTON, JOANNE L. SLAVIN, and JON DEVRIES

Contents

3.1 Summary

In November 2008, the Codex Committee on Nutrition and Foods for Special Dietary Uses (CCNFSDU) reached a landmark decision after some 16 years of debate when it agreed on a definition of dietary fiber (DF). The Codex Alimentarius Commission (CAC) adopted the recommendation of the committee in July 2009. The decision was not without some compromise, and while it is a major step in establishing a global standard for DF, issues remain that need to be considered on the path to implementing a single, global definition of DF. The Ninth Vahouny Symposium gave an opportunity to consider these issues with distinguished scientific and regulatory experts in the field. Session 10 part 1 was chaired by Dr. Lisa Sanders, Tate & Lyle PLC, and its purpose was to review these issues from a global perspective. Dr. Sanders was joined by the following speakers: Dr. Joanne R. Lupton, Distinguished Professor, Department of Nutrition and Food Science, Texas A&M University, who gave an overview of the Codex definition and future implementation issues; Dr. Jonathan W. DeVries, Senior Principal scientist, General Mills, and senior technical manager, Medallion Laboratories, who presented on Dietary Fiber Analyses—Moving from Definition to Practice; Dr. Joanne Slavin, professor in the Department of Food Science and Nutrition, the University of Minnesota, who spoke on Determining the Physiological Benefits of Dietary Fiber; and Wim Caers, Manager of Regulatory Affairs, Beneo Group, who concluded part 1 with European and International Perspectives of the Dietary Fiber Definition.

The objectives of this session were to review the key issues affecting implementation from the perspective of establishing a global standard and to consider avenues toward a solution. The issues discussed were as follows: Footnote 2 of the definition allowing that national authorities may decide how to classify those oligosaccharides with a degree of polymerization (DP) from 3 to 9, analytical processes for the measurement of DF with particular emphasis on the Codex definition, and determining the beneficial physiological effects.

Failure to agree on the inclusion, or not, of non-digestible oligosaccharides (NDOs) that fall within the DP 3–9 range would mean two DF definitions, and failure to have some consensus on determining beneficial physiological effects would compound the problem further. Consistent implementation is necessary to maintain the value of the definition as a global standard and thereby provide a single definition for use in research and product development, facilitate harmonized application in food labeling and intake assessments, and ultimately lead to a healthier food supply for the consumer. Scientific consensus on how to tackle the issues of implementation would be progress toward this goal to the benefit of all stakeholders: the consumer, the scientific community, food companies, and regulatory and health authorities.

Part 1 of the session on Dietary Fiber Definition and Analysis considered possible ways to tackle these issues and gave the background for part 2, sponsored by the International Life Sciences Institute (ILSI), which provided the forum for a live debate on the issues, the proceedings from which you will also find in this manual.

3.2 Introduction

3.2.1 Overview of the Codex Definition and Future Implementation Issues

The Codex Alimentarius (CA) was created in 1963 jointly by FAO and WHO to develop food standards, guidelines, and related texts. The document "Understanding the CA" states that "The CA system presents a unique opportunity for all countries to join the international community in formulating and harmonizing food standards and ensuring their global implementation." The CCNFSDU is the subcommittee within CA that has been dealing with the DF definition since the early 1990s. Although the finalization of the Codex definition of DF was a significant accomplishment and the result of a collaborative effort over 16 years, a number of critical elements have been left to the decision of national authorities and may, if left unresolved, represent a missed opportunity to support global harmonization and implementation.

Codex Definition of Dietary Fiber (CAC 2009 Appendix II)
DF means carbohydrate polymers* with 10 or more monomeric units,[†] which are not hydrolyzed by the endogenous enzymes in the small intestine of humans and belong to the following categories:

- Edible carbohydrate polymers naturally occurring in the food as consumed
- Carbohydrate polymers which have been obtained from food raw material by physical, enzymatic, or chemical means and which have been shown to have a physiological effect of benefit to health as demonstrated by generally accepted scientific evidence to competent authorities
- Synthetic carbohydrate polymers which have been shown to have a physiological effect of benefit to health as demonstrated by generally accepted scientific evidence to competent authorities

The definition offers the benefit of a worldwide standard which can be used as a basis for measurement, food labeling, reference nutrient values, nutrition claims, and health claims. The elements of the definition that were amended during the final discussions in Cape Town 2008, include the decision to introduce Footnote 2 by which national authorities can decide on inclusion of those carbohydrate polymers of chain lengths that fall within the range of DP 3–9 (CAC 2009) and the simplification of the definition which included removal of the non-exclusive list of beneficial physiological effects (CAC 2009). In addition, there is ongoing discussion on relevant analytical considerations for the effective, reproducible measurement of DFs in foods in a manner that supports the definition. In order to maintain the value of the Codex definition as a global standard, these issues warrant further consideration as failure to do so risks undermining the harmonized implementation of a single global definition.

---

* When derived from a plant origin, DF may include fractions of lignin and/or other compounds associated with polysaccharides in the plant cell walls. These compounds also may be measured by certain analytical method(s) for DF. However, such compounds are not included in the definition of DF if extracted and reintroduced into a food (CAC 2010 Appendix II).

[†] Decision on whether to include carbohydrates from 3 to 9 monomeric units should be left to national authorities.

3.3 International Context

To consider these issues, it would seem sensible to look at how the Codex definition fits within a more international context, and to this end, an overview is given of the most prominent existing DF definitions.

3.3.1 European Scene

Within the European Union (EU) regulatory arena, a first reference to fiber is found in Council Directive 90/496 of September 24, 1990, on Nutritional Labeling for Foodstuffs (European Community 1990). In the recitals, it states that "for the benefit of the consumer on the one hand, and to avoid any possible technical barriers to trade on the other, nutrition labeling should be represented in a standardized form applying throughout the community." Clearly, a standardized approach is envisaged throughout the member states' territories, in the interest of both consumer and industry. In addition, a clear reference is made to the CA guidelines on nutrition labeling, which should be taken into account when rules are laid down. Although fiber is included as one out of six types of nutrients that can be declared on the "nutrition labeling" under Article 4, it is further stated in Article 1 of the Directive that "'fiber' means the material to be defined in accordance with the procedure laid down in Article 10 and measured by the method of analysis to be determined in accordance with that procedure."

Interestingly, it took 18 years, until October 29, 2008, before the European Commission succeeded in officially defining fiber (European Commission 2008). Around 1 year earlier, the European Food Safety Authority (EFSA) published, on request from the Commission, a statement related to DF (EFSA 2007). It was clearly stated in the Commission's request that the EFSA advice on the DF definition was to be used when preparing the community position for the CCNFSDU meeting in November 2007.

In conclusion, EFSA states that the definition should include all carbohydrate components occurring in foods that are nondigestible in the human small intestine. The main types include the following:

- Non-starch polysaccharides, cellulose, hemicellulose, pectins, and hydrocolloids (i.e., gums, mucilages, β-glucans)
- Resistant starch
- Resistant oligosaccharides with three (3) or more monomeric units
- Other non-digestible but quantitatively minor compounds when naturally associated with DF polysaccharides, especially lignin

The previously mentioned October 2008 DF definition was published in Commission Directive 2008/100/EC, amending Council Directive 910/496/EEC on nutrition labeling for foodstuffs as regards recommended daily allowances, energy conversion factors, and definitions. The definition reads as follows:

For the purposes of this Directive "fiber" means carbohydrate polymers with three or more monomeric units, which are neither digested nor absorbed in the human intestine and belong to the following categories:

- Edible carbohydrate polymers naturally occurring in the food as consumed;
- Edible carbohydrate polymers which have been obtained from food raw material by physical, enzymatic or chemical means and which have a beneficial physiological effect demonstrated by generally accepted scientific evidence;
- Edible synthetic carbohydrate polymers which have a beneficial physiological effect demonstrated by generally accepted scientific evidence.

When comparing this definition by the European Commission (and by extension that of EFSA) to the one adopted by CA, the overlap is nearly 100%, providing the option in Footnote 2 is taken up, meaning non-digestible carbohydrates with a DP in the range of 3–9 are part of the DF definition.

3.3.2 Broader International Scene

In addition to the CA, the European Commission, and EFSA, several other panels of scientific experts have evaluated the DF question and provided their views on a definition. Although in some cases there are significant differences in wording and approach, they do have one thing in common: they all include NDOs. A brief summary of the most prominent ones is provided in the following:

3.3.2.1 Institute of Medicine, National Academy of Sciences, United States (IOM 2005)

- DF consists of non-digestible carbohydrates and lignin that are intrinsic and intact in plants.

As examples of DF, the Institute of Medicine (IOM) provides cellulose, pectin, gums, hemicelluloses, β-glucans, and fibers contained in oat and wheat bran, plant carbohydrates that are not recovered by alcohol precipitation (e.g., inulin, oligosaccharides, and fructans), lignin, and some resistant starch. Excluded are non-digestible mono- and disaccharides and polyols, some resistant starch, and non-digestible animal carbohydrates.

- Functional fiber consists of isolated, nondigestible carbohydrates that have beneficial physiological effects in humans.

As examples of potential functional fibers, the IOM provides isolated nondigestible plant (e.g., resistant starch, pectins, gums), animal (chitin, chitosan), or commercially produced (e.g., resistant starch, polydextrose, inulin, indigestible dextrins) carbohydrates.

- Total dietary fiber (TDF) is the sum of dietary and functional fiber.

3.3.2.2 American Association of Cereal Chemists   In November 1998, the president of the American Association of Cereal Chemists (AACC) appointed a scientific review committee and charged it with the task of reviewing, and if necessary, updating the definition of DF. The outcome was published in 2001 (AACC 2001).
The definition is stated as follows:

> Dietary fiber is the edible parts of plants or analogous carbohydrates that are resistant to digestion and absorption in the human small intestine with complete or partial fermentation in the large intestine. Dietary fiber includes polysaccharides, oligosaccharides, lignin and associated plant substances. Dietary fibers promote beneficial physiological effects including laxation, and/or blood cholesterol attenuation, and/or glucose attenuation.

The publication further states the following: "The updated definition includes the same food components as the historical working definition used for almost 30 years (a very important point, considering that most of the research of the past 30 years delineating the positive health effects of dietary fiber is based on that working definition)." In the list of constituents of DF, oligosaccharides, such as oligofructans, polydextrose, and galacto-oligosaccharides, are explicitly mentioned.

3.3.2.3 Australia and New Zealand: FSANZ   The following DF definition has been published within Standard 1.2.8 (FSANZ 2001):

> Dietary fiber means that fraction of the edible part of plants or their extracts, or synthetic analogues, that
>
> • are resistant to digestion and absorption in the small intestine, usually with complete or partial fermentation in the large intestine; and
> • promotes one or more of these beneficial physiological effects: laxation, reduction in blood cholesterol, and/or modulation of blood glucose.
>
> and includes polysaccharides, oligosaccharides (DP > 2), and lignins.

Further, as an example, oligofructose with DP 3–9 was the subject of a separate evaluation and was confirmed to be a DF: Application A227 (Amendment 55, Gazetted 2001).

3.3.2.4 Agence Française de Securité Sanitaire des Aliments, France   Agence Française de Securité Sanitaire des Aliments (AFSSA) conducted an in-depth evaluation and review of the science related to DF. In the report of the Specialist Expert Committee on Human Nutrition (AFSSA 2002), the definition is stated as follows:

> Dietary fiber consists of:
>
> • Carbohydrate polymers (Polymerization degree (PD) $\geq$ 3) of plant origin, which may or may not be associated in the plant with lignin or other non-carbohydrate components (polyphenols, waxes, saponins, cutin, phytates, phytosterols, etc.);

or:

- Carbohydrate polymers (PD $\geq$ 3) processed (by physical, enzymatic, or chemical means) or synthetic, included in the attached list whose components may change on the basis of AFSSA recommendations.

In addition dietary fiber is neither digested nor absorbed in the small intestine. It has at least one of the following properties:

- Increase stools production;
- Stimulate colonic fermentation;
- Reduce post-prandial cholesterol levels;
- Reduce post-prandial blood sugar and/or insulin levels.

3.3.2.5 International Life Sciences Institute (ILSI) In its concise monograph on DF (ILSI 2006), ILSI emphasizes the importance of a physiological definition:

Physiological properties of dietary fiber determine its importance in the human body and its requirement in the human diet. Therefore, most scientists now agree that the definition of dietary fiber should be physiologically based.

Throughout the publication, different oligosaccharides (with a range of chain lengths from DP $\geq$ 3) are given as examples of DF.

3.3.2.6 Association of Official Analytical Chemists Association of Official Analytical Chemists (AOAC) states (AOAC 1997) that "Most scientists working in the dietary fiber field support the inclusion of non-digestible (resistant) oligosaccharides for quantification of dietary fiber because the properties of the oligosaccharides fit the definition of dietary fiber."

3.3.2.7 Mexico In April 2010, the Mexican Authorities updated the national standard NOM-051-SCFI/SSA1-2010, establishing the general specifications for the labeling of prepackaged foods and non-alcoholic beverages—commercial and sanitary information. Mexico adapted the DF definition from Codex and included DP $\geq$ 3.

3.3.2.8 Confirmations by National Authorities During the past, several oligo-/polysaccharides with a variety of chain lengths at or below the DP 10 "threshold" (e.g., fructo-oligosaccharides) and both below and above (e.g., inulin and polydextrose) have been the subject of written confirmation by national authorities—that for food labeling purposes, they may be labeled as DF.

3.4 Can We Come to a Resolution on DP 3–9?

To answer this, there are both analytical and physiological considerations.

In some countries, for labeling purposes, the analytical method determines what is or is not DF (IOM 2001). In such countries, the most commonly accepted methods, such as AOAC 985.29, include an ethanol precipitation step, and DF is defined according to what is, and what is not, soluble in ethanol/water. Oligo-/polysaccharides, with chain lengths both below and above the DP 10 threshold, do not precipitate in ethanol as solubility in ethanol is dependent on the type of fiber being analyzed and its precise solubility in ethanol/water mixtures. They would therefore not measure as DF by these methods, regardless of chain length, and to include them would require additional procedures in regulations and, in some cases, the development of new procedures. Definitions based solely on analytical methods are dependent entirely on the parameters of the method chosen and pay no regard to physiological considerations.

Lower molecular weight components may not have the same mechanism of action, for example, for laxation, as the higher molecular weight substances. For lower molecular weight components, there may be a more rapid and greater degree of fermentation leading to increased microbial mass and fecal bulking, or there may be more of an osmotic effect as compared to the bulking effect of higher molecular weight fibers. These carbohydrate polymers being soluble in water, however, provide greater opportunity for greater consumption of DFs, for example, in beverages. Moreover, there are non-digestible carbohydrates with chain lengths in the range of 3–9, such as fructo-oligosaccharides, that would be considered DF by most formal definitions by virtue of the physiological effects they exert.

3.5 Determining Beneficial Physiological Effects

The lack of an agreed list of qualifying physiological effects presents challenges to any harmonized roll-out of the Codex Standard. In hindsight, removal of the previously agreed non-exhaustive list at Codex to "simplify" the definition potentially risks the reverse happening. The achievement in Cape Town in 2008 set a landmark in defining DF according to its physiological properties. If we are not to lose momentum toward a global standard, we need to consider classifying the potential beneficial physiological effects according to the evidence available and move toward defining criteria for the purpose of compliance.

3.5.1 Which Fibers Need to "Prove" a Beneficial Physiological Effect?

The Codex definition identifies three categories of DFs:

1. Naturally occurring in the food as consumed
2. Obtained from food raw material by physical, enzymatic, or chemical means
3. Synthetic carbohydrate polymers

The last two categories are required to prove a beneficial physiological effect. The Codex definition is close in this respect to that of the EU (European Commission 2008) which identifies the same three categories of DFs. The IOM defines fiber in two categories: (1) DF (carbohydrates and lignin that are intrinsic and intact in plants) and (2) functional fiber (isolated or purified carbohydrates not digested and absorbed that confer beneficial physiological effects) (IOM 2001, 2002).

When combined, they would equate to total fiber for nutritional labeling purposes. As with the Codex definition and that of the EU, the second category is required to confer a beneficial physiological effect.

The rationale behind this is that the phrase "dietary fiber" has a positive association among consumers in that they expect DF to be "good for them," i.e., they expect it to have a beneficial physiological effect. If the fiber is endogenous to the food, there is a history of the physiological benefits associated with high-fiber *foods*—whether associated with the fiber itself or other components in these foods is not entirely certain—and therefore, there is no requirement to re-prove the benefits for these foods.

3.5.2 Which Physiological Effects Are Beneficial?

The issues to resolve are what constitute beneficial physiological effects and what might be the requirements necessary to prove them for the so-termed "added" DFs.

A number of regulatory authorities and institutions have considered the issue of beneficial physiological effects. The European Commission, in defining DF for legislation (European Commission 2008), stipulates that "Fiber has.....one or more beneficial physiological effects such as: decrease intestinal transit time, increase stool bulk, is fermentable by colonic microflora, reduce blood total cholesterol, reduce blood LDL cholesterol levels, reduce post-prandial blood glucose or reduce blood insulin levels." This legislation reflects the work of the EFSA (EFSA 2007, 2010) on DF. This list is reflective of the consensus achieved on beneficial physiological effects at CCNFSDU and was included in the Codex definition from 2004 (CAC 2005) until its finalization in Cape Town in 2008 when the list was removed to "simplify" the definition (CAC 2009). While removing the list has the benefit of ensuring that the definition is open to inclusion of additional DF components subject to substantiation of their beneficial effects, it risks undermining the harmonized implementation of the definition if competent authorities have different views on what constitutes a beneficial physiological effect.

In its report of Dietary Reference Intakes (IOM 2001, 2002), the IOM panel considered a number of physiological effects for different fibers, notably laxation, normalization of blood lipid levels, and attenuation of blood glucose response, together with a number of other effects, such as weight management (satiety, lower fat absorption, weight loss), blood pressure control, and gut environment (microflora, fermentation, transit time) which it considered in the context of individual fiber components.

The potential physiological effects of DFs are varied with weight of evidence ranging from "well-established" to "probable" and "possible." In some cases, evidence is based on large, prospective, epidemiologic studies showing a protective effect of DF foods against coronary heart disease (CHD) via the lowering of serum cholesterol. It is this that forms the basis for the dietary reference intakes from the National Academy of Science for fiber (38 and 25 g/day for young men and women, respectively, based on an intake of 14 g fiber per 1000 kcal), though it is not entirely certain whether the benefit to CHD is from the DF itself or phytochemicals that accompany the fiber. In other cases, evidence suggests that DF decreases gut transit time, increases stool bulk/laxation, and can attenuate blood glucose response (Health Canada 1997, FSANZ 2001, IOM 2001/2002, European Commission 2008, EFSA 2007) and that fiber fermentation provides physiological benefits (AFSSA 2002, ILSI 2006, European Commission 2008, EFSA 2010), such as increased mineral absorption, stimulation of beneficial microbes (prebiotic, selective colonic fermentation), decreased survival of pathogenic bacteria through reduction in pH, provision of nourishment to colonocytes (SCFAs, butyrate) for increased cell growth and maintenance, and a possible influence on satiety. While an impact on satiety is not included in the previously agreed list of beneficial physiological effects at Codex, the IOM acknowledges that evidence of impact on satiety exists for certain fibers (e.g., viscous fibers like psyllium gum, β-glucans), though is not yet strong enough to support its effect on food intake.

In summary, there are data to support a list of physiological benefits, although there is a need for standardized methodology and agreement on endpoints for some of them. Establishing a core list that leaves room for the addition of others, as and when their physiological benefits are substantiated, would therefore seem a sensible place to start, and this was further debated during the symposium in part 2 of this session.

3.6 Dietary Fiber Analysis

3.6.1 Moving from Definition to Practice

A key aspect to the effective implementation of the Codex definition is consensus on methodology to support the definition and thereby to validate labeling declarations and claims. The relationship between the methodology, specifically its capability or not to measure fiber on the basis of chain length alone (the DP issue), and the development of a validated procedure to combine AOAC methods accurately to determine TDF is an issue that requires further consideration to support a global standard.

The history of development of analytical procedures can be mapped alongside the progress of the definition. During the "dietary fiber hypothesis" years (Trowell et al. 1972–1976), initially the term dietary fiber was used to describe the remnants of plant cell wall components that were resistant to hydrolysis by human alimentary enzymes. These included cellulose, hemicellulose, lignin, and associated minor substances (such as waxes, cutin, and suberin). By 1976, the definition was broadened to include analogous indigestible polysaccharides from other plant sources including gums, modified celluloses, mucilages, oligosaccharides, and pectins, as they were found to have physiological actions attributed to DF.

The growing knowledge of the physiological benefits of DF led to increased research in both nutrition and analysis. To assist in the research by most accurately quantifying DF, the AOAC/Prosky worldwide surveys were conducted, achieving scientific consensus on the 1976 definition of DF and facilitating the pursuit of the methodology necessary to quantify it. The resultant landmark method completed official validation in 1985 as AOAC 985.29 (AACC 32.05).

3.6.1.1 Landmark Method Capable of Measuring Components Insoluble in Alcohol/Water Mixtures   The definition had led the development of 985.29, the method still known today as the Prosky method, and it would serve as the basis for DF and the health state relationships that have since been developed. The method depended on precipitation in a water/alcohol mixture and captured only those polymers that were insoluble in the mixture. In other words, it could not yet sufficiently capture all the components potentially covered by the definition, such as NDOs and certain polysaccharides.

3.6.1.2 Development in Methods Capable of Measuring Those Components That Do Not Precipitate in a Water/Alcohol Mixture: Including Nondigestible Oligosaccharides   Progress through the consensus on the DF definition expanded arenas of DF nutrition research and led to the development of additional enzymatic gravimetric methods including 991.43 (AACC 32.07), allowing separate determination of insoluble and soluble fractions. Following subsequent AOAC worldwide surveys on NDOs between 1991 and 1993, and scientific consensus at the AOAC Workshop in 1995, a variety of methods (AOAC and AACC validated) were developed to measure these specific DF components which do not precipitate in a water/alcohol mixture. These included AOAC 997.08 (AACC 32-31) and AOAC 999.03 (AACC 32-32) for fructans, AOAC 2000.11 (AACC 32-28) for polydextrose, AOAC 2001.02 (AACC 32-33) for galacto-oligosaccharides, AOAC 2001.03 (AACC 32-41) for resistant maltodextrins and higher and lower molecular weight fibers of all types in foods where resistant starch is not present, and AOAC 2006.08 for modified celluloses. These and other methods used enzymes and added techniques such as liquid chromatography to quantify the specific fiber components. While care has to be taken when using combinations of these methods to avoid "double counting" of components of the TDF, these individual component methods remain fully relevant today for the components they measure.

3.6.1.3 Resolving Resistant Starch   No single method yet measured all components considered DF, and while a majority of resistant starch is included in the quantities measured by AOAC 985.29 or 991.43, some portions of resistant starch were not accurately included. The direct measurement of resistant starch came with the development of AOAC 2002.02 (AACC 32-40), although since part of the resistant starch is quantitated using 985.29 or 991.43, the results of AOAC 2002.02 cannot be added to the results of those two methods to obtain an accurate DF quantity because double counting will occur. However, AOAC 2002.02 was designed to give results that match physiological studies, and it is useful for measuring resistant starch in ingredients and plants. It would become a critical step in the move toward the development of a new method for TDF. Resistant starch levels often change with processing, and for this reason, the finished product needs to be analyzed.

3.6.1.4 New Method for Total Dietary Fiber   The lack of a validated procedure to combine AOAC methods to determine total fiber content frequently raised concerns during the lengthy process to finalize the definition of DF at the CCNFSDU. In response to this lack, development began on a new method of analysis that would result in an integrated method capable of measuring TDF with carbohydrates of DP > 2. The new method combined the features of 985.29, 991.43, 2001.03, and 2002.02 and was adopted in October 2009 after the first interlaboratory collaborative study as AOAC 2009.01 (AACC 32-45) to quantitate TDF as defined by Codex/EU definitions. Combining enzymatic digestion under conditions that match physiological study results, gravimetric isolation of ethanol/water insoluble DFs, and liquid chromatography to quantitate ethanol/water soluble DFs, the new method is better able to simulate the human digestive system, is applicable to foods as they will be consumed, and recovers amounts of degraded resistant starches and other fibers that were not quantitated in older TDF methods.

The Codex definition aligns with research and the definition going back to the early years of Trowell et al. including those components with a DP of >2. Methodology has consistently aligned with state of the science to provide a base for advancing DF research. The new TDF 2009.01 method involves a two-step process that enables the measurement of insoluble and soluble higher molecular weight DFs via alcohol precipitation from an aqueous medium in a first step and a second step that recovers all fibers that are not precipitated in ethanol/water mixtures including higher molecular weight soluble fibers and lower molecular weight soluble fibers with three or more monomeric units.

3.7 Discussion

There are numerous advantages and arguments that can be offered to support the incorporation of Footnote 2 into the body of the DF definition, or in other words to support the inclusion of DP 3–9, or to modify the main body of the definition to remove the limitation to DP 10 or greater. These include, but may not be limited to, the following:

- It supports correct consumer information and understanding.
- It supports accurate labeling with a correct, related caloric value.
- It supports global harmonization and implementation consistent with many existing DF definitions (thus addressing one of the main missions of Codex).
- It supports global harmonization and implementation consistent with many existing individual national approvals.
- NDOs, regardless of chain length, exert physiological properties which are associated with DFs.

- These physiological properties do not suddenly change as the carbohydrate chain length goes from DP 9 to 10 (or higher).
- The DP 3–9 issue versus DP 10 cut-off was extensively discussed during the Codex meetings, and the inclusion of DP 3–9 thereof confirmed.
- It will help to bridge the gap between the recommended and the actual DF intake.
- No actual AOAC reference method (or any other) is available to correctly separate or distinguish fibers on the basis of a cut-off at DP 10.
- It will encourage product innovation and will increase the range of healthy functional foods for the consumer to choose from.

3.8 Conclusion

The adoption of the Codex definition represents a significant step forward in the establishment of a global standard for DF, but it falls short of providing a fully harmonized, implementable standard because it allows mutually exclusive interpretations at the national level as to the chemical identity of what constitutes fiber, and it leaves open the question of what constitutes a beneficial physiological effect. In the view of the authors, the harmonizing force of the definition would have been much improved if the default option had been to include nondigestible carbohydrates with DP 3–9 and if it had provided a core list of beneficial physiological effects upon which there is general agreement to provide greater certainty to those using the definition for nutrition information, scientific, and trading purposes.

Tate & Lyle would like to acknowledge the hard work of Dr. Lisa Sanders in the preparation and chairing of this session.

References

AACC. (2001). American Association of Cereal Chemists. Definition of dietary fiber. Report of the dietary fiber definition committee to the board of directors of the American Association of Cereal Chemists. *Cereal Foods World* 46(3), 112–126.

AFSSA. (2002). Agence Française de Securité Sanitaire des Aliments. Dietary fiber: Definitions, analysis and nutrition claims—Report of the Specialist Expert Committee on Human Nutrition, Maisons-Alfort, France, September 2002.

AOAC. (1997). Association of Official Analytical Chemists. *Dietary Fiber Analysis and Applications*. AOAC International, Gaithersburg, MD.

CAC. (2005). Codex Alimentarius Commission. Report of the 26th session of the Codex Committee on Nutrition and Foods for special dietary uses. ALINORM 05/28/26 November 2004, Rome, Italy.

CAC. (2009). Codex Alimentarius Commission. Report of the 30th session of the Codex Committee on Nutrition and Foods for special dietary uses. ALINORM 09/32/26 November 2008, Appendix II, p. 46; Guidelines for the use of nutrition claims: Draft table of conditions for nutrient content (Part B containing provision on dietary fiber) at Step 7, Rome, Italy.

CAC. (2010). Codex Alimentarius Commission. Report of the 31st session of the Codex Committee on Nutrition and Foods for Special Dietary Uses. ALINORM 10/33/26 November 2009, Appendix II, p. 45, Rome, Italy.

European Commission. (2008). Commission directive 2008/100/EC of 28 October 2008 amending council directive 90/496/EEC on nutrition labelling for foodstuffs as regards recommended daily allowances, energy conversion factors and definitions. *Official Journal of the European Union* No. L 285, October 29, 2008, p. 9.

European Community. (1990). Council directive 90/496/EEC of 24 September 1990 on nutrition labelling for foodstuffs. *Official Journal of the European Communities* No. L 276, October 6, 1990, p. 40.

EFSA. (2007). European Food Safety Authority. Statement of the scientific panel on dietetic products, nutrition and allergies on request from the European Commission related to dietary fiber (request No. EFSA–Q-2007-121), expressed on July 6, 2007.

EFSA. (2010). European Food Safety Authority. Panel on dietetic products, nutrition and allergies. Scientific opinion on dietary reference values for carbohydrates and dietary fiber. On request from the European Commission (question No EFSA-Q-2008-467) adopted on December 4, 2009. *EFSA Journal* 2010, 8(3), 1462. Available online: www.efsa.europa.eu

FSANZ. (2001). Food Standards Australia New Zealand Code, Amendment 55, August 2001: *Definition of Dietary Fiber Standard 1.2.8 Nutrition Information Requirements.*

Health Canada. (1997). Guideline concerning the safety and physiological effects of novel fiber sources and food products containing them. Food directorate health protection branch, Ottawa, Ontario, Canada.

ILSI. (2006). International Life Science Institute. ILSI Europe concise monograph series; Dietary Fiber, Brussels, Belgium.

IOM. (2001). Institute of Medicine. *Dietary Reference Intakes: Proposed Definition of Dietary Fiber.* National Academies Press, Washington, DC.

IOM. (2002). Institute of Medicine. *Dietary Reference Intakes for Energy, Fiber, Fat, Fatty Acids, Cholesterol, Protein and Amino Acids.* National Academies Press, Washington, DC.

IOM. (2005). Institute of Medicine. *Dietary Reference Intakes for Energy, Fiber, Fat, Fatty Acids, Cholesterol, Protein and Amino Acids.* National Academies Press, Washington, DC.

Trowell H., Southgate D.A.T., Wolever T.M.S., Leeds A.R., Gassull M.A., and Jenkins D.J.A. (1976). Dietary fibre redefined. The Lancet, 307(7966), 967.

4

Regulations for the Food Labeling of Dietary Fiber

PAULA R. TRUMBO

Contents

4.1 Introduction

Claims that can be used on conventional foods and dietary supplement labels fall into three general regulatory categories: nutrient content claims, structure/function claims, and health claims. The responsibility for ensuring the validity of these claims rests with the manufacturer or the U.S. Food and Drug Administration (FDA). In addition to claims, the FDA regulates other aspects of food labeling, including the nutrition facts label. This chapter provides an overview of these various categories of food labeling, with an emphasis on the labeling of dietary fiber.

4.2 Nutrient Content Claims

The FDA requires the premarket review of nutrient content claims. Nutrient content claims are used on food products to directly or by implication characterize the level of a nutrient in the food.[1] A "good source" claim may be made when a food contains 10%–19% of the reference amount customarily consumed (RACC) of the Daily Value for the nutrient that is subject of the nutrient content claim. A "high" or "excellent source of" claim may be made when a food contains 20% or more of the Daily Value per RACC. When a nutrient content claim is made and the food contains one or more of the following nutrients in excess per RACC, per labeled serving, or for foods with small serving sizes, a disclosure statement must be made for total fat, 13 g; saturated fat, 4 g; cholesterol, 60 g; and sodium, 480 mg.[1] A disclosure statement calls the consumer's attention to one or more of these nutrients in the food that may increase the risk of a disease or health-related condition. For example, if a fiber nutrient content claim is made and the food is not low in total fat, then the label must disclose the amount of total fat per labeled serving (e.g., "contains [x amount] of total fat per serving. See nutrition information for fat content"). Based on the current Daily Value for dietary fiber (25 g/2000 kcal), an excellent source of fiber would be greater than or equal to 5 g/RACC and a good source is at least 2.5 g/RACC and less than 5 g/RACC. Furthermore, terms such as "more," "fortified," or "enriched" can be used for the labeling of foods that contain 10% or more of the Daily Value per RACC of dietary fiber.

4.3 Structure/Function Claims

Structure/function claims are statements that describe the role of a nutrient or dietary ingredient intended to affect the structure or function in humans or that characterize the documented mechanism by which a nutrient or dietary ingredient acts to maintain such structure or function. Structure/function claims for the labeling of dietary supplements may also describe a benefit related to a nutrient deficiency disease (e.g., vitamin C and scurvy), as long as the statement also tells how widespread such a disease is in the United States.[2] While structure/function claims do not undergo premarket review, the law states that FDA must be notified about the claim on dietary supplements within 30 days of first marketing the product and there must be substantiation that the claims are truthful and not misleading. FDA has guidance on the substantiation of structure/function claims for the labeling of dietary supplements.[3] Dietary supplements that bear a structure/function claim must include a mandatory disclaimer statement that is provided for in the law. This disclaimer indicates that FDA has not evaluated the claim and must also state that the dietary supplement product is not intended to "diagnose, treat, cure or prevent any disease," because only a drug can legally make such a claim.[4] A structure/function claim often used for dietary fiber is "fiber maintains bowel regularity."

4.4 Health Claims

Health claim means any claim made on the label or in labeling of a food, including a dietary supplement, that expressly or by implication, including "third party" references, written statements (e.g., a brand name including a term such as "heart"), symbols (e.g., a heart symbol), or vignettes, characterizes the relationship of any substance to a disease or health-related condition.[5] Implied health claims include those statements, symbols, vignettes, or other forms of communication that suggest, within the context in which they are presented, that a relationship exists between the presence or level of a substance (food or food component) and a disease or health-related condition. Further, health claims are limited to claims about disease risk reduction and cannot be claims about the diagnosis, cure, mitigation, or treatment of disease.

4.4.1 Health Claims That Meet the Significant Scientific Agreement Standard

Health claims are required to be reviewed and evaluated by FDA prior to use. The scientific evidence to support a health claim that is authorized must meet the significant scientific agreement standard as described in the Code of Federal Regulations (CFR).[5] Specifications for each of the 12 authorized health claims are provided in the CFR. There are several health claims related to dietary fiber that have been authorized by the FDA (Table 4.1).[6–9] The substance of these claims is considered to be the eligible foods within each specified food category. Dietary fiber was identified as a "marker" for each claim because it is considered to be a component of these foods that is associated with reduced risk of coronary heart disease or cancer. A specific example of an authorized health claim is as follows: "Three grams of soluble fiber from oatmeal daily in a diet low in saturated fat and cholesterol may reduce the risk of heart disease. This cereal has 2 grams per serving."[10]

4.4.2 Food and Drug Administration Modernization Act Health Claims

The Food and Drug Administration Modernization Act (FDAMA) permits health claims based on current, published authoritative statements from "a scientific body of the United States with official responsibility for public health protection or research directly related to human nutrition or the National Academy of Sciences (NAS) or any of its subdivisions."[10] FDAMA upholds the significant scientific agreement standard that is applied to authorized health claims.

In 1999, an FDAMA notification containing a prospective claim about the relationship of whole-grain foods and heart disease and certain cancers was submitted to the FDA. The notification cited the following statement from

Table 4.1 Authorized Health Claims Related to Dietary Fiber

Regulation	Claim	Marker
21 CFR 101.76[6]	Diets low in fat and rich in fiber-containing grain products, fruits, and vegetables and cancer	Good source of fiber
21 CFR 101.77[7]	Diets low in saturated fat and cholesterol and rich in fruits, vegetables, and grain products that contain fiber, particularly soluble fiber, and risk of coronary heart disease	At least 0.6 g soluble fiber per RACC
21 CFR 101.78[8]	Diets low in fat and high in fruits and vegetables that contain fiber (vitamins A and C) and cancer	Good source of fiber, vitamin A or C
21 CFR 101.81[9]	Diets low in saturated fat and cholesterol and that include soluble fiber from certain foods and risk of coronary heart disease	Soluble fiber

the Executive Summary of the NAS report, Diet and Health: Implications for Reducing Chronic Disease Risk[11] as an authoritative statement: "Diets high in plant foods—that is, fruits, vegetables, legumes, and whole-grain cereals—are associated with a lower occurrence of coronary heart disease and cancers of the lung, colon, esophagus, and stomach." For purposes of bearing the prospective claim, the notification defined "whole-grain foods" as foods that contain 51% or more whole-grain ingredient(s) by weight per RACC. The notification proposed that compliance with this definition could be assessed by reference to the dietary fiber level of whole wheat, the predominant grain in the U.S. diet. Whole wheat contains 11 g of dietary fiber per 100 g; thus, the qualifying amount of dietary fiber required for a food to bear the prospective claim could be determined by the following formula: 11 g × 51% × RACC/100. FDA did not prohibit this notification, and therefore, manufacturers can use the following claim on the label and in labeling of any product that meets the eligibility criteria described in the notification: "Diets rich in whole-grain foods and other plant foods and low in total fat, saturated fat, and cholesterol, may help reduce the risk of heart disease and certain cancers."

4.4.3 Qualified Health Claims

Qualified health claims are health claims that include qualifying language about the level of scientific evidence since the evidence to support the claim is not as strong and does not meet the significant scientific agreement standard.[12] Qualified health claims also require premarket review prior to use. Currently, there are no qualified health claims for dietary fiber.

4.5 Nutrition Facts Label

4.5.1 Current Regulations

The nutrition facts label has been required on conventional foods since 1994, and any changes to the label require changes to the current regulations by the FDA.[13] Mandatory labeling of dietary fiber was considered to be warranted based on its beneficial role in human health, including improved laxation and reduced risk of coronary heart disease. The label must provide the weight amount and percent Daily Value per serving. The current Daily Value for dietary fiber is 25 g/2000 kcal. There is individual labeling of soluble and insoluble fiber since each type of fiber has unique physiological benefits. The labeling of soluble and insoluble fiber is voluntary except when a claim is made on the label or in labeling about either type of fiber. Only the weight amount is provided since there are no Daily Values for soluble or insoluble fiber.

Currently, FDA does not have a regulatory definition for dietary fiber and relies on the Association of Official Analytical Chemists (AOAC) International methods for quantifying dietary fiber on the label. Analytical methods recognized by the FDA[13] are provided in the AOAC International 15th edition[14] or are subsequent modifications or publications of the same method. The methods include AOAC 985.29[15] and 991.43[16] for total fiber, AOAC 993.19[17] and 991.43[16] for soluble fiber, and AOAC 991.42[18] and 991.43[16] for insoluble fiber. The utility of the AOAC methods is limited since food components that are isolated as fiber by these methods may not necessarily provide the physiological or health benefits associated with consuming naturally occurring fiber found in foods. Furthermore, dietary fibers, or portions of them, that provide physiological or health benefits may not be isolated by these methods.

4.5.2 Recent Reports by the Institute of Medicine

The FDA requested the Institute of Medicine (IOM) to define dietary fiber for labeling purposes. Based on the panel's deliberations, the following definitions were proposed:[19]

Dietary fiber consists of nondigestible carbohydrates and lignin that are intrinsic and intact in plants.

Added fiber consists of isolated, nondigestible carbohydrates that have beneficial physiological effects in humans. Included in this definition are isolated or extracted fibers, as well as synthetically manufactured fibers.

Total fiber is the sum of dietary fiber and added fiber.

These definitions include oligosaccharides that have 3–9 degrees of polymerization. The IOM[20] later changed the term "added fiber" to "functional fiber" because "added fiber" on the label is a nutrient content claim that requires 10% or more of the Daily Value per RACC. The IOM panel recognized that there were analytical limitations in measuring dietary fiber separately from functional fiber. The IOM fiber report did not identify which isolated or synthetic fibers provided physiological benefits and therefore did not identify food components that met the definition of functional fiber.

The IOM set Adequate Intake (AI) levels for dietary fiber, primarily based on intake levels associated with the greatest reduced risk of cardiovascular disease.[19] For adults, the AI is 14 g/1000 kcal. Although decisions have not been made about modifying the nutrient Daily Values, if the Daily Value for dietary fiber were to change from 25 to 28 g/2000 kcal, then this change could affect those foods that can bear a "good source" or "excellent source" fiber claim. Furthermore, a potential change in the Daily Value for dietary fiber, as well vitamin A, vitamin C, calcium, protein, and iron, could change which foods bear an authorized or qualified health claim, since 10% of the Daily Value for one of these nutrients must be met.

4.5.3 Advance Notice of Proposed Rulemaking

Because the IOM set Dietary Reference Intakes for various nutrients, including the AI for dietary fiber, the FDA issued an Advance Notice of Proposed Rulemaking (ANPRM)[21] in 2007 for seeking public comments to questions that the agency had for future rulemaking on modernizing the regulation related to the nutrition facts label (21 CFR 101.9).[13] The ANPRM asked four questions specific to dietary fiber. A question was asked about the IOM definitions for dietary fiber. The majority of the public comments supported a definition that was similar to the IOM definition for total fiber, as well as a draft Codex definition for dietary fiber which resembled the IOM total fiber definition (e.g., the potential for inclusion of isolated and synthetic fibers that have a physiological benefit and nondigestible oligosaccharides [3–9 monomeric units]). The draft Codex definition was modified, and the final definition is part of Codex's Guidelines on Nutrition Labeling.[22] One major change made to the final definition was the exclusion of nondigestible oligosaccharides. The definition, however, is footnoted to indicate that the inclusion of nondigestible oligosaccharides is left to national authorities. National authorities will also need to determine how to substantiate the physiological effect(s) of isolated and synthetic fibers.

In the 2007 ANPRM, FDA also asked a question on the term that should be used for dietary fiber, considering that a new definition could be developed. The majority of comments supported the continued use of the term "dietary fiber" even though the definition of fiber could be based on a new definition, rather than analytical methods.

The IOM fiber report[20] recommended phasing out the terms "soluble" and "insoluble" fiber on the label with physicochemical terms related to viscosity and fermentability for distinguishing between fibers that modulate gastric and small bowel function from those that provide substantial fecal bulk. The vast majority of comments supported keeping the terms "soluble" and "insoluble." Reasons given in these comments were that there are not validated methods for measuring viscosity, viscosity cannot be used to predict fermentability, and it is not known at which level of viscosity that fiber begins to have a physiological benefit.

Finally, the 2007 ANPRM asked about the process that FDA should use to determine whether a food component met the criteria for a "functional" fiber (e.g., demonstrate a physiological benefit). The only comment received suggested a postmarket notification similar to structure/function claims made on dietary supplements. As discussed earlier, structure/function claims do not require premarket scientific review. Modifications to the nutrition facts label, however, have required changes to the regulation by the FDA.

All of the public comments and supportive scientific information to the 2007 ANPRM, as well as more recent evidence and reports relevant to the labeling of dietary fiber, will be considered in drafting the proposed rule on updating the nutrition facts label. Following this, public comments to the proposed rule will be considered for publication of a final rule and amendments to 21 CFR 101.9.[21]

References

1. 21 Code of Federal Regulations 101.13. 2010. *Nutrient Content Claims—General Principles*. Washington, DC: U.S. Government Printing Office.
2. Federal Food, Drug and Cosmetic Act, Section 403 (r) (6) http://www.fda.gov/RegulatoryInformation/Legislation/FederalFoodDrugandCosmeticActFDCAct/default.htm (accessed January 30, 2012).
3. Guidance for Industry: Substantiation for Dietary Supplement Claims Made under Section 403(r) (6) of the Federal Food, Drug, and Cosmetic Act. 2008. http://www.fda.gov/Food/GuidanceComplianceRegulatoryInformation/GuidanceDocuments/DietarySupplements/ucm073200.htm (accessed January 30, 2012).

4. 21 Code of Federal Regulations 101.93. 2010. *Specific Requirements for Descriptive Claims That Are neither Nutrient Content nor Health Claims.* Washington, DC: U.S. Government Printing Office.
5. 21 Code of Federal Regulations 101.14. 2010. *Health Claims: General Requirements.* Washington, DC: U.S. Government Printing Office.
6. 21 Code of Federal Regulations 101.76. 2010. *Health Claims: Fiber-Containing Grain Products, Fruits, and Vegetables and Cancer.* Washington, DC: U.S. Government Printing Office.
7. 21 Code of Federal Regulations 101.77. 2010. *Health Claims: Fruits, Vegetables, and Grain Products That Contain Fiber, Particularly Soluble Fiber, and Risk of Coronary Heart Disease.* Washington, DC: U.S. Government Printing Office.
8. 21 Code of Federal Regulations 101.78. 2010. *Health Claims: Fruits and Vegetables and Cancer.* Washington, DC: U.S. Government Printing Office.
9. 21 Code of Federal Regulations 101.81. 2010. *Health Claims: Soluble Fiber from Certain Foods and Risk of Coronary Heart Disease (CHD).* Washington, DC: U.S. Government Printing Office.
10. Guidance for Industry: Notification of a Health Claim or Nutrient Content Claim Based on an Authoritative Statement of a Scientific. 1998. http://www.fda.gov/Food/GuidanceComplianceRegulatoryInformation/GuidanceDocuments/FoodLabelingNutrition/ucm056975.htm (accessed January 30, 2012).
11. National Research Council. 1989. *Diet and Health: Implications for Reducing Chronic Disease Risk.* Washington, DC: National Research Council/National Academy Press.
12. Guidance for Industry: Evidence-Based Review System for the Scientific Evaluation of Health Claims—Final. 2009. http://www.fda.gov/Food/GuidanceComplianceRegulatoryInformation/GuidanceDocuments/FoodLabelingNutrition/ucm073332.htm (accessed January 30, 2012).
13. 21 Code of Federal Regulations 101.9. 2010. *Nutrition Labeling of Food.* Washington, DC: U.S. Government Printing Office.
14. AOAC. 1990. *Official Methods of Analysis of the AOAC International.* 15th edn. Washington, DC: Association of Official Analytical Chemists.
15. Prosky, L. et al. Determination of total dietary fiber in foods and food products: Collaborative study. *J. Assoc. Off. Anal. Chem.*, 68, 677, 1985.
16. Lee, S.C., Prosky, L., and DeVries, J.W. Determination of total, soluble, and insoluble dietary fiber in foods—Enzymatic-gravimetric method, MES-TRIS buffer: Collaborative study. *J. AOAC Int.*, 75, 395, 1992.
17. Prosky, L. et al. Determination of insoluble and soluble dietary fiber in foods and food products: Collaborative study. *J. AOAC Int.*, 75, 360, 1992.
18. Prosky, L. et al. Determination of soluble dietary fiber in foods and food products: Collaborative study. *J. AOAC Int.*, 77, 690, 1994.
19. Institute of Medicine. 2001. *Dietary Reference Intakes Proposed Definition of Dietary Fiber.* Washington, DC: National Academy Press.
20. Institute of Medicine. 2002. *Dietary Reference Intakes for Energy, Carbohydrate, Fiber, Fat, Fatty Acids, Cholesterol, Protein, and Amino Acids.* Washington, DC: National Academies Press.
21. U.S. Food and Drug Administration. 2007. *Food Labeling: Revision of Reference Values and Mandatory Nutrients.* Advance Notice of proposed rulemaking. Federal Register 72. pp. 62149–62175. http://heinonline.org/HOL/Page?public=false&handle=hein.fedreg/072212&men_hide=false&men_tab=citnav&collection=fedreg&page=62149 (accessed January 30, 2012).
22. Codex Alimentarius. 2010. *Guidelines on Nutrition Labeling.* www.codexalimentarius.net/download/standards/34/CXG_002e.pdf (accessed January 30, 2012).

5

Resistant Starch

Measurement, Intakes, and Dietary Targets

ANTHONY R. BIRD, SYLVIA USHER, BRUCE MAY,
DAVID L. TOPPING, and MATTHEW K. MORELL

Contents

5.1 Introduction

Resistant starches (RSs) are starches and their digestion products which escape small intestinal digestion in healthy humans and enter the large bowel [1], thereby contributing to total dietary fiber (TDF) intake. Historically, most of the interest in dietary fiber has focused on nonstarch polysaccharides (NSP), but RS is acquiring much greater recognition for its potential to improve human health. Food Standards Australia New Zealand was the first regulatory authority to include RS in the definition of dietary fiber. RS has a range of properties which in and of themselves suggest it may be more important not just for improving large bowel health, including risk of colorectal cancer [2–7], but for enhancing systemic health as well [5,8–12]. Understandably, RS is attracting increasing widespread attention, and nowadays, in addition to health professionals, cereal breeders and food designers and manufacturers are realizing the potential of RS to improve the nutritional and health-promoting attributes of their products. This interest is also driving demand for reliable, fast, and cost-effective assays for commercial, regulatory, and research use.

5.2 Resistant Starches

Unlike NSP and oligosaccharides (OS), RS is not a distinct chemical entity but the end result of a series of integrated physical and chemical processes in the upper gut. Exposure of starchy foods to salivary and pancreatic amylases and small intestinal brush border hydrolases releases glucose which is absorbed rapidly and effectively. Under most circumstances, there is an excess of hydrolytic and absorptive capacity relative to the amount of starch habitually consumed so that little escapes into the large bowel [13–15]. However, starch can (and does) escape digestion and absorption for various reasons. One of the major determinants of the passage of starch out of the terminal ileum is the rate at which digesta moves through the upper gut. The more rapid the rate of transit, the less is the time of exposure of ingested starch to small intestinal hydrolases so that factors which slow or hasten passage rate of starch along the bowel play a major role in determining the RS content of a food or meal.

Particle size is an important element in controlling the rate of passage, with larger particles moving more rapidly than smaller ones [16]. It follows that the extent to which an individual chews their food, and, hence, dentition, is a determinant of the amount of starch which makes it through to the terminal ileum. The importance of the functional capacity of the upper intestinal tract with respect to starch assimilation is clearly evident in individuals with a shortened small bowel (see Table 5.1). Intrinsic factors, notably physical form of the food, how it is prepared and stored, characteristics of coconsumed foods as well as the physicochemical properties of starch itself, the proportion of amylose and amylopectin, and degree of gelatinization, for instance, also play a major role in determining its susceptibility to hydrolysis by α-amylases in the gut lumen [17].

NSP owe their indigestibility to their polymeric structure, but starch differs in that the two major forms (amylose and amylopectin) are digestible. This digestibility is increased by cooking, especially with water, so that RS is comparatively more labile and can be destroyed completely by conventional food processing and cooking methods. Conversely, there are food processing techniques, e.g., repeated cooking and cooling, which result in the formation of RS. Collectively, these diverse physicochemical properties present considerable technical challenges for the accurate determination of RS in foods.

5.3 Measurement of Resistant Starch

5.3.1 In Vivo Methods

RS is a physiological construct so that *in vivo* methods for its determination are the most relevant. However, there is no standardized *in vivo* testing procedure at present, but various physiological approaches have been used. These include the application of animal models, the strategy for which has been to perform digestibility trials in which the confounding effects of large bowel starch fermentation are removed through antibiotic administration or surgical preparation. The latter primarily encompasses ileal cannulation in pigs [18] and ileorectal anastomosis and cecectomy/colectomy in rodents [9,19–21]. While these may be useful research tools, the relevance of the results to humans has not been established.

Table 5.1 RS Content of Test Foods as Determined in a Volunteer with a Short Small Bowel

Food	Short-Bowel Subject[a]	Main Group[b] (Intact Small Bowel)
	RS Content (g/100 g, as Eaten)	
Cornflakes	5.6	2.3
Muesli	24.8	2.9
Breakfast drink	1.7	0.2
Bread (white)	12.6	2.1
Cornish pasty	2.9	0.6
Fries	4.8	0.5

[a] Volunteer had undergone surgical removal of an extensive section of their small bowel for treatment of Crohn's disease.

[b] Values are means of five ileostomy volunteers with minimally resected small bowels.

Daily stomal excretion of ileal digesta in the main group was within the range of that reported for ileostomates with known minimal SI resection (<100 mm) (Sandberg et al. [73]; Lia et al. [74]). Wet and dry matter stomal excretion of the short-bowel subject was several-fold greater than that of the other volunteers, although effluent moisture content was not markedly different, nor were digesta pH, SCFA concentrations, and bacterial numbers. Accordingly, the amount of starch recovered in stomal effluent was markedly larger, for instance, averaging about six times more than that excreted by volunteers with normal digestive function, equating to 10–25 g/day extra starch per day depending on the test food or diet. Day-to-day variation in the data was comparable to that of the other volunteers. These observations demonstrate that the functional capacity of the small intestine of a given individual, and by inference the residence time of chyme in that region of the gut, is a critical determinant of the RS content of foods they consume.

Clearly, measurement of RS using human subjects is the ideal choice, and several procedures have been developed. The first of these is the hydrogen breath test which relies on H_2 evolution through the fermentation of undigested carbohydrate by the large bowel microflora [22,23]. While it has considerable appeal on account of its simplicity and noninvasiveness, it is an indirect measure and is semiquantitative at best. The data are considered to be generally unreliable and unsuitable, especially for food labeling purposes. Small intestinal intubation, either via the nasogastric or retrograde routes, represents a direct approach to quantifying RS [24], but it too has several major deficiencies. Aside from its invasiveness and, hence, risk to the volunteers, the technique itself interferes with the process of starch digestion and, as such, overestimates the amount of RS present in test foods.

The human ileostomy model is the most commonly used *in vivo* method for RS determination and is widely considered the "gold standard." It is essentially a mass-balance technique in which ileostomates consume a test food and the proportion of starch exiting the terminal ileum is then determined and RS calculated. In addition to being direct, quantitative, noninvasive, and relatively straightforward, the model is useful for providing detailed information on the morphological and molecular architecture and other properties of RS [25].

Despite its practical advantages, it is claimed the ileostomy model may suffer from several possible shortcomings which would impact on the accuracy of RS determinations. The most important of these is that upper gut function may not be normal through the absence of the ileocolonic brake. This is a feedback control mechanism whereby large bowel fermentation products slow the transit of food through the ileocecal valve. These products are the short-chain fatty acids (SCFA) which play a key role in modulating large bowel and terminal ileum motility. This criticism seems to be relatively unimportant as the gastric emptying of liquids is comparable to that in individuals with an intact gastrointestinal tract; however, the rate of release of solids may be somewhat slower in ileostomists [26]. However, mouth-to-ileum transit time of ileostomists and normal subjects appears similar [27–29]. These findings suggest that the ileal brake remains functional in ileostomists [30], possibly through the quite small levels of SCFA which are found in these subjects following the passage of food. Most importantly for RS determination, small intestinal starch digestibility has been shown to be independent of starch intake as indicated by a positive linear relationship between starch consumption and ileal stomal output [27,31].

Possible bacterial overgrowth in the ileum and digesta collection bags has been raised as a concern with this model [9]; however, microbial numbers and activity are low in digesta effluent of healthy recruits [32]. Consistent with this observation are the near-neutral pH and low SCFA concentrations in ileal digesta of volunteers who meet the usual study selection criteria. Of the individual major SCFA, acetate predominates (molar ratio usually >0.80) in ileal digesta [33]. In our studies (Bird, Topping and Usher, unpublished results), total SCFA concentrations in stomal collections from eligible volunteers were never high ($\leq 10\,mM$) and similar to those published in the literature (e.g., [28,34]). Furthermore, regression analysis demonstrated that bacterial metabolic activity in stomal collections (as evidenced by low SCFA concentration and excretion as well a slightly acidic pH) did not influence ileal starch excretion or RS determination significantly. Administration of antibiotics to ileostomists had no effect on subsequent ileal starch recovery [28], providing further direct evidence that bacterial activity, either in the small intestine or ileostomy bag, does not interfere greatly with RS determination. It seems reasonable to assume that bacterial hydrolysis of starch in the small intestinal lumen of ileostomists is unlikely to differ greatly from that in subjects with an intact intestinal system. Frequent collection and immediate freezing of stomal collections further ensure that bacterial degradation of starch is negligible.

Provided stringent testing criteria and study conditions are met, the model yields reliable RS data. Recruitment of "healthy" volunteers (i.e., without active disease) with "minimally" resected small bowel and well-established, normal functioning stoma are deemed an imperative, as is intensive management of volunteers and a postprandial stomal effluent collection period no shorter than 24 h.

However, ileostomy studies are becoming increasingly challenging because of the difficulty in recruiting ileostomates who fulfill the necessary selection criteria. For instance, the volunteers often do not know the extent of their terminal ileal resection (preferably <10 cm). Measurement of stomal bile acid excretion provides a direct gauge of functional integrity of the upper gut in these individuals. Ulcerative colitis (UC) is a common cause for stomal surgery, but sometimes it is necessary to enlist ileostomates whose total colectomy was performed for other conditions (e.g., cancer). In our experience, provided that the recruits have a well-established, normally functioning stoma and intestinal inflammation is not evident, their digestibility data are no different from ileostomates diagnosed previously with UC.

5.3.2 Laboratory Methods

By definition, *in vivo* methods are essential for RS determination, but they, as such, are prone to serious technical, practical, and ethical constraints. They are also slow, costly to perform and require stringent testing conditions in order to achieve acceptable levels of precision and, as such, they are quite incompatible with routine or high volume testing. This along with other shortcomings has prompted the development of laboratory methods which ostensibly offer a practical solution to screen foods for RS.

Englyst and colleagues [35] were the first to use the term "resistant starch" to describe starch which resists enzymatic amylolysis *in vitro*. Since then, numerous *in vitro* procedures have been developed, all of which essentially attempt to simulate, to varying degrees of complexity, starch digestion as occurs in humans [17,36]. The general analytical principle is based on an incubation system combined with conventional enzymatic and spectrophotometric methods of quantifying end products of digestion (glucose). The relative strengths and shortcomings of these methods have been reviewed elsewhere (see [9,12,36]). Most methods derive from Berry's [37] modification of Englyst's original method. The earlier assays tended to use harsh laboratory methods which did not mimic conditions or processes that occur in the gut, whereas subsequent methods, such as those of Englyst et al. [38], Muir and O'Dea [39], Champ et al. [40] and McCleary and Monaghan [41], employ protocols more consistent with the fundamental nature of the RS concept. Furthermore, these investigators have attempted to validate their assays against results obtained from human studies. Champ et al. [36] have evaluated the defining features and performance of some of these analytical methods comprehensively.

Generally, most *in vitro* RS assays are relatively easy to perform and yield precise and reproducible results, but their physiological relevance is a vexed question because *in vivo* validation is either nonexistent or inadequate. The *in vitro* results for RS tend to be method specific, and comparative studies have demonstrated large discrepancies between *in vitro* methods in their estimation of the RS content of various foods [42–44]. Of the published laboratory-based methods, those of McCleary and Monaghan [41] and Muir and O'Dea [39] appear to be the best in that they are direct techniques for which there has been some attempt to validate their accuracy. Unfortunately, the number and range of foods tested were limited and included uncommon or experimental foods. Both methods have, in addition, various practical limitations. For instance, Muir and O'Dea's use of volunteers to preprocess test food samples is clearly unviable for routine analyses [45]. McCleary and Monaghan [41] instead use laboratory milling, but this approach is not in keeping with the physiological concept of RS. There is also concern that *in vitro* techniques fail to account for products of partial starch degradation that may escape digestion in the upper gut and potentially contribute to starch-derived α-glucan efflux from the ileum of healthy individuals [42].

The method of McCleary and Monaghan [41] has achieved international accreditation (AOAC Method 2002.02 and AACC Method [32–40]) and can be performed using a commercial assay kit. However, as with other RS assays, it is labor intensive and takes several days to complete. Conversely, Englyst's assay [38] has shorter incubation times more in keeping with human small intestinal digesta passage rates [46], but it still has the disadvantage of being an indirect analytical procedure which is generally considered difficult to perform.

A quantitative high-throughput bench-scale method for predicting the RS content of human foods has been developed by CSIRO Food Futures National Research Flagship. Essentially, the procedure mimics the starch digestion processes of the human upper gastrointestinal tract. Samples of foods in a form ready to be eaten are prepared for testing first by chopping using a simple mechanical device that disrupts the physical structure of the food matrix to mimic mastication. The test foods are then mixed with artificial saliva and the resultant digesta incubated at physiological pH and temperature with a suite of hydrolases to simulate gastric and pancreatic phases of digestion. Residual starch is subsequently isolated, dispersed and digested enzymatically to completion using high-purity α-amylase and amyloglucosidase. Glucose is quantified by standard laboratory techniques and the (resistant) starch yield calculated.

Accuracy of the CSIRO *in vitro* method was assessed by assaying a wide variety of foods and the results were compared with those obtained *in vivo* in ileostomy effluent. The method of food preparation was identical for both *in vivo* and *in vitro* determinations. Starchy foods selected for validation studies were typical of those eaten in industrialized countries, required minimal if any preparation for consumption, and were shelf stable so as to minimize food preparation and storage effects on RS content. The foods analyzed encompassed a broad range of food types and RS contents. Many of the reference foods were commercially manufactured products sold through local supermarkets and other retail outlets and were chosen because they account for a large share of total starch intake of adult consumers in Australia. In the validation studies, it was ensured that total α-glucan content of ileal digesta was quantified. A fundamental criticism of

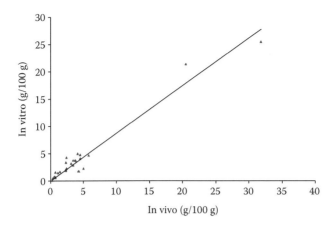

Figure 5.1 Relationship between the resistant starch content of a variety of everyday foods determined in vivo in ileostomates and in vitro using the CSIRO assay.

many RS methodologies is that they do not accord with the (physiological) definition of RS. Specifically, only starch contained in intact and broken granules is captured, whereas small-molecular-weight starch derivatives (i.e., glucooligosaccharides, maltose, and glucose) escaping digestion and absorption in the upper gut and reaching the terminal ileum of healthy volunteers are overlooked [40,47]. It has been reported that free glucose and glucooligosaccharides represent about 10%–20% of starch in ileal digesta [42,48–50]; however, studies in our laboratory indicate that starch-derived glucose and maltodextrins together often contribute no more than 10% of the total RS content of common starchy foods.

In vitro values were within the range obtained with ileostomates and demonstrate the validity of the CSIRO assay for RS determination. The relationship between *in vitro* and *in vivo* values was strong ($r^2 = 0.953$, n = 28; Figure 5.1). The CSIRO assay also demonstrates acceptable precision as evidenced by coefficients of variation of about 5% or less, which were achieved regularly for homogeneous foods, as well as specificity and sensitivity. Furthermore, analytical precision is achieved for foods with low levels of RS which is important because customarily starchy foods contain little RS, usually <1% (Bird, Topping, and Usher, unpublished results; [51]). The low-cost predictive method has utility for expediting development of new cereal lines as well as foods and food ingredients containing reduced digestibility starches of benefit to the health and well-being of consumers.

5.3.3 Resistant Starch Analyzer

The CSIRO laboratory assay has now been fully automated, and a compact, robotics-based prototype instrument has been fabricated, which is capable of rapidly and reliably predicting the RS content of human foods. Reaction cycles and digestion are computer controlled, and the conditions are programmed by the operator. The instrument has undergone extensive validation to verify its predictive accuracy, and the results generated for foods spanning a broad range of RS values and food groups are in close agreement with those obtained from human ileostomy studies. Using the instrument, the time taken to complete RS testing is markedly shortened to about one-third that of the manual RS method. Results for a given test food can now be produced within 1 working day.

5.4 Resistant Starch Consumption

The aggregated intake data suggest that in most middle- and high-income countries, little RS is consumed and per capita intakes are estimated to be in the order of no more than 10 g per day [2,51–53]. The low intakes are explained by relatively recent changes in dietary patterns with a decline in total starch consumption as a consequence of rising economic status [2,54]. It appears also that the starch in modern processed foods is comparatively highly digestible through the introduction of high-speed steel roller grain mills and other technologies for producing extensively processed, highly refined starchy foods. Existing food databases are only a rough guide to the true amount of RS consumed by different populations because they have been derived largely using unsubstantiated analytical methods. Aside from the well-established limitations of measuring food consumption accurately, estimates of RS intakes have been often calculated simply as a fixed proportion (e.g., 5%) of total starch intake (see Baghurst et al. [2]). More sophisticated methods using food databases coupled to nutrition survey data of large populations have produced similar estimates (e.g., approximately 9 g/day, Roberts et al. [53]).

We have used the CSIRO assay to construct an RS database encompassing an extensive range of everyday starchy foods commonly eaten by many Australians. These and other data (Bird, Topping, and Usher, unpublished data; [55]) suggest that RS intake for Australians as well as that of many other comparable populations should be revised downward to <5 g RS/day for adults. Accurate population-wide RS consumption data for populations at low risk of chronic diseases, such as colorectal cancer, are limited. An estimate of RS intakes for one such population (black South Africans) suggested intakes of >20 g/day [6]. Other estimates suggest that RS intakes in rural agrarian populations are likely to be almost an order of magnitude higher than in high-risk Western populations [52]. Reliable data on RS intakes in children and adolescents are not presently available.

5.5 Dietary Sources of RS

The majority of modern starchy foods are low in RS, the exceptions being legumes and pulses [38,36] along with a limited range of manufactured foods which have been formulated with RS-rich ingredients such as high-amylose maize starch. As with other types of fiber, cereals and cereal-based products contribute the largest share of RS in various Western diets ([2,51,53]; see Table 5.2). For most people, wheat is the predominant dietary cereal. However, conventional wheat cultivars are low in RS. Only about 1% of starch in commonly used wheat lines is RS (Bird, Topping, Usher, and Morell, unpublished results), and modern flour

Table 5.2 Intake and Dietary Sources of RS for Various Populations

Population	Food Source (Major Foods)	Contribution to Total RS Intake (%)	Estimated Average RS Intake	Methodology	Reference
Italy	Cereals (white bread, breakfast cereals)	71	8.5 g/day	Direct (*in vitro*) analysis of representative foods; national dietary survey data	Brighenti et al. [75]
	Vegetables (potatoes)	7			
	Legumes	13			
Australia	Cereals (white bread, breakfast cereals)	38	5 g/day		Baghurst et al. [2], Roberts et al. [53]
	Vegetables (potatoes)	26			
	Fruit (bananas)	22			
United States	Cereals (cereal-based foods, breads)	40	5 g/day (range 3–8 g/day)	Database on RS content of foods compiled using published *in vitro* and *in vivo* values; population dietary profile based on NHANES	Murphy et al. [51]
	Vegetables	19			
	Bananas	14			
China	Cereals (wheat and rice, porridge, pancakes, biscuits)	53	15	*In vitro* analysis of selected foods and methods; Goni et al. [77], Akerberg et al. [78], Danjo et al. [47], and dietary survey data	Chen et al. [76]
	Tubers (potato and sweet potato; deep-fried, roasted foods; cooked and cooled)	11			

milling and food processing methods deplete further the amount of starch escaping digestion in the upper gut. Although vegetables, principally potato and other tubers, account for about 20% of dietary RS, our analyses show that potatoes, especially instant preparations, contain negligible amounts of RS. Markedly greater amounts (up to 12%) of starch escape digestion when potato is cooked and cooled [56]. Bananas are probably the richest fruit source of RS; however, the amount present varies with stage of ripeness which essentially dictates the starch content ([57]; Bird et al., unpublished data).

5.6 Intake Targets

Understandably, there are no broad-based public health recommendations for RS consumption as yet. Even for dietary fiber, the information available to health authorities is considered inadequate to establish firm targets such as Recommended Dietary Intakes or Estimated Average Requirements. Instead, an Adequate Intake (AI) of about 30–40 g/day for adults is currently recommended (see NHMRC [58]). Australian authorities have established AIs for fiber according to life stage and gender. For men and women, the current recommended fiber intakes are 30 and 25 g/day, and these were derived based on median population intakes from the latest nutrition survey results [58]. Allowance has been made for RS intakes of 3–4 g/day which are not as yet captured in food database values for TDF.

Dietary targets for adults of 20 g RS per day have been proposed [2], but the reliable epidemiological data needed to provide a set point estimate remain to be gathered. Population data from Cassidy et al. [52] documenting estimated RS consumption and prevalence of colorectal cancer among and between diverse populations suggest that low risk of large bowel cancer, as occurs in rural-based, low-income countries, corresponds to eating about 15 g RS per day. However, the reliability of the intake data is another matter. Unfortunately, quantitative information from controlled feeding trials in humans is inconsistent, often inaccurate, and concerned mainly with evaluating high doses of a narrow range of RS sources. In many studies, the actual amount of RS that is administered is unknown or erroneously documented as simply the amount of high-amylose starch ingested by volunteers. As a consequence, actual RS intakes would have been quite modest and perhaps not surprisingly failed to bring satisfactory or anticipated improvements in physiological endpoints [59]. Even more problematic is interpretation of results from controlled feeding trials owing to the possibility of interactions between RS and other sources of fiber in study foods and meals [5,60]. Nevertheless, numerous feeding trials have demonstrated that daily intakes of RS on the order of 20 g elicit meaningful physiological responses in adults [3,5,6,13]. In animal studies, health benefits have been achieved at RS intakes that equate proportionately by metabolic body weight to those proposed for people (20 g/day). Toden et al. [61] established a clear dose response in rats, demonstrating that RS attenuates colonocyte DNA damage at dietary levels which would be readily achievable in humans. Given that most contemporary starchy foods supply little RS, especially those common in high-income countries, achieving the proposed four- to fivefold increase in dietary levels through dietary change poses a significant challenge.

5.7 Strategies for Increasing RS Intake

Consumption of minimally processed starchy foods, especially whole grains containing rolled, flaked, cracked, or kibbled kernels or coarsely milled flour made from the entire grain (wholemeal flour), is the most obvious means for raising the average consumption of RS. Birkett et al. [55] showed that a diet based on wholegrain breads, cereals, and legumes delivered almost 12 g of starch daily to the terminal ileum of ileostomates, an amount two- to threefold greater than that achieved on a typical Western diet providing about 120 g of starch. However, diets containing a large proportion of minimally processed cereals, grains, and seeds lack mass appeal because they fail to meet consumer preferences for taste, appearance, mouthfeel, and/or convenience. Wholemeal foods such as breads and pasta, while more appealing to consumers, contribute little RS because they are derived from cereal cultivars with highly digestible starch (see Table 5.1). Recent food processing and cereal breeding efforts have led to the development of high-amylose maize starches which produce foods with more RS than conventional varieties. These food ingredients are now available in many markets, and there is an expanding scientific literature as to the health benefits they offer [3,6,13,62]. We have shown recently that RS in the form of high-amylose maize starch abrogates DNA damage and mucus barrier thinning in the colon of rats fed high-protein diets [63,64], and subsequent studies are under way to determine whether these benefits translate to humans (Le Leu, Conlon, Bird, Young, and Topping, unpublished results). Although high-amylose maize starches have proven effective as a source of RS (Table 5.1), various technological and commercial factors limit their range of application as a food ingredient [62].

CSIRO is using both conventional and genetic modification technologies to develop new lines of staple cereals, principally wheat, barley, and rice. These are substantially more concentrated in RS than conventional cultivars and have considerable potential for the production of convenience foods, delivering substantiated health benefits as well as having taste and texture attributes which appeal to broad sections of the population [65–67]. Integral to expediting this process has been the development and application of reliable, high-throughput methods for discriminating high-amylose cereal lines and prototype foods on the basis of their RS content. Novel methods for processing low-digestibility starches are also being established to augment further the RS content of foods derived from these ingredients.

A novel hull-less, high-amylose barley (BARLEYmax™) has been produced, grown on a commercial scale, and the grain processed into new consumer foods with substantiated health benefits [68,69]. Wholemeal flour from this cereal incorporates readily into a range of acceptable processed foods which are two to three times higher in RS and contain substantially more soluble and insoluble dietary fiber than other commercially available barley products. Dietary intervention trials in various animal models and humans have demonstrated improvements in established indices of metabolic and bowel health relative to conventional cereal lines [70,71].

High-amylose wheat (HAW) has been produced using genetic technologies involving RNA interference, which was used to silence expression of two starch branching enzymes in wheat endosperm to produce a line that is high in amylose [66]. Laboratory testing has established that this novel wheat is high in RS. A short-term feeding trial in rats, in which the novel grain was incorporated into the diet as wholemeal flour, has demonstrated positive effects on various physiological and biochemical biomarkers of gut health [66]. A subsequent study in which rats were fed HAW in conjunction with a high-risk Western diet for 3 months confirms and builds on earlier findings showing that the new wheat variety attenuated high levels of DNA damage induced by the Western diet. In this study, the three sources of RS—HAW, conventional, and butyrylated high-amylose maize starches—that were used all reduced DNA damage to approximately the same extent [72].

Cereal foods are basic dietary commodities for most humans, and so foods produced using low-digestibility starchy endosperms may be particularly helpful in preventing and managing metabolic syndrome and as a useful adjunct in the battle against the global epidemic of noncommunicable diseases, such as type II diabetes. It is anticipated that in the long term, these low-digestibility starches will be used in formulations that result in the creation of healthier modern convenience foods acceptable to consumers while contributing to improved public health through a lowering of diet-related morbidity and mortality.

References

1. Asp, N.-G., Resistant starch, *Eur. J. Clin. Nutr.*, 46(Suppl 2), S1, 1992.
2. Baghurst, P.A., Baghurst, K.I., and Record, S.J., Dietary fibre, non-starch polysaccharides and resistant starch: A review, *Food Aust.*, 48(Suppl), S3–S35, 1996.
3. Bird, A.R. and Topping, D.L., Resistant starch, fermentation, and large bowel health, in *Handbook of Dietary Fiber*, Cho, S.S. and Dreher, M.L., Eds., Marcel Dekker, New York, 2001, Chapter 9.
4. Young, G.P. and Le Leu, R.K., Resistant starch and colorectal neoplasia, *J. AOACI.*, 87, 775, 2004.
5. Bird, A.R., Lopez-Rubio, A., Shrestha, A.K., and Gidley, M.J., Resistant starch in vitro and in vivo: Factors determining yield, structure, and physiological relevance, in *Modern Biopolymer Science: Bridging the Divide between Fundamental Treatise and Industrial Application*, Kasapsis, S., Norton, I.T., and Ubbink, J.B., Eds., Academic Press, Burlington, MA, Chapter 14, 2009.
6. Topping, D.L., Segal, I., Regina, A., Conlon, M.A., Bajka, B.H., Toden, S., Clarke, J.M., Morell, M.K., and Bird, A.R., Resistant starch and human health, in *Dietary Fibre: New Frontiers in Food and Health*, van der Kamp, J.W., Jones, J., McCleary, B., and Topping, D., Eds., Wageningen Academic Publishers, Wageningen, the Netherlands, 2010, pp. 311–321.
7. Bird, A.R., Conlon, M.A., Christophersen, C.T., and Topping, D.L., Resistant starch, large bowel fermentation and a broader perspective of prebiotics and probiotics, *Benef. Microbes*, 1, 43, 2010.

8. Brouns, F., Kettlitz, B., and Arrigoni, E., Resistant starch and the butyrate revolution, *Trends Food Sci. Technol.*, 13, 251, 2002.
9. Champ, M.M., Physiological aspects of resistant starch and in vivo measurements, *J. AOAC Int.*, 87, 749, 2004.
10. Higgins, J.A., Resistant starch: Metabolic effects and potential health benefits, *J. AOAC Int.*, 87, 761, 2004.
11. Kendall, C.W., Emam, A., Augustin, L.S., and Jenkins, D.J., Resistant starches and health, *J. AOAC Int.*, 87, 769, 2004.
12. Nugent, A.P., Health properties of resistant starch, *Nutr. Bull.*, 30, 27, 2005.
13. Bird, A.R., Brown, I.L., and Topping, D.L., Starches, resistant starches, the gut microflora and human health, *Curr. Issues Intest. Microbiol.*, 1, 25, 2000.
14. Diamond, J.M. and Karasov, W.H., Adaptive regulation of intestinal nutrient transporters, *Proc. Natl. Acad. Sci. USA*, 84, 2242, 1987.
15. Moran, A.W., Al-Rammahi, M.A., Arora, D.K., Batchelor, D.J., Coulter, E.A., Ionescu, C., Bravo, D., and Shirazi-Beechey, S.P., Expression of Na+/glucose co-transporter 1 (SGLT1) in the intestine of piglets weaned to different concentrations of dietary carbohydrate, *Br. J. Nutr.*, 104, 647, 2010.
16. Heaton, K.W., Dietary fibre, *BMJ*, 300, 1479, 1990.
17. Woolnough, J.W., Monro, J.A., Brennan, C.S., and Bird, A.R., Simulating human carbohydrate digestion in vitro: A review of methods and the need for standardisation, *Int. J. Food Sci. Technol.*, 43, 2245, 2008.
18. Zhang, Y.C., Jorgensen, H., Fernandez, J.A. et al., Digestibility of carbohydrates in growing pigs: A comparison between the t-cannula and the steered ileo-caecal valve cannula, *Arch. Anim. Nutr.*, 58, 219, 2004.
19. Hildebrandt, L.A. and Marlett, J.A., Starch bioavailability in the upper gastrointestinal-tract of colectomized rats, *J. Nutr.*, 121, 679, 1991.
20. Marlett, J.A. and Longacre, M.J., Comparison of in vitro and in vivo measures of resistant starch in selected grain products, *Cereal Chem.*, 73, 63, 1996.
21. Morita, T., Kasoka, S., Kiriyama, S., Brown, I.L., and Topping, D.L., Comparative effects of acetylated and unmodified high amylomaize starch in rats, *Starch-Stärke*, 57, 246, 2005.
22. Olesen, M., Critical review of hydrogen breath test methods in resistant starch and dietary fiber research, in *Handbook of Dietary Fiber*, Cho, S.S. and Dreher, M.L., Eds., Marcel Dekker, New York, 2001, Chapter 11.
23. Symonds, E.L., Kritas, S., Omari, T.I., and Butler, R.N., A combined 13CO2/H2 breath test can be used to assess starch digestion and fermentation in humans, *J. Nutr.*, 134, 1193, 2004.
24. Stephen, A.M., Starch and dietary fibre: Their physiological and epidemiological interrelationships, *Can. J. Physiol. Pharmacol.*, 69, 116, 1991.
25. Zhou, Z.K., Topping, D.L., Morell, M.K., and Bird, A.R., Changes in starch physical characteristics following digestion of foods in the human small intestine, *Br. J. Nutr.*, 104, 573, 2010.
26. Robertson, M.D. and Mathers, J.C., Gastric emptying rate of solids is reduced in a group of ileostomy patients, *Dig. Dis. Sci.*, 45, 1285, 2000.
27. Chapman, R.W., Sillery, J.K., Graham, M.M. et al., Absorption of starch by healthy ileostomates: Effect of transit time and of carbohydrate load, *Am. J. Clin. Nutr.*, 41, 1244, 1985.
28. Englyst, H.N. and Cummings, J.H., Digestion of the polysaccharides of some cereal foods in the human small intestine, *Am. J. Clin. Nutr.*, 42, 778, 1985.
29. Schweizer, T.P., Anderson, H., Langkilde, A.M. et al., Nutrients excreted in ileostomy effluents after consumption of mixed diets with beans or potatoes. II. Starch, dietary fibre and sugars, *Eur. J. Clin. Nutr.*, 44, 567, 1990.

30. Soper, N.J., Chapman, N.J., Kelly, K.A. et al., The 'ileal brake' after ileal pouch-anal anastomosis, *Gastroenterology*, 98, 111, 1990.

31. Langkilde, A.M., Champ, M., and Andersson, H., Effects of high-resistant-starch banana flour (RS(2)) on in vitro fermentation and the small-bowel excretion of energy, nutrients, and sterols: An ileostomy study, *Am. J. Clin. Nutr.*, 75, 104, 1992.

32. Berghouse, L., Hori, S., Hill, M., Hudson, M., Lennard-Jones, J.E., and Rogers, E., Comparison between the bacterial and oligosaccharide content of ileostomy effluent in subjects taking diets rich in refined or unrefined carbohydrate, *Gut*, 25, 1071, 1984.

33. Nordgaard, I., Mortensen, P.B., and Langkilde, A.M., Small intestinal malabsorption and colonic fermentation of resistant starch and resistant peptides to short-chain fatty acids, *Nutrition*, 11, 129, 1995.

34. Newton, C.R., Comparison of bowel function after colectomy and ileostomy or ileo-rectal anastomosis for inflammatory bowel disease, *Gut*, 13, 85, 1972.

35. Englyst, H., Wiggins, H.S., and Cummings, J.H., Determination of the non-starch polysaccharides in plant foods by gas-liquid chromatography of constituent sugars as alditol acetates, *Analyst*, 107, 307, 1982.

36. Champ, M., Langkilde, A.M., Brouns, F. et al., Advances in dietary fibre characterisation. 2. Consumption, chemistry, physiology and measurement of resistant starch; implications for health and food labelling, *Nutr. Res. Rev.*, 16, 143, 2003.

37. Berry, C.S., Resistant starch: Formation and measurement of starch that survives exhaustive digestion with amylolytic enzymes during the determination of dietary fibre, *J. Cereal Sci.*, 4, 301, 1986.

38. Englyst, H.N., Kingman, S.M., and Cummings, J.H., Classification and measurement of nutritionally important starch fractions, *Eur. J. Clin. Nutr.*, 46(Suppl. 2), S33, 1992.

39. Muir, J.G. and O'Dea, K., Measurement of resistant starch: Factors affecting the amount of starch escaping digestion in vitro, *Am. J. Clin. Nutr.*, 56, 123, 1992.

40. Champ, M., Martin, L., Noah, L., and Gratas, M., Analytical methods for resistant starch, in *Complex Carbohydrates in Foods*, Cho, S.S., Prosky, L., and Dreher, M.L., Eds., Marcel Dekker, New York, 1999, p. 169, Chapter 14.

41. McCleary, B.V. and Monaghan, D.A., Measurement of resistant starch, *J. AOAC Int.*, 85, 665, 2002.

42. Champ, M.M., Molis, C., Flourie, B., Bornet, F., Pellier, P., Colonna, P., Galmiche, J.P., and Rambaud, J.C., Small-intestinal digestion of partially resistant cornstarch in healthy subjects, *Am. J. Clin. Nutr.*, 68, 705, 1998.

43. Madrid, J. and Arcot, J., Comparison of two in vitro analysis of resistant starch of some carbohydrate containing foods, *Proc. Nutr. Soc. Aust.*, 24, 208, 2000.

44. Walter, M., da Silva, L.P., and Denardin, C.C., Rice and resistant starch: Different content depending on chosen methodology, *J. Food Comp. Anal.*, 18, 279, 2005.

45. Muir, J.G. and O'Dea, K., Validation of an in vitro assay for predicting the amount of starch that escapes digestion in the small intestine of humans, *Am. J. Clin. Nutr.*, 57, 540, 1993.

46. Read, N.W., Al-Janabi, M.N., Holgate, A.M., Barber, D.C., and Edwards, C.A., Simultaneous measurement of gastric emptying, small bowel residence and colonic filling of a solid meal by the use of the gamma camera, *Gut*, 27, 300, 1986.

47. Danjo, K., Nakaji, S., Fukuda, S., Shimoyama, T., Sakamoto, J., and Sugawara, K., The resistant starch level of heat moisture–treated high amylose cornstarch is much lower when measured in the human terminal ileum than when estimated in vitro, *J. Nutr.*, 133, 2218–2221, 2003.

48. Faisant, N., Buleon, A., Colonna, P., Molis, C., Lartigue, S., Galmiche, J.P., and Champ, M., Digestion of raw banana starch in the small intestine of healthy humans: Structural features of resistant starch, *Br. J. Nutr.*, 73, 111, 1995.

49. Silvester, K.R., Englyst, H.N., and Cummings, J.H., Ileal recovery of starch from whole diets containing resistant starch measured in vitro and fermentation of ileal effluent, *Am. J. Clin. Nutr.*, 62, 403, 1995.

50. Noah, L., Guillon, F., Bouchet, B., Buleon, A., Molis, C., Gratas, M., and Champ, M., Digestion of carbohydrate from white beans (*Phaseolus vulgaris* L.) in healthy humans. *J. Nutr.*, 128, 977, 1998.

51. Murphy, M.M., Douglass, J.S., and Birkett, A., Resistant starch intakes in the United States, *J. Am. Diet. Assoc.*, 108, 67, 2008.

52. Cassidy, A., Bingham, S.A., and Cummings, J.H., Starch intake and colorectal-cancer risk: An international comparison, *Br. J. Cancer*, 69, 937, 1994.

53. Roberts, J., Jones, G.P., Rutihauser, I.H.E., Birkett, A., and Gibbons, C., Resistant starch in the Australian diet, *Nutr. Diet.*, 61, 98, 2004.

54. Barnard, N.D., Trends in food availability, 1909–2007, *Am. J. Clin. Nutr.*, 91(Suppl), 1530S, 2010.

55. Birkett, A.M., Mathers, J.C., Jones, G.P. et al., Changes to the quantity and processing of starchy foods in a western diet can increase polysaccharides escaping digestion and improve in vitro fermentation variables, *Br. J. Nutr.*, 84, 63, 2000.

56. Englyst, H.N. and Cummings, J.H., Digestion of polysaccharides of potato in the small intestine of man, *Am. J. Clin. Nutr.*, 45, 423, 1987.

57. Englyst, H.N. and Cummings, J.H., Digestion of the carbohydrates of banana (*Musa paradisiaca sapientum*) in the human small intestine, *Am. J. Clin. Nutr.*, 44, 42, 1986.

58. Australian Government Department of Health and Aging. National Health and Medical Research Council, Nutrient reference values for Australia and New Zealand including recommended dietary intakes. September 2005. http://www.nhmrc.gov.au

59. Penn-Marshall, M., Holtzman, G.I., and Barbeau, W.E., African Americans may have to consume more than 12 grams a day of resistant starch to lower their risk for type 2 diabetes, *J. Med. Food*, 13, 999, 2010.

60. Muir, J.G., Yeow, E.G.W., Keogh, J., Pizzey, C., Bird, A.R., Sharpe, K., O'Dea, K., and Macrae, F.A., Combining wheat bran with resistant starch raised faecal butyrate and lowered phenols in humans. *Am. J. Clin. Nutr.*, 79, 1020–1028, 2004.

61. Toden, S., Bird, A.R., Topping, D.L., and Conlon, M.A., Dose-dependent reduction of dietary protein-induced colonocyte DNA damage by resistant starch in rats correlates more highly with caecal butyrate than with other short chain fatty acids, *Cancer Biol. Ther.*, 6, 253, 2007.

62. Brown, I.L., Applications and uses of resistant starch, *J. AOAC Int.*, 87, 727, 2004.

63. Toden, S., Bird, A.R., Topping, D.L., and Conlon, M.A., Differential effects of dietary whey and casein on colonic DNA damage in rats, *Aust. J. Dairy Technol.*, 60, 146, 2005.

64. Toden, S., Bird, A.R., Topping, D.L., and Conlon, M.A., Resistant starch prevents colonic DNA damage induced by high dietary cooked red meat or casein in rats, *Cancer Biol. Ther.*, 5, 267, 2006.

65. Rahman, S., Bird, A., Regina, A. et al., Resistant starch in cereals: Exploiting genetic engineering and genetic variation, *J. Cereal Sci.*, 46, 251, 2007.

66. Regina, A., Bird, A., Li, Z., Rahman, S. et al., Bioengineering cereal carbohydrates to improve human health, *Cereal Foods World*, 52, 182, 2007.

67. Topping, D., Bird, A., Toden, S., Conlon, M. et al., Resistant starch as a contributor to the health benefits of whole grains, in *Whole Grains and Health*, Marquardt, L., Jacobs, D., McIntosh, G., Poutanen, K., and Reicks, D., Eds., Blackwell Publishing, Ames, IA, 2007, Chapter 17.

68. Bird, A.R., Vuaran, M.S., King, R.A. et al., Wholegrain foods made from a novel high amylose barley variety (Himalaya 292) improve indices of bowel health in human subjects, *Br. J. Nutr.*, 99, 1032, 2008.

69. King, R.A., Noakes, M., Bird, A.R. et al., An extruded breakfast cereal made from a high amylose barley cultivar has a low glycemic index and lower plasma insulin response than one made from a standard barley, *J. Cereal Sci.*, 48, 526, 2008.
70. Bird, A.R., Flory, C., Davies, A., Usher, S., and Topping, D.L., A novel barley cultivar (Himalaya 292) with a specific gene mutation in starch synthetase IIa resulting in altered grain starch and non-starch polysaccharide composition raises large bowel starch and short chain fatty acids in rats, *J. Nutr.*, 134, 831, 2004.
71. Bird, A.R., Jackson, M., King, R.A., Davies, A., Usher, S., and Topping, D.L., A novel high amylose barley cultivar (Himalaya 292) lowers plasma cholesterol and alters indices of large bowel fermentation in pigs, *Br. J. Nutr.*, 92, 607, 2004.
72. Conlon, M.A., Bird, A.R., Regina, A. et al., Resistant starches lower calorie DNA damage and alter coloric gene expression and microflova profiles in rat fed on western diet. *J. Nutr.*, 2012 (in press).
73. Sandberg, A.S., Hasselblad, C., Hasselblad, K. et al., The effect of wheat bran on the absorption of minerals in the small intestine, *Br. J. Nutr.*, 48, 185, 1982.
74. Lia, A., Sundberg, B., Aman, P. et al., Substrates available for colonic fermentation from oat, barley and wheat bread diets. A study in ileostomy subjects, *Br. J. Nutr.*, 76, 797, 1996.
75. Brighenti, F., Casiraghi, M.C., and Baggio, C., Resistant starch in the Italian diet, *Br. J. Nutr.*, 80, 333, 1998.
76. Chen, L., Liu, R., Qin, C., Meng, Y., Zhang, J., Wang, Y., and Xu, G., Sources and intake of resistant starch in the Chinese diet, *Asia Pac. J. Clin. Nutr.*, 19, 274, 2010.
77. Goni, I., Garcia-Diz, L., Manas, E., and Saura-Calixto, F., Analysis of resistant starch: A method for foods and food products, *Food Chem.*, 56, 445, 1996.
78. Akerberg, A.K.E., Liljeberg, H.G.M., Granfeldt, Y.E., Drews, A.W., and Bjorck, I.M.E., An in vitro method, based on chewing, to predict resistant starch content in foods allows parallel determination of potentially available starch and dietary fiber, *J. Nutr.*, 128, 651, 1998.

6
Measurement Techniques for Insulin Sensitivity

KEVIN C. MAKI

Contents

6.1 Introduction

Insulin resistance is an impaired ability of insulin to effectively lower blood glucose. It is a contributing factor in a number of metabolic abnormalities that increase risk for type 2 diabetes mellitus and atherosclerotic cardiovascular disease.[1] As such, measurement of insulin resistance has important applications for evaluating the efficacy of interventions aimed at prevention.

The term insulin sensitivity describes the ability of a given circulating level of insulin to promote a reduction in blood glucose concentration, which can result from enhanced cellular glucose uptake and/or suppression of hepatic glucose output. Diabetes prevention trials have shown that interventions which increase insulin sensitivity significantly reduce the rate of conversion to diabetes in high-risk individuals.[2-6] In the Diabetes Prevention Program, a lifestyle intervention with targets of 150 min per week of physical activity and weight loss of 7% reduced the rate of progression to diabetes by 58% relative to placebo without lifestyle intervention,[3] which was greater than the 31% reduction in new-onset diabetes with metformin treatment. Thiazolidinediones which activate peroxisome-proliferator-activated receptors (PPAR), specifically PPAR-gamma, also reduce insulin resistance and have been shown to lower the risk of diabetes by as much as 80% when administered alone or combined with metformin.[6-8] The goal of this review is to describe several methods for measuring insulin sensitivity, the advantages and limitations associated with each approach, and considerations for their use in clinical trials.

6.2 Direct Methods for Assessing Insulin Sensitivity

Direct and indirect methods for assessing insulin sensitivity are available.[9–11] Direct methods, including the euglycemic, hyperinsulinemic glucose clamp and the insulin suppression test (IST), assess insulin-mediated glucose under steady-state conditions.[12–14]

6.2.1 Euglycemic, Hyperinsulinemic Glucose Clamp

The euglycemic, hyperinsulinemic glucose clamp, often referred to simply as the glucose clamp, is considered the reference standard for measuring insulin sensitivity. The procedure for administering the euglycemic, hyperinsulinemic glucose clamp has been described in detail.[14] Briefly, after an overnight fast, insulin is infused intravenously (IV) at a constant rate to produce a new steady-state insulin level, typically well above the fasting concentration (hyperinsulinemia). Bedside glucose is then measured at 5–10 min intervals while a 10%–20% glucose solution is administered IV at a variable rate to "clamp" the blood glucose concentration in the normal range, in other words, euglycemia. To prevent hypokalemia, which can result from hyperinsulinemia, potassium phosphate may be concurrently infused. Following approximately 2 h of constant insulin infusion, a steady-state glucose infusion rate is typically achieved. When the hyperinsulinemic state is sufficient to completely suppress hepatic glucose production, the glucose infusion rate will equal the glucose disposal rate (M). M in mg per kg of body weight (or per kg of fat-free mass) is a measure of insulin sensitivity. If insulin (I) levels are found to vary within (via repeat testing) or between individuals, it is sometimes necessary to adjust for this by calculating the M/I ratio.

While most glucose clamp studies are completed with a single insulin infusion rate, some have employed two or more insulin infusion rates, which allow greater characterization of the insulin dose-response curve (Figure 6.1).[9] This procedure also allows calculation of an insulin sensitivity index (S_I) derived from clamp data with two or more insulin levels ($SI_{Clamp} = \Delta M/\Delta I$), which is conceptually similar to the S_I derived from minimal model analysis of data from an IV glucose tolerance test (discussed in the following text). Radiolabeled glucose tracers ("hot clamp" methods) are also sometimes used to measure hepatic glucose production, allowing characterization of both hepatic and peripheral (mostly skeletal muscle) insulin sensitivity.[15–17]

The validity of the glucose clamp depends on the achievement of steady-state conditions and that hepatic glucose production is completely suppressed by steady-state hyperinsulinemia. This method measures whole-body glucose disposal directly at a given level of insulinemia under steady-state conditions. However, the glucose clamp method does not reflect hepatic or adipose tissue insulin sensitivity, which are important in the pathophysiology of diabetes and in the development of cardiovascular disease risk factors associated with insulin resistance (e.g., the metabolic syndrome).[18] Furthermore, this method is time consuming, labor intensive, and expensive.

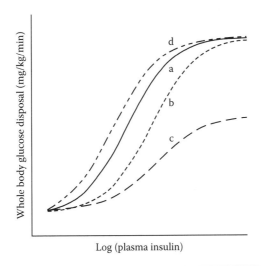

Figure 6.1 Clamp-derived measures of concentration response relationships between plasma insulin concentrations and insulin-mediated whole-body glucose disposal. Curve a = normal insulin sensitivity and responsiveness, curve b = rightward shift in insulin concentration-response curve (decreased insulin sensitivity with normal insulin responsiveness), curve c = decreased insulin sensitivity and reduced insulin responsiveness, and curve d = leftward shift in insulin-concentration response curve (increased insulin sensitivity with normal insulin responsiveness). (Reprinted from Muniyappa, R. et al., *Am. J. Physiol. Endocrinol. Metab.*, 294, E15, 2008. With permission. Copyright 2008 American Physiological Society.)

6.2.2 Insulin Suppression Test

The IST is another direct method for measurement of the ability of exogenous insulin to mediate glucose disposal under steady-state conditions, where endogenous insulin (and glucagon) secretion and hepatic glucose output are fully suppressed (Figure 6.2).[19] The IST procedure was first introduced by Shen et al.[12] and later modified by Harano et al.[13] After an overnight fast, somatostatin (or the somatostatin analog, octreotide), insulin, and glucose are infused simultaneously at constant rates for 3 h. Glucose and insulin concentrations are measured every 10 min during the final 30 min of the test and averaged. The steady-state plasma glucose (SSPG) level is a direct measure of insulin sensitivity. The validity of the IST result depends on the achievement of a steady-state condition with constant levels of plasma glucose (SSPG) and plasma insulin (SSPI), and assumes that the somatostatin infusion is sufficient to completely suppress endogenous insulin and glucagon secretion. However, the standard infusion rates may not be ideal for every population. In very insulin-sensitive individuals, there is some risk of hypoglycemia, and in very insulin-resistant individuals, the glucose level may rise to the point where renal spillover occurs. Also, SSPI levels may vary within or between subjects. If marked differences occur, it may be necessary to calculate SSPG/SSPI, similar to the M/I ratio adjustment used with the euglycemic, hyperinsulinemic clamp.

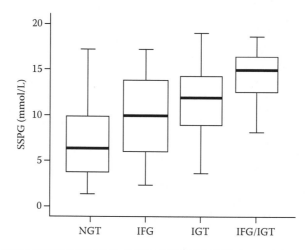

Figure 6.2 SSPG concentrations in glucose tolerance categories assessed by an IST. NGT, normal glucose tolerance; IFG, impaired fasting glucose; IGT, impaired glucose tolerance; and IFG/IGT, combined IFG and IGT. (Reprinted from Kim, S.H. and Reaven, G.M., *Diabetes Care*, 31, 347, 2008. With permission. Copyright 2008 American Diabetes Association.)

Because the IST has no variable infusion, steady-state conditions are more easily achieved than during the glucose clamp method. SSPG from the IST is highly reproducible, and estimates of insulin sensitivity from the IST method correlate well with those from the reference euglycemic, hyperinsulinemic glucose clamp method in subjects with either normal glucose tolerance ($r = 0.93$) or type 2 diabetes ($r = 0.91$).[20,21] However, there are limitations to this method, including the fact that SSPG measures peripheral insulin sensitivity and does not reflect differences in hepatic insulin sensitivity. The IST is significantly less labor intensive than the glucose clamp procedure and requires less technical expertise to administer, but it is still both time consuming and expensive and thus impractical in population and large clinical studies.

6.3 Indirect Methods for Assessing Insulin Sensitivity

Due to the expense and complexity of direct measures of insulin sensitivity, lower cost and simpler indirect measures have great potential utility for clinical and population studies. Indirect measures commonly utilized include the frequently sampled IV glucose tolerance test (FSIVGTT) with minimal model analysis, indices derived from oral glucose tolerance test (OGTT) or meal tolerance test (MTT), and fasting markers for insulin sensitivity.[9–11]

6.3.1 Frequently Sampled Intravenous Glucose Tolerance Test

In the FSIVGTT, following an overnight fast, an IV bolus of glucose is given. IV insulin (or tolbutamide) is infused 20 min after the IV glucose bolus to produce a second peak in plasma insulin, which helps to distinguish between insulin

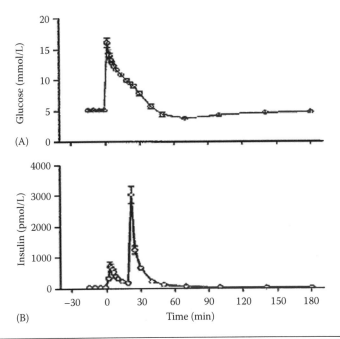

Figure 6.3 Fasting glucose (Panel A) and insulin (Panel B) in a FSIVGTT. (Reprinted from Steil, G.M. et al., *Diabetes*, 53, 1201, 2004. With permission. Copyright 2004 American Diabetes Association.)

and non-insulin-dependent glucose disappearance.[22,23] Blood samples for measurement of plasma glucose and insulin are taken prior to the initial IV glucose bolus and then at frequent postload time points over 180 min (Figure 6.3).[24] Data are evaluated via minimal model analysis using the MINMOD software[25,26] to generate an S_I, which is an indication of the ability of insulin to promote disappearance from the circulation resulting from enhancement of glucose disposal and suppression of hepatic glucose production. MINMOD also generates an index of glucose effectiveness (S_G), which is a measure of the ability of a rise in plasma glucose to increase the rate of glucose disappearance, independent of insulin (Figure 6.4).[9,24–27] The test–retest coefficient of variation for S_I with FSIVGTT is comparable to the glucose clamp method, and the method of glucose delivery is more physiologic than those of the glucose clamp and IST methods. Furthermore, because this test is dynamic, it can also provide information about β-cell function via calculation of a disposition index (Figures 6.5 and 6.6)[28,29]:

Disposition index[28] = Insulin sensitivity index (S_I) × Acute insulin response

The disposition index is a measure of the appropriateness of insulin secretion for a given level of insulin sensitivity. A review of the interplay between insulin resistance and beta-cell function in the development of glucose intolerance and type 2 diabetes mellitus is beyond the scope of this chapter. The interested reader is referred to a review of this topic by Kahn and colleagues.[30]

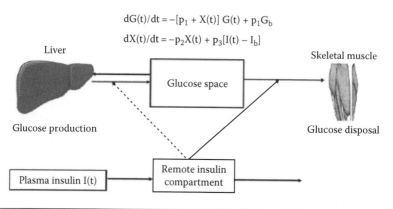

Figure 6.4 Minimal model analysis of FSIVGTT. Differential equations describing glucose dynamics [G(*t*)] in a monocompartmental "glucose space" and insulin dynamics in a "remote compartment" [X(*t*)] are shown at the *top*. Glucose leaves or enters its space at a rate proportional to the difference between plasma glucose level, G(*t*), and the basal fasting level, G_b. In addition, glucose also disappears from its compartment at a rate proportional to insulin levels in the "remote" compartment [X(*t*)]. In this model, *t* = time; G(*t*) = plasma glucose at time *t*; I(*t*) = plasma insulin concentration at *time t*; X(*t*) = insulin concentration in "remote" compartment at time *t*; G_b = basal plasma glucose concentration; I_b = basal plasma insulin concentration; G(0) = G_0 (assuming instantaneous mixing of the IV glucose load); p_1, p_2, p_3, and G_0 = unknown parameters in the model that are uniquely identifiable from FSIVGTT; glucose effectiveness = p_1; and insulin sensitivity = p_3/p_2. (Reprinted from Muniyappa, R. et al., *Am. J. Physiol. Endocrinol. Metab.*, 294, E15, 2008. With permission. Copyright 2008 American Physiological Society.)

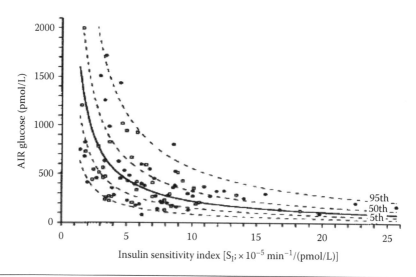

Figure 6.5 Disposition index [relationship between the acute insulin secretory response (AIR) and the S_I (the effects of insulin to promote glucose disposal and suppress hepatic glucose production generated from minimal model analysis of the FSIVGTT)] in healthy subjects. (Reprinted from Kahn, S.E. et al., *Diabetes*, 42, 1663, 1993. With permission. Copyright 1993 American Diabetes Association.)

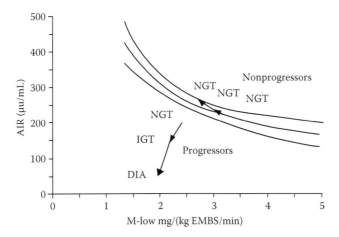

Figure 6.6 Disposition index [relationship between the acute insulin secretory response (AIR) and the rate of total insulin (low dose)-stimulated glucose disposal (M-low)] in 11 Pima Indian subjects in whom glucose tolerance deteriorated from normal (NGT) to impaired (IGT) to diabetic (DIA) (progressors) and in 23 subjects who retained NGT (nonprogressors). The lines represent the prediction line and the lower and upper limits of the 95% confidence interval of the regression between AIR and M-low as derived from a reference population of 277 Pima Indians with NGT. (Reprinted from Weyer, C. et al., *J. Clin. Invest.*, 104, 787, 1999. With permission from the American Society for Clinical Investigation.)

There are some limitations of the FSIVGTT method. The minimal model requires several assumptions including that there is an instantaneous distribution of the glucose bolus, that the disappearance of glucose in response to the glucose or insulin occurs at a monoexponential rate, and that insulin promotes glucose disappearance from a "remote" extravascular compartment.[9,31] This monocompartmental representation of glucose dynamics may result in overestimation of S_G and underestimation of S_I and occasional nonsensical negative values for S_I in subjects with marked insulin resistance.[9,32] Although the FSIVGTT is less complex to administer than the glucose clamp, because steady-state conditions with precise infusion rate adjustments are not required, IV infusions with numerous blood sample collections are still necessary and may be impractical for large epidemiologic and clinical studies. A reduced sampling schedule with 12 rather than 30 samples has been employed for some population studies (e.g., the Insulin Resistance and Atherosclerosis Study[33]), which sacrifices some precision in exchange for lower cost and a less demanding measurement protocol.

6.3.2 Oral Glucose and Meal Tolerance Tests

The indirect methods most often utilized in clinical studies to assess insulin sensitivity under dynamic conditions are the OGTT and the MTT.[9–11] The OGTT typically administers a 75 or 100 g glucose load and then measures glucose and insulin responses at various time points over a 2–4 h interval. The MTT uses a standardized liquid or solid meal, followed by collection of blood samples for measurements of glucose and insulin over 2–4 h. A modification of the minimal model procedure has been used to estimate insulin sensitivity from an OGTT or MTT.[34,35] More commonly, empirically derived surrogate indices of insulin sensitivity such as the Matsuda index (shown in the following) are calculated from glucose and insulin data obtained during the OGTT or MTT:

$$\text{Matsuda index}^{36} = 10,000/[(G_{\text{fasting}} \times I_{\text{fasting}}) \times (G_{\text{Pmean}} \times I_{\text{Pmean}})]^{0.5}$$

where

G_{fasting} and I_{fasting} are preload values for plasma glucose and insulin
G_{Pmean} and I_{Pmean} are mean postload values from samples collected at 30, 60, 90, and 120 min after the start of the glucose load or test meal

The Matsuda index is one of several empirically derived indices of insulin sensitivity. It reflects a composite estimate of hepatic and peripheral (mainly skeletal muscle) insulin sensitivity. It has been shown to correlate reasonably well with whole-body insulin sensitivity estimates determined by the glucose clamp or minimal model methods (Figure 6.7).[36–39] Oral glucose or meal consumption mimics glucose and insulin dynamics of physiological conditions more closely than either of the direct methods previously described.[27] Noteworthy limitations of the OGTT and MTT methods include the fact that they do not directly measure insulin-mediated glucose utilization and that factors other than insulin sensitivity (e.g., variations in the glucose absorption rate, splanchnic glucose uptake, and incretin effects) have the potential to influence the results.[40]

A mixed MTT (liquid or solid) has a number of potential advantages over the OGTT. Insulin-resistant states not only reflect disorders in carbohydrate

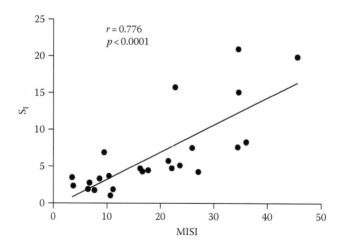

Figure 6.7 Pearson correlations between IV glucose tolerance test S_I and Matsuda insulin sensitivity index (MISI) ($r = 0.776$, $p < 0.0001$). (Reprinted from Maki, K.C. et al., *Diabetes Technol. Ther.*, [Epub ahead of print], April 2, 13, 331, 2011. With permission. Copyright 2011 Mary Ann Liebert, Inc.)

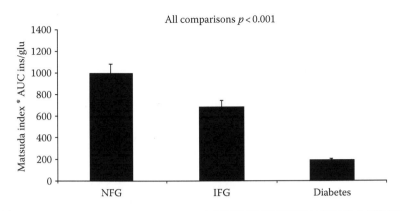

Figure 6.8 Oral disposition index (product of the Matsuda index and the ratio of the areas under the curve for insulin to glucose over 120 min following a liquid MTT) according to categories of fasting glucose tolerance (normal, NFG and impaired, IFG). (From Maki, K.C. et al., *Nutr. J.*, 8, 22, 2009.)

metabolism but are also typically associated with disturbances in fasting and postprandial lipid levels.[1] A mixed MTT provides a physiologic stimulus for simultaneous assessment of postload lipids and for measurement of incretin responses.[41] In addition, some subjects experience nausea or reactive hypoglycemia after a glucose load, which, in the author's experience, is quite rare with a mixed meal.

Solid food meals are difficult to standardize in multisite research studies because food ingredients and meal preparation vary among regions and countries, and subjects differ in the degree to which they chew foods. We recently examined the ability to estimate insulin sensitivity from a liquid MTT which provided a commercially available liquid meal product (Ensure®, Abbott Nutrition, Columbus, OH) that requires no preparation.[42,43] Our studies demonstrated that the Matsuda index and an oral disposition index, calculated as the product of the Matsuda index and the ratio of the total areas under the curves for insulin and glucose from premeal to 120 min after the start of the liquid meal, appropriately ranked categories of fasting glucose status (Figure 6.8).[42,43] The repeatability profiles of the liquid MTT suggested its usefulness in population studies and moderately sized clinical trials requiring repeated measurements.[43]

6.3.3 Fasting Indices

Simple surrogate indices calculated from fasting glucose and/or insulin values including the homeostasis model assessment of insulin resistance (HOMA-IR),[44–46] the quantitative insulin sensitivity check index (QUICKI),[47,48] and 1/fasting insulin[49,50] are also commonly used to evaluate insulin sensitivity.[9,11] These are inexpensive and easily applied in most settings. Of the simple surrogate methods, the most extensively validated for calculating insulin sensitivity are HOMA-IR and QUICKI.[51] The HOMA calculator (available at www.dtu.ox.ac.uk) allows calculation of both an index of insulin sensitivity (HOMA-IR or HOMA-%S) and an index of pancreatic beta-cell function (HOMA-%B) from fasting insulin and glucose concentrations. It should be noted that there are two versions of the HOMA (www.dtu.ox.ac.uk).[44,45] The original version and the updated version (which we refer to as HOMA2) produce similar, but not identical, results. While simple fasting indicators such as HOMA-IR, QUICKI, and 1/fasting insulin are useful in population studies and very large clinical trials,[52–58] they have low precision and thus have limited value as measures of insulin sensitivity in most clinical studies.[46]

6.4 Conclusion

Numerous methods for estimating insulin sensitivity are available. This chapter has provided an overview of some of the methods most commonly employed in clinical research. The preferred method for estimating insulin sensitivity in a particular clinical study depends on many factors. Investigators need to consider accuracy and precision, cost, staff expertise and availability, and subject burden when deciding which method to employ for a particular study.

References

1. Reaven, G., Abbasi, F., and McLaughlin, T., Obesity, insulin resistance, and cardiovascular disease, *Recent Prog. Horm. Res.*, 59, 207, 2004.
2. Tuomilehto, J. et al., Prevention of type 2 diabetes mellitus by changes in lifestyle among subjects with impaired glucose tolerance, *N Engl J Med.*, 344, 1343, 2001.
3. Diabetes Prevention Program Research Group, Reduction in the incidence of type 2 diabetes with lifestyle intervention or metformin, *N Engl J Med.*, 346, 393, 2002.
4. Cherian, B. et al., Therapeutic implications of diabetes in cardiovascular disease, *Am. J. Ther.*, 15, e51, 2009.
5. Hanna-Moussa, A. et al., Dysglycemia/prediabetes and cardiovascular risk factors, *Rev. Cardiovasc. Med.*, 10, 202, 2009.
6. Zinman, B. et al., Low-dose combination therapy with rosiglitazone and metformin to prevent type 2 diabetes mellitus (CANOE trial): A double-blind randomized controlled study, *The Lancet*, 376(9735), 103–111, 2010. 3 June 2010, doi:10.1016/S0140-6736(10)60746-5.
7. Snitker, S. et al., Changes in insulin sensitivity in response to troglitazone do not differ between subjects with and without the common, functional Pro12Ala peroxisome proliferator-activated receptor-gamma2 gene variant: Results from the troglitazone in prevention of diabetes (TRIPOD) study, *Diabetes*, 27, 1365, 2004.
8. DeFronzo, R.A. et al., Determinants of glucose tolerance in impaired glucose tolerance at baseline in the Actos Now for Prevention of Diabetes (ACT NOW) study, *Diabetologia*, 53, 435, 2010.
9. Muniyappa, R. et al., Current approaches for assessing insulin sensitivity and resistance in vivo: Advantages, limitations, and appropriate usage, *Am. J. Physiol. Endocrinol. Metab.*, 294, E15, 2008.
10. Matsuda, M., Measuring and estimating insulin resistance in clinical and research settings, *Nutr. Metab. Cardiovasc. Dis.*, 20, 79, 2010.
11. Singh, B. and Saxena, A., Surrogate markers of insulin resistance: A review, *World J. Diabetes*, 1, 36, 2010.
12. Shen, S.W., Reaven, G.M., and Farquhar, J.W., Comparison of impedance to insulin-mediated glucose uptake in normal subjects and in subjects with latent diabetes, *J. Clin. Invest.*, 49, 2151, 1970.

13. Harano, Y. et al., Glucose, insulin, and somatostatin infusion for the determination of insulin sensitivity in vivo, *Metabolism*, 27, 1449, 1978.
14. DeFronzo, R.A., Tobin, J.D., and Andres, R., Glucose clamp technique: A method for quantifying insulin secretion and resistance, *Am. J. Physiol. Endocrinol. Metab.*, 237, E214, 1979.
15. Rizza, R.A., Mandarino, L.J., and Gerich, J.E., Dose-response characteristics for effects of insulin on production and utilization of glucose in man, *Am. J. Physiol.*, 240, E630, 1981.
16. Finegood, D.T., Bergman, R.N., and Vranic, M., Estimation of endogenous glucose production during hyperinsulinemic-euglycemic glucose clamps. Comparison of unlabeled and labeled exogenous glucose infusates, *Diabetes*, 36, 914, 1987.
17. Campbell, P.J., Mandarino, L.J., and Gerich, J.E., Quantification of the relative impairment in actions of insulin on hepatic glucose production and peripheral glucose uptake in non-insulin-dependent diabetes mellitus, *Metabolism*, 37, 15, 1988.
18. DeFronzo, R.A., Pathogenesis for type 2 diabetes: Metabolic and molecular implications for identifying diabetes genes, *Diabetes Rev.*, 5, 177, 1997.
19. Kim, S.H. and Reaven, G.M., Isolated impaired fasting glucose and peripheral insulin sensitivity: Not a simple relationship, *Diabetes Care*, 31, 347, 2008.
20. Greenfield, M.S. et al., Assessment of insulin resistance with the insulin suppression test and the euglycemic clamp, *Diabetes*, 30, 387, 1981.
21. Mimura, A. et al., Insulin sensitivity test using a somatostatin analogue, octreotide (Sandostatin), *Horm. Metab. Res.*, 26, 184, 1994.
22. Bergman, R.N. et al., Quantitative estimation of insulin sensitivity, *Am. J. Physiol.*, 236, E667, 1979.
23. Bergman, R.N., Lilly lecture 1989. Toward physiological understanding of glucose tolerance. Minimal-model approach, *Diabetes*, 38, 1512, 1989.
24. Steil, G.M. et al., Evaluation of insulin sensitivity and β-cell function indexes obtained from minimal model analysis of a meal tolerance test, *Diabetes*, 53, 1201, 2004.
25. Pacini, G. and Bergman, R.N., MINMOD: A computer program to calculate insulin sensitivity and pancreatic responsivity from the frequently sampled intravenous glucose tolerance test, *Comput. Methods Programs Biomed.*, 23, 113, 1986.
26. Boston, R.C. et al., MINMOD Millennium: A computer program to calculate glucose effectiveness and insulin sensitivity from the frequently sampled intravenous glucose tolerance test, *Diabetes Technol. Ther.*, 5, 1003, 2003.
27. Cobelli, C. et al., Assessment of β-cell function in humans, simultaneously with insulin sensitivity and hepatic extraction, from intravenous and oral glucose tests, *Am. J. Physiol. Endocrinol. Metab.*, 293, E1, 2007.
28. Kahn, S.E. et al., Quantification of the relationship between insulin sensitivity and beta-cell function in human subjects. Evidence for a hyperbolic function, *Diabetes*, 42, 1663, 1993.
29. Weyer, C. et al., The natural history of insulin secretory dysfunction and insulin resistance in the pathogenesis of type 2 diabetes mellitus, *J. Clin. Invest.*, 104, 787, 1999.
30. Kahn, S.E. et al., The relative contributions of insulin resistance and beta-cell dysfunction to the pathophysiology of type 2 diabetes, *Diabetologia*, 46, 3, 2003.
31. Bergman, R.N., Banting Lecture 2006. Orchestration of glucose homeostasis: From a small acorn to the California oak, *Diabetes*, 56, 1489, 2007.
32. Cobelli, C., Caumo, A., and Omenetto, M., Minimal model SG overestimation and SI underestimation: Improved accuracy by a Bayesian two-compartment model, *Am. J. Physiol. Endocrinol. Metab.*, 277, E481, 1999.
33. Howard, G. et al., Insulin sensitivity and atherosclerosis. The Insulin Resistance Atherosclerosis Study (IRAS) investigators, *Circulation* 93, 1809, 1996.
34. Caumo, A., Bergman, R.N., and Cobelli, C., Insulin sensitivity from meal tolerance tests in normal subjects: A minimal model index, *J. Clin. Endocrinol. Metab.*, 85, 4396, 2000.

35. Breda, E. et al., Oral glucose tolerance test minimal model indexes of beta-cell function and insulin sensitivity, *Diabetes*, 50, 150, 2001.

36. Maki, K.C. et al., Validation of insulin sensitivity and secretion indices derived from the liquid meal tolerance test, *Diabetes Technol. Ther.*, 13, 661, 2011.

37. Matsuda, M. and DeFronzo, R.A., Insulin sensitivity indices obtained from oral glucose tolerance testing: Comparison with the euglycemic insulin clamp, *Diabetes Care*, 22, 1462, 1999.

38. Soonthornpun, S. et al., Novel sensitivity index derived from oral glucose tolerance test, *J. Clin. Endocrinol. Metab.*, 88, 1019, 2003.

39. Aloulou, I., Brun, J.F., and Mercier, J., Evaluation of insulin sensitivity and glucose effectiveness during a standardized breakfast test: Comparison with the minimal model analysis of an intravenous glucose tolerance test, *Metabolism*, 55, 676, 2006.

40. Hücking, K. et al., OGTT-derived measures of insulin sensitivity are confounded by factors other than insulin sensitivity itself, *Obesity*, 16, 1938, 2008.

41. Vollmer, K. et al., Predictors of incretin concentrations in subjects with normal, impaired, and diabetic glucose tolerance, *Diabetes*, 57, 678, 2008.

42. Maki, K.C. et al., Indices of insulin sensitivity and secretion from a standard liquid meal test in subjects with type 2 diabetes, impaired or normal fasting glucose, *Nutr. J.*, 8, 22, 2009.

43. Maki, K.C. et al., Repeatability of indices of insulin sensitivity and secretion from standard liquid meal tests in subjects with type 2 diabetes mellitus or normal or impaired fasting glucose, *Diabetes Technol. Ther.*, 12, 895, 2010.

44. Matthews, D.R. et al., Homeostasis model assessment: Insulin resistance and beta-cell function from fasting plasma glucose and insulin concentrations in man, *Diabetologia*, 28, 412, 1985.

45. Levy, J.C., Matthews, D.R., and Hermans, M.P., Correct homeostasis model assessment (HOMA) evaluation uses the computer program, *Diabetes Care*, 21, 2191, 1998.

46. Wallace, T.M., Levy, J.C., and Matthews, D.R., Use and abuse of HOMA modeling, *Diabetes Care*, 27, 1487, 2004.

47. Katz, A. et al., Quantitative insulin sensitivity check index: A simple, accurate method for assessing insulin sensitivity in humans, *J. Clin. Endocrinol. Metab.*, 85, 2402, 2000.

48. Bastard, J.P. et al., Is quantitative insulin sensitivity check index, a fair insulin sensitivity index in humans? *Diabetes Metab.*, 27, 69, 2001.

49. Laakso, M., How good a marker is insulin level for insulin resistance? *Am. J. Epidemiol.*, 137, 959, 1993.

50. de Rooij, S.R. et al., Fasting insulin has a stronger association with an adverse cardiometabolic risk profile than insulin resistance: The RISC study, *Eur. J. Endocrinol.*, 161, 223, 2009.

51. Chen, H., Sullivan, G., and Quon, M.J., Assessing the predictive accuracy of QUICKI as a surrogate index for insulin sensitivity using a calibration model, *Diabetes*, 54, 1914, 2005.

52. Hanley, A.J.G. et al., Prediction of type 2 diabetes using simple measures of insulin resistance. Combined results from the San Antonio Heart Study, the Mexico City Diabetes Study, and the Insulin Resistance Atherosclerosis Study, *Diabetes*, 52, 463, 2003.

53. Torréns, J.I. et al., Ethnic differences in insulin sensitivity and beta-cell function in premenopausal or early perimenopausal women without diabetes: The Study of Women's health Across the Nation (SWAN), *Diabetes Care*, 27, 354, 2004.

54. Kahn, S.E. et al., Glycemic durability of rosiglitazone, metformin, or glyburide monotherapy, *N. Engl. J. Med.*, 355, 2427, 2006.

55. Bertoni, A.G. et al., Insulin resistance, metabolic syndrome, and subclinical athero-sclerosis: The multi-ethnic study of atherosclerosis (MESA), *Diabetes Care*, 30, 3951, 2007.

56. Song, Y. et al., Insulin sensitivity and insulin secretion determined by homeostasis model assessment and risk of diabetes in a multiethnic cohort of women: The Women's Health Initiative observational study, *Diabetes Care*, 30, 1747, 2007.

57. Festa, A. et al., Beta-cell dysfunction in subjects with impaired glucose tolerance and early type 2 diabetes: Comparison of surrogate markers with first-phase insulin secretion from an intravenous glucose tolerance test, *Diabetes*, 57, 1638, 2008.

58. Barr, E.L. et al., HOMA insulin sensitivity index and the risk of all-cause mortality and cardiovascular disease events in the general population: The Australian diabetes, obesity and lifestyle study (AusDiab) study, *Diabetologia*, 53, 79, 2010.

Website:

HOMA Calculator. www.dtu.ox.ac.uk

7

Consumption of Total Fiber and Types of Fiber Are Associated with a Lower Prevalence of Obesity and Abdominal Adiposity in U.S. Adults

NHANES 1999–2006

THERESA A. NICKLAS, CAROL E. O'NEIL,
JOANNE L. SLAVIN, and SUSAN S. CHO

Contents

7.1 Introduction

Dietary fiber is defined as carbohydrate and lignin that are intrinsic and intact in plants [1]. The recommended intake of dietary fiber is 14 g/1000 kcal [1,2] which is based on protection against cardiovascular disease in prospective, cohort studies. Dietary fiber also has accepted health benefits [3] of optimizing gut health [4–6], reducing serum lipids [7–13], and modulating blood glucose [14]. Dietary fiber is linked to lower body weight and protection against weight gain [15–17]. More than 90% of Americans do not meet the fiber recommendation [18].

Dietary fiber promotes a healthy body weight through different physiologic mechanisms [19–21] related to intrinsic, colonic, and hormonal effects. Fiber-rich foods are relatively low in energy and tend to be more satiating than foods low in fiber. Dietary fiber could slow down digestion which facilitates the release of gut hormones that promote satiety. Dietary fiber may slow digestion and absorption of foods and lead to a reduced postprandial blood glucose response, which could improve insulin sensitivity, thus favoring fat oxidation [19–21].

The physiologic effects of dietary fiber on body weight depend on the type of fiber. Higher intakes of fiber from fruit [22] and cereal [9,22–26], but not from vegetables, were associated with a lower weight gain in epidemiologic studies. A recent study found total fiber and cereal fiber were inversely associated with changes in body weight and waist circumference (WC) in adults [23]. However, fruit and vegetable fiber was not associated with changes in body weight but was associated with changes in WC. In contrast, in older adults 60–80 years of age (y), no association was found between intake of total fiber, vegetable fiber, or fruit fiber and body mass index (BMI) and body composition measurements [26]. Individuals with higher intakes of cereal fiber had lower abdominal obesity [26]. The findings from these studies are inconsistent and warrant further investigation. The goal of this study was to evaluate the effect of consumption of total dietary fiber and types of fiber on weight and abdominal obesity in U.S. adults using data from the National Health and Nutrition Examination Survey (NHANES) 1999–2006.

7.2 Subjects and Methods

The NHANES is a continuous surveillance program that collects nationally representative information on the nutrition and health status of the civilian, non-institutionalized U.S. population. Conducted by the National Center for Health Statistics, NHANES data are collected using a complex, stratified, multistage probability cluster sampling design. Data are collected via an in-home interview for demographic and basic health information, and a comprehensive health examination is conducted in a mobile examination center. Detailed descriptions of the sample design, interview procedures, and physical examinations conducted are available [27]. As recommended by NHANES, the data sets from 1999 to 2000, 2001 to 2002, 2003 to 2004, and 2005 to 2006 were combined [28] to increase sample size.

7.2.1 Subjects and Fiber Consumption Categories

The NHANES data collected from 1999 to 2006 were used to compare fiber consumption and weight parameters in adults 19+ y (n = 16,590). The sample was dichotomized into two age groups, 19–50 y (n = 9168) and 51+ y (n = 7422). Only individuals with complete demographic data, body measurements, and whose dietary interview data were deemed reliable by the Food Surveys Research Group were included. Pregnant and lactating females were excluded. Due to the nature of the analysis (secondary data analysis) and the lack of personal identifiers, this study was exempted by the Institutional Review Board of Baylor College of Medicine.

To obtain dietary data, trained interviewers conducted in-person 24 h dietary recalls using a multiple-pass method [29]. For data collection years, 1999–2002, only one interview-administered 24 h dietary recall was conducted. In 2003–2006, 2 days of intake were collected; however, for this study, only day 1 interview-administered recalls were included in the analysis to assure consistency with the 1999–2002 dietary data. Detailed descriptions of these methods are provided in the NHANES Dietary Interviewer's Training Manual [30].

The MyPyramid Equivalents Database (MPED) for USDA Survey Food Codes, versions 1 [31] and 2 [32], was used in NHANES 1999–2002 and 2003–2006, respectively, to calculate fiber intake. The MPED food data files contain the number of servings (or ounce equivalents) per 100 g of food by 32 MyPyramid food groups [33–35]. Participants were categorized into quartiles for total dietary fiber intake: quartile 1 = <9 g of total fiber; quartile 2 = ≥9 g and <13.8 g; quartile 3 = ≥13.8 g and <20 g; and quartile 4 = ≥20 g. Five fiber types were examined in the analyses: cereal, vegetable, grain, fruit, and other. All fiber groups were categorized with nonconsumers (0 intake) as the first group and quartiles of intake for consumers. Cereal fiber included all food codes for ready-to-eat cereals (RTEC); grain fiber included RTEC grains in addition to yeast breads, rolls, quick breads, cakes, cookies, pies, pastries, salty snacks, pancakes, waffles, pastas, and cooked cereals; fruit fiber includes whole fruits, fruit juices, dried fruits, and fruit mixtures; vegetable fiber included all vegetables and vegetable mixtures; and other fiber included other foods where grains, fruits, and vegetables were not a major ingredient, such as chocolate milk and nuts and seeds.

7.2.2 Anthropometric Measures

The Anthropometry Procedures Manual [36] used in the 1999–2006 NHANES provides information about equipment, calibration, methods, and quality control. BMIs were calculated as weight in kilograms divided by height in meters squared (kg/m^2). Overweight was defined as a BMI ≥25, and obese was defined as a BMI ≥30. Increased WC was defined as ≥102 cm in men and ≥88 cm in women.

7.2.3 Statistical Analysis

Data were analyzed using SAS (Release 9.1.3) and SUDAAN (Release 10.0, RTI, Research Triangle Park, NC) software programs. All analyses included sample weights that account for the unequal probabilities of selection due to oversampling and nonresponse. Sample-weighted data were used, and all analyses to adjust the variance for the complex sample design. For the 1999–2006, an 8 year sample weight variable was created by assigning ½ of the 4 year sample weight for 1999–2002 and ½ of the 4 year sample weight for 2003–2006. The 8 year sample weight was used in all analyses [37].

Least square means and standard errors were generated. P for trend was calculated using linear regression, modeling the dependent variable (weight outcomes) on intake of total fiber or the five types of fiber as linear variables in the independent regression models. A p-value <0.05 was considered significant. For total fiber intake, covariates used were age, gender, ethnicity, the poverty income ratio, energy, smoking status, alcohol intake, and physical activity. The same covariates were included in the regression models for each fiber type controlling for the other four fiber components.

7.3 Results

The sample consisted of 55.3% of 19–50 years and 44.7% 51+ years; 47.7% were males, 51.1% whites, 19.7% blacks, 25.5% Hispanics, and 3.6% other (Table 7.1). Mean fiber intake was 15.8 g ± 0.1 g, and only 9.4% of adults met the adequate

Table 7.1 Demographics of the Sample

Demographic Variables	Age Group		
	19–50 Years	51+ Years	19+ Years
Total n (%)	9,168 (55.3%)	7,422 (44.7%)	16,590 (100%)
Gender			
Males n (%)	4,201 (25.3%)	3,711 (22.4%)	7,912 (47.7%)
Females n (%)	4,967 (29.9%)	3,711 (22.4%)	8,678 (52.3%)
Ethnicity/race			
Whites n (%)	4,157 (25.1%)	4,321 (26.0%)	8,478 (51.1%)
Blacks n (%)	1,970 (11.9%)	1,305 (7.9%)	3,275 (19.7%)
Hispanics n (%)	2,653 (16.0%)	1,582 (9.5%)	4,235 (25.5%)
Other n (%)	388 (2.3%)	214 (1.3%)	602 (3.6%)
Total dietary fiber intake			
Mean (g) ± SE	15.76 ± 0.13	15.72 ± 0.14	15.75 ± 0.10
% meeting AI	7.1% ± 0.3%	13.4% ± 0.5%	9.4% ± 0.3%
Intake by type of fiber			
Grain fiber (mean $\bar{x}$ ± SE)	7.14 ± 0.08	6.51 ± 0.08	6.92 ± 0.06
% of total fiber	46.2% ± 0.3%	42.7% ± 0.4%	44.9% ± 0.3%
Vegetable fiber (mean $\bar{x}$ ± SE)	3.41 ± 0.05	3.69 ± 0.05	3.51 ± 0.04
% of total fiber	23.3% ± 0.3%	24.9% ± 0.3%	23.9% ± 0.2%
Fruit fiber (mean $\bar{x}$ ± SE)	1.48 ± 0.03	2.25 ± 0.04	1.75 ± 0.03
% of total fiber	8.39% ± 0.2%	13.2% ± 0.2%	10.1% ± 0.1%
Cereal fiber (mean $\bar{x}$ ± SE)	0.74 ± 0.03	1.15 ± 0.05	0.88 ± 0.03
% of total fiber	3.8% ± 0.1%	5.85% ± 0.2%	4.5% ± 0.1%
Other fibers (mean $\bar{x}$ ± SE)	3.73 ± 0.07	3.26 ± 0.07	3.56 ± 0.05
% of total fiber	22.1% ± 0.3%	19.2% ± 0.3%	21.1% ± 0.2%

intake (AI) for fiber. Most of the fiber consumed was grain fiber (44.9%), followed by vegetable fiber (23.9%), other fiber (21.1%), fruit fiber (10.1%), and cereal fiber (4.5%) (Table 7.1).

The association between total fiber intake and weight is shown in Figure 7.1. There was a significant (p = 0.0001) linear decrease in BMI and WC with increasing total fiber intake. BMI decreased from 28.8 (quartile 1) to 27.6 (quartile 4). WC decreased from 98.0 (quartile 1) to 95.0 (quartile 4).

The association between percent overweight, percent obese, and percent with high WC and total fiber intake is shown in Figure 7.1. No significant association was found between total fiber intake and percent overweight. A significant (p = 0.0001) linear trend was found between total fiber intake and percent obese and percent with elevated WC. The percent obese decreased from 36.5% (quartile 1) to 27.9% (quartile 4). The percent with high WC decreased from 54.6% (quartile 1) to 45.6% (quartile 4).

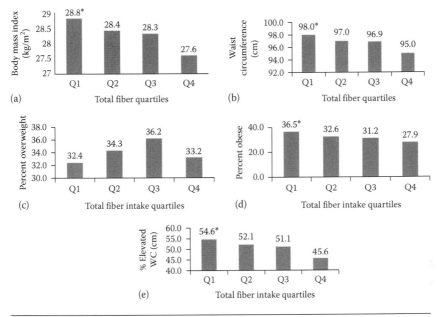

Figure 7.1 Association between (a) body mass index and total fiber intake (19+ years old), (b) waist circumference and total fiber intake (19+ years old), (c) percent overweight and total fiber intake (19+ years old), (d) percent obese and total fiber intake (19+ years old), and (e) percent with elevated waist circumference and total fiber intake. *p for trend = 0.0001.

The association between the type of fiber and weight is shown in Table 7.2. There was a significant (p < 0.05) linear decrease in BMI, WC, percent obese, and percent with high WC with increased intakes of grain fiber, cereal fiber, fruit fiber, and other fiber. BMI decreased from 28.7 to 27.9 (grain fiber), 28.4 to 27.5 (cereal fiber), 28.8 to 27.4 (fruit fiber), and 28.8 to 27.9 (other fiber) for quartiles 1 and 4, respectively. WC decreased from 97.8 to 96.0 (grain fiber), 97.1 to 95.5 (cereal fiber), 98.0 to 94.7 (fruit fiber), and 98.1 to 95.7 (other fiber) for quartiles 1 and 4, respectively. The percent with high WC decreased from 51.8% to 49.1% (grain fiber), 51.9% to 47.8% (cereal fiber), 54.4% to 44.1% (fruit fiber), and 53.7% to 47.7% (other fiber) for quartiles 1 and 4, respectively. No association was seen between the types of fiber consumed and the percent overweight. No association was found between vegetable fiber and any of the weight measures studied.

7.4 Discussion

In this cross-sectional study, an inverse association was found between intakes of total dietary fiber and five types of fiber with BMI, WC, and percent obese and with increased WC. Intake of vegetable fiber was not associated with any of the weight measures. All of the significant associations between types of fiber and weight were attenuated after controlling for the other types of fiber in the model. Total fiber intake and types of fiber were not associated with percent overweight.

Table 7.2 Association between Type of Fiber Consumed and Weight

Weight Measures	Nonconsumer LSM ± SE	Q1 LSM ± SE	Q2 LSM ± SE	Q3 LSM ± SE	Q4 LSM ± SE
			Consumers of grain fiber		
BMI (kg/m²)[a]	28.7 ± 0.4	28.4 ± 0.1	28.4 ± 0.1	28.2 ± 0.1	27.9 ± 0.1[A]
WC (cm)	97.8 ± 1.0	97.1 ± 0.3	97.1 ± 0.3	96.7 ± 0.3	96.0 ± 0.3[A]
% overweight	32.5 ± 2.7	32.7 ± 1.0	34.1 ± 0.9	33.5 ± 0.9	35.9 ± 1.0
% obese	33.9 ± 2.7	33.5 ± 1.0	33.4 ± 0.9	31.6 ± 0.9	29.6 ± 1.0[C]
% ↑ WC	51.8 ± 2.8	52.0 ± 1.0	52.6 ± 1.0	49.6 ± 0.9	49.1 ± 1.0[A]
			Consumers of cereal fiber		
BMI (kg/m²)[b]	28.4 ± 0.1	27.8 ± 0.3	27.5 ± 0.3	27.3 ± 0.3	27.5 ± 0.3[D]
WC (cm)	97.1 ± 0.2	96.5 ± 0.6	95.1 ± 0.7	94.7 ± 0.6	95.5 ± 0.6[D]
% overweight	33.8 ± 0.5	35.9 ± 2.0	32.4 ± 1.9	33.9 ± 2.0	37.2 ± 2.1
% obese	33.3 ± 0.5	31.1 ± 2.0	26.3 ± 1.8	25.7 ± 1.8	25.7 ± 1.8[D]
% ↑ WC	51.9 ± 0.5	50.3 ± 2.1	44.3 ± 1.9	44.2 ± 2.0	47.8 ± 2.1[C]
			Consumers of fruit fiber		
BMI (kg/m²)[c]	28.8 ± 0.1	27.9 ± 0.2	28 ± 0.2	27.6 ± 0.2	27.4 ± 0.2[D]
WC (cm)	98.0 ± 0.2	95.8 ± 0.4	96.4 ± 0.4	95.7 ± 0.4	94.7 ± 0.4[D]
% overweight	33.6 ± 0.7	34.2 ± 1.3	34 ± 1.3	33.6 ± 1.2	35.7 ± 1.3
% obese	35.7 ± 0.7	30.1 ± 1.2	30.4 ± 1.2	29.1 ± 1.2	25.4 ± 1.2[D]
% ↑ WC	54.4 ± 0.7	48.5 ± 1.3	49.2 ± 1.3	48.8 ± 1.3	44.1 ± 1.3[D]
			Consumers of vegetable fiber		
BMI (kg/m²)[d]	28.5 ± 0.2	28.1 ± 0.1	28.4 ± 0.1	28.2 ± 0.1	28.1 ± 0.2
WC (cm)	97.3 ± 0.4	96.5 ± 0.3	97.3 ± 0.3	96.8 ± 0.3	96.1 ± 0.3
% overweight	34.4 ± 1.2	33.2 ± 1.0	34.4 ± 1.0	34.6 ± 1.0	33.5 ± 1.0
% obese	33.7 ± 1.1	31.5 ± 1.0	33.3 ± 1.0	31.7 ± 1.0	30.4 ± 1.0
% ↑ WC	51.8 ± 1.2	50.1 ± 1.1	52.2 ± 1.0	51.1 ± 1.0	49.2 ± 1.1
			Consumers of other fiber		
BMI (kg/m²)[d]	28.8 ± 0.2	28.3 ± 0.1	28.3 ± 0.1	28.2 ± 0.1	27.9 ± 0.1[B]
WC (cm)	98.1 ± 0.4	96.9 ± 0.3	96.8 ± 0.3	96.7 ± 0.3	95.7 ± 0.3[C]
% overweight	33.6 ± 1.2	34.8 ± 1.0	34.5 ± 1.0	34.0 ± 1.0	33.0 ± 1.0
% obese	34.9 ± 1.2	32.0 ± 1.0	32.5 ± 1.0	31.4 ± 1.0	30.3 ± 1.0[B]
% ↑ WC	53.7 ± 1.3	51.3 ± 1.1	52.1 ± 1.0	50.1 ± 1.0	47.7 ± 1.1[D]

[a] Controlling for vegetable, fruit, and other fibers.
[b] Controlling for vegetable, noncereal grain, fruit, and other fibers.
[c] Controlling for grain, vegetable, and other fibers.
[d] Controlling for grain, vegetable, and fruit fibers.
LSM (SE) = least square means and standard error.
WC = waist circumference.
Trend: [A]$p < 0.05$; [B]$p < 0.01$; [C]$p < 0.001$; [D]$p < 0.0001$.

This lack of association between fiber and percent overweight could be due to decreased sensitivity of detecting relationships using categorical data compared to continuous data. It may be that it is at the extremes (i.e., normal weight vs. obese) that associations with fibers can be detected. The use of categorical data loses some of the variance in the data, whereas the use of continuous data (i.e., BMI) is more likely to detect stronger relationships. In this study, BMI and WC decreased significantly with increased fiber intake. These results are consistent with other published studies conducted on adults [13,16,17,23,26].

Observational and intervention studies with adults support a beneficial role of total dietary fiber and types of fiber in maintaining body weight [26], promoting weight loss [17,23], and preventing weight gain [13,16,22]. In observational studies, fiber intake was inversely associated with body weight [38,39] and adiposity [40]. In the Seven Countries Study, dietary fiber was inversely related to subscapular skinfold thickness [5]. Populations that reported higher fiber consumption also demonstrated lower obesity rates [6].

In a prospective study with 89,432 European adults who were followed for an average of 6.5 years, total fiber intake was associated with subsequent decreases in weight and WC [23]. In the Nurse's Health Study, women with higher fiber intake gained less weight over 12 years [16]. In the Coronary Artery Risk Development in Young Adults Study, high fiber intake was associated with lower weight gain over a 10 year period [13].

Few studies have compared different fiber types and their association with weight [22,23,26]. A prospective cohort study among 27,082 male U.S. health professionals compared the effects of cereal and fruit fiber with subsequent weight change [22]. Significant inverse associations were found between weight change and concurrent change in the intake of total fiber, cereal fiber, and fruit fiber, but not vegetable fiber. These findings corroborate with another study of adult males and females for total and cereal fiber [23]. The inverse association between fiber intake and weight appears to be more pronounced for cereal fiber compared with fruit and vegetable fiber.

There are several possible explanations for this finding. Most fiber consumed in the American diet is cereal fiber. Cereal fiber is likely to be a marker for whole grain foods [41] which are associated with a lower BMI and adiposity in cross-sectional or cohort studies with adults [42]. The inverse association between fruit fiber and weight may be due to the displacement of energy-dense foods and the satiating effect of fiber, resulting in less energy consumed [43]. The lack of an association between intake of vegetable fiber and weight may reflect the low consumption of vegetables by Americans [44,45] regardless of body weight.

A recent systematic review was conducted on the relationship of fruit and vegetable intake with adiposity [46]. Of the 11 longitudinal and experimental studies on adults, 8 showed that higher fruit and vegetable intake was related to weight loss while 3 did not. Three of the seven longitudinal studies in adults found an inverse association between fruit and vegetable intake and adiposity, one found no association, and three obtained mixed results. The authors of the review concluded that the inverse association between fruit and vegetable intake and adiposity among overweight adults appeared weak and the findings were inconsistent.

Physiologic mechanisms by which dietary fiber helps in maintaining body weight have been summarized previously [19–21]. Briefly, foods high in fiber tend to be more satiating because digestion is slowed down and can lead to reduced energy intake, high fiber intakes may prevent enzymatic digestion of other macronutrients in the small intestine, and high fiber intakes may lead to a reduced postprandial blood glucose response that improves insulin sensitivity, thus favoring fat oxidation. What is less clear is whether these mechanisms apply equally to all types of fiber.

Analysis of NHANES data is limited by the cross-sectional design that precludes any causal inferences. Participants relied on their memory to self-report dietary intakes; therefore, data were subject to nonsampling errors, such as over- and underreporting of energy and examiner effects.

To our knowledge, this is the most recent analysis looking at intake of total fiber and types of fiber on weight and adiposity in a nationally representative sample of adults. The findings support earlier studies for total fiber and cereal fiber but not for vegetable and fruit fiber. Longitudinal studies are needed to better understand the associations between types of fiber and weight and the mechanisms for those associations.

Acknowledgments

This work is a publication of the U.S. Department of Agriculture (USDA/ARS) Children's Nutrition Research Center, Department of Pediatrics, Baylor College of Medicine in Houston, Texas, and was also funded in part with federal funds from the USDA/Agricultural Research Service under Cooperative Agreement No. 58-6250-6-003. The contents of this publication do not necessarily reflect the views or policies of the USDA, nor does the mention of trade names, commercial products, or organizations imply endorsement from the U.S. government. Partial support was also received from the USDA HATCH project LAB 93951. The authors thank Bee Wong for help in obtaining research articles and Nisha Jamal for typing the manuscript.

References

1. National Academy of Sciences, Institute of Medicine of the National Academies. *Dietary Reference Intakes for Energy, Carbohydrate, Fiber, Fat, Fatty Acids, Cholesterol, Protein, and Amino Acids. Panel on Macronutrients.* Washington, DC: National Academy Press, 2002.
2. Dietary Guidelines Advisory Committee. Nutrition and your health: Dietary guidelines for Americans. 2005 Dietary Guidelines Advisory Committee Report. U.S. Department of Agriculture, Agricultural Research Service, Washington, DC, 2005.
3. Anderson JW, Baird P, Davis RH, Jr. et al. Health benefits of dietary fiber. *Nutr Rev* 2009;67:188–205.

4. Wong JM, de Souza R, Kendall CW, Emam A, Jenkins DJ. Colonic health: Fermentation and short chain fatty acids. *J Clin Gastroenterol* 2006;40:235–243.

5. Macfarlane S, Macfarlane GT, Cummings JH. Review article: Prebiotics in the gastro-intestinal tract. *Aliment Pharmacol Ther* 2006;24:701–714.

6. Watzl B, Girrbach S, Roller M. Inulin, oligofructose and immunomodulation. *Br J Nutr* 2005;93(Suppl 1):S49–S55.

7. Van Horn L. Fiber, lipids, and coronary heart disease. A statement for healthcare pro-fessionals from the Nutrition Committee, American Heart Association. *Circulation* 1997;95:2701–2704.

8. Flight I, Clifton P. Cereal grains and legumes in the prevention of coronary heart disease and stroke: A review of the literature. *Eur J Clin Nutr* 2006;60:1145–1159.

9. Newby PK, Maras J, Bakun P, Muller D, Ferrucci L, Tucker KL. Intake of whole grains, refined grains, and cereal fiber measured with 7-d diet records and associations with risk factors for chronic disease. *Am J Clin Nutr* 2007;86:1745–1753.

10. He M, van Dam RM, Rimm E, Hu FB, Qi L. Whole-grain, cereal fiber, bran, and germ intake and the risks of all-cause and cardiovascular disease-specific mortality among women with type 2 diabetes mellitus. *Circulation* 2010;121:2162–2168.

11. Rimm EB, Ascherio A, Giovannucci E, Spiegelman D, Stampfer MJ, Willett WC. Vegetable, fruit, and cereal fiber intake and risk of coronary heart disease among men. *J Am Med Assoc* 1996;275:447–451.

12. Mozaffarian D, Kumanyika SK, Lemaitre RN, Olson JL, Burke GL, Siscovick DS. Cereal, fruit, and vegetable fiber intake and the risk of cardiovascular disease in elderly individuals. *JAMA* 2003;289:1659–1666.

13. Ludwig DS, Pereira MA, Kroenke CH et al. Dietary fiber, weight gain, and cardiovas-cular disease risk factors in young adults. *JAMA* 1999;282:1539–1546.

14. Anderson JW, Randles KM, Kendall CW, Jenkins DJ. Carbohydrate and fiber rec-ommendations for individuals with diabetes: A quantitative assessment and meta-analysis of the evidence. *J Am Coll Nutr* 2004;23:5–17.

15. Slavin JL. Dietary fiber and body weight. *Nutrition* 2005;21:411–418.

16. Liu S, Willett WC, Manson JE, Hu FB, Rosner B, Colditz G. Relation between changes in intakes of dietary fiber and grain products and changes in weight and development of obesity among middle-aged women. *Am J Clin Nutr* 2003;78:920–927.

17. Tucker LA, Thomas KS. Increasing total fiber intake reduces risk of weight and fat gains in women. *J Nutr* 2009;139:576–581.

18. Moshfegh A, Goldman J, Cleveland L. What we eat in America, NHANES 2001–2002: Usual nutrient intakes from food compared to Dietary Reference Intakes. U.S. Department of Agriculture, Agricultural Research Service, 2005.

19. Howarth NC, Saltzman E, Roberts SB. Dietary fiber and weight regulation. *Nutr Rev* 2001;59:129–139.

20. Heaton KW. Food fiber as an obstacle to energy intake. *Lancet* 1973;2:1418–1421.

21. Pereira MA, Ludwig DS. Dietary fiber and body-weight regulation. Observations and mechanisms. *Pediatr Clin North Am* 2001;48:969–980.

22. Koh-Banerjee P, Franz M, Sampson L et al. Changes in whole-grain, bran, and cereal fiber consumption in relation to 8-y weight gain among men. *Am J Clin Nutr* 2004;80:1237–1245.

23. Du H, van der AD, Boshuizen HC et al. Dietary fiber and subsequent changes in body weight and waist circumference in European men and women. *Am J Clin Nutr* 2010;91:329–336.

24. Gaesser GA. Carbohydrate quantity and quality in relation to body mass index. *J Am Diet Assoc* 2007;107:1768–1780.

25. van de Vijver LP, van den Bosch LM, van den Brandt PA, Goldbohm RA. Whole-grain consumption, dietary fiber intake and body mass index in the Netherlands cohort study. *Eur J Clin Nutr* 2009;63:31–38.
26. McKeown NM, Yoshida M, Shea MK et al. Whole-grain intake and cereal fiber are associated with lower abdominal adiposity in older adults. *J Nutr* 2009;139:1950–1955.
27. National Center for Health Statistics. NHANES 1999–2000 public data release file documentation. Available from: http://www.cdc.gov/nchs/data/nhanes/gendoc.pdf. Accessed August 18, 2009.
28. The National Health and Nutrition Examination Survey (NHANES) Analytic and Reporting Guidelines. Last update December, 2005; Last correction, December, 2006. http://www.cdc.gov/nchs/data/nhanes/nhanes_03_04/nhanes_analytic_guidelines_dec_2005.pdf. Accessed January 20, 2011.
29. Blanton CA, Moshfegh AJ, Baer DJ, Kretsch MJ. The USDA automated multiple-pass method accurately estimates group total energy and nutrient intake. *J Nutr* 2006;136:2594–2599.
30. National Health and Nutrition Examination Survey. MEC interviewer's procedure manual. http://www.cdc.gov/nchs/data/nhanes/c1-4_int.pdf. Accessed January 20, 2011.
31. U.S. Department of Agriculture. Agricultural Research Service. USDA food and nutrient database for dietary studies, 1.0. http://www.ars.usda.gov/Services/docs.htm?docid=8498. Accessed January 20, 2011.
32. U.S. Department of Agriculture. Agricultural Research Service. USDA food and nutrient database for dietary studies, 2.0. http://www.ars.usda.gov/Services/docs.htm?docid=17563. Accessed January 20, 2011.
33. Friday JE, Bowman SA. *MyPyramid Equivalents Database for USDA Survey Food Codes, 1994–2002, Version 1.0* [On-line]. Beltsville, MD: USDA, Agricultural Research Service, Beltsville Human Nutrition Research Center, Community Nutrition Research Group, 2006.
34. Bowman SA, Friday JE, Moshfegh A. *MyPyramid Equivalents Database, 2.0 for USDA Survey Foods, 2003–2004* [Online]. Beltsville, MD: Food Surveys Research Group, Beltsville Human Nutrition Research Center, Agricultural Research Service, US Department of Agriculture, 2008. http://www.ars.usda.gov/Services/docs.htm?docid=12083. Accessed June 6, 2010.
35. U.S. Department of Agriculture, Agricultural Research Service. *USDA Food and Nutrient Database for Dietary Studies, 3.0.* 2008 [cited June 6, 2010]. Available from: http://www.ars.usda.gov/Services/docs.htm?docid=17031. Accessed June 6, 2010.
36. National Center for Health Statistics. *The NHANES Anthropometry Procedures Manual.* Revised 2004. Available at: http://www.cdc.gov/nchs/data/nhanes/nhanes_03_04/BM.pdf. Accessed December 19, 2009.
37. Specifying weighting parameters in NHANES III. In: Prevention CDC, ed. *NHANES III Web Tutorial*, 2010. http://www.cdc.gov/nchs/tutorials/Nhanes/SurveyDesign/Weighting/intro.htm. Accessed January 20, 2011.
38. Alfieri MA, Pomerleau J, Grace DM, Anderson L. Fiber intake of normal weight, moderately obese and severely obese subjects. *Obes Res* 1995;3:541–547.
39. Appleby PN, Thorogood M, Mann JI, Key TJ. Low body mass index in non-meat eaters: The possible roles of animal fat, dietary fiber and alcohol. *Int J Obes Rel Metab Dis* 1998;22:454–460.
40. Nelson LH, Tucker LA. Diet composition related to body fat in a multivariate study of 203 men. *J Am Diet Assoc* 1996;96:771–777.
41. Schulze MB, Schulz M, Heidemann C, Schienkiewitz A, Hoffmann K, Boeing H. Fiber and magnesium intake and incidence of type 2 diabetes: A prospective study and meta-analysis. *Arch Intern Med* 2007;167:956–965.

42. Harland JI, Garton LE. Whole-grain intake as a marker of healthy body weight and adiposity. *Public Health Nutr* 2008;11:554–563.
43. Rolls BJ, Ello-Martin JA, Tohill BC. What can intervention studies tell us about the relationship between fruit and vegetable consumption and weight management? *Nutr Rev* 2004;62:1–17.
44. Guenther PM, Dodd KW, Reedy J, Krebs-Smith SM. Most Americans eat much less than recommended amounts of fruits and vegetables. *J Am Diet Assoc* 2006;106:1371–1379.
45. Kimmons J, Gillespie C, Seymour J, Serdula M, Blanck HM. Fruit and vegetable intake among adolescents and adults in the United States: Percentage meeting individualized recommendations. *Medscape J Med* 2009;11(1):26.
46. Ledoux TA, Hingle MD, Baranowski T. Relationship of fruit and vegetable intake with adiposity: A systematic review. *Obes Rev* 2010;12:e143–e150.

8

Fiber and Satiety

CATHERINE LEFRANC-MILLOT, VALÉRIE MACIOCE,
LAETITIA GUÉRIN-DEREMAUX, ALBERT W. LEE, and SUSAN S. CHO

Contents

8.1 Clinical Methods for Measuring Satiety

Although there is no universally standardized methodology for satiety testing, most studies use either subjective visual analog scale (VAS) scores, direct measurements of food intake (FI), or a combination of both. Studies typically present one of several test meals of varying nutrient content to each subject on several occasions (Porrini et al., 1995). Satiety is measured at specific times after consumption of test meals. The VAS provides subjective ratings of hunger, satiety, prospective food consumption, and palatability of meals. VAS is typically 100 or 150 mm long and anchored at either end with "the least" and "the most." Subjects are asked such questions as "how hungry do you feel, how satisfied do you feel, how full do you feel, or how much do you think you can eat?" (Willis et al., 2009).

When FI metrics are required, subjects are given free access to food and instructed to eat until they feel comfortably full. The timing of ad libitum FIs varies from 1 to 8 h postpreload, but certain studies have monitored FI and/or energy intake (EI) well into the next day (Nilsson et al., 2008). Most satiety investigations use a crossover design, so participants receive both test meals on separate occasions and, thus, act as their own controls. In some experiments, plasma concentrations of glucose, lactate, and satiety-related gut hormones are also collected.

8.2 Satiety and Satiation

Intrinsic, hormonal, and colonic effects of dietary fiber decrease FI by promoting satiation and/or satiety (Pereira and Ludwig, 2001) (Figure 8.1). Satiation is defined as the satisfaction of appetite that develops during the course of eating and eventually results in the cessation of eating; satiety refers to the state in which further eating is inhibited and occurs as a consequence of having eaten (Slavin, 2005) (Figure 8.2).

Dietary fiber is an essential constituent of a healthy diet and is well known for its satiety impact (Karhunen et al., 2010). It had been recommended by the Scientific Panel on Dietetic Products, Nutrition and Allergies of the European Food Safety Authority (2010) that dietary fiber should include all nondigestible carbohydrates (CHOs) in accordance with the proposal for a Codex definition of dietary fiber. According to the Annex II of the Commission Directive 2008/100/EC of October 28, 2008 (European Commission, 2008), dietary fiber is now

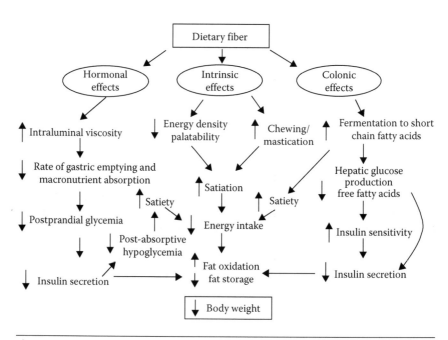

Figure 8.1 Summarizes physiologic mechanisms by which dietary fiber affects body weight regulation. Intrinsic, hormonal, and colonic effects of dietary fiber decrease food intake by promoting satiation and/or satiety. Satiation is defined as the satisfaction of appetite that develops during the course of eating and eventually results in the cessation of eating. (From Slavin, J.L., *Nutrition*, 21, 411, 2005. Adapted with permission from Pereira and Ludwig (2001).)

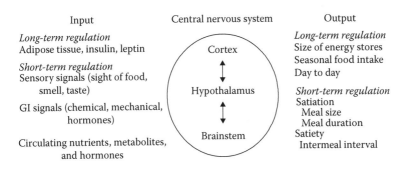

Input	Central nervous system	Output

Long-term regulation
Adipose tissue, insulin, leptin

Short-term regulation
Sensory signals (sight of food, smell, taste)

GI signals (chemical, mechanical, hormones)

Circulating nutrients, metabolites, and hormones

Cortex
↑
Hypothalamus
↑
Brainstem

Long-term regulation
Size of energy stores
Seasonal food intake
Day to day

Short-term regulation
Satiation
  Meal size
  Meal duration
Satiety
  Intermeal interval

Figure 8.2 Food intake is regulated in the central nervous system, which receives input from sensory properties of food, mechanical and chemical receptors in the gut, circulating metabolites, and hormones. (From Anderson, G.H. et al., Physiology of food intake regulation: Interaction with dietary components, in *Complementary Foods*, Rigo, J. and Ziegler, E.E. (eds.), Protein and energy requirements in infancy and childhood, *Nestlé Nutr Workshop Ser Pediatr Program*, vol. 58, pp. 133–145, Nestec Ltd., Vevey/S. Karger AG, Basel, Switzerland, 2006.)

defined in the European Union as follows: "carbohydrate polymers with three or more monomeric units, which are neither digested nor absorbed in the human small intestine and belong to the following categories:

- Edible carbohydrate polymers naturally occurring in the food as consumed.
- Edible carbohydrate polymers which have been obtained from food raw material by physical, enzymatic or chemical means and which have a beneficial physiological effect demonstrated by generally accepted scientific evidence.
- Edible synthetic carbohydrate polymers which have a beneficial physiological effect demonstrated by generally accepted scientific evidence." Dietary fiber includes a wide range of compounds, and although it generally affects satiety, not all fibers are equally effective (Slavin, 2008). Large variations that exist in the physical and chemical characteristics of dietary fiber influence physiological responses in humans (Carabin et al., 2009; Lyly et al., 2010).

Slavin and Green (2007) found that the viscosity-forming capacity of water-soluble fibers, such as guar gum and β-glucan, is crucial for their impact on satiety-related attributes. Lyon and Reichart (2010) report that dietary fiber might promote satiety by reducing postprandial glycemia. Similarly, Bodinham et al. (2010) found that short-term consumption of resistant starch dietary fiber enhances satiety by improving postprandial glucose metabolism in healthy individuals.

8.3 Dietary Fiber and Satiety

The addition of dietary fiber to foods as well as beverages has been associated with greater satiety (Bolton et al., 1981; Perrigue et al., 2009; Tsuchiya et al., 2006) and reduced EI in the short term (Pereira and Ludwig, 2001). In longer-term studies, high-fiber diets have been linked with greater weight loss (Ledikwe et al., 2007). Systematic reviews on the health implications of dietary fiber show that high-fiber diets provide bulk, are satiating, and have been related to lower body weight (Slavin, 2008; U.S. Department of Agriculture, Center for Nutrition Policy and Promotion, 2010).

A review by Howarth et al. (2001) summarized the effects of dietary fiber on hunger, satiety, EI, and body weight. Under conditions of fixed EI, the majority of studies indicate that an increase in dietary fiber improves postmeal satiety and decreases subsequent hunger. With *ad libitum* EI, the average effect of increasing dietary fiber across all the studies indicated that an additional 14 g of fiber per day resulted in a 10% decrease in EI and body weight loss of more than 1.9 kg through approximately 3.8 months of intervention. The effect was even more pronounced among obese individuals. These outcomes were seen regardless of whether the fiber came from high-fiber foods or fiber supplements, or soluble or insoluble dietary fibers.

In the prospective Nurses Health study, women who consumed more fiber weighed less than women who consumed less fiber (Liu et al., 2003). In addition, women in the highest quintile of dietary fiber intake had a 49% lower risk of major weight gain. Maskarinec et al. (2006) reported that plant-based foods and dietary fiber were most protective against excess body weight in a large ethnically diverse population. Howarth et al. (2005) examined the association of dietary composition variables with body mass index (BMI) among U.S. adults aged 20–59 years in the Continuing Survey of Food Intakes by Individuals, 1994–1996. For women, a low-fiber, high-fat diet was associated with the greatest risk in overweight or obesity compared with a high-fiber, low-fat diet.

Davis et al. (2006) matched 52 normal-weight women to 52 overweight/obese women and found that the normal-weight subjects had higher fiber and fruit intake than the overweight subjects. In the Coronary Artery Risk Development in Young Adults (CARDIA) study, Ludwig et al. (1999b) observed more than 2900 black and white participants 18–30 years of age and found a linear relation from lowest to highest quintile of dietary fiber intake with body weight. They also reported that regardless of fat intake, those who consumed the most fiber gained less weight than those who consumed the least amount of fiber. More recently, Du et al. (2010) followed a cohort of 89,432 European participants aged 20–78 years for an average of 6.5 years. Data showed that total fiber was inversely associated with subsequent changes in weight and waist circumference. For a 10 g/day higher total fiber intake, the pooled estimate was −39 g/year for weight change and 0.08 cm/year for change in waist circumference.

Numerous studies have examined not only body weight but also body composition (Astrup et al., 2010). In a report on the relation between dietary composition and body fat in 293 men, Nelson and Tucker (1996) found an inverse association between fiber intake and body fat. In the Seven Countries Study, a cross-cultural investigation of 12,763 middle-aged men, Kromhout et al. (2001) reported a strong inverse relationship between the average population physical activity index and dietary fiber intake and mean subscapular skinfold thickness.

More recently, Tucker and Thomas (2009) conducted a 20 month prospective cohort study in 252 women and found that fiber intake decreased weight and reduced percent of body fat independent of several potential confounding factors, including physical activity. Outcomes showed that for each 1 g increase in total fiber consumed, weight decreased by 0.25 kg and fat decreased by a 0.25 kg percentage point. Similarly, a longitudinal study in 85 overweight Latino adolescents by Davis et al. (2009) showed that increases in total dietary fiber and insoluble fiber were associated with decreases in visceral adipose tissue (VAT). The authors concluded that small reductions in dietary fiber intake over 1–2 years can have profound effects on increasing visceral adiposity in a high-risk Latino population.

8.4 Mechanisms of Action

Dietary fiber increases satiety, reduces EI, and improves weight control via several mechanisms (Bodinham et al., 2010). These include effects that are intrinsic (e.g., viscosity and sensory properties), colonic, hormonal, and related to glycemic control (Pereira and Ludwig, 2001). Proposed mechanisms include lower energy density of high-fiber foods, delayed gastric emptying (GE) that can prolong feelings of fullness, slower glucose absorption (Pereira and Ludwig, 2001), and increased chewing, which promotes the secretion of saliva and gastric juices that expand the stomach and increase satiety (Howarth et al., 2001). A recent study found that short-term consumption of dietary resistant starch increased satiety by improving postprandial glucose in healthy individuals (Robertson et al., 2005).

8.4.1 Viscosity

According to Burton-Freeman (2000) and Howarth et al. (2001), increased viscosity of chyme in the gut slows GE time, lengthens small intestine passage time, and delays the absorption of nutrients—effects that increase feelings of fullness by enhancing satiety-mediating signals to the central nervous system. Tucker and Thomas (2009) report that fiber's influence occurs as a result of changes in appetite-suppressing gut hormone levels that decrease FI at subsequent meals. Ghrelin is positively correlated with hunger (Kojima and Kangawa, 2008), while glucagon-like peptide-1 (GLP-1) and peptide YY_{3-36} have inverse relationships (Holst, 2007; Neary and Batterham, 2009). However, very few studies have evaluated how these three hormones change in response to fiber intake (Essah et al., 2007; Karhunen et al., 2010; Stock et al., 2005).

8.4.2 Colonic Effects

Research suggests that the biologic actions of fiber in the large intestine may also have implications for body weight regulation (Pereira and Ludwig, 2001). Fibers and certain types of starch are resistant to enzymatic digestion in the small intestine and are therefore susceptible to fermentation by bacteria in the colon. The products of this fermentation process (e.g., short-chain fatty acids [SCFAs], butyrate, and propionate) enter the portal circulation and affect glucose homeostasis in a variety of ways (Lu et al., 2000; Pereira and Ludwig, 2001; Thornburn et al., 1993). SCFAs, for example, influence upper gut motility (Cherbut, 2003). They also decrease hepatic output of glucose and circulating concentrations of free fatty acids (Pereira and Ludwig, 2001; Thornburn et al., 1993) and stimulate secretion of GLP-1 (Pereira and Ludwig, 2001)—actions that alter insulin sensitivity, insulin secretion patterns, the partitioning of metabolic fuels, and regulation of satiety.

8.4.3 Hormonal Effects Including Glycemic Control

By decreasing GE and/or slowing energy and nutrient absorption, dietary fiber reduces postprandial glucose levels. Pereira and Ludwig (2001) reviewed 16 studies comparing the effects of glycemic response (GR) with changes in weight regulation parameters, such as hunger, satiety, or EI. In 15 of the studies, at least one weight regulation parameter was positively modified by changing the glycemic index (GI) of foods. For example, low-GI foods increased satiety in five studies, decreased hunger in four, and reduced EI in six.

GI was first defined by Jenkins et al. (1981) as an indicator of the potential of glycemic CHOs in different types of food to raise blood glucose levels within 2 h of ingestion (Niwano et al., 2009). The index is based on the increase in blood glucose levels (the AUC [area under the curve] for blood glucose levels) after the ingestion of 50 g of CHO from a test food compared with a standard amount (50 g) of reference CHO (glucose or white bread (Hu, 2008)). GI is therefore a measure of blood glucose excursion per unit of CHO.

Researchers report that low-GI foods enhance satiety responses more than high-GI foods (Ebbeling et al., 2007; Ludwig and Roberts, 2006; Thomas et al., 2007). Foods with high GI are rapidly digested, absorbed, and transformed into glucose. These processes cause accelerated and transient surges in blood glucose and insulin, usually postprandial hypoglycemia and earlier return of hunger sensation, therefore excessive calorie intake (Kong et al., 2010).

Conversely, low-GI diets decrease blood glucose and insulin excursion, induce less consecutive hypoglycemia, promote greater fat oxidation, decrease lipogenesis, and increase satiety (Kong et al., 2010). In a small cohort of healthy adults ($n = 15$) taking evening meals with low-GI foods, glucose response was inversely correlated with colonic fermentation, GLP-1, and satiety at breakfast. This finding suggests that the observed effects of reduced satiety after taking low-GI foods may be due to higher levels of incretin hormones related to increased colonic fermentation (Nilsson et al., 2008). Holt et al. (1992) found that glycemic and insulin responses to CHO foods are inversely proportional to the cholecystokinin (CCK) response and satiety.

In a systematic review (Roberts, 2000), most of the short-term feeding studies in humans (lasting for a single meal or a single day) demonstrated a direct association between consumption of high-GI foods/liquids and increased subsequent hunger and/or decreased satiety. Voluntary EI increased after consumption of high-GI meals compared with low-GI meals. Four short-term human intervention studies also showed that ingestion of test meals with high GI increased the level of FI, suggesting that meals with low GI prolong satiety (Arumugam et al., 2008; Ball et al., 2003; Ludwig et al., 1999a; Warren et al., 2003).

A Cochrane review (Thomas et al., 2007) found that overweight or obese people on a low-GI diet lost more weight and had greater improvement in lipid profiles than those receiving high-GI or other diets. Body mass, total fat mass, BMI, total cholesterol, and LDL-cholesterol all decreased significantly more in the low-GI group. In studies comparing ad libitum low-GI diets to conventional restricted energy low-fat diets, participants fared as well or better on the low-GI diet, even though they could eat as much as desired. The authors concluded that lowering the glycemic load of the diet appears to be an effective way to promote weight loss and improve lipid profiles, as well as an option that can be simply incorporated into a person's lifestyle. These findings are consistent with those from Ball et al.; based on time to request for additional food, prolonged satiety was observed after a low-GI meal replacement compared to a high-GI meal replacement (Ball et al., 2003).

A study in preadolescent boys and girls (9–12 years of age) by Warren et al. (2003) demonstrated that those who had a low-GI breakfast ate less at lunch and had a lower hunger rating than those who ate a high-GI breakfast. The gender of the child, or whether they were of normal weight or overweight/obese, did not alter the effect of the breakfast GI on the subsequent lunch intake. Similarly, Ludwig et al. (1999a) found that rapid absorption of glucose after the consumption of high-GI meals induced a sequence of hormonal and metabolic changes that promoted excessive FI in obese teenage boys.

Flint et al. (2006) report that after the intake of a typical European breakfast (including bread, cookies, cereals, and porridge) by healthy male subjects, the insulinemic response (IR), but not the glycemic response, was positively associated with subsequent EI at lunch, although no significant relations were found between glycemic response and appetite sensations.

These short-term studies indicate that both glycemic and IRs are associated with hunger and/or satiety irrespective of age, gender, or weight. The relatively early and sharp decline to below baseline in blood glucose seems to be a key to the quicker loss of satiety and the faster return of appetite and hunger (Niwano et al., 2009). In contrast to the short-term studies, there is no clear evidence that meals with a low GI prolong satiety or reduce appetite and/or hunger over a long period of time (Niwano et al., 2009). Further research with longer-term follow-up is needed to determine whether improvement continues long term and improves quality of life.

8.5 Types of Fibers

8.5.1 Viscous Fibers

Alginate is a linear polysaccharide with a gel-forming property, especially in the presence of calcium ions (Panouille and Larreta-Garde, 2009). Its monomers are mannuronic and guluronic acids. A review of three studies on alginate indicates that the seaweed-derived fiber (Paxman et al., 2008) consistently promotes satiety, most likely through its gel-forming capacity. The mechanisms underlying this effect may include slowed gastric clearance and attenuated nutrient uptake from the small intestine, which contributes to slower GE (Hoad et al., 2004; Paxman et al., 2008; Pelkman et al., 2007). The minimum intake needed to decrease EI is 1.5 g/dose.

Paxman et al. (2008) randomly assigned 68 normal-weight adults with an average age of 24.6 years to a beverage with 1.5 g/day of sodium alginate (C BioPolymer, Philadelphia, PA) or an 18.2 g/day dose of SlimFast (Unilever, Englewood Cliffs, NJ) for 7 days. Preprandial ingestion of the sodium alginate formulation produced a significant 134.8 kcal (7%) reduction in mean daily EI. The alginate test beverage had a guluronate content of 65%–75%. Its other ingredients included 0.7 g calcium carbonate, 2.8 g glucono-delta-lactone, 0.5 g sodium bicarbonate, 0.05 g malic acid, 0.24 g vanilla flavor, and 7 g fructose. The composition is reportedly patented under patent number WO2007039294. Although this carboxylic polymer can contribute to increase viscosity in the gastrointestinal tract by either acid-induced gelation or calcium-induced cross-linking (with coingestion of calcium), high material cost and difficult handling properties may limit food uses of this hydrocolloid.

Guar gum is a high-molecular-weight natural polymer that consists of a polymannan backbone with single galactose and glucose unit side chains. It is highly soluble and viscous in aqueous solutions (Chauhan et al., 2009). Overall, guar gum tends to promote satiety when over 2.5 g/dose is administered. This is most likely due to its gel-forming properties (Adam and Westerterp-Plantenga, 2005a,b; Chow et al., 2007; French and Read, 1994; Heini et al., 1998; Hoad et al., 2004; Krotkiewski, 1984; Lavin and Read, 1995; Pasman et al., 1997; Van de Ven et al., 1994). However, six studies found no effects of guar gum on measures of satiety (Ellis et al., 1981; Heini et al., 1998; Kovacs et al., 2001; Kovacs et al., 2002; Mattes, 2007; van Nieuwenhoven et al., 2001).

Psyllium mucilage is obtained from the seed coat by mechanical milling/grinding of the outer layer of the seeds and has a gel-forming property in aqueous solutions. The gel-forming fraction of the alkali-extractable polysaccharides is composed of arabinose, xylose, and traces of other sugars (Singh and Chauhan, 2009). All studies using more than 7 g of psyllium fiber report positive effects on controlling satiety (Bergmann et al., 1992; Delargy et al., 1997; Nguyen et al., 1982; Rigaud et al., 1998; Stevens et al., 1987; Turnbull and Thomas, 1995). However, two studies using less than 5 g of psyllium showed no effects on measures of satiety (Bianchi and Capurso, 2002; Frost et al., 2003).

Oat β-glucan is a water-soluble viscous polysaccharide (Lyly et al., 2010) that consists of a mixture of β-(1,3)- and β-(1,4)-glycosidic bonds. It has been linked with many health benefits, such as reduced cholesterol levels and balanced blood glucose and insulin levels (Juvonen et al., 2010). Soluble fibers, such as β-glucan, influence appetite by physical and chemical properties (particularly their bulking action) and increased viscosity in the gastrointestinal tract (Burton-Freeman, 2000). But despite its high viscosity, which is affected by concentration and molar mass (Wood et al., 2000), two studies on oat β-glucan (over 4 g/dose) report that it has no effect on satiety (Hlebowicz et al., 2008; Juntunen et al., 2002). Results from more recent reports, however, are mixed. Beck et al. (2009) found that β-glucan improves satiety, increases postprandial CCK levels, decreases insulin response, and extends subjective satiety in overweight subjects. In a study with seven male and seven female subjects with BMI 25–36 kg/m², subsequent meal intake decreased by greater than 400 kJ with higher β-glucan dose (>5 g). Lyly et al. (2010) also found that the addition of an oat ingredient rich in β-glucan and high viscosity of beverages enhanced postprandial satiety induced by beverages. Conversely, a study in 20 healthy, normal-weight subjects by Juvonen et al. (2010) found that oat β-glucan decreased postprandial plasma glucose and serum insulin responses, yet had no significant effects on GI peptide responses or appetite ratings.

Studies on pectin reported inconsistent results. Administration of pectin at a dosage of 15 g for 1 day delayed GE time and/or significantly increased satiety in obese adults as compared to the same dosage/same duration of methyl cellulose ingestion (di Lorenzo et al., 1988) and healthy U.S. Army adults (Pelkman et al., 2007; Tiwary et al., 1997), and it was also reported that consumption of 5.6 g/day pectin-alginate mixture for 7 days significantly decreased EI by 12%–22% in overweight and obese women. However, Howarth et al. (2003) reported that administration of 27 g/day fermentable fiber (a mixture of pectin and β-glucan) for 3 weeks did not alter hunger and satiety.

There is no published study on the effect of acacia gum on satiety or EIs.

8.5.2 Nonviscous Insoluble Fibers

Soy fiber and oat hull fiber have become important food ingredients due to their high fiber content (about 90%). The results of two studies using oat hull fiber found that it accelerated or gastric inhibitory peptide (GIP), glucagon-like peptide-1 (GLP-1), and peptide YY (PYY) responses without affecting hunger scores, suggesting that it has little effect on satiety (Weickert et al., 2005, 2006).

Similarly, studies on soy fiber show no effects on GE (Bouin et al., 2001; Morgan et al., 1993; Zarling et al., 1994). GE and gastric acid secretion in healthy adults were unaffected by an enteral diet supplemented with 7.5 g of soy polysaccharides (500 kcal, 250 mL/h) (Bouin et al., 2001). Morgan et al. (1993) also reported that 10 g of soy fiber in a test meal containing 100 g CHOs had no effect on GIP response and GE. Similarly, Zarling et al. (1994) found that a mixture of soy fiber and oat hull fiber (28.8 g/day for 10 days) showed no effect on GE in medically stable residents of a chronic care facility.

8.5.3 Nonviscous Soluble Fibers

Nonviscous soluble fibers include resistant dextrins (RDs), inulin, oligofructose (OF), and polydextrose. Among them, some show inconsistent outcomes on the ability to affect satiety. Polydextrose and inulin have demonstrated no effect. OF has shown promise; RD, a significantly positive impact on satiety.

Inulin: Three studies on inulin showed no effects on GE (Archer et al., 2004; Den Hond, 2000; Geboes et al., 2003). However, Archer et al. (2004) reported that supplementation of 24 g of inulin/day had no effect on satiety at breakfast but reduced EI during the test day. The authors suggested that a late postabsorptive satiety may be related to the fermentation of inulin.

Oligofructose: Cani et al. (2006) reported that supplementation of 16 g of OF/day for 2 weeks increased short-term satiety measures. In this study, subjects were included in two 2 week experimental phases during which they received either 16 g of OF (8 g with breakfast and 8 g with dinner) or a placebo (dextrin maltose). The OF treatment increased satiety following breakfast and dinner and reduced hunger and prospective food consumption after dinner. EIs at breakfast and lunch were significantly lower after OF treatment than after placebo. Total daily EI was 5% lower when subjects received OF rather than placebo.

Parnell and Reimer (2009) examined the effects of OF supplementation on body weight and satiety hormone concentrations in 48 otherwise healthy overweight and obese adults in a randomized, double-blind, placebo-controlled trial. Subjects were randomly assigned to receive 21 g of OF/day or placebo (maltodextrin) for 12 weeks. The researchers found a reduction in body weight in the OF group versus an increase in body weight in the controls. A lower AUC for ghrelin and a higher AUC for PYY with OF coincided with a reduction in self-reported caloric intake. Between the initial and final tests, glucose decreased in the OF group and increased in the controls. Insulin concentrations mirrored that pattern. Although most digestive side symptoms subsided with adaptation to the fiber regimen, a VAS administered on the final test day indicated that 45% ± 8% of the time subjects in the OF group experienced negative side effects, which would deter them from consuming the product at the current dosage compared with the placebo group (11% ± 4%; *p*, 0.01).

Differences between inulin and OF may be partly explained by intestinal properties. Long-chain inulin is largely fermented in the distal colon, whereas OF is fermented in the proximal colon. Thus, inulin may be unable to produce the same amount of GLP-1 as OF (Cani et al., 2006).

Polydextrose: Few studies have been done on the satiating effects of polydextrose, with mixed findings. King et al. (2005) assessed the independent and combined effects of polydextrose and xylitol on appetite. Subjects received either placebo or yogurt supplemented with 25 g xylitol, 25 g polydextrose, or a combination of 12.5 g of both. Findings showed that when the energy content of the preloads was accounted for, polydextrose caused a significant suppression of EI compared with control. Conversely, a randomized controlled trial conducted by Willis et al. (2009) showed that when fasting subjects consumed either a low-fiber muffin (1.6 g fiber) or one of four high-fiber muffins (8.0–9.6 g fiber) for breakfast on five separate visits, satiety differed among treatments. Resistant starch and corn bran had the greatest impact on satiety, but polydextrose had little effect.

Resistant starch: Bodinham et al. (2010) studied the effects of resistant starch on FI in 20 young, healthy adult males, aged 19–31 years, with a mean BMI of 23.2 kg/m². An acute, randomized, single-blind crossover study showed that the nonviscous starch significantly lowered EI following consumption of the supplement compared to placebo during both an ad libitum test meal and over 24 h. These findings suggest that an increased intake of resistant starch may have positive implications in weight management.

8.6 Resistant Dextrin

8.6.1 Definition and Characterization of Resistant Dextrin (RD)

The net energy value of RDs is an estimated 2.1 kcal/g, which is in agreement with the approximate caloric value for other soluble dietary fibers (Livesey, 1992; Vermorel et al., 2004). Among water soluble fibers, NUTRIOSE® (Roquette Freres, Lestrem, France) is a glucose polymer that is largely resistant to digestion and absorption in the small intestine, and is therefore considered an RD. Because it is fermented in the colon, it meets the criteria for a dietary fiber and has therefore a caloric value of 2 kcal/g in EU according to the Commission Directive 2008/100/EC of October 28, 2008 (European Commission, 2008). RDs can be made from either wheat (NUTRIOSE® FB) or maize starch (NUTRIOSE® FM).

NUTRIOSE® is obtained by heating starch at high temperature and adjusting it to a low moisture level in the presence of an acid catalyst (Vermorel et al., 2004). During a highly controlled process of dextrinization, the starch undergoes a degree of hydrolysis followed by repolymerization that converts it to fiber (Lefranc-Millot, 2008). In addition to the typical starch α-1,4 and α-1,6 glucosidic linkages, the presence of α-1,2 and α-1,3 glycosidic linkages makes the RD resistant to hydrolysis by human alimentary enzymes (Table 8.1).

According to Pasman et al. (2006), approximately 15% of RD is enzymatically digested in the small intestine (range, 8.7%–19%). The rest passes to the colon, where about 75% of the initial amount is slowly and progressively fermented in the large intestine (Vermorel et al., 2004) and 10% is excreted (van den Heuvel et al., 2004). In a study of fecal residue of RD, van den Heuvel et al. (2005) found that it increases in a nonlinear fashion with dose. The authors recovered approximately 2% of 10 g/day and 13% of 80 g/day in the feces (assuming a constant excretion of RD in feces per 24 h). Vermorel et al. (2004) have estimated an apparent digestibility of RD of 90.8%. This figure is consistent with van den Heuvel et al. (2005) estimation that more than 87% of RD is digested or fermented in the

Table 8.1 Indicative Values of Glycosidic Bond Distributions (%), Respectively, in (1) NUTRIOSE® 06, (2) Standard Maltodextrin GLUCIDEX® (ROQUETTE, Lestrem, France), and (3) Starch

Type of Osidic Linkages	(1)	(2)	(3)
(1,4)	41	95	95
(1,6)	32	5	5
(1,2)	13	0	0
(1,3)	14	0	0

human gastrointestinal tract (van den Heuvel et al., 2005). Furthermore, unlike most of other fibers, the RD is outstandingly tolerated in the gut, whether in a short- or a long-term tolerance study, which allows a concrete utilization of this dietary product in meals (van den Heuvel et al., 2004; Pasman et al., 2006).

Soluble dietary fibers, such as OF and NUTRIOSE®, may have a positive impact on total daily energy expenditure through colonic fermentations and viscosity of the gut contents. With RD, activity of α-glucosidase improves fermentation, leading to production of SCFAs. A daily dose of 30 g and over of RD increases the concentration of α-glucosidase, and daily doses of 10–80 g/day induce significant changes in the concentration of β-glucosidases (van den Heuvel et al., 2005). SCFAs, which are a source of energy for tissues, have been linked to satiety control (Pereira and Ludwig, 2001).

8.6.2 Resistant Dextrins and Satiety

van den Heuvel et al. (2004) investigated the effects of RD supplementation on satiety and EI compared to usual diets. In this study, initially designed to evaluate the short-term digestive tolerance of the RD, meals contained similar amounts of energy as subject's habitual breakfasts or dinners. Subjects (average BMI = 22.3 kg/m²) ate standard breakfast, lunch, and afternoon snacks. Hunger and satiety were measured just before breakfast (time point 0) and at 30, 60, 90, 120, 150, 180, 240 (just before lunch), 270, and 480 min. On day 7 of treatment, feelings of hunger and satiety were rated by a 10 cm VAS on such variables as appetite for a meal, appetite for something sweet, appetite for something savory, satiety (fullness), and feeble/weak with hunger. Only the AUC of the rating on "feeble or weak with hunger" was lower with 15 g/day of RD compared to 15 g/day of placebo. These findings suggested that RD may have a satiating effect in subjects on unrestricted energy diets.

A recent study (Guerin-Deremaux et al., 2011b) on the addition of NUTRIOSE® FB to a beverage found that the soluble, nonviscous dietary fiber increased short-term satiety. Healthy overweight factory workers consumed orange juice twice daily for 9 weeks either alone (placebo) or supplemented with NUTRIOSE® at different dosages (8, 14, 18, and 24 g/day). A significant increase in satiation was demonstrated by a drop in VAS hunger scores by 5.4–5.7 points within 10 min of taking the study product. Short-term satiety, as measured by the delay of return of hunger after the beverage consumption, was significantly greater in the NUTRIOSE® groups compared with placebo. Subjects who received the highest dose (24 g) had the earliest and most robust responses, suggesting a dose-response relationship (Figure 8.3). Moreover, regular consumption of a given dosage of NUTRIOSE® induced an increase in short-term satiety (expressed as perception dimension of hunger ratings) over time (Figure 8.4) as well as mean time to hunger after the last meal. This might be explained by a modification of gut microbiota composition due to RD colonic fermentations, possibly leading to a better yield of energy thanks to these higher fermentations. Compared to placebo, the NUTRIOSE® groups ate significantly fewer kcal at subsequent meals (Table 8.2).

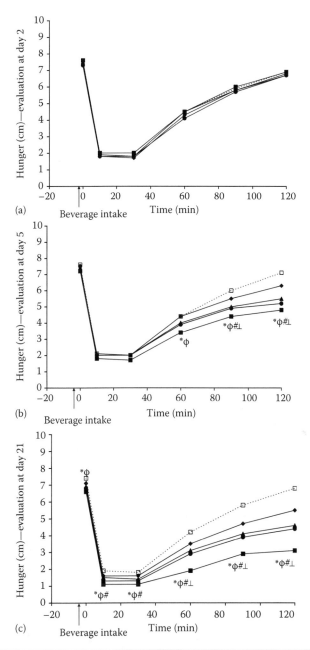

Figure 8.3 Perception dimension of hunger ratings on the VAS from the beverage intake to the lunch on the different days of evaluation. Each point represents mean ratings in cm for placebo (□), 8 g of NUTRIOSE® (♦), 14 g of NUTRIOSE® (▲), 18 g of NUTRIOSE® (●) and 24 g of NUTRIOSE® (■). The symbols represent the statistical differences compared to the placebo group ($p < 0.05$): NUTRIOSE® 8 g (⊥), NUTRIOSE® 14 g (φ), NUTRIOSE® 18 g (#) and NUTRIOSE® 24 g (*). (a) At day 2, (b) at day 5, and (c) at day 21. (From Guerin-Deremaux, L. et al., *Nutr. Res.*, 31, 665, 2011b.)

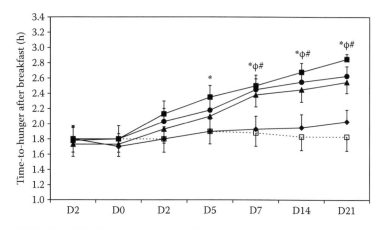

Figure 8.4 Mean VAS score by subject group over time from baseline until day 21, the last day of this side of the study. Time to return of hunger after the last meal was significantly greater in the NUTRIOSE® FB06 groups compared to placebo. Subjects who received the highest dose (24 g) had the earliest and most robust response. (From Guerin-Deremaux, L. et al., *Nutr. Res.*, 31, 665, 2011b.)

BMI decreased significantly in the 14, 18, and 24 g groups ($p < 0.05$) (Figure 8.5), as did mean body fat in the 18 and 24 g fiber groups.

Another investigation (Guérin-Deremaux et al., 2011a) on the effect of NUTRIOSE® tested EI, body weight, BMI, and body fat in overweight Chinese adults who consumed twice daily a 17 g dosage of NUTRIOSE® or a placebo in orange juice. Study products were orally consumed twice daily, 3 h after breakfast and 4 h after lunch. In this 12 week randomized, double-blind, placebo-controlled clinical trial, 120 adult males and females were stratified by BMI and caloric intake. Significant decreases in body weight ($p < 0.001$), BMI ($p < 0.001$), body fat ($p < 0.001$), and hunger feeling ($p < 0.001$) associated with a decreased caloric intake ($p < 0.001$) were observed throughout the study in the NUTRIOSE® group, as well as a final significant reduction in waist circumference as measured by abdominal scans ($p < 0.001$), while no changes were observed in the placebo group. Moreover, secondary outcomes of this studied revealed significant improvements of some biomarkers of the metabolic syndrome (Li et al., 2011) (Table 8.3).

During and immediately after eating, afferent information provides the major control over appetite (Blundell, 1999). Physiological events are triggered as responses to the ingestion of food and form the inhibitory processes, which stop eating and then prevent its reoccurrence until another meal is triggered. These physiological events are termed satiety signals. Satiation is the process that leads to the termination of FI. Termination of the period of satiety leads to the resurgence of the feeling of hunger and a consequent resumption of the FI cycle (Blundell et al., 1999). It appears that RD has a more powerful satiating effect in subjects compared to a maltodextrin placebo. The modulation of the microbial ratios in the gut flora composition may partly explain this result (Ley et al., 2005, 2006). Moreover, the prolonged production of SCFAs all along the colon may

Table 8.2 Total Daily Calorie Intake over the 9 Week Study Period in Subjects Taking NUTRIOSE® FB06 in a Beverage Twice a Day

Week	0 g	8 g	14 g	18 g	24 g
0	2705.2 ± 336.5	2705.2 ± 332.6	2708.0 ± 336.8	2716.5 ± 337.2	2713.7 ± 332.2
1	2711.5 ± 299.5	2706.3 ± 259.4	2697.4 ± 254.2	2695.3 ± 305.1	2688.1 ± 274.4
2	2730.1 ± 283.5	2703.8 ± 257.0	2661.1 ± 232.6*	2649.7 ± 287.9*	2620.4 ± 214.8*
3	2714.7 ± 297.1	2699.8 ± 253.6	2625.9 ± 239.3*	2614.6 ± 290.5*	2565.9 ± 260.5[*a]
4	2772.4 ± 290.9	2691.7 ± 246.3	2531.9 ± 233.2[*a]	2625.5 ± 2 31.7[*a]	2495.8 ± 241.3 [*a]
5	2772.4 ± 290.9	2691.7 ± 246.3	2531.9 ± 233.2[*a]	2625.5 ± 31.7[*a]	2495.8 ± 41.3[*a]
6	2728.4 ± 300.0	2689.3 ± 244.2	2520.9 ± 277.3[*a]	2514.0 ± 44.2[*a]	2461.7 ± 250.0[*a]
7	2719.4 ± 304.8	2680.4 ± 248.9	2477.7 ± 236.7[*a]	2469.2 ± 23.0[*a]	2417.4 ± 230.2[*a]
8	2719.4 ± 304.8	2675.3 ± 245.4	2449.7 ± 188.4[*a]	2438.5 ± 188.9[*a]	2373.1 ± 170.1[*a]
9	2725.4 ± 301.5	2667.3 ± 244.8*	2440.4 ± 143.8[*a]	2380.3 ± 151.2[*a]	2334.0 ± 110.8[*a]

Note: Meals were ad libitum.

* $P < .05$ comparing different dosages within the same week.

[a] $P < .05$ comparing time effects within the same treatment group.

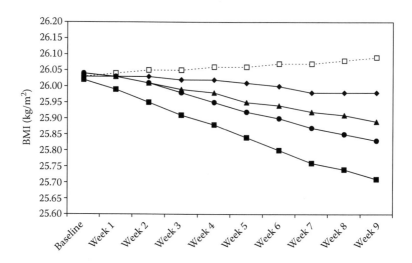

Figure 8.5 Mean BMI of study groups between baseline and week 9. Each point represents mean BMI (kg/m²) of the placebo (□), 8 g of NUTRIOSE® (♦), 14 g of NUTRIOSE® (▲), 18 g of NUTRIOSE® (●), and 24 g of NUTRIOSE® (■). BMI in the 24 g group fell by 0.41 ± 0.04 kg/m² ($p = 0.03212$) between baseline and week 9; during the same period for the 18 and 14 g groups, the declines were 0.21 ± 0.04 kg/m² ($p = 0.03720$) and 0.15 ± 0.03 kg/m² ($p = 0.0421$). The outcomes suggest a dose–response relationship. (From Guerin-Deremaux, L. et al., *Nutr. Res.*, 31, 665, 2011b.)

Table 8.3 Mean BMI (in kg/m²) of Study Groups over the Study Period

	Placebo	NUTRIOSE® 8 g	NUTRIOSE® 14 g	NUTRIOSE® 18 g	NUTRIOSE® 24 g
Baseline	26.03 ± 1.13	26.03 ± 1.28	26.04 ± 1.05	26.04 ± 0.82	26.02 ± 1.07
Week 1	26.04 ± 1.13	26.03 ± 1.27	26.03 ± 1.04	26.03 ± 0.83	25.99 ± 1.08
Week 2	26.05 ± 1.13	26.03 ± 1.27	26.01 ± 1.04	26.01 ± 0.84	25.95 ± 1.07
Week 3	26.05 ± 1.13	26.02 ± 1.27	25.99 ± 1.03	25.98 ± 0.85	25.91 ± 1.07
Week 4	26.06 ± 1.13	26.02 ± 1.27	25.98 ± 1.03	25.95 ± 0.85	25.88 ± 1.07
Week 5	26.06 ± 1.12	26.01 ± 1.27	25.95 ± 1.03	25.92 ± 0.85	25.84 ± 1.07
Week 6	26.07 ± 1.07	26.00 ± 1.31	25.94 ± 1.03	25.90 ± 0.86	25.80 ± 1.07
Week 7	26.07 ± 1.07	25.98 ± 1.29	25.92 ± 1.02	25.87 ± 0.87	25.76 ± 1.08
Week 8	26.08 ± 1.07	25.98 ± 1.30	25.91 ± 1.01	25.85 ± 0.89	25.74 ± 1.09
Week 9	26.09 ± 1.07	25.98 ± 1.31	25.89 ± 1.00	25.83 ± 0.88	25.71 ± 1.09
Change at week 9 relative to baseline (*P*-value)	+0.06 ± 0.03 (0.7340)	−0.05 ± 0.04 (0.6532)	−0.15 ± 0.03 (0.0421)	−0.21 ± 0.04 (0.03720)	−0.41 ± 0.04 (0.03212)

Source: Li, S. et al., *Appl Physiol Nutr Metabol*, 35, 773, 2010.
P values are for differences between week 9 and baseline.

provide long-lasting energy and delay the return of hunger. It is also in line with more recent results showing that the butyrate might be involved in inducing the production of some gut peptides such as PYY and GLP1 that play an important role in the control of energy homeostasis and are secreted in response to ingested nutrients (Zhou et al., 2006). Butyrate in particular (Hamer et al., 2008), but also other SCFAs, may therefore promote satiety, even if more human studies are needed to clearly understand the underlying mechanisms.

8.6.3   *Resistant Dextrins, Caloric Intake, and Body Weight Management*

Nonviscous fibers can help reduce body weight and/or body fat by substituting for fats and CHOs that increase caloric intake value. But they also do so by promoting satiety through improved glucose control (Lefranc-Millot, 2008). In vitro, the 15% of NUTRIOSE® FB 2006 that is slowly digested in the small intestine (Vermorel et al., 2004) induces a low glycemic response (GR = 25) and a low IR (IR = 13) (Donazzolo et al., 2003). Compared to glucose, the low IR of RD might contribute to greater satiety. The fiber can therefore be used as a slow-energy-release CHO that can partially or totally replace other CHOs, such as sugars and starches. With dietary starch, postprandial blood glucose and insulin responses are directly related to the rate of starch digestion (Wolf et al., 2001), which depends on intrinsic and extrinsic factors (Englyst et al., 1992). Chemical modification of starch may affect the rate and decrease the extent of its hydrolysis (Wolf et al., 1999). The combination of heat and enzyme treatments (dextrinization) can result in a CHO that is more resistant to digestion: less glucose is available to enzymes because, on the one hand, the newly formed linkages are resistant to digestive enzymes, and, on the other hand, the spatial rearrangement of the molecule makes it less accessible to enzymes (Flickinger et al., 2000; Pereira and Ludwig, 2001). In this way, the modification allows for the production of CHOs that induce a lower postprandial GRs (Wolf et al., 2001).

In two studies, Lefranc-Millot et al. (Lefranc-Millot, 2008; Lefranc-Millot et al., 2006) demonstrated that incorporation of RD into foods such as pasta, biscuits, and syrups induced very low glycemic responses. Data showed that peak glycemia was 7.6 mmol/L for glucose and 5.3 mmol/L for the pasta containing RD. Mean AUC for RD pasta was significantly lower than that of glucose (42.0 vs. 123.6, *p* < 0.01), likewise for biscuits (66.6 vs. 137.0, *p* < 0.01). When used in a concentrated fruit drink and consumed after dilution with water, syrups made with NUTRIOSE 06 elicited a glucose response of only 10% of the equivalent product made with sugar (Lefranc-Millot, 2008) (Figure 8.6).

Because low-GI foods are characterized by a slower rate of digestion and absorption, they provide prolonged feedback (most likely through satiety signals) to the hunger/satiety center in the brain via nutrient receptors in the gastrointestinal tract. In a study with 26 males (mean BMI = 23.4 ± 2.2 kg/m²), Pasman et al. (2003) reported that consumption of a simple CHO breakfast resulted in higher glucose and insulin levels 30 min after breakfast. Satiety scores were higher after consumption of a complex CHO breakfast for the first 90 min after intake.

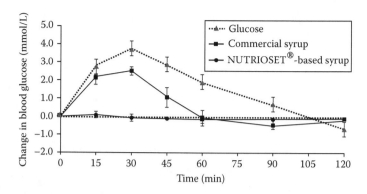

Figure 8.6 Mean change in human blood glucose concentrations after the ingestion of either NUTRIOSE® 06-based syrup (based on concentrated fruit syrup including 18.3 g per 100 g NUTRIOSE 06), commercial syrup reference (both products being similarly diluted, as directed by the manufacturer), or 50 g anhydrous glucose injection. Compared with glucose, the mean glycemic response (GR) value for the commercial syrup (51 ± 6) was significantly higher ($p = 0.001$) than the mean GR value for the NUTRIOSE 06-based syrup (6 ± 3). (From Lefranc-Millot, C., *Nutr. Bull.*, 33, 234, 2008.)

8.7 Conclusion

Given the extreme variance in viscosity, solubility in the gut, fermentation profiles, and hormonal responses, dietary fibers vary widely in the degree of satiety they provide. In general, consumption of viscous fibers is associated with increased satiety and nonviscous fibers with less consistent effects on satiety. But RDs, such as NUTRIOSE, effectively promote satiety by firstly inducing low glycemic and IRs, secondly promoting long-lasting colonic fermentations without digestive side effects, possibly contributing to prolonging satiety and delaying the return of hunger.

References

Adam, T. C. and Westerterp-Plantenga, M. S. (2005a). Glucagon-like peptide-1 release and satiety after a nutrient challenge in normal-weight and obese subjects. *Br J Nutr, 93*, 845–851.

Adam, T. C. and Westerterp-Plantenga, M. S. (2005b). Nutrient-stimulated GLP-1 release in normal-weight men and women. *Horm Metab Res, 37*, 111–117.

Anderson, G. H., Aziz, A., and Samra, R. A. (2006). Physiology of food intake regulation: Interaction with dietary components. In: *Complementary Foods.* Rigo J. and Ziegler E.E. (eds): Protein and energy requirements in infancy and childhood. *Nestlé Nutr Workshop Ser Pediatr Program*, vol. 58, pp. 133–145, Lausanne, Switzerland, Nestec Ltd., Vevey/S. Karger AG, Basel, © 2006.

Archer, B. J., Johnson, S. K., Devereux, H. M., and Baxter, A. L. (2004). Effect of fat replacement by inulin or lupin-kernel fiber on sausage patty acceptability, post-meal perceptions of satiety and food intake in men. *Br J Nutr, 91*, 591–599.

Arumugam, V., Lee, J. S., Nowak, J. K., Pohle, R. J., Nyrop, J. E., Leddy, J. J. et al. (2008). A high-glycemic meal pattern elicited increased subjective appetite sensations in overweight and obese women. *Appetite, 50*, 215–222.

Astrup, A., Kristensen, M., Gregersen, N. T., Belza, A., Lorenzen, J. K., Due, A. et al. (2010). Can bioactive foods affect obesity? *Ann NY Acad Sci, 1190*, 25–41.

Ball, S., Keller, K. R., Moyer-Mileur, L. J., Ding, Y. W., Donaldson, D., and Jackson, W. D. (2003). Prolongation of satiety after low versus moderately high glycemic index meals in obese adolescents. *Pediatrics, 111,* 488–494.

Beck, E. J., Tosh, S. M., Batterham, M. J., Tapsell, L. C., and Huang, X. F. (2009). Oat beta-glucan increases postprandial cholecystokinin levels, decreases insulin response and extends subjective satiety in overweight subjects. *Mol Nutr Food Res, 53,* 1343–1351.

Bergmann, J. F., Chassany, O., Petit, A., Triki, R., Caulin, C., and Segrestaa, J. M. (1992). Correlation between echographic gastric emptying and appetite: Influence of psyllium. *Gut, 33,* 1042–1043.

Bianchi, M. and Capurso, L. (2002). Effects of guar gum, ispaghula and microcrystalline cellulose on abdominal symptoms, gastric emptying, orocaecal transit time and gas production in healthy volunteers. *Dig Liver Dis, 34*(Suppl 2), S129–S133.

Blundell, J. E. (1999). The control of appetite: Basic concepts and practical implications. *Schweiz Med Wochenschr, 129,* 182–188.

Bodinham, B. L., Frost, G. S., and Robertson, M. D. (2010). Acute ingestion of resistant starch reduces food intake in healthy adults. *Br J Nutr, 103,* 917–922.

Bolton, R. P., Heaton, K. W., and Burroughs, L. F. (1981). The role of dietary fiber in satiety, glucose, and insulin: Studies with fruit and fruit juices. *Am J Clin Nutr, 34,* 211–217.

Bouin, M., Savoye, G., Hervé, S., Hellot, M. F., Denis, P., and Ducrotté, P. (2001). Does the supplementation of the formula with fiber increase the risk of gastro-oesophageal reflux during enteral nutrition? A human study. *Clin Nutr, 20,* 307–312.

Burton-Freeman, B. (2000). Dietary fiber and energy regulation. *J Nutr, 130*(2S Suppl), 272S–275S.

Cani, P. D., Joly, E., Horsmans, Y., and Delzenne, N. M. (2006). Oligofructose promotes satiety in healthy human: A pilot study. *Eur J Clin Nutr, 60,* 567–572.

Carabin, I. G., Lyon, M. R., Wood, S., Pelletier, X., Donazzolo, Y., and Burdock, G. A. (2009). Supplementation of the diet with the functional fiber PolyGlycoplex is well tolerated by healthy subjects in a clinical trial. *Nutr J, 8,* 9.

Chauhan, K., Chauhan, G. S., and Ahn, J. H. (2009). Synthesis and characterization of novel guar gum hydrogels and their use as Cu2+ sorbents. *Bioresour Technol, 100,* 3599–3603.

Cherbut, C. (2003). Motor effects of short-chain fatty acids and lactate in the gastrointestinal tract. *Proc Nutr Soc, 62,* 95–99.

Chow, J., Choe, Y. S., Noss, M. J., Robinson, K. J., Dugle, J. E., Acosta, S. H. et al. (2007). Effect of a viscous fiber-containing nutrition bar on satiety of patients with type 2 diabetes. *Diabetes Res Clin Pract, 76,* 335–340.

Davis, J. N., Alexander, K. E., Ventura, E. E., Toledo-Corral, C. M., and Goran, M. I. (2009). Inverse relation between dietary fiber intake and visceral adiposity in overweight Latino youth. *Am J Clin Nutr, 90,* 1160–1166.

Davis, J. N., Hodges, V. A., and Gillham, M. B. (2006). Normal-weight adults consume more fiber and fruit than their age- and height-matched overweight/obese counterparts. *J Am Diet Assoc, 106,* 833–840.

Delargy, H. J., O'Sullivan, K. R., Fletcher, R. J., and Blundell, J. E. (1997). Effects of amount and type of dietary fiber (soluble and insoluble) on short-term control of appetite. *Int J Food Sci Nutr, 48,* 67–77.

Den Hond, E. D. (2000). Effect of high performance chicory inulin on constipation. *Nutr Res, 5,* 731–736.

Donazzolo, Y., Pelletier, X., Cristiani, I., and Wils, D. (2003). Glycemic and insulinemic indexes of NUTRIOSE® FB in healthy subjects. Paper presented at the Proceedings of the Dietary Fiber Conference, Noordwijkerhout, the Netherlands.

Du, H., van der, A. D. L., Boshuizen, H. C., Forouhi, N. G., Wareham, N. J., Halkjaer, J. et al. (2010). Dietary fiber and subsequent changes in body weight and waist circumference in European men and women. *Am J Clin Nutr, 91,* 329–336.

Ebbeling, C. B., Leidig, M. M., Feldman, H. A., Lovesky, M. M., and Ludwig, D. S. (2007). Effects of a low-glycemic load vs low-fat diet in obese young adults: A randomized trial. *JAMA, 297,* 2092–2102.

Ellis, P. R., Apling, E. C., Leeds, A. R., and Bolster, N. R. (1981). Guar bread: Acceptability and efficacy combined. Studies on blood glucose, serum insulin and satiety in normal subjects. *Br J Nutr, 46,* 267–276.

Englyst, H. N., Kingman, S. M., and Cummings, J. H. (1992). Classification and measurement of nutritionally important starch fractions. *Eur J Clin Nutr, 46*(Suppl 2), S33–S50.

Essah, P. A., Levy, J. R., Sistrun, S. N., Kelly, S. M., and Nestler, J. E. (2007). Effect of macronutrient composition on postprandial peptide YY levels. *J Clin Endocrinol Metab, 92,* 4052–4055.

EFSA Panel on Dietetic Products, Nutrition, and Allergies (NDA) (2010). Scientific opinion on dietary reference values for carbohydrates and dietary fibre. *EFSA Journal,* 8, 1462, pp. 77, www.efsa.europa.eu

European Commission. (2008). Draft commission directive: Amending directive 90/496/EEC. Available at http://www.food.gov.uk/multimedia/pdfs/consultation/cwd (accessed February 23, 2012.)

Flickinger, E. A., Wolf, B. W., Garleb, K. A., Chow, J., Leyer, G. J., Johns, P. W. et al. (2000). Glucose-based oligosaccharides exhibit different in vitro fermentation patterns and affect in vivo apparent nutrient digestibility and microbial populations in dogs. *J Nutr, 130,* 1267–1273.

Flint, A., Møller, B. K., Raben, A., Sloth, B., Pedersen, D., Tetens, I. et al. (2006). Glycemic and insulinemic responses as determinants of appetite in humans. *Am J Clin Nutr, 84,* 1365–1373.

French, S. J. and Read, N. W. (1994). Effect of guar gum on hunger and satiety after meals of differing fat content: Relationship with gastric emptying. *Am J Clin Nutr, 59,* 87–91.

Frost, G. S., Brynes, A. E., Dhillo, W. S., Bloom, S. R., and McBurney, M. I. (2003). The effects of fiber enrichment of pasta and fat content on gastric emptying, GLP-1, glucose, and insulin responses to a meal. *Eur J Clin Nutr, 57,* 293–298.

Geboes, K. P., Luypaerts, A., Rutgeerts, P., and Verbeke, K. (2003). Inulin is an ideal substrate for a hydrogen breath test to measure the orocaecal transit time. *Aliment Pharmacol Ther, 18,* 721–729.

Guerin-Deremaux, L., Li, S., Pochat, M., Wils, D., Mubasher, M., Reifer, C., and Miller, L. E. (2011a). Effects of NUTRIOSE® dietary fiber supplementation on body weight, body composition, energy intake, and hunger in overweight men. *Int. J. Food Sci. Nutr., 62*(6), 628–635.

Guerin-Deremaux, L., Pochat, M., Reifer, C., Wils, D., Cho, S., and Miller, L. E. (2011b). The soluble fiber NUTRIOSE® induces a dose-dependent beneficial impact on satiety over time in humans. *Nutr. Res., 31,* 665–672.

Hamer, H. M., Jonkers, D., Venema, K., Vanhoutvin, S., Troost, F. J., and Brummer, R. J. (2008). The role of butyrate in colonic function. *Aliment Pharmacol Ther, 27,* 104–119.

Heini, A. F., Lara-Castro, C., Schneider, H., Kirk, K. A., Considine, R. V., and Weinsier, R. L. (1998). Effect of hydrolyzed guar fiber on fasting and postprandial satiety and satiety hormones: A double-blind, placebo-controlled trial during controlled weight loss. *Int J Obes Relat Metab Disord, 22,* 906–909.

van den Heuvel, E. G., Wils, D., Pasman, W. J., Bakker, M., Saniez, M. H., and Kardinaal, A. F. (2004). Short-term digestive tolerance of different doses of NUTRIOSE FB, a food dextrin, in adult men. *Eur J Clin Nutr, 58,* 1046–1055.

van den Heuvel, E. G., Wils, D., Pasman, W. J., Saniez, M. H., and Kardinaal, A. F. (2005). Dietary supplementation of different doses of NUTRIOSE FB, a fermentable dextrin, alters the activity of faecal enzymes in healthy men. *Eur J Nutr, 44,* 445–451.

Hlebowicz, J., Darwiche, G., Björgell, O., and Almér, L. O. (2008). Effect of muesli with 4 g oat beta-glucan on postprandial blood glucose, gastric emptying and satiety in healthy subjects: A randomized crossover trial. *J Am Coll Nutr, 27*, 470–475.

Hoad, C. L., Rayment, P., Spiller, R. C., Marciani, L., Alonso Bde, C., Traynor, C. et al. (2004). In vivo imaging of intragastric gelation and its effect on satiety in humans. *J Nutr, 134*, 2293–2300.

Holst, J. (2007). The physiology of glucagon-like peptide 1. *Physiol Rev, 87*, 1409–1439.

Holt, S., Brand, J., Soveny, C., and Hansky, J. (1992). Relationship of satiety to postprandial glycaemic, insulin and cholecystokinin responses. *Appetite, 18*, 129–141.

Howarth, N. C., Huang, T. T., Roberts, S. B., and McCrory, M. A. (2005). Dietary fiber and fat are associated with excess weight in young and middle-aged US adults. *J Am Diet Assoc, 105*, 1365–1372.

Howarth, N. C., Saltzman, E., McCrory, M. A., Greenberg, A. S., Dwyer, J., Ausman, L., Kramer, D. G., and Roberts, S. B. (2003). Fermentable and nonfermentable fiber supplements did not alter hunger, satiety or body weight in a pilot study of men and women consuming self-selected diets. *J. Nutr., 133*, 3141–3144.

Howarth, N. C., Saltzman, E., and Roberts, S. B. (2001). Dietary fiber and weight regulation. *Nutr Rev, 59*, 129–139.

Hu, F. B. (2008). *Obesity Epidemiology*. Oxford University Press, New York.

Jenkins, D. J., Wolever, T. M., Taylor, R. H., Barker, H., Fielden, H., Baldwin, J. M. et al. (1981). Glycemic index of foods: A physiological basis for carbohydrate exchange. *Am J Clin Nutr, 34*, 362–366.

Juntunen, K. S., Niskanen, L. K., Liukkonen, K. H., Poutanen, K. S., Holst, J. J., and Mykkänen, H. M. (2002). Postprandial glucose, insulin, and incretin responses to grain products in healthy subjects. *Am J Clin Nutr, 75*, 254–262.

Juvonen, K., Salmenkallio-Marttila, M., Lyly, M., Liukkonen, K. H., Lähteenmäki, L., Laaksonen, D. et al. (2011). Semisolid meal enriched in oat bran decreases plasma glucose and insulin levels, but does not change gastrointestinal peptide responses or short-term appetite in healthy subjects. *Nutr Metab Cardiovasc Dis, 21*, 74–75.

Karhunen, L. J., Juvonen, K. R., Flander, S. M., Liukkonen, K. H., Lähteenmäki, L., Siloaho, M. et al. (2010). A psyllium fiber-enriched meal strongly attenuates postprandial gastrointestinal peptide release in healthy young adults. *J Nutr, 140*, 737–744.

King, N. A., Craig, S. A., Pepper, T., and Blundell, J. E. (2005). Evaluation of the independent and combined effects of xylitol and polydextrose consumed as a snack on hunger and energy intake over 10 d. *Br J Nutr, 93*, 911–915.

Kojima, M. and Kangawa, K. (2008). Structure and function of ghrelin. *Results Probl Cell Differ, 46*, 89–115.

Kong, A. P., Chan, R. S., Nelson, E. A., and Chan, J. C. (2011). Role of low-glycemic index diet in management of childhood obesity. *Obes Rev, 12*, 492–498.

Kovacs, E. M., Westerterp-Plantenga, M. S., Saris, W. H., Goossens, I., Geurten, P., and Brouns, F. (2001). The effect of addition of modified guar gum to a low-energy semisolid meal on appetite and body weight loss. *Int J Obes Relat Metab Disord, 25*, 307–315.

Kovacs, E. M., Westerterp-Plantenga, M. S., Saris, W. H., Melanson, K. J., Goossens, I., Geurten, P. et al. (2002). The effect of guar gum addition to a semisolid meal on appetite related to blood glucose, in dieting men. *Eur J Clin Nutr, 56*, 771–778.

Kromhout, D., Bloemberg, B., Seidell, J. C., Nissinen, A., and Menotti, A. (2001). Physical activity and dietary fiber determine population body fat levels: The seven countries study. *Int J Obes Relat Metab Disord, 25*, 301–306.

Krotkiewski, M. (1984). Effect of guar gum on body-weight, hunger ratings and metabolism in obese subjects. *Br J Nutr, 52*, 97–105.

Lavin, J. H. and Read, N. W. (1995). The effect on hunger and satiety of slowing the absorption of glucose: Relationship with gastric emptying and postprandial blood glucose and insulin responses. *Appetite, 25,* 89–96.

Ledikwe, J. H., Rolls, B. J., Smiciklas-Wright, H., Mitchell, D. C., Ard, J. D., Champagne, C. et al. (2007). Reductions in dietary energy density are associated with weight loss in overweight and obese participants in the PREMIER trial. *Am J Clin Nutr, 85,* 1212–1221.

Lefranc-Millot, C. (2008). NUTRIOSE 06: A useful soluble fiber for added nutritional value. *Nutr Bull, 33,* 234–239.

Lefranc-Millot, C., Wils, D., Henry, J., Lightowler, H., and Saniez-Degrave, M.-H. (2006). NUTRIOSE®, a resistant dextrin, and MALTISORB®, a sugar alcohol, two key ingredients for healthy diets and obesity management. *Obes Rev, 7*(Suppl 2), 269.

Ley, R. E., Bäckhed, F., Turnbaugh, P., Lozupone, C. A., Knight, R. D., and Gordon, J. I. (2005). Obesity alters gut microbial ecology. *Proc Natl Acad Sci USA, 102,* 11070–11075.

Ley, R. E., Turnbaugh, P. J., Klein, S., and Gordon, J. I. (2006). Microbial ecology: Human gut microbes associate with obesity. *Nature, 444,* 1022–1023.

Li, S., Guerin-Deremaux, L. G., Pochat, M., Wils, D., Reifer, C., and Miller, L. E. (2010). NUTRIOSE® dietary fiber supplementation improves insulin resistance and determinants of metabolic syndrome in overweight men: A double blind, randomized, placebo-controlled study. *Appl Physiol Nutr Metabol, 35,* 773–782.

Liu, S., Willett, W. C., Manson, J. E., Hu, F. B., Rosner, B., and Colditz, G. (2003). Relation between changes in intakes of dietary fiber and grain products and changes in weight and development of obesity among middle-aged women. *Am J Clin Nutr, 78,* 920–927.

Livesey, G. (1992). The energy values of dietary fiber and sugar alcohols for man. *Nutr Res Rev, 5,* 61–84.

di Lorenzo, C., Williams, C. M., Hajnal, F., and Valenzuela, J. E. (1988). Pectin delays gastric emptying and increases satiety in obese subjects. *Gastroenterology, 95,* 1211–1215.

Lu, Z. X., Gibson, P. R., Muir, J. G., Fielding, M., and O'Dea, K. (2000). Arabinoxylan fiber from a by-product of wheat flour processing behaves physiologically like a soluble, fermentable fiber in the large bowel of rats. *J Nutr, 130,* 1984–1990.

Ludwig, D. S., Majzoub, J. A., Al-Zahrani, A., Dallal, G. E., Blanco, I., and Roberts, S. B. (1999a). High glycemic index foods, overeating, and obesity. *Pediatrics, 103,* E26.

Ludwig, D. S., Pereira, M. A., Kroenke, C. H., Hilner, J. E., Van Horn, L., Slattery, M. L. et al. (1999b). Dietary fiber, weight gain, and cardiovascular disease risk factors in young adults. *JAMA, 282,* 1539–1546.

Ludwig, D. S. and Roberts, S. B. (2006). Influence of glycemic index/load on glycemic response, appetite, and food intake in healthy humans. *Diabetes Care, 29,* 474.

Lyly, M., Ohls, N., Lähteenmäki, L., Salmenkallio-Marttila, M., Liukkonen, K. H., Karhunen, L. et al. (2010). The effect of fiber amount, energy level and viscosity of beverages containing oat fiber supplement on perceived satiety. *Food Nutr Res, 54,* doi: 10.3402/fnr.v3454i3400.2149.

Lyon, M. R. and Reichert, R. G. (2010). The effect of a novel viscous polysaccharide along with lifestyle changes on short-term weight loss and associated risk factors in overweight and obese adults: An observational retrospective clinical program analysis. *Altern Med Rev, 15,* 68–75.

Maskarinec, G., Takata, Y., Pagano, I., Carlin, L., Goodman, M. T., Le Marchand, L. et al. (2006). Trends and dietary determinants of overweight and obesity in a multiethnic population. *Obesity (Silver Spring), 14,* 717–726.

Mattes, R. D. (2007). Effects of a combination fiber system on appetite and energy intake in overweight humans. *Physiol Behav, 90,* 705–711.

Morgan, L. M., Tredger, J. A., Shavila, Y., Travis, J. S., and Wright, J. (1993). The effect of non-starch polysaccharide supplementation on circulating bile acids, hormone and metabolite levels following a fat meal in human subjects. *Br J Nutr, 70,* 491–501.

Neary, M. T. and Batterham, R. L. (2009). Peptide YY: Food for thought. *Physiol Behav, 97*, 616–619.

Nelson, L. H. and Tucker, L. A. (1996). Diet composition related to body fat in a multivariate study of 203 men. *J Am Diet Assoc, 96*, 771–777.

Nguyen, K. N., Welsh, J. D., Manion, C. V., and Ficken, V. J. (1982). Effect of fiber on breath hydrogen response and symptoms after oral lactose in lactose malabsorbers. *Am J Clin Nutr, 35*, 1347–1351.

van Nieuwenhoven, M. A., Kovacs, E. M., Brummer, R. J., Westerterp-Plantenga, M. S., and Brouns, F. (2001). The effect of different dosages of guar gum on gastric emptying and small intestinal transit of a consumed semisolid meal. *J Am Coll Nutr, 20*, 87–91.

Nilsson, A. C., Ostman, E. M., Holst, J. J., and Björck, I. M. (2008). Including indigestible carbohydrates in the evening meal of healthy subjects improves glucose tolerance, lowers inflammatory markers, and increases satiety after a subsequent standardized breakfast. *J Nutr, 138*, 732–739.

Niwano, Y., Adachi, T., Kashimura, J., Sakata, T., Sasaki, H., Sekine, K. et al. (2009). Is glycemic index of food a feasible predictor of appetite, hunger, and satiety? *J Nutr Sci Vitaminol (Tokyo), 55*, 201–207.

Panouille, M. and Larreta-Garde, V. (2009). Gelation behaviour of gelatin and alginate mixtures. *Food Hydrocolloids, 23*, 1074–1080.

Parnell, J. A. and Reimer, R. A. (2009). Weight loss during oligofructose supplementation is associated with decreased ghrelin and increased peptide YY in overweight and obese adults. *Am J Clin Nutr, 89*, 1751–1759.

Pasman, W., Wils, D., Saniez, M. H., and Kardinaal, A. (2006). Long-term gastrointestinal tolerance of NUTRIOSE FB in healthy men. *Eur J Clin Nutr, 60*, 1024–1034.

Pasman, W. J., Blokdijk, V. M., Bertina, F. M., Hopman, W. P., and Hendriks, H. F. (2003). Effect of two breakfasts, different in carbohydrate composition, on hunger and satiety and mood in healthy men. *Int J Obes Relat Metab Disord, 27*, 663–668.

Pasman, W. J., Saris, W. H., Wauters, M. A., and Westerterp-Plantenga, M. S. (1997). Effect of one week of fiber supplementation on hunger and satiety ratings and energy intake. *Appetite, 29*, 77–87.

Paxman, J. R., Richardson, J. C., Dettmar, P. W., and Corfe, B. M. (2008). Daily ingestion of alginate reduces energy intake in free-living subjects. *Appetite, 51*, 713–719.

Pelkman, C. L., Navia, J. L., Miller, A. E., and Pohle, R. J. (2007). Novel calcium-gelled, alginate-pectin beverage reduced energy intake in nondieting overweight and obese women: Interactions with dietary restraint status. *Am J Clin Nutr, 86*, 1595–1602.

Pereira, M. A. and Ludwig, D. S. (2001). Dietary fiber and body-weight regulation. Observations and mechanisms. *Pediatr Clin North Am, 48*, 969–980.

Perrigue, M. M., Monsivais, P., and Drewnowski, A. (2009). Added soluble fiber enhances the satiating power of low-energy-density liquid yogurts. *J Am Diet Assoc, 109*, 1862–1868.

Porrini, M., Crovetti, R., Testolin, G., and Silva, S. (1995). Evaluation of satiety sensations and food intake after different preloads. *Appetite, 25*, 17–30.

Rigaud, D., Paycha, F., Meulemans, A., Merrouche, M., and Mignon, M. (1998). Effect of psyllium on gastric emptying, hunger feeling and food intake in normal volunteers: A double blind study. *Eur J Clin Nutr, 52*, 239–245.

Roberts, S. B. (2000). High-glycemic index foods, hunger, and obesity: Is there a connection? *Nutr Rev, 58*, 163–169.

Robertson, M. D., Bickerton, A. S., Dennis, A. L., Vidal, H., and Frayn, K. N. (2005). Insulin-sensitizing effects of dietary resistant starch and effects on skeletal muscle and adipose tissue metabolism. *Am J Clin Nutr, 82*, 559–567.

Singh, B. and Chauhan, N. (2009). Modification of psyllium polysaccharides for use in oral insulin delivery. *Food Hydrocolloids, 23*, 928–935.

Slavin, J. and Green, H. (2007). Dietary fiber and satiety. *Nutr Bull, 32*, 32–42.

Slavin, J. L. (2005). Dietary fiber and body weight. *Nutrition, 21*, 411–418.

Slavin, J. L. (2008). Position of the American Dietetic Association: Health implications of dietary fiber. *J Am Diet Assoc, 108*, 1716–1731.

Stevens, J., Levitsky, D. A., VanSoest, P. J., Robertson, J. B., Kalkwarf, H. J., and Roe, D. A. (1987). Effect of psyllium gum and wheat bran on spontaneous energy intake. *Am J Clin Nutr, 46*, 812–817.

Stock, S., Leichner, P., Wong, A. C., Ghatei, M. A., Kieffer, T. J., Bloom, S. R. et al. (2005). Ghrelin, peptide YY, glucose-dependent insulinotropic polypeptide, and hunger responses to a mixed meal in anorexic, obese, and control female adolescents. *J Clin Endocrinol Metab, 90*, 2161–2168.

Thomas, D., Elliott, E. J., and Baur, L. (2007). Low glycaemic index or low glycaemic load diets for overweight and obesity. *Cochrane Database Syst Rev,* Jul 18, (3), CD005105.

Thornburn, A., Muir, J., and Proietto, J. (1993). Carbohydrate fermentation decreases hepatic glucose output in healthy subjects. *Metabolism, 42*, 780–785.

Tiwary, C. M., Ward, J. A., and Jackson, B. A. (1997). Effect of pectin on satiety in healthy US Army adults. *J Am Coll Nutr, 16*, 423–428.

Tsuchiya, A., Almiron-Roig, E., Lluch, A., Guyonnet, D., and Drewnowski, A. (2006). Higher satiety ratings following yogurt consumption relative to fruit drink or dairy fruit drink. *J Am Diet Assoc, 106*, 550–557.

Tucker, L. A. and Thomas, K. S. (2009). Increasing total fiber intake reduces risk of weight and fat gains in women. *J Nutr, 139*, 576–581.

Turnbull, W. H. and Thomas, H. G. (1995). The effect of a Plantago ovata seed containing preparation on appetite variables, nutrient and energy intake. *Int J Obes Relat Metab Disord, 19*, 338–342.

US Department of Agriculture, Center for Nutrition Policy and Promotion. (2010). Dietary guidelines for Americans. Report of the Dietary Guidelines Advisory Committee on the Dietary Guidelines for Americans, 2010. Retrieved on July 20, 2010, from http://www.cnpp.usda.gov/DGAs2010-DGACReport.htm

Van de Ven, M. L., Westerterp-Plantenga, M. S., Wouters, L., and Saris, W. H. (1994). Effects of liquid preloads with different fructose/fiber concentrations on subsequent food intake and ratings of hunger in women. *Appetite, 23*, 139–146.

Vermorel, M., Coudray, C., Wils, D., Sinaud, S., Tressol, J. C., Montaurier, C. et al. (2004). Energy value of a low-digestible carbohydrate, NUTRIOSE FB, and its impact on magnesium, calcium and zinc apparent absorption and retention in healthy young men. *Eur J Nutr, 43*, 344–352.

Warren, J. M., Henry, C. J., and Simonite, V. (2003). Low glycemic index breakfasts and reduced food intake in preadolescent children. *Pediatrics, 112*, e414.

Weickert, M. O., Mohlig, M., Koebnick, C., Holst, J. J., Namsolleck, P., Ristow, M. et al. (2005). Impact of cereal fiber on glucose-regulating factors. *Diabetologia, 48*, 2343–2353.

Weickert, M. O., Spranger, J., Holst, J. J., Otto, B., Koebnick, C., Möhlig, M. et al. (2006). Wheat-fiber-induced changes of postprandial peptide YY and ghrelin responses are not associated with acute alterations of satiety. *Br J Nutr, 96*, 795.

Willis, H. J., Eldridge, A. L., Beiseigel, J., Thomas, W., and Slavin, J. L. (2009). Greater satiety response with resistant starch and corn bran in human subjects. *Nutr Res, 29*, 100–105.

Wolf, B. W., Bauer, L. L., and Fahey, G. C., Jr. (1999). Effects of chemical modification on in vitro rate and extent of food starch digestion: An attempt to discover a slowly digested starch. *J Agric Food Chem, 47*, 4178–4183.

Wolf, B. W., Wolever, T. M. S., Bolognesi, C., Zinker, B. A., and Garleb, K. A. (2001). Glycemic response to a rapidly digested starch is not affected by the addition of an indigestible dextrin in humans. *Nutr Res, 21*, 1099–1106.

Wood, P. J., Beer, M. U., and Butler, G. (2000). Evaluation of role of concentration and molecular weight of oat beta-glucan in determining effect of viscosity on plasma glucose and insulin following an oral glucose load. *Br J Nutr, 84*, 19–23.

Zarling, E. J., Edison, T., Berger, S., Leya, J., and DeMeo, M. (1994). Effect of dietary oat and soy fiber on bowel function and clinical tolerance in a tube feeding dependent population. *J Am Coll Nutr, 13*, 565–568.

Zhou, J., Hegsted, M., McCutcheon, K. L., Keenan, M. J., Xi, X., Raggio, A. M., and Martin, R. J. (2006). Peptide YY and proglucagon mRNA expression patterns and regulation in the gut. *Obesity, 14*, 683–689.

9

Viscous Dietary Fiber Reduces Adiposity and Plasma Adipokines and Increases Gene Expression Related to Fat Oxidation in Rats

DANIEL D. GALLAHER, AJMILA ISLAM, ANTHONY E. CIVITARESE, LAURA KOTOWSKI, JULIE-ANNE NAZARE, and ROBERT HESSLINK

Contents

9.1 Introduction

The prevalence of obesity in the human population has reached unprecedented levels. It is estimated that as of 2005, over 23% of the world's adult population was overweight, a figure that is projected to increase to 57.8% by 2030 [1]. Within the United States, in 2003–2004, the combined prevalence of overweight and obesity was estimated at 66.3% of adults [2]. As of 2008, the Centers for Disease Control reported that 32 states had a prevalence of obesity $\geq$25% [3]. The etiology of obesity is complex but certainly involves several factors such as reduced physical activity and overconsumption of energy-dense, highly palatable foods [4]. The primary health concern for obesity is the increased risk for a number of comorbidities, including insulin resistance, hypertension, type 2 diabetes, coronary heart disease, and certain cancers.

To combat this epidemic of obesity, considerable effort and expense has been put forth in developing drugs that facilitate a reduction in body weight. Currently, only the lipase inhibitor orlistat (Xenical®) is approved by the U.S. Food and Drug Administration for long-term body weight reduction [5]. However, it is only modestly effective and has a number of gastrointestinal side effects.

Thus, dietary approaches to reducing body fat would be highly desirable. A number of studies now report that diets reducing the glycemic response reduce adiposity relative to a diet producing a greater glycemic response. For example, rats fed a high-amylose-based diet for 7 weeks, which leads to a low glycemic response, had a significantly reduced epididymal fat pad weight and a lower concentration of plasma leptin, both markers of total body fat, when compared to rats fed a waxy-cornstarch-based diet, which has a high glycemic response [6].

Similarly, rats fed mung-bean starch, which has a low glycemic response, for 5 weeks had a strong trend toward a lighter epididymal fat pad, fewer adipocytes, and smaller adipocyte volume compared to rats fed a high glycemic response wheat-starch-based diet [7]. Thus, dietary interventions that reduce the glycemic response to a meal may be a useful strategy for reducing adiposity.

One of the best established physiological effects of viscous dietary fibers is the ability to blunt the postprandial plasma glucose and insulin response to a meal (see [8,9] for reviews). Viscous dietary fibers with this property include β-glucans [10,11], glucomannan [12], psyllium [13], and hydroxypropyl methylcellulose (HPMC) [14]. Therefore, viscous polysaccharides, by slowing glucose absorption after a meal, have the potential to reduce adiposity.

9.2 Intestinal Contents Viscosity Inversely Correlates with Adiposity

We first examined this potential for viscous fiber to reduce adiposity in a study in which rats were fed viscous fibers that were either fermentable or nonfermentable (experiment 1). We employed β-glucan concentrates as a source of fermentable viscous fiber and HPMC as a nonfermentable viscous fiber. Three different dietary concentrations of the β-glucan concentrate and two different mixtures of different viscosity grades of HPMC were used to produce a range of viscosity within the intestinal contents. Cellulose, which has no viscosity, was used as a control. The diets were closely balanced in terms of macronutrient concentration and therefore were essentially isoenergetic. In a first study, plasma leptin concentration was used as a marker of whole body adiposity, since leptin concentrations are proportional to total body fat, both in humans [15,16] and rats [17]. The animals were fed their respective diets for 4 weeks, fasted overnight, and then presented with 5 g of their respective diets. Two hours later, the animals were killed, blood collected, and their intestinal contents collected. Intestinal contents supernatant viscosity was determined, as previously described [18].

Body weight gain did not differ between the cellulose control group and the low and medium-viscosity β-glucan groups or the medium-viscosity HPMC group (Table 9.1). Both the high-viscosity β-glucan group and the high-viscosity HPMC (HV-HPMC) group had a significantly lower body weight compared to

Table 9.1 Body Weight Gain and Food Intake: Experiment 1[1]

	Cellulose	Low-Viscosity β-Glucan	Medium-Viscosity β-Glucan	High-Viscosity β-Glucan	Medium-Viscosity HPMC[2]	High-Viscosity-HPMC
Body weight gain, g	296 ± 10[a]	287 ± 9[a]	284 ± 9[ab]	264 ± 13[bc]	297 ± 10[a]	249 ± 5[c]
Daily food intake, g/day	18.1 ± 0.6	20.1 ± 0.9	18.8 ± 0.8	19.7 ± 0.5	19.2 ± 0.4	18.5 ± 0.6

[1] Values are means ± SEM, n = 10–11 per group. Values within a row that do not share a common superscript are significantly different, p < 0.05.
[2] HPMC, hydroxypropyl methylcellulose.

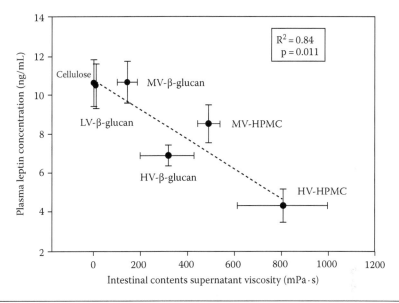

Figure 9.1 Correlation between plasma leptin concentration and intestinal contents supernatant viscosity in rats 2 h after a meal—experiment 1. Values represent means ± SEM, n = 10 for each group. The correlation was statistically significant. *Abbreviations:* LV, low viscosity; MV, medium viscosity; HV, high viscosity; HPMC, hydroxypropyl methylcellulose.

the cellulose group. Interestingly, daily food intake was not different among the groups. Plasma leptin concentration was found to inversely correlate with the intestinal contents supernatant viscosity (Figure 9.1); that is, as contents viscosity increased, total body fat decreased. This correlation remained significant even after correcting for differences in body weight.

In order to confirm and extend this finding of decreased adiposity with viscous fiber intake, with no change in food intake, a second animal study was carried out (experiment 2). The design of this study was substantially similar to the previous study, except that a medium-viscosity β-glucan group was not included. As before, the animals were fed their respective diets for 4 weeks, fasted overnight, and then presented with 7.5 g of their respective diets. Two hours later, the animals were killed, blood collected, and their intestinal contents collected and viscosity determined. In addition, epididymal fat pads were excised and weighed to give a more direct measure of body fat, as fat pad weights are highly correlated with total body fat in rats [19]. Body weight gains were slightly less in the low-viscosity β-glucan, medium-viscosity HPMC, and HV-HPMC groups, compared to the cellulose control group, but these differences were not statistically significant (Table 9.2). Only the high-viscosity β-glucan group had a significantly lower body weight compared to the cellulose group. This pattern was mirrored in the daily food intake; only the high-viscosity β-glucan group had a significantly lower food intake compared to the cellulose group. Once again, there was an inverse correlation between plasma leptin concentration and intestinal contents supernatant

Table 9.2 Body Weight Gain and Food Intake: Experiment 2[1]

	Cellulose	Low-Viscosity β-Glucan	High-Viscosity β-Glucan	Medium-Viscosity HPMC[2]	High-Viscosity HPMC
Body weight gain, g	227 ± 8[a]	208 ± 8[ab]	197 ± 8[b]	210 ± 8[ab]	203 ± 6[ab]
Daily food intake, g/day	18.4 ± 0.8[a]	16.5 ± 0.8[ab]	15.8 ± 0.6[b]	17.5 ± 0.7[ab]	16.3 ± 0.4[ab]

[1] Values are means ± SEM, n = 10 per group. Values within a row that do not share a common superscript are significantly different, p < 0.05.
[2] HPMC, hydroxypropyl methylcellulose.

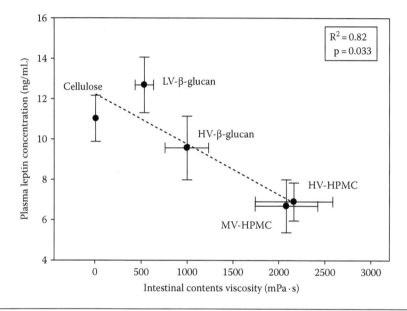

Figure 9.2 Correlation between plasma leptin concentration and intestinal contents supernatant viscosity in rats 2 h after a meal—experiment 2. Values represent means ± SEM, n = 10–11 for each group. The correlation was statistically significant. *Abbreviations*: LV, low viscosity; MV, medium viscosity; HV, high viscosity; HPMC, hydroxypropyl methylcellulose.

viscosity (Figure 9.2). Fat pad weight, as a % of body weight, also correlated with intestinal contents viscosity (Figure 9.3), although this correlation did not quite achieve statistical significance. Thus, these results confirmed the previous study and further supported the ability of viscous dietary fiber to reduce adiposity.

9.3 Viscous Fiber Consumption Increases Markers of Fat Oxidation

An additional study was carried out to investigate the effect of viscous fiber on body composition and to define changes in liver and skeletal muscle energetics as a way to understand the mechanism by which viscous fiber may be reducing

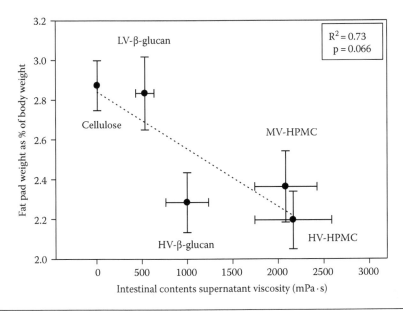

Figure 9.3 Correlation between fat pad weight (as a % of final body weight) and intestinal contents supernatant viscosity—experiment 2. Values represent means ± SEM, n = 10–11 for each group. *Abbreviations*: LV, low viscosity; MV, medium viscosity; HV, high viscosity; HPMC, hydroxypropyl methylcellulose.

adiposity (experiment 3). In this study, animals were fed either cellulose or an HV-HPMC for 6 weeks. Body composition was determined by dual x-ray absorptiometry (DXA) just prior to beginning the feeding study and after 5 weeks of feeding. Also in the 5th week of feeding, animals were fasted overnight, and a blood sample collected the following morning. At the end of the 6th week, animals were fasted overnight and then presented with 5 g of their respective diets. Two hours later, the animals were killed; blood collected; liver, soleus muscle, and fat pads excised; and intestinal contents collected and viscosity determined.

In this third experiment, body weight gain was less in the HV-HPMC group than the cellulose group (Table 9.3). However, there was no difference in daily food intake. Adiposity was examined in three different ways—by DXA, fat pad weight, and the plasma concentration of adipokines that vary in proportion to total body fat. Two adipokines were measured in this regard—leptin and resistin. As stated

Table 9.3 Body Weight Gain and Food Intake: Experiment 3[a]

	Cellulose	High-Viscosity HPMC[b]
Body weight gain, g	251 ± 8	220 ± 6*
Daily food intake, g/day	23.3 ± 0.6	22.8 ± 0.5

[a] Values represent mean ± SEM, n = 13 for cellulose and 26–27 for HV-HPMC. * $p < 0.05$ compared to cellulose group.

[b] HPMC, hydroxypropyl methylcellulose.

Table 9.4 Indicators of Adiposity in Rats Fed Cellulose or High-Viscosity HPMC for 6 Weeks: Experiment 3[a]

Parameter[b]	Cellulose	High-Viscosity HPMC[c]
Adipose tissue gain, g	83.9 ± 3.6	65.5 ± 2.4***
Adipose tissue, % of final body weight	(29.3 ± 0.8)	(26.3 ± 0.5)*
Lean tissue gain, g	192.1 ± 5.7	185.0 ± 4.3
Lean tissue, % of final body weight	(75.5 ± 1.1)	(80.5 ± 0.6)**
Epididymal fat pad, g	7.73 ± 0.43	5.49 ± 0.28***
Weight as % of final body weight	(1.81 ± 0.09)	(1.41 ± 0.06)**
Plasma leptin, fed, ng/mL	4.27 ± 0.61	2.61 ± 0.33*
Plasma leptin, fasted, ng/mL	1.83 ± 0.13	1.00 ± 0.08***
Plasma resistin, fed, ng/mL	90.71 ± 4.45	68.14 ± 4.78**

[a] Values represent mean ± SEM, n = 13 for cellulose and 26–27 for HV-HPMC. * $p < 0.05$; ** $p < 0.01$; *** $p < 0.001$ compared to cellulose group.

[b] Adipose and lean tissue gain were determined by DXA in the 5th week of feeding, as was fasted plasma leptin. Epididymal fat pad weight and plasma leptin and resistin concentrations were determined at the end of the feeding trial, 2 h after a meal.

[c] HPMC, hydroxypropyl methylcellulose.

previously, it is well established that plasma leptin concentration is proportional to total body fat. Plasma resistin is increased in genetic models of obesity and in diet-induced obesity [20], suggesting that the plasma concentration of this adipokine is also an indicator of total body fat. Adipose tissue gain, as measured by DXA, was less in the group fed HV-HPMC, whether expressed as the absolute amount of tissue gain or as a % of final body weight (Table 9.4). Lean tissue gain, as the absolute amount, did not differ between the two groups. However, lean tissue, as a % of the final body weight, was greater in the HV-HPMC group than the cellulose group, indicating a decrease in the proportion of fat to lean tissue with feeding of a viscous fiber. Epididymal fat pads, both as an absolute weight and as a % of final body weight, were lighter in the HV-HPMC group compared to the cellulose group. Finally, the plasma concentration of the two adipokines leptin and resistin was lower in the HV-HPMC group relative to the cellulose group. In the case of plasma leptin, this difference was found in both the fasted and fed states. Thus, all three measures of adiposity were in agreement in indicating a lower degree of adiposity in animals fed a highly viscous dietary fiber.

As an explanation for this reduced adiposity, we hypothesized that consumption of viscous fiber altered fuel utilization in liver and muscle. As a first step toward examining this hypothesis, we determined the activation of AMP-activated protein kinase (AMPK). AMPK is a sensor and master regulator of cellular energetics [21]. Under conditions of low intracellular ATP concentrations that accompany stresses such as nutrient deprivation or hypoxia, AMPK is activated by phosphorylation, primarily by the kinase LKB1 [22]. Overall, activation of AMPK leads to phosphorylation of many targets, including transcription

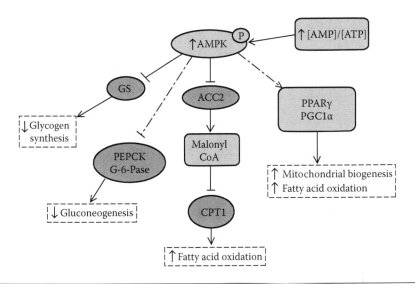

Figure 9.4 AMPK signaling. → direct stimulatory modification; ⊣ direct inhibitory modification; ⤑ transcriptional stimulation; ⊣ transcriptional inhibition. *Abbreviations:* GS, glycogen synthase; PEPCK, phosphoenolpyruvate carboxykinase; G-6-Pase, glucose-6-phosphatase; ACC2, acetyl-CoA carboxylase 2; CPT1, carnitine palmitoyltransferase 1; PPARγ, peroxisome proliferator–activated receptor γ; PGC1α, PPARγ coactivator 1α.

factors and coactivators, resulting in the downregulation of expression of biosynthetic genes and upregulation of genes involved in catabolism. A few of these targets relevant to the current discussion are shown in Figure 9.4. As shown, increased AMPK activity inhibits glycogen synthase activity, decreasing glycogen synthesis while decreasing the expression of the rate-limiting enzymes for gluconeogenesis: phosphoenolpyruvate carboxykinase (PEPCK) and glucose-6-phosphatase (G-6-Pase) [23]. AMPK also decreases the activity of acetyl-CoA carboxylase 2 (ACC2), thereby reducing the concentration of its product, malonyl-CoA. The decreased concentration of malonyl-CoA relieves inhibition of carnitine palmitoyltransferase 1B (CPT1B), the enzyme responsible for transport of fatty acids into the mitochondria, and the rate-limiting step for fatty acid oxidation, thus stimulating this energy-yielding pathway [24,25]. Finally, AMPK activation leads to increased expression of PPARγ coactivator 1α (PGC1α) [26]. PGC1α is a transcriptional coactivator that binds to and transactivates several nuclear hormone receptors, including the PPARs, to increase expression of genes involved in mitochondrial fatty acid oxidation, including CPT1B [27].

Greater phosphorylation, and therefore activation of AMPK, was found in both the liver and soleus muscle of the group fed HV-HPMC compared to the cellulose group (Table 9.5), suggesting a shift in fuel utilization toward greater fatty acid oxidation. As activation of AMPK has also been shown to be associated with a decrease in fat mass [28], this is consistent with our findings of reduced fat mass with consumption of viscous fiber.

Table 9.5 Ratio of Phosphorylated to Total AMPK in Liver and Soleus Muscle of Rats Fed HPMC for 6 Weeks: Experiment 3[a]

	Cellulose	High-Viscosity HPMC[b]
Liver	2.27 ± 0.24	2.98 ± 0.11*
Soleus muscle	3.19 ± 0.40	6.79 ± 1.02**

[a] Values represent mean ± SEM, n = 13 for cellulose and 26–27 for HV-HPMC. * p = 0.004; ** p = 0.022 compared to cellulose group.
[b] HPMC, hydroxypropyl methylcellulose.

Given the greater activation of AMPK with viscous fiber feeding, we next examined the expression of genes related to mitochondrial biogenesis, lipid oxidation, and oxidative fiber-type conversion in soleus muscle. As shown in Figure 9.5, the expression in soleus muscle of the genes for CPT1B, PGC1α, PPARβ/δ, and uncoupling protein 3 (UCP3) was all significantly greater in the HV-HPMC group compared to the cellulose group. PPARα expression did not differ between the two groups. The greater expression in soleus muscle of CPT1B and PGC1α is consistent with our finding of greater activation of AMPK in this tissue and further supports an increase in fatty acid oxidation in muscle with viscous fiber feeding. Increased expression of PGC1α in muscle leads to increased type I fibers [29], which have greater mitochondrial number and a higher oxidative metabolism than type II fibers. Thus, greater expression of PGC1α in the HV-HPMC group suggests that viscous fiber may increase fatty acid oxidation in muscle by increasing the proportion of type I muscle fibers. This concept is

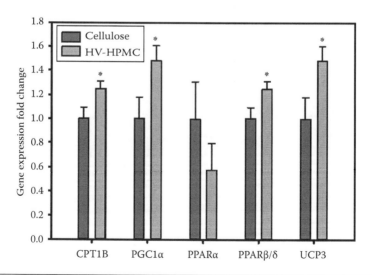

Figure 9.5 Gene expression in soleus muscle related to fatty acid oxidation, expressed as a fold change from the cellulose group—experiment 3. Values represent means ± SEM, n = 13 for cellulose and 26–27 for HV-HPMC. * p < 0.05 compared to the cellulose group.

further supported by the finding of greater expression of PPARβ/δ in the soleus muscle of the HV-HPMC group. PPARα and PPARβ/δ are abundant in oxidative tissue such as muscle and liver and function as catabolic regulators of energy [30], particularly in regulating fatty acid catabolism. PPARβ/δ, the predominant form of PPAR in muscle, is expressed to a much greater degree in type I muscle fiber [31] than type II fibers. PPARβ/δ is also known to activate UCP3 [31], consistent with our finding of greater UCP3 expression in the HV-HPMC group. Although the exact metabolic role of UCP3 remains uncertain, it is upregulated in situations of increased lipid supply to the muscle and may be involved in preventing mitochondrial oxidative stress [32]. Finally, citrate synthase activity (a marker of mitochondrial mass and TCA cycle activity) was greater in the HV-HPMC group compared to the cellulose group (9.01 ± 0.44 vs. $7.35 \pm 0.68\,\mu mol/min/mg$ protein, respectively, $p < 0.05$). Thus, the gene expression profile in the soleus muscle, combined with the greater citrate synthase activity, points to an increase in mitochondria and in fatty acid oxidation in the soleus muscle in the HV-HPMC group compared to the cellulose group.

We also examined hepatic gene expression related to energetics as well as to gluconeogenesis. As shown in Figure 9.6, PGC1α expression was greater in the HV-HPMC group than the cellulose group. There was also a trend toward greater expression of PPARα in the HV-HPMC group. This is of interest, as feeding activators of PPARα to mice has been shown to prevent increases in body weight due to a high-fat diet, with no change in caloric intake [33], similar to our findings after feeding HV-HPMC. There was no significant difference in PPARβ/δ expression between the groups, in contrast to the finding in muscle. Expression of PEPCK,

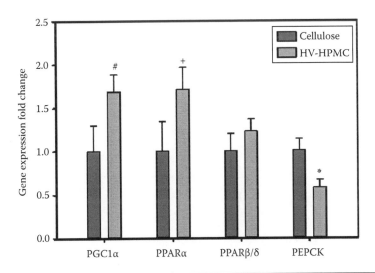

Figure 9.6 Gene expression in liver related to fatty acid oxidation, expressed as a fold change from the cellulose group—experiment 3. Values represent means ± SEM, n = 13 for cellulose and 26–27 for HV-HPMC. *, p = 0.014; #, p = 0.053; +, p = 0.103 compared to the cellulose group.

the rate-limiting enzyme for gluconeogenesis, was decreased in the HV-HPMC, suggesting a decrease in glucose production by the liver. This decreased expression of PEPCK is consistent with the greater hepatic activation of AMPK in the HV-HPMC group. Interestingly, PGC1α is known to induce transcription of PEPCK [34]. However, in this situation, the greater activation of liver AMPK in the HV-HPMC group seems to predominate over the effect of PGC1α in terms of hepatic PEPCK expression. Regardless, these results, taken together, are consistent with an increase in hepatic fatty acid oxidation in the HV-HPMC group relative to the cellulose group.

9.4 Conclusions

Taken together, our results suggest that consumption of viscous dietary fiber leads to a shift in fuel utilization, in which there is increased fatty acid oxidation. This shift is accompanied by a decrease in adiposity and, with the highest viscosity fibers, a modest decrease in body weight, but with little or no decrease in food intake.

Viscous dietary fibers have two well-established physiological effects. These are (1) decreasing the postprandial glucose concentration and (2) reducing of serum cholesterol. Our studies suggest a third physiological effect, which is reducing adiposity. This reduction in adiposity is not accompanied by a reduction in food intake and cannot be attributed to reductions in body weight, since the reductions in adiposity remain statistically significant after adjustment for differences in body weight. Examination of changes in AMPK activation, a master regulator of energy utilization, and of gene expression related to energy metabolism, suggests that viscous fiber causes a shift in fuel utilization, leading to an increase in fatty acid oxidation in both muscle and liver. We suggest that consumption of viscous fiber may be a useful dietary approach to assist with maintaining or achieving normal levels of body fat.

References

1. Kelly, T. et al. Global burden of obesity in 2005 and projections to 2030. *Int. J. Obes. (Lond.)*, 32, 1431, 2008.
2. Ogden, C. L. et al. Prevalence of overweight and obesity in the United States, 1999–2004. *JAMA*, 295, 1549, 2006.
3. Centers for Disease Control and Prevention. U.S. Obesity Trends. http://www.cdc.gov/nccdphp/dnpa/obesity/trend/maps/index.htm. Accessed January 12, 2010.
4. Hill, J. O. and Peters, J. C. Environmental contributions to the obesity epidemic. *Science*, 280, 1371, 1998.
5. U.S. Department of Health and Human Services, N.I.H. Prescription medications for the treatment of obesity. NIH Publication No. 07-4191, December 2010.
6. Pawlak, D. B. et al. High glycemic index starch promotes hypersecretion of insulin and higher body fat in rats without affecting insulin sensitivity. *J. Nutr.*, 131, 99, 2001.
7. Lerer-Metzger, M. et al. Effects of long-term low-glycaemic index starchy food on plasma glucose and lipid concentrations and adipose tissue cellularity in normal and diabetic rats. *Br. J. Nutr.*, 75, 723, 1996.

8. Jenkins, D. J. et al. Viscous and nonviscous fibers, nonabsorbable and low glycaemic index carbohydrates, blood lipids and coronary heart disease. *Curr. Opin. Lipidol.*, 11, 49, 2000.

9. Wursch, P. and Pi-Sunyer, F. X. The role of viscous soluble fiber in the metabolic control of diabetes. A review with special emphasis on cereals rich in beta-glucan. *Diabetes Care*, 20, 1774, 1997.

10. Wood, P. J. et al. Effect of dose and modification of viscous properties of oat gum on plasma glucose and insulin following an oral glucose load. *Br. J. Nutr.*, 72, 731, 1994.

11. Liljeberg, H. G., Akerberg, A. K., and Bjorck, I. M. Effect of the glycemic index and content of indigestible carbohydrates of cereal-based breakfast meals on glucose tolerance at lunch in healthy subjects. *Am. J. Clin. Nutr.*, 69, 647, 1999.

12. Venter, C. S., Vorster, H. H., and Van der Nest, D. G. Comparison between physiological effects of konjac-glucomannan and propionate in baboons fed "Western" diets. *J. Nutr.*, 120, 1046, 1990.

13. Wolever, T. M. et al. Effect of method of administration of psyllium on glycemic response and carbohydrate digestibility. *J. Am. Coll. Nutr.*, 10, 364, 1991.

14. Reppas, C., Greenwood, D. E., and Dressman, J. B. Longitudinal versus radial effects of hydroxypropylmethylcellulose on gastrointestinal glucose absorption in dogs. *Eur. J. Pharm. Sci.*, 8, 211, 1999.

15. Maffei, M. et al. Leptin levels in human and rodent: Measurement of plasma leptin and ob RNA in obese and weight-reduced subjects. *Nat. Med.*, 1, 1155, 1995.

16. Considine, R. V. et al. Serum immunoreactive-leptin concentrations in normal-weight and obese humans. *N. Engl. J. Med.*, 334, 292, 1996.

17. Wolden-Hanson, T. et al. Cross-sectional and longitudinal analysis of age-associated changes in body composition of male Brown Norway rats: Association of serum leptin levels with peripheral adiposity. *J. Gerontol. A Biol. Sci. Med. Sci.*, 54, B99, 1999.

18. Gallaher, C. M. et al. Cholesterol reduction by glucomannan and chitosan is mediated by changes in cholesterol absorption and bile acid and fat excretion in rats. *J. Nutr.*, 130, 2753, 2000.

19. Luu, Y. et al. In vivo quantification of subcutaneous and visceral adiposity by micro-computed tomography in a small animal model. *Med. Eng. Phys.*, 31, 34, 2009.

20. Steppan, C. M. et al. The hormone resistin links obesity to diabetes. *Nature*, 409, 307, 2001.

21. Kahn, B. B. et al. AMP-activated protein kinase: Ancient energy gauge provides clues to modern understanding of metabolism. *Cell Metab.*, 1, 15, 2005.

22. Hardie, D. G. AMP-activated/SNF1 protein kinases: Conserved guardians of cellular energy. *Nat. Rev. Mol. Cell Biol.*, 8, 774, 2007.

23. Foretz, M. et al. Short-term overexpression of a constitutively active form of AMP-activated protein kinase in the liver leads to mild hypoglycemia and fatty liver. *Diabetes*, 54, 1331, 2005.

24. Kaushik, V. K. et al. Regulation of fatty acid oxidation and glucose metabolism in rat soleus muscle: Effects of AICAR. *Am. J. Physiol. Endocrinol. Metab.*, 281, E335, 2001.

25. Thomson, D. M. and Winder, W. W. AMP-activated protein kinase control of fat metabolism in skeletal muscle. *Acta Physiol. (Oxf.)*, 196, 147, 2009.

26. Zong, H. et al. AMP kinase is required for mitochondrial biogenesis in skeletal muscle in response to chronic energy deprivation. *Proc. Natl. Acad. Sci. USA*, 99, 15983, 2002.

27. Vega, R. B., Huss, J. M., and Kelly, D. P. The coactivator PGC-1 cooperates with peroxisome proliferator-activated receptor alpha in transcriptional control of nuclear genes encoding mitochondrial fatty acid oxidation enzymes. *Mol. Cell. Biol.*, 20, 1868, 2000.

28. Narkar, V. A. et al. AMPK and PPARδ agonists are exercise mimetics. *Cell*, 134, 405, 2008.

29. Lin, J. et al. Transcriptional co-activator PGC-1 alpha drives the formation of slow-twitch muscle fibers. *Nature*, 418, 797, 2002.

30. Pyper, S. R. et al. PPARalpha: Energy combustion, hypolipidemia, inflammation and cancer. *Nucl. Recept. Signal.*, 8, E002, 2010.

31. Wang, Y. X. et al. Regulation of muscle fiber type and running endurance by PPARdelta. *PLoS Biol.*, 2, E294, 2004.

32. Seifert, E. L. et al. Essential role for uncoupling protein-3 in mitochondrial adaptation to fasting but not in fatty acid oxidation or fatty acid anion export. *J. Biol. Chem.*, 283, 25124, 2008.

33. Guerre-Millo, M. et al. Peroxisome proliferator-activated receptor alpha activators improve insulin sensitivity and reduce adiposity. *J. Biol. Chem.*, 275, 16638, 2000.

34. Yoon, J. C. et al. Control of hepatic gluconeogenesis through the transcriptional coactivator PGC-1. *Nature*, 413, 131, 2001.

10

Epidemiological Studies of Dietary Fiber and Cardiovascular Disease

JAMES W. ANDERSON and MANAN JHAVERI

Contents

10.1 Introduction

Dietary fiber intake is associated with significant reductions in risk for cardiovascular disease (CVD).[1,2] Early Vahouny Fiber Symposium participants—Denis Burkitt, Hugh Trowell, and Alex Walker—stimulated and inspired interest in this important area.[3–5] Specifically, consumption of high-fiber foods reduces risk for coronary heart disease (CHD), stroke, peripheral vascular disease, and hypertension.[2,6,7] High-fiber intakes also reduce risk for major risk factors for CVD, especially dyslipidemia, diabetes, and obesity.[2]

Trowell forwarded the "ischemic heart disease (IHD) and dietary fiber hypothesis" in 1972, which he supported using strong epidemiologic data, country comparator data, and clinical observations. He stated, "high consumption of natural starchy carbohydrates, taken with their full component of fiber, is protective against hyperlipidemia and IHD."[4] In 1977 Morris et al., in a remarkably prescient study, reported that cereal fiber, but not fruit/vegetable fiber, was associated with a dramatic reduction in CHD events. They noted that intakes of brown bread and breakfast cereals were major contributors to the protective effects of dietary fiber (Table 10.1).[8] In 1982 Kromhout et al. reported from a prospective cohort study that CHD deaths were 74% lower for men who consumed the highest level of total dietary fiber (TDF) compared to those who were in the lowest quintile for TDF intake.[9] Concurrently, Lui et al. reported data from a cross-sectional study that CHD deaths were significantly lower for men and women with the highest level of TDF consumption than for those with the lowest fiber intake.[10] However, the randomized, controlled trial (RCT) reported by Burr et al.[11] noted that increased cereal fiber intake was not associated with a significant effect on CHD events for men following a myocardial infarction; the 2 year duration of this study may not have allowed the increased fiber consumption to exert a protective effect. In a subsequent RCT, Burr reported that recommending an increased intake of fruit and vegetables to men with CHD did not have a significant effect on CHD events over a 3–9 year period, probably related to poor compliance.[12]

Over the past two decades, many prospective cohort studies have examined the association between dietary fiber intakes and CVD. The purpose of this chapter is to review these reports to assess the strength of associations for CVD between TDF from all foods and the intake of different types of dietary fiber and different food sources of dietary fiber.

10.2 Dietary Fiber Characteristics

Dietary fiber is contained in most plant foods that are consumed by humans. Fibers from different foods can have very different chemical and physiological properties. Current research is examining the effects of fibers from different foods and dietary fibers with different specific physicochemical properties.[2] Simplistically, fibers can be classified as insoluble (e.g., cellulose), soluble and viscous (e.g., β-glucan), and soluble and nonviscous (e.g., resistant starches and inulin).[13] Since soluble and viscous fibers (such as oat β-glucan) have greater effects on serum low-density lipoproteins than insoluble fibers, one might expect that sources of this type of soluble fiber (such as fibers contained in oats, barley, beans, and fruits) might have the greatest effects on CVD risk because of their favorable effects on these lipoprotein risk factors.[13] However, whole grain fibers, largely from wheat and largely insoluble fibers, have the strongest associations with reduced CVD events.[1] These relationships will be further examined in this chapter.

10.2.1 Insoluble Fiber

Wheat bran, the fiber made famous by Burkitt[14]—also known as the "Bran Man"[15]—is about 90% insoluble fiber.[16] It is the prototypic fiber for improving laxation and increasing fecal bulk.[17] However, it does not reduce serum low-density-lipoprotein (LDL)-cholesterol values in animals or humans.[13,18] Wheat bran and most other insoluble fibers do appear to have favorable effects on serum

Table 10.1 Dietary Fiber and CVD: Clinical Studies

Author	Number of Subjects	Sex	Population Characteristics	Type Study	Outcome	Duration (Years)	Fiber Source	RR	Comments
Morris[8]	337	M	Middle age	ProCohort	CHD events	14	TDF	0.32	Unadjusted tertile comparison
Morris[8]	337	M	Middle age	ProCohort	CHD events	14	F/V fiber	0.93	Unadjusted tertile comparison
Morris[8]	337	M	Middle age	ProCohort	CHD events	14	Cereal fiber	0.20	Unadjusted tertile comparison
Morris[8]	337	M	Middle age	ProCohort	CHD events	14	Cereal fiber	0.18	Age, duration adjusted
Kromhout[9]	871	M	Middle age	ProCohort	CHD death	10	TDF	0.26	Highest quintile, lower CHD deaths
Liu[10]	Multicountry	MF	Low lipid score	Cross-sectional	CHD death	na	TDF	0.77	Higher fiber intake, lower CHD deaths
Burr[11]	2,033	M	Post-MI	RCT	CHD events	2	Increased cereal fiber	1.23	95% CI, 0.97–1.57
Gramenzi[23]	938	F	Post-MI	Case control	Association	na	Vegetables, fruit, wholemeal bread	0.40–1.10	Fresh fruit, carrots, green vegetables, protection; WM bread, no effect
Bolton-Smith[24]	2,058	MF	With and without CHD	Cross-sectional	CHD events	na	TDF	0.63	95% CI, 0.55–1.14
Humble[25]	1,801	M	Hyperchol	ProCohort	CHD events	9.6	Crude fiber	0.64	CHD risk lower with high fiber intake

(continued)

Table 10.1 (continued) Dietary Fiber and CVD: Clinical Studies

Author	Number of Subjects	Sex	Population Characteristics	Type Study	Outcome	Duration (Years)	Fiber Source	RR	Comments
Pietinen[30]	21,930	M	Smokers	ProCohort	CHD events	6.1	Soluble fiber	0.61	95% CI, 0.46–0.79
Pietinen[30]	21,930	M	Smokers	ProCohort	CHD events	6.1	Insoluble fiber	0.71	95% CI, 0.55–0.93
Wu[88]	573	MF	Age 40–60	ProCohort	Carotid IMT	3	TDF, viscous fiber, pectin	na	TDF, ns slowing of thickness; viscous fiber and pectin, significant slowing
Dauchet[62]	232,049	MF	Seven studies	Meta-analysis	Stroke	na	Fruit and vegetables	0.95/ serving	Stroke risk decreased significantly for each serving of fruit or vegetables
Dauchet[63]	221,080	MF	Nine studies	Meta-analysis	CHD events	na	Fruit and vegetables	0.93/ serving	CHD event risk decreased significantly for each serving of fruit or vegetables
Streppel[38]	1,373	M	Middle age	ProCohort	CHD mort	40	TDF—recent	0.83	Dietary fiber, significantly lower
Streppel[38]	1,373	M	Middle age	ProCohort	CHD mort	40	TDF—long-term	0.87	Dietary fiber intake, no significant changes

Abbreviations: ProCohort, prospective cohort; CHD, coronary heart disease; CVD, cardiovascular disease; TDF, total dietary fiber; F/V, fruit/vegetable; na, not applicable; MI, myocardial infarction; RCT, randomized, controlled trial; WM, wholemeal; hyperchol, hypercholesterolemic; IMT, intima-media thickness, ns, nonsignificant; CI, confidence intervals.

triglycerides, blood pressure, and weight management.[2,13] As Slavin reviews, whole grain foods deliver many phytochemicals, antioxidants, and probably anti-inflammatory factors that may protect from CVD.[19]

10.2.2 Soluble Viscous Fiber

Soluble viscous fibers—such as β-glucan from barley or oats, pectin, and guar— have substantial hypocholesterolemic effects.[2,20] These fibers selectively decrease serum LDL-cholesterol values without affecting serum high-density-lipoprotein (HDL) cholesterol or triglycerides.[21] In addition, many of these fibers have favorable effects on postprandial glycemia, blood pressure, weight management, and, possible, immune function.[13] Whole grain wheat products, the predominant grain consumed in many countries, have very limited amounts of this soluble viscous fiber, but oat and barley products have generous amounts.[16]

10.2.3 Soluble Nonviscous Fiber

The soluble nonviscous fibers can be classified as resistant starches and oligofructoses (such as inulin). The resistant starches, in large doses, decrease postprandial glycemia, and some have bifidogenic effects. The main effects of inulin and the oligofructoses are their important bifidogenic effects and probably immune-enhancing properties.[13] Their effects related to CVD risk have not been specifically examined.

10.3 Cardiovascular Disease

10.3.1 Coronary Heart Disease

CHD is the major cause of death in Western countries and is emerging as a major health problem in most of the world.[22] The early reports of Morris et al.,[8] Kromhout et al.,[9] and Liu et al.[10] pointed to the protective relationship between TDF intake and CHD and suggested that cereal fiber provided the greatest protection (Table 10.1). Case control[23] and cross-sectional[24] studies confirmed these observations as did a prospective cohort study utilizing crude fiber estimates[25] (Table 10.1). Since then the effects of different types and sources of dietary fiber have been extensively examined. The different sources (TDF, grain fibers, fruit and vegetables) have been aggregated and analyzed (Tables 10.2 through 10.4). Fixed-effects meta-analyses[26,27] have been done to obtain estimates of the effects of these different sources and compare their relative protective effects. When possible, CHD events were selected for analyses because this category captured the largest number of individuals specifically affected by coronary events. CHD mortality was the second choice. When these estimates were not available, CVD events (that included strokes) and finally CVD mortality were used for estimates. Most studies calculated relative risk (RR) by comparing those in the highest quintile for dietary fiber intake to those in the lowest quintile. Where different groups—such as men and women—were reported, values were weighted to achieve composite means.

Table 10.2 TDF and CVD: Prospective Cohort Studies

Reference	Number of Subjects	Sex	Age or Characteristics	Outcome	Years Follow-Up	Fiber Type	RR	LCI	UCI
Kushi[28]	1,001	M	Middle age	CHD mortality	20	TDF[1]	0.57	0.33	0.97
Khaw[29]	859	MF	Middle age	CHD mortality	12	TDF	0.35	0.12	1.05
Pietinen[30]	21,930	M	Smokers	CHD events	6.1	TDF	0.68	0.52	0.88
Rimm[31]	43,757	M	No CHD, DM	CHD events	6	TDF	0.64	0.47	0.87
Todd[32]	7,869	MF	40–59 years	CHD events	7.7	TDF	0.60	0.37	0.99
Wolk[33]	68,782	F	37–64 years	CHD events	10	TDF	0.77	0.57	1.04
Mozaffarrian[34]	3,588	MF	≥65 years	CVD events	8.6	TDF	0.84	0.66	1.07
Sum, average, weighted mean	147,786	MF		CVD or CHD events or death	10.1	TDF	0.69	0.49	0.89

Abbreviations, see Table 10.1.

Table 10.3 Grains and CVD: Prospective Cohort Studies

Reference	Number of Subjects	Sex	Age or Characteristics	Outcome	Years Follow-Up	Fiber Type	RR	LCI	UCI
Fraser[35]	31,208	MF	Seventh-Day Adventist	CHD events	6	Whole wheat bread	0.56	0.35	0.89
Jacobs[36]	38,740	F	Age 55–69	CHD mortality	9	Whole grains	0.82	0.63	1.06
Liu[39]	75,521	F	Age 38–63	CHD events	10	Whole grains	0.79	0.62	1.01
Steffen[40]	15,792	MF	Age 45–64	CHD events	11	Whole grains	0.72	0.53	0.97
Jensen[41]	42,850	M	Age 40–75	CHD events	14	Whole grains	0.82	0.70	0.96
Nettleton[37]	5,316	MF	Age 45–84	CVD events	4.6	Whole grains/fruit pattern	0.54	0.33	0.91
He[42]	7,822	F	Diabetic	CVD mortality	26	Whole grains	0.89	0.69	1.14
Sum, average, weighted mean	217,249	MF		CVD or CHD events or death	11.5	Whole grains	0.77	0.60	0.94
Pietinen[30]	21,930	M	Smokers	CHD events	6.1	Cereal fiber	0.77	0.59	1.00
Rimm[31]	43,757	M	No CHD, DM	CHD events	6	Cereal fiber	0.71	0.54	0.92
Wolk[33]	68,782	F	Age 37–64	CHD events	10	Cereal fiber	0.66	0.49	0.88
Mozaffarrian[34]	3,588	MF	≥65	CVD events	8.6	Cereal fiber	0.79	0.62	0.99

(continued)

Table 10.3 (continued) Grains and CVD: Prospective Cohort Studies

Reference	Number of Subjects	Sex	Age or Characteristics	Outcome	Years Follow-Up	Fiber Type	RR	LCI	UCI
He[42]	7,822	F	Diabetic	CVD mort	26	Cereal fiber	0.86	0.66	1.12
Sum, average, weighted mean	145,879	MF		CVD or CVD events or death	11.3	Cereal fiber	0.75	0.55	0.95
Liu[39]	75,521	F	Age 38–63	CHD events	10	Bran	0.63	0.42	0.95
Jensen[41]	42,850	M	Age 40–75	CHD risk	14	Bran	0.70	0.60	0.82
He[42]	7,822	F	Diabetic	CVD mort	26	Bran	0.72	0.56	0.92
Sum, average, weighted mean	126,193	MF		CVD or CHD events or death	16.7	Bran	0.70	0.50	0.89
Liu[39]	75,521	F	Age 38–63	CHD events	10	Germ	0.41	0.15	1.10
Jensen[41]	42,850	M	Age 40–75	CHD risk	14	Germ	0.98	0.85	1.13
He[42]	7,822	F	Diabetic	CVD mort	26	Germ	0.99	0.78	1.26
Sum, average, weighted mean	126,193			CVD or CHD events or death	16.7	Germ	0.95	0.66	1.27
Jacobs[36]	38,740	F	Age 55–69	CHD mortality	9	Refined grain	1.15	0.84	1.56
Steffen[40]	15,792	MF	Age 45–64	CHD events	11	Refined grain	1.17	0.82	1.66
Sum, average, weighted mean	54,532			CHD events or death	10.0	Refined grain	1.16	0.55	1.77

Abbreviations, see Table 10.1.

Table 10.4 Fruit/Vegetable and CVD: Prospective Cohort Studies

Reference	Number of Subjects	Sex	Age or Characteristics	Outcome	Years Follow-Up	Fiber Type	RR	LCI	UCI
Gaziana[43]	1,299	MF	Elderly	CHD deaths	4.8	Fruit and vegetables	0.25	0.09	0.67
Liu[44]	39,876	F	Healthy	CHD events	5	Fruit and vegetables	0.63	0.38	1.17
Joshipura[45]	126,399	MF	Age 34–75	CHD events	11	Fruit and vegetables	0.80	0.69	0.93
Bazzano[46]	9,608	MF	Age 25–74	CHD events	19	Fruit and vegetables	1.01	0.84	1.21
Steffen[40]	15,792	MF	Age 45–64	CHD events	11	Fruit and vegetables	0.82	0.57	1.17
Sum, average, weighted mean	192,974			Events or death	10.2	Fruit and vegetables	0.78	0.58	0.97
Knekt[47]	5,133	MF	Age 30–69	CHD deaths	14	Fruit	0.72	0.44	1.17
Pietinen[30]	21,930	M	Smokers	CHD events	6.1	Fruit fiber	0.82	0.67	1.07
Liu[44]	39,876	F	Healthy	CHD events	5	Fruit	0.66	0.36	1.22
Joshipura[45]	126,399	MF	Age 34–75	CHD events	11	Fruit	0.80	0.69	0.92
Mozaffarrian[34]	3,588	MF	≥65	CVD events	8.6	Fruit fiber	0.99	0.78	1.25
Sum, average, weighted mean	196,926			Events or death	8.9	Fruit and fruit fiber	0.82	0.62	1.07
Knekt[47]	5,133	MF	Age 30–69	CHD deaths	14	Vegetables	0.66	0.41	1.09
Liu[44]	39,876	F	Healthy	CHD events	5	Vegetables	0.88	0.50	1.48
Joshipura[45]	126,399	MF	Age 34–75	CHD events	11	Vegetables	0.82	0.71	0.92
Mozaffarrian[34]	3,588	MF	≥65	CVD events	8.6	Vegetable fiber	1.08	0.86	1.36
Average, weighted mean	174,996			Events or death	9.7	Vegetables or fiber	0.84	0.64	1.04
Bazzano[48]	9,632	MF	No CVD	CHD events	19	Legumes	0.78	0.68	0.90
Joshipura[45]	126,399		Age 34–75	CHD events	11	Legumes	1.06	0.91	1.24
Sum, average, weighted mean	136,031			CHD events	15.0	Legumes	0.88	0.65	1.11

Abbreviations, see Table 10.1.

10.3.1.1 Total Dietary Fiber   Between 1985 and 2003, seven prospective cohort studies[28-34] confirmed the very strong protective association between TDF intake and protection from CHD or CVD (Table 10.2). Data for more than 147,000 men and women, usually middle-aged at baseline without evidence of CHD, followed for a mean period of 10 years were analyzed. Those individuals with the highest intake of TDF had an RR of 0.69 (95% confidence interval [CI], 0.49–0.89) for CVD compared to those with the lowest level of total fiber intake. The data of Streppel et al.[38] (Table 10.1) comparing effects of short-term and long-term TDF use were not included in these analyses. Thus, high dietary fiber consumption appears to reduce rates of CVD events by approximately 31%.

10.3.1.2 Grains

10.3.1.2.1 Whole Grains   In 1992, Fraser et al.[35] reported that Seventh-Day Adventist men or women who had the highest consumption of whole wheat bread had a lower frequency of CHD events than those who had the lowest intake. In 1998, Jacobs et al.[1] presented persuasive data that whole grain intake was associated with a substantial reduction in CHD risk. Subsequent prospective cohort studies confirmed that whole grain intake was associated with a significant reduction in CHD events (Table 10.3). When two reports are available from the same group—like the two reports from Jacobs et al.[1,36]—we selected the studies that provided the most complete or focused comparisons—Jacobs et al.[36] and Nettleton et al.[37] Seven studies that included over 217,000 men and women, mostly middle aged without CHD at baseline, were followed for 12 years.[35-37,39-42] Those individuals with the highest consumption of whole grains had an RR for CVD of 0.77 (95% CI, 0.60–0.94) compared to those with the lowest consumption. Thus, a generous intake of whole grains appears to reduce risks of CVD events by approximately 23%.

10.3.1.2.2 Cereal Fiber   The analyses of Pietinen et al.[30] and of Rimm et al.[31] in 1996 reinforced the earlier observations of Morris et al.[8] indicating that cereal fiber intake was associated with lower rates of CHD. Subsequent reports confirmed and strengthened these observations.[33,34,42] Five studies that included about 145,000 men and women, middle aged or elderly with varying risk factors, were followed for 11 years. Those individuals with the highest consumption of cereal fiber had an RR for CVD events of 0.75 (95% CI, 0.55–0.95) compared to those with the lowest cereal fiber intake (Table 10.3). Thus, higher intakes of cereal fiber appear to reduce risk for CVD by approximately 25%.

10.3.1.2.3 Bran, Germ, and Refined Grain   The whole grain studies raise the question of whether the cardioprotective effects are related to the complex carbohydrate, the fiber, or the phytonutrients in whole grains. Examination of the associations with bran, germ, or refined grains sheds some light on this question. Bran, rich in fiber, was associated with significant protection, while germ, rich in phytonutrients, and refined grains, delivering complex carbohydrates, had no association with CVD events. Three studies included about 126,000 men and women who were followed for 17 years.[39,41,42] Those individuals with the highest intake of bran—largely from wheat—had an RR of 0.70 (95% CI, 0.50–0.89) for CVD compared to those with the lowest consumption. Germ intake (RR, 0.95) or refined grain intake (RR, 1.16) was not associated with significant differences in CVD (Table 10.3). Thus, higher intakes of bran appear to reduce risk for CVD by 30%.

10.3.1.3 Fruit and Vegetables   Associations between consumption of fruit, vegetables, or their combination and CHD have been inconsistent (Table 10.4). Most prospective cohort studies have noted a suggestion of a protective association between fruit and or vegetable intake and CHD that has not been statistically significant. The availability of four or five studies provides the power from meta-analyses to suggest that there are protective associations between fruit, vegetables, and their combination with respect to CHD.

Five prospective cohort studies have assessed the association between the combination of fruit and vegetable intake and CHD.[40,43–46] These studies have assessed about 192,000 participants followed for an average of 10 years. Those individuals with the highest intake of fruit and vegetable consumption had an RR of 0.78 (95% CI, 0.58–0.97) for CHD compared to those with the lowest level of fruit and vegetable intake.

Five prospective cohort studies have assessed the association between fruit or fruit fiber intake and CVD.[30,34,44,45,47] These studies have assessed more than 196,000 participants followed for an average of 9 years. Those individuals with the highest fruit or fruit fiber consumption had an RR of 0.82 (95% CI, 0.62–01.07) for CHD compared to those with the lowest level of fruit intake.

Four prospective cohort studies have assessed the association between vegetable or vegetable fiber intake and CHD.[34,44,45,47] These studies have assessed around 174,000 participants followed for an average of 10 years. Those individuals with the highest level of vegetable or vegetable fiber consumption had an RR of 0.84 (95% CI, 0.64–1.04) for CHD compared to those with the lowest level of vegetable intake.

The consumption of dry beans or legumes is so low in most Western countries that it is difficult to assess the independent effects or associations with CHD. Two prospective cohort studies have been able to assess the association between legume intake and CHD.[45,48] These studies have assessed more than 136,000 participants followed for an average of 15 years. Those individuals with the highest intake of legumes had an RR of 0.88 (95% CI, 0.65–1.11) for CHD compared to those with the lowest level of legume consumption.

In the aggregate, these studies suggest that fruit and vegetable consumption is associated with a reduction in CVD risk of approximately 18% and that legume consumption may be somewhat less protective from CVD.

10.3.2 Stroke

Stroke is the second most common form of CVD—after CHD—among most Western people, and stroke ranks third as cause of death in the United States after CHD and cancer.[22] While data supporting the protective effect of dietary fiber consumption for CHD have been available for almost 40 years,[4] evidence supporting the protective effects of fiber related to stroke has only been available for about 15 years.[51] Four prospective cohort studies assessing TDF or whole grain consumption have included more than 113,000 participants that have been followed for an average of 10 years (Table 10.5).[36,40,49,50] Those individuals with the highest consumption of dietary fiber or whole grains had an RR of 0.72 (95% CI, 0.38–1.06) for stroke events compared to those with the lowest fiber or whole grain intake.

Four prospective cohort studies have also assessed fruit and vegetable consumption and included over 182,000 participants followed for an average of 13 years.[51-54] Those individuals with the highest consumption of the combination of fruit and vegetables had an RR of 0.74 (95% CI, 0.52–0.96) for stroke events compared to those with the lowest fruit and vegetable intake. Thus, higher intakes of dietary fiber appear to be associated with a risk reduction from stroke events of approximately 27%.

10.3.3 Peripheral Arterial Disease

Peripheral arterial disease (PAD), also termed peripheral vascular disease, represents atherosclerotic disease of vessels to the lower extremities and shares pathophysiologic etiologies with CHD and stroke. Just as dietary fiber is associated with reductions in cardiovascular events, one would anticipate that high-fiber intakes would reduce risk for PAD. Only limited prospective cohort data are available to specifically examine the relationship of dietary fiber intake to PAD.[6,55,56] Merchant et al. reported a prospective cohort study of 46,032 men followed for 12 years; the incidence of PAD was noted in only 308 men. Unadjusted comparison of the highest quintile for TDF, cereal fiber, fruit fiber, and vegetable fiber indicated that all these sources of fiber were significantly associated with a reduction in PAD. When adjusted for multiple covariate, especially smoking, only cereal fiber (RR 0.67; 95% CI, 0.47–0.97) remained significant.[6] Hung et al. reported the association between fruit and vegetable intake from the same study. Men in the highest quintile for fruit or vegetable consumption had significantly lower risk for PAD than those in the lowest quintile; with adjustment for covariates, especially smoking, these associations were not significant.[55] Antonelli-Incalzi et al. performed a cross-sectional assessment of PAD defined as an ankle-brachial index of <0.90 for 1251 home-dwelling subjects; 125 participants had PAD. The RR indicated that dietary fiber intake had a protective effect (0.64; 95% CI, 0.40–1.03; P = 0.062).[56] The Merchant[6] and Antonelli-Incalzi[56] studies can be aggregated to give a composite variance-weighted mean RR estimate of approximately 0.72 (95% CI, 0.25–1.20).

Table 10.5 Dietary Fiber and Stroke: Prospective Cohort Studies*

Reference	Number of Subjects	Sex	Age or Characteristics	Outcome	Years Follow-Up	Fiber Type	RR	LCI	UCI
Ascherio[49]	43,738	M	Age 40–75	Stroke events	8	Total fiber	0.70	0.48	1.00
Jacobs[36]	38,740	F	Age 55–69	Stroke deaths	9	Whole grains	0.87	0.52	1.48
Liu[50]	15,104	F	Age 38–63	Stroke events	12	Whole grains	0.69	0.50	0.98
Steffen[40]	15,792	MF	Age 45–64	Stroke events	11	Whole grains	0.75	0.46	1.22
Sum, average, weighted mean	113,374				10.0	Whole grains or TDF	0.72	0.38	1.06
Gillman[51]	832	M	Age 45–65	Stroke events	20	Fruit and vegetables	0.78	0.62	0.98
Joshipura[52]	117,249	MF	Age 34–75	Stroke events	11	Fruit and vegetables	0.69	0.52	0.92
Bazzano[53]	9,608	MF	Age 25–74	Stroke events	19	Fruit and vegetables	0.73	0.57	0.95
Johnsen[54]	54,506	MF	Age 50–64	Stroke events	3.1	Fruit and vegetables	0.72	0.47	1.12
Sum, average, weighted mean	182,195				13.3	Fruit and vegetables	0.74	0.52	0.96

* Abbreviations, see Table 10.1.

These three reports indicate that dietary fiber intake, especially cereal fiber intake, is associated with a reduced risk for PAD of approximately 30%. Smoking seems to be the predominant risk factor, and these fiber effects were not significant when adjusted for smoking in the small number of subjects with PAD. These observations are consistent with those reported for CHD again suggesting that cereal fiber, and indirectly pointing to whole grains, is protective against PVD.

10.3.4 All-Cause Mortality

Several prospective cohort studies have assessed the association between dietary fiber consumption and all-cause mortality (Table 10.6). Two studies including over 46,000 individuals were followed for an average of 8 years; individuals consuming the largest amount of TDF or whole grains had an RR for all-cause mortality of 0.84 (95% CI, 0.61–1.06) compared to those with the lowest intake.[32,36] Two studies including about 25,000 individuals were followed for an average of 15 years; individuals consuming the largest amount of fruit and vegetables had an RR for all-cause mortality of 0.82 (95% CI, 0.57–1.07) compared to those who had the lowest intakes.[40,46] These observations suggest that higher levels of dietary fiber intake are associated with a reduction in all-cause mortality rates of approximately 17%. Of interest, Bazzano et al.[46] reported that fruit and vegetable intake did not significantly affect non-CVD mortality rates (RR 0.95, Table 10.6).

10.4 Risk Factors for Cardiovascular Disease

10.4.1 Dyslipidemia

The LDLs—estimated by LDL-cholesterol measurements—appear to be the most atherogenic blood lipid particles, while the very LDLs—estimated by fasting serum triglyceride measures—are also atherogenic. Selected HDL particles—estimated by HDL-cholesterol measures—are cardiovascular protective.[21] Short term (1–3 months), intermediate term (3–12 months), and long term (>12 months) have documented that a number of foods rich in viscous soluble fiber decrease serum LDL-cholesterol values[2,21]; these foods include beans, oats, oat bran, and barley beta-glucan.[57–59] Long-term studies using large doses of guar gum document sustained reductions in LDL-cholesterol values.[2] Long-term consumption of generous amounts of oat bran is associated with increases in serum HDL-cholesterol values.[60] Wheat bran consumption is associated with significant reductions in serum triglyceride values.[61]

Pietinen et al.[30] specifically assessed the associations of soluble and insoluble fiber consumption and CHD events in a prospective cohort study of 21,930 male cigarette smokers (Table 10.1). Individuals in the highest quintile compared to the lowest quintile had these associations with CHD events: soluble fiber, RR 0.61 (95% CI, 0.46–0.79), and insoluble fiber, RR 0.71 (95% CI, 0.55–0.93).

Table 10.6 Dietary Fiber and All-Cause Mortality and Non-CVD Mortality: Prospective Cohort Studies

Reference	Number of Subjects	Sex	Age or Characteristics	Outcome	Years Follow-Up	Fiber Type	RR	LCI	UCI
Todd[32]	7,869	MF	Age 40–59	All-cause mortality	7.7	TDF	0.64	0.39	1.07
Jacobs[36]	38,740	F	Age 55–69	All-cause mortality	9	Whole grains	0.86	0.76	0.97
Sum, average, weighted mean	46,609	MF		All-cause mortality	8.4	TDF or whole grains	0.84	0.61	1.06
Bazzano[46]	9,608	MF	Age 25–74	All-cause mortality	19	Fruit and vegetables	0.85	0.72	1.00
Steffen[40]	15,792	MF	Age 45–64	All-cause mortality	11	Fruit and vegetables	0.77	0.61	0.97
Sum, average, weighted mean	25,400	MF		All-cause mortality	15	Fruit and vegetables	0.82	0.57	1.07
Bazzano[46]	9,608	MF	Age 25–74	Non-CVD mortality	19	Fruit and vegetables	0.95	0.76	1.18

Abbreviations, see Table 10.1.

The effects of specific foods that affect serum lipoproteins and CVD risk have not been well characterized. The viscous soluble fiber content of fruit, vegetables, and legumes could contribute importantly to the 18% reduction in CVD events (Table 10.4). The two meta-analyses of Dauchet and colleagues (Table 10.1)[62,63] are consistent with our observations (Tables 10.4 and 10.5) that fruit and vegetable consumption is inversely associated with risk for CVD events and stroke.

10.4.2 Hypertension

Hypertension is a major risk factor for CHD and stroke.[64] Early clinical trials indicated that increased consumption of dietary fiber decreased systolic and diastolic blood pressure.[65,66] The available epidemiological data support the hypothesis that generous dietary fiber consumption prevents development of hypertension.[67,68] Two prospective cohort studies[64,69] noted that the RR for development of hypertension was significantly and inversely related to whole grain intake (RR 0.83; 95% CI, 0.78–0.88) (Table 10.7). In a cross-sectional study, Lairon et al.[70] noted that TDF intake was associated with a significantly lower incidence of hypertension (RR 0.71; 95% CI, 0.54–0.93).

Streppel et al.[7] performed meta-analyses of placebo-controlled, randomized clinical trials related to dietary fiber supplementation and blood pressure. Incorporation of an average of 11.5 g of fiber supplementation was accompanied by a small favorable changes in systolic and diastolic blood pressures, respectively, of −1.1 and −1.3 mmHg. Concurrently, Whelton et al.[71] performed a meta-analysis of RCTs related to fiber supplementation and reported very similar results with net changes in systolic (−1.2 mmHg) and diastolic blood pressure (−1.7 mmHg). Based on my own meta-analysis, in progress, and the

Table 10.7 Dietary Fiber and Cardiovascular Risk Factors: Prospective Cohort Studies

Author	Years	Number of Subjects (Number of Studies)	Outcome	Fiber Type	RR	LCI	UCI
Steffen,[69] Flint[64]	2005, 2009	35,988 (2)	Hypertension	Whole grains	0.83	0.78	0.88
Anderson[73]	2008	427,935 (11)	Diabetes	Whole grains or cereal fiber	0.71	0.67	0.75
Eight reports[78–85] (see text)	1999–2007	119,595 (8)	Obesity	Dietary fiber	0.91	0.85	0.97

Note: Onset of conditions for highest quintile of fiber intake compared with those with the lowest quintile of fiber consumption.

epidemiologic observations, these two reports[7,71] probably underestimate the effects of increased dietary fiber consumption on blood pressure.

10.4.3 Diabetes

Generous intakes of TDF, cereal fiber, and whole grains are associated with a significantly lower risk for diabetes than low levels of consumption.[72,73] The overall reduction in risk for diabetes, as we reported earlier,[73] is approximately 29% (Table 10.7). Available data do not indicate that fruit or vegetable fibers are associated with a lower risk for developing diabetes.[72] In a cross-sectional analysis, Newby et al.[74] reported that higher levels of whole grain intake were associated with lower 2 h glucose values than were lower levels of consumption. Recently Lindstrom et al.,[75] from the Finnish Diabetes Study, reported that individuals with the highest consumption of dietary fiber had a 62% reduction in progression of prediabetes to diabetes over a 4 year period.

Clinical trials with viscous soluble fibers indicate that consumption of these fibers decreases postprandial glycemia acutely and, over longer periods, fiber intake decreases fasting and postprandial plasma glucose values.[2] We have also recently observed that intake of barley beta-glucan by individuals with high risk for diabetes over a 12 week period is associated with a net reduction in post-glucose plasma glucose values and an improvement in insulin sensitivity.[76] The data from all these studies suggest that higher levels of dietary fiber consumption are likely to slow the progression of prediabetes to diabetes and improve blood glucose control in diabetic individuals.[77]

10.4.4 Obesity

The epidemiologic evidence strongly supports an inverse relationship between dietary fiber intake and obesity. Eight prospective cohort studies including 119,000 individuals noted that those with the highest fiber intake had significantly less likelihood to gain weight than those with lower fiber consumption.[78-86] The overall risk reduction was 9% (RR 0.91; 95% CI, 0.85–0.97) for studies comparing these fiber components: TDF, whole grains, or fruit and vegetables (Table 10.7). Since the definition of weight gain differed across studies, this variance-weighted estimate is not as precise as estimates of CHD events, for example. However, the five studies[78-82] examining TDF or whole grains evidenced similar reductions in weight gain (RR 0.91; 95% CI, 0.85–0.97) to the three studies[83-85] that used estimated of fruit and vegetable intake (RR 0.79; 95% CI, 0.71–0.87).

Four cross-sectional studies have compared TDF or whole grain intake related to body mass index (BMI) for 112,676 subjects.[70,74,87,88] The RR values ranged from 0.70 to 0.98. The composite-weighted mean RR was virtually identical to that reported by Maskarinec[89] (RR 0.79; 95% CI, 0.67–0.94). Thus, consumption of high-fiber foods may be associated with a reduction in weight gain or obesity of approximately 15%.

In randomized clinical trials, including fiber supplements compared to placebo is associated with significantly less weight gain.[2] As summarized previously, in 15 RCTs including 423 subjects on fiber supplements and 391 control subjects followed for 12 weeks, those randomized to the fiber arm of the trial lost significantly more weight than those on the control arm; all subjects were instructed in similar energy-restricted diets and lifestyle changes.[2] These studies are consistent with countless animal studies indicating that including fiber in the diet results in significantly less weight gain than with non-fiber-supplemented diets. Extensive research in animals and humans also provides evidence that fiber consumption favorably affects gastrointestinal hormones acting to regulate food intake.[2,73] Thus, consumption of high-fiber foods is one of the most effective strategies for weight management.[89]

10.5 Mechanisms

Most high-fiber foods deliver a wide array of nutrients and phytonutrients. Common to most grains, legumes, fruits, and vegetables are soluble and insoluble fibers, vitamins, minerals, antioxidants, and anti-inflammatory components.[19,90–92] Some high-fiber foods—those rich in soluble fibers—have bifidogenic properties that appear to enhance immune function.[13] Refining whole grain cereals removes the following amounts of components presumed to have cardioprotective effects: vitamin E, 95%; magnesium, 85%; fiber, 78%; and potassium, 74%.[92] Wheat bran, cereal fibers, and whole grain cereal consumption, in order listed, are more consistently reported to lower CVD risks than other sources of plant fiber (Tables 10.3 and 10.4). Slavin,[19] Liu,[92] and Jones[91] have carefully reviewed the components of whole grains and proposed mechanisms for how they may be associated with reduced CVD risk; data are not available to carefully assess the role of individual components and possible synergistic actions.

The best documented effects of dietary fiber intake on risk factors for CVD relate to favorable effects on serum lipoprotein risk factors.[2] Viscous soluble fiber intake—such as β-glucan from oats or barley and psyllium—significantly decreases serum LDL-cholesterol levels.[2] Intermediate or long-term consumption of oat bran is accompanied by sustained increases in HDL-cholesterol values.[60] Wheat bran intake is accompanied by significant decreases in serum triglycerides,[61] and increasing fiber intake from a variety of sources leads to significant reductions in serum triglycerides.[93] The observations of Wu et al.[94] that higher fiber intake is associated with slower progression of thickening of the intima-media of carotid arteries suggest that dietary fiber consumption may lower risk for CVD by slowing the atherosclerotic process but the complementary mechanisms are not delineated.

As summarized in a previous section and elsewhere,[2] higher levels of dietary fiber intake decrease other extremely important risk factors for CVD including hypertension, risk for diabetes, insulin resistance, and obesity (Table 10.7).[95] There is clear evidence that restoring acceptable blood pressure levels reduces risk for CVD[64] but the effects of improved diabetes control,[96] improved insulin sensitivity, and weight loss on CVD events are not well established.

10.6 Discussion

Among specific dietary descriptors, "dietary fiber" has one of the strongest associations with protection from CVD. Another descriptor, "Mediterranean diet," is widely heralded as the most protective nutrition plan for protection from CVD. Relative contributors of these Mediterranean diet components were as follows: moderate alcohol intake (median of 3.5 units or drinks per day), 24%; low consumption of meat and meat products, 17%; high vegetable consumption, 16%; high fruit and nut consumption, 11%; high monounsaturated to saturated lipid ratio, 11%; and high legume consumption, 10%.[97] This study, consistent with many other reports,[98,99] indicates that high levels of alcohol intake—far above the recommended 1 unit/day for women and 2 units for men,[100]—low intake of animal fat, and high intake of fruit, vegetables, and legumes outweigh the "flag-bearing" effects of olive oil intake in the Mediterranean diet. The epidemiological data supporting the cardioprotective effects of olive oil (RR 0.96; 95% CI, 0.83–1.10)[101] are dwarfed by those herein cited for dietary fiber. It seems likely that the dietary fiber intake may be the most protective component of the Mediterranean diet, if alcohol intake is not included in the assessment.

Because CHD is the most common cause of death in Western countries, search for the "heart-healthy diet" has been the Holy Grail for many years.[102] In their recommendations for optimal diets, Hu and Willett[102] conclude that three dietary strategies are effective for preventing CHD: substitute nonhydrogenated unsaturated fats for saturated and trans fats; consume omega-3 fatty acids; and consume a diet high in fruits, vegetables, nuts, and whole grains. In their comprehensive review of the epidemiology and purported mechanisms, Flight and Clifton[103] conclude that, "the intake of whole grain foods clearly protects from heart disease and stroke but the exact mechanism is not clear." Fiber, magnesium, folate, and vitamin B6 and vitamin E may be important. In a study of white, black, Hispanic, and Chinese adults in six U.S. cities, the whole grain and fruit dietary pattern was associated with an RR for CVD of 0.54 (95% CI, 0.33–0.91) compared to a fats and processed meats dietary pattern.[37] Based on the data summarized in this chapter and data cited by others, the American Heart Association Nutrition Committee had these positive dietary recommendations: "consume a diet rich in vegetables and fruits; choose whole grain, high-fiber foods; consume fish, especially oily fish, at least twice a week."[100]

10.7 Conclusions

CVDs are the leading cause of death in most Western countries. Generous intakes of dietary fiber appear to have a protective effect for CHD, stroke, peripheral artery disease, and hypertension. A generous intake of TDF is associated with an estimated 31% lower risk for developing CVD than is a low consumption level.

Wheat bran consumption appears to have a protective association that is similar to that of whole grains. A high level of consumption of fruit and vegetables is associated with a reduced risk for CVD, which is approximately 18%. With respect to strokes, individuals who consume the largest amounts of dietary fiber have an estimated reduction in risk for CVD of approximately 27% compared to those who consume modest amounts of fiber. The risk for peripheral artery disease also is reduced by about 30% for individuals who consume the largest amounts of dietary fiber.

Reductions in serum LDL-cholesterol values are the best documented mechanism related to dietary fiber and CVD. Viscous soluble fibers such as oat or barley β-glucans and psyllium have significant hypocholesterolemic effects, and limited epidemiologic data indicate that those individuals who consume the largest amounts of soluble fiber have 39% lower rates to CVD than those who consume limited amounts.

Major risk factors for CVD are hypertension, diabetes, and obesity. The estimated reductions in risk for these risk factors for high-level-fiber consumers compared to low-level users are as follows: hypertension, 17%; diabetes, 29%; and obesity, 15%. In the Finnish Diabetes Study, those individuals with the highest level of dietary fiber intake had a 62% lower progression rate from prediabetes to diabetes over a 4 year period. Encouraging preliminary clinical trials also suggest that viscous, soluble fiber intake slows the progression of prediabetes to diabetes when compared to placebo groups. Soluble and insoluble fiber intake has significantly enhanced weight loss in clinical trials of obese individuals when fiber supplements are compared to placebo controls.

The available evidence strongly indicates that increased dietary fiber intake should be strongly recommended for individuals at risk for CVD. The evidence suggests that dietary fiber from plant foods, wheat bran, and viscous, soluble fiber supplements will reduce risk for CVD.

References

1. Jacobs, D.R., Jr. et al., Whole-grain intake may reduce the risk of ischemic heart disease death in postmenopausal women: The Iowa Women's Health Study, *Am. J. Clin. Nutr.*, 68, 248, 1998.
2. Anderson, J.W. et al., Health benefits of dietary fiber, *Nutr. Rev.*, 67, 188, 2009.
3. Burkitt, D.P. and Trowell, H.C., *Refined Carbohydrate Foods and Diseases: Some Implications of Dietary Fibre,* London, U.K.: Academic Press, 1975.
4. Trowell, H., Ischemic heart disease and dietary fiber, *Am. J. Clin. Nutr.*, 25, 926, 1972.
5. Walker, A.R.P., The effects of recent changes of food habits and bowel motility, *S. Afr. Med. J.*, 21, 590, 1947.
6. Merchant, A.T. et al., Dietary fiber reduces peripheral arterial disease risk in men, *J. Nutr.*, 133, 3658, 2003.
7. Streppel, M.T. et al., Dietary fiber and blood pressure: A meta-analysis of randomized placebo-controlled trials, *Arch. Intern. Med.*, 165, 150, 2005.
8. Morris, J.N., Marr, J.W., and Clayton, D.G., Diet and heart: A postscript, *Brit. Med. J.*, 2, 1307, 1977.

9. Kromhout, D., Bosschieter, E.B., and De Lezenne Coulander, C., Dietary fiber and 10-year mortality from coronary heart disease, cancer and all causes, *Lancet*, 2, 518, 1982.

10. Liu, K. et al., Dietary lipids, sugar, fiber and mortality from coronary heart disease. Bivariate analysis of international data, *Arteriosclerosis*, 2, 221, 1982.

11. Burr, M.L. et al., Effects of changes in fat, fish, and fibre intakes on death and myocardial reinfarction: Diet and reinfarction trial (DART), *Lancet*, 2, 757, 1989.

12. Burr, M.L., Secondary prevention of CHD in UK men: The diet and reinfarction trial and its sequel, *Proc. Nutr. Soc.*, 66, 9, 2007.

13. Anderson, J.W., All fibers are not created equal, *J. Med.*, 2, 87, 2009.

14. Burkitt, D., *Don't Forget Fibre in Your Diet: To Help Avoid Many on Our Commonest Diseases*, London, U.K.: Martin Dunitz, Ltd., 1979.

15. Kellock, B., *The Fibre Man: The Life-Story of Dr. Denis Burkitt*, Herts, England: Lion Publishing, plc, 1985.

16. Anderson, J.W., *Plant Fiber in Foods*, Lexington, KY: HCF Nutrition Research Foundation, Inc., 1990.

17. Cummings, J.H., The effect of dietary fiber on fecal weight and composition, in: Spiller, G, ed. *Dietary Fiber in Human Nutrition*, Boca Raton, FL: CRC Press, 2001, p. 183.

18. Chen, W.J. and Anderson, J.W., Effects of guar gum and wheat bran on lipid metabolism of rats, *J. Nutr.*, 109, 1028, 1979.

19. Slavin, J., Why whole grains are protective: biological mechanisms, *Proc. Nutr. Soc.*, 62, 129, 2003.

20. Anderson, J.W., Jones, A.E., and Riddell-Mason, S., Ten different dietary fibers have significantly different effects on serum and liver lipids of cholesterol-fed rats, *J. Nutr.*, 124, 78, 1994.

21. Sirtori, C.R., Anderson, J.W., and Arnoldi, A., Nutritional and nutraceutical considerations for dyslipidemia, *Future Lipidol.*, 3, 313, 2007.

22. Lloyd-Jones, D. et al., Heart disease and stroke statistics—2009 update: A report from the American Heart Association Statistics Committee and Stroke Statistics Subcommittee, *Circulation*, 119, e21, 2009.

23. Gamenzi, A. et al., Association between certain foods and risk of acute myocardial infarction in women, *Brit. J. Med.*, 300, 771, 1990.

24. Bolton-Smith, C. et al., The Scottish Heart Health Study. Dietary intake by food frequency questionnaire and odds ratios for coronary heart disease risk. The antioxidant vitamins and fiber, *Eur. J. Clin. Nutr.*, 46, 85, 1992.

25. Humble, H.G., Malarcher, A.M., and Tyroler, H.A., Dietary fiber and coronary heart disease in middle-aged hypercholesterolemic men, *Am. J. Prev. Med.*, 9, 197, 1993.

26. Anderson, J.W., Johnstone, B.M., and Cook-Newell, M.E., Meta-analysis of the effects of soy protein intake on serum lipids, *N. Engl. J. Med.*, 333, 276, 1995.

27. Anderson, J.W., Liu, C., and Kryscio, R.J., Blood pressure response to transcendental meditation: A meta-analysis, *Am. J. Hypertens.*, 21, 310, 2008.

28. Kushi, L.H. et al., Diet and 20-year mortality from coronary heart disease. The Ireland-Boston Diet-Heart Study, *N. Engl. J. Med.*, 312, 811, 1985.

29. Khaw, K.T. and Barrett-Conner, E., Dietary fiber and reduced ischemic heart disease mortality rates in men and women: A 12-year prospective study, *Am. J. Epidemiol.*, 126, 1093, 1987.

30. Pietinen, P. et al., Intake of dietary fiber and risk of coronary heart disease in a cohort of Finnish men: The alpha-tocopherol, beta-carotene cancer prevention study, *Circulation*, 94, 2720, 1996.

31. Rimm, E.B. et al., Vegetable, fruit, and cereal fiber intake and risk of coronary heart disease among men, *J. Am. Med. Assoc.*, 275, 447, 1996.

32. Todd, S. et al., Dietary antioxidant vitamins and fiber in the etiology of cardiovascular disease and all-causes mortality: Results from the Scottish Heart Health Study, *Am. J. Epidemiol.*, 150, 1073, 1999.

33. Wolk, A. et al., Long-term intake of dietary fiber and decreased risk of coronary heart disease among women, *J. Am. Med. Assoc.*, 281, 1998, 1999.

34. Mozaffarian, D. et al., Cereal, fruit, and vegetable fiber intake and the risk of cardiovascular disease in elderly individuals, *J. Am. Med. Assoc.*, 289, 1659, 2003.

35. Fraser, G.E. et al., A possible protective effect of nut consumption on risk of coronary heart disease. The Adventist Health Study, *Arch. Intern. Med.*, 152, 1416, 1992.

36. Jacobs, D.R. et al., Is whole grain intake associated with reduced total and cause-specific death rates in older women? The Iowa Women's Health Study, *Am. J. Public Health*, 89, 322, 1999.

37. Nettleton, J.A. et al., Dietary patterns and incident cardiovascular disease in the multi-ethnic study of atherosclerosis, *Am. J. Clin. Nutr.*, 90, 647, 2009.

38. Streppel, M.T. et al., Dietary fiber intake in relation to coronary heart disease and all-cause mortality over 40 y: The Zutphen Study, *Am. J. Clin. Nutr.*, 88, 1119, 2008.

39. Liu, S. et al., Whole-grain consumption and risk of coronary heart disease: Results from the Nurses' Health Study, *Am. J. Clin. Nutr.*, 70, 412, 1999.

40. Steffen, L.M. et al., Associations of whole-grain, refined-grain, and fruit and vegetable consumption with risks of all-cause mortality and incident coronary artery disease and ischemic stroke: The Atherosclerosis Risk in Communities (ARIC) Study, *Am. J. Clin. Nutr.*, 78, 383, 2003.

41. Jensen, M.K. et al., Intakes of whole grains, bran, and germ and the risk of coronary heart disease in men, *Am. J. Clin. Nutr.*, 80, 1492, 2004.

42. He, M. et al., Whole-grain, cereal fiber, bran, and germ intake and the risks of all-cause and cardiovascular disease-specific mortality among women with type 2 diabetes mellitus, *Circulation*, 121, 2162, 2010.

43. Gaziano, J.M. et al., A prospective study of consumption of carotenoids in fruits and vegetables and decreased cardiovascular mortality in the elderly, *Ann. Epidemiol.*, 5, 255, 1995.

44. Liu, S. et al., Fruit and vegetable intake and risk of cardiovascular disease: The Women's Health Study, *Am. J. Clin. Nutr.*, 72, 922, 2000.

45. Joshipura, K.J. et al., The effect of fruit and vegetable intake on risk for coronary heart disease, *Ann. Intern. Med.*, 134, 1106, 2001.

46. Bazzano, L.A. et al., Fruit and vegetable intake and risk of cardiovascular disease in US adults: The first National Health and Nutrition Examination Survey Epidemiologic Follow-up Study, *Am. J. Clin. Nutr.*, 76, 93, 2002.

47. Knekt, P. et al., Antioxidant vitamin intake and coronary mortality in a longitudinal population study, *Am. J. Epidemiol.*, 139, 1180, 1994.

48. Bazzano, L.A. et al., Legume consumption and risk of coronary heart disease in US men and women: NHANES I Epidemiologic Follow-up Study, *Arch. Int. Med.*, 161, 2573, 2001.

49. Ascherio, A. et al., Intake of potassium, magnesium, calcium, and fiber and risk of stroke among US men, *Circulation*, 98, 1198, 1998.

50. Liu, S. et al., Whole grain consumption and risk of ischemic stroke in women: A prospective study. *J. Am. Med. Assoc.*, 284, 1534, 2000.

51. Gillman, M.W. et al., Protective effect of fruits and vegetables on development of stroke in men, *J. Am. Med. Assoc.*, 273, 1113, 1995.

52. Joshipura, K.J. et al., Fruit and vegetable intake in relation to risk of ischemic stroke, *J. Am. Med. Assoc.*, 282, 1233, 1999.

53. Bazzano, L.A. et al., Dietary intake of folate and risk of stroke in US men and women: NHANES I Epidemiologic Follow-up Study. National Health and Nutrition Examination Survey, *Stroke*, 33, 1183, 2002.

54. Johnsen, S.P. et al., Intake of fruit and vegetables and the risk of ischemic stroke in a cohort of Danish men and women, *Am. J. Clin. Nutr.,* 78, 57, 2003.
55. Hung, H.C. et al., The association between fruit and vegetable consumption and peripheral arterial disease, *Epidemiology,* 14, 659, 2003.
56. Antonelli-Incalzi, R. et al., Association between nutrient intake and peripheral artery disease: Results from the InCHIANTI study, *Atherosclerosis,* 186, 200, 2006.
57. Sirtori, C.R. et al., Nutritional and nutraceutical approaches to dyslipidemia and atherosclerosis prevention: Focus on dietary protein, *Atherosclerosis,* 203, 8, 2009.
58. Andon, M. and Anderson, J.W., The oatmeal-cholesterol connection: 10 years later, *Am. J. Lifestyle Med.,* 2, 51, 2008.
59. Anderson, J.W. and Gustafson, N.J., Hypocholesterolemic effects of oat and bean products, *Am. J. Clin. Nutr.,* 48, 749, 1998.
60. Anderson, J.W. et al., Hypocholesterolemic effects of high-fibre diets rich in water-soluble plant fibres, *J. Canad. Dietet. Assoc.,* 45, 140, 1984.
61. Anderson, J.W. et al., Lipid responses of hypercholesterolemic men to oat-bran and wheat-bran intake, *Am. J. Clin. Nutr.,* 54, 678, 1991.
62. Dauchet, L., Amouyel, P., and Dallongeville, J., Fruit and vegetable consumption and risk of stroke: A meta-analysis of cohort studies, *Neurology,* 65, 1193, 2005.
63. Dauchet, L. et al., Fruit and vegetable consumption and risk of coronary heart disease: A meta-analysis of cohort studies, *J. Nutr.,* 136, 2588, 2006.
64. Flint, A.J. et al., Whole grains and incident hypertension in men, *Am. J. Clin. Nutr.,* 90, 493, 2009.
65. Anderson, J.W., Plant fiber and blood pressure, *Ann. Int. Med.,* 98, 842, 1983.
66. Krotkiewski, M., Effect of guar gum on the arterial blood pressure, *Acta Med. Scand.,* 222, 43, 1987.
67. Ascherio, A. et al., Prospective study of nutritional factors, blood pressure, and hypertension among US women, *Hypertension,* 27, 1065, 1996.
68. Hallfrisch, J. et al., Fiber intake, age, and other coronary risk factors in men of the Baltimore Longitudinal Study (1959–1975), *J. Gerontol.,* 4, M64, 1988.
69. Steffen, L.M. et al., Associations of plant food, dairy product, and meat intakes with 15-y incidence of elevated blood pressure in young black and white adults: The Coronary Artery Risk Development in Young Adults (CARDIA) Study, *Am. J. Clin. Nutr.,* 82, 1169, 2005.
70. Lairon, D. et al., Dietary fiber intake and risk factors for cardiovascular disease in French adults, *Am. J. Clin. Nutr.,* 82, 1185, 2005.
71. Whelton, S.P. et al., Effect of dietary fiber intake on blood pressure: A meta-analysis of randomized, controlled clinical trials, *J. Hypertens.,* 23, 475, 2005.
72. Anderson, J.W. and Conley, S.B., Whole grains and diabetes, in: Marquart, L. et al., eds., *Whole Grains and Health,* Ames, IA: Blackwell Publishing Professional, 2007, p. 29.
73. Anderson, J.W., Dietary fiber and associated phytochemicals in prevention and reversal of diabetes, in: Pasupuleti, V.K. and Anderson, J.W., eds., *Nutraceuticals, Glycemic Health and Type 2 Diabetes,* Ames, IA: Blackwell Publishing Professional, 2008, p. 97.
74. Newby, P.K. et al., Intake of whole grains, refined grains, and cereal fiber measured with 7-d diet records and associations with risk factors for chronic disease, *Am. J. Clin. Nutr.,* 86, 1745, 2007.
75. Lindstrom, J. et al., High-fibre, low-fat diet predicts long-term weight loss and decreased type 2 diabetes risk: The Finnish Diabetes Prevention Study, *Diabetologia,* 49, 912, 2006.
76. Anderson, J.W. et al., Barley beta-glucan beverage improves insulin sensitivity at 12 weeks for individuals at high risk for diabetes, Abstract. IFT Program Abstracts, 2011.

77. Anderson, J.W. et al., Carbohydrate and fiber recommendations for individuals with diabetes: A quantitative assessment and meta-analysis of the evidence, *J. Am. Coll. Nutr.*, 23, 5, 2004.
78. Ludwig, D.S. et al., Dietary fiber, weight gain, and cardiovascular disease risk factors in young adults, *J. Am. Med. Assoc.*, 282, 1539, 1999.
79. Liu, S. et al., Relation between changes in intakes of dietary fiber and grain products and changes in weight and development of obesity among middle-aged women, *Am. J. Clin. Nutr.*, 78, 920, 2003.
80. Koh-Banerjee, P. et al., Changes in whole-grain, bran, and cereal fiber consumption in relation to 8-y weight gain among men, *Am. J. Clin. Nutr.*, 80, 1237, 2004.
81. Bazzano, L.A. et al., Dietary intake of whole and refined grain breakfast cereals and weight gain in men, *Obes. Res.*, 13, 1952, 2005.
82. Sahyoun, N.R. et al., Whole-grain intake is inversely associated with the metabolic syndrome and mortality in older adults, *Am. J. Clin. Nutr.*, 83, 124, 2006.
83. He, K. et al., Changes in intake of fruits and vegetables in relation to risk of obesity and weight gain among middle-aged women, *Int. J. Obes. (Lond.)*, 28, 1569, 2004.
84. Sanchez-Villegas, A. et al., Adherence to a Mediterranean dietary pattern and weight gain in a follow-up study: The SUN cohort, *Int. J. Obes. (Lond.)*, 30, 350, 2006.
85. Vioque, J. et al., Intake of fruits and vegetables in relation to 10-year weight gain among Spanish adults, *Obesity (Silver Spring)*, 16, 664, 2008.
86. Buijsse, B. et al., Fruit and vegetable intakes and subsequent changes in body weight in European populations: Results from the project on Diet, Obesity, and Genes (DiOGenes), *Am. J. Clin. Nutr.*, 90, 202, 2009.
87. McKeown, N.M. et al., Whole-grain intake is favorably associated with metabolic risk factors for type 2 diabetes and cardiovascular disease in the Framingham Offspring Study, *Am. J. Clin. Nutr.*, 76, 390, 2002.
88. Maskarinec, G. et al., Trends and dietary determinants of overweight and obesity in a multiethnic population, *Obesity*, 14, 717, 2006.
89. Anderson, J.W., Konz, E.C., and Jenkins, D.J., Health advantages and disadvantages of weight-reducing diets: A computer analysis and critical review, *J. Am. Coll. Nutr.*, 19, 578, 2000.
90. Liu, S., Intake of refined carbohydrates and whole grain foods in relation to risk of type 2 diabetes mellitus and coronary heart disease, *J. Am. Coll. Nutr.*, 21, 298, 2002.
91. Jones, J.M., Grain-based foods and health, *Cereal Food World*, 50, 108, 2006.
92. Liu, R.H., Whole grain phytochemicals and health, *J. Cereal Sci.*, 46, 207, 2007.
93. Anderson, J.W., Dietary fiber prevents carbohydrate-induced hypertriglyceridemia, *Curr. Atheroscler. Rep.*, 2, 536, 2000.
94. Wu, H. et al., Dietary fiber and progression of atherosclerosis: The Los Angeles Atherosclerosis Study, *Am. J. Clin. Nutr.*, 78, 1085, 2003.
95. Fung, T.T. et al., Association between dietary patterns and plasma biomarkers of obesity and cardiovascular disease risk, *Am. J. Clin. Nutr.*, 73, 61, 2001.
96. Duckworth, W. et al., Glucose control and vascular complications in veterans with type 2 diabetes, *N. Engl. J. Med.*, 360, 129, 2009.
97. Trichopoulou, A., Bamia, C., and Trichopoulos, D., Anatomy of health effects of Mediterranean diet: Greek EPIC prospective cohort study, *Brit. Med. J.*, 338, b2337, 2009.
98. Knoops, K.T. et al., Mediterranean diet, lifestyle factors, and 10-year mortality in elderly European men and women: The HALE project, *J. Am. Med. Assoc.*, 292, 1433, 2004.

99. Psaltopoulou, T. et al., Olive oil, the Mediterranean diet, and arterial blood pressure: The Greek European Prospective Investigation into Cancer and Nutrition (EPIC) study, *Am. J. Clin. Nutr.,* 80, 1012, 2004.
100. Lichtenstein, A.H. et al., Diet and lifestyle recommendations revision 2006: A scientific statement from the American Heart Association Nutrition Committee, *Circulation,* 114, 82, 2006.
101. Trichopoulou, A. et al., Adherence to a Mediterranean diet and survival in a Greek population, *N. Engl. J. Med.,* 348, 2599, 2003.
102. Hu, F.B. and Willett, W.C., Optimal diets for prevention of coronary heart disease, *J. Am. Med. Assoc.,* 288, 2569, 2002.
103. Flight, I. and Clifton, P., Cereal grains and legumes in the prevention of coronary heart disease and stroke: A review of the literature, *Eur. J. Clin. Nutr.,* 60, 1145, 2006.

11

Fasting Glucose Turnover but Not Peripheral Insulin Resistance Is Reduced after Acetogenic and Non-Digestible Carbohydrate Ingestion in Metabolic Syndrome Patients

ETIENNE POUTEAU, VÉRONIQUE FERCHAUD-ROUCHER,
YASSINE ZAIR, MORINE PAINTIN, MARC ENSLEN, LAURENT FLET,
NICOLAS AURIOU, KATHERINE MACÉ, JEAN-PHILIPPE GODIN,
OLIVIER BALLÈVRE, and MICHEL KREMPF

Contents

11.1 Introduction

The prevalence of metabolic syndrome has dramatically increased worldwide. The metabolic syndrome is characterized by central abdominal obesity associated primarily with insulin resistance (IR) and possibly hypertriglyceridemia, reduced HDL cholesterol, elevated blood pressure, and/or raised glycemia. An excess of abdominal fat is associated with higher plasma free fatty acids (FFAs) and enhanced lipotoxicity in the whole body. Insulin action in hepatic and peripheral tissues, as well as insulin suppression of FFA release from adipose tissues, is thereby inhibited by lipotoxicity. FFA and glucose concentrations rise over time [1]. One of the strategies for the treatment of such metabolic disorders and possibly type 2 diabetes mellitus is to constrain lipolysis and reduce plasma FFA [2]. Acipimox, a nicotinic acid–like drug, was used as an antilipolytic agent to reduce dyslipidemia for diabetes treatment. It beneficially lowered plasma FFA, which was accompanied by decreased IR in short-term clinical studies [2,3].

An improvement of insulin sensitivity has been reported in insulin-resistant middle-aged men [4] as well as in healthy adults [5] with moderate alcohol consumption. Abramson and Arky [6] have shown that plasma acetate derived from ethanol inhibits lipolysis and decreases plasma FFA. Since colonic fermentation of dietary fibers yields large amounts of acetate [7], our working hypothesis was that intake of acetogenic, indigestible, fermentable carbohydrates, or fibers would

1. Enhance the concentration and turnover of acetate in the systemic circulation
2. Reduce lipolysis and plasma FFA
3. Beneficially improve insulin sensitivity

In a first-step study, we observed that acute lactulose (an acetogenic indigestible disaccharide) ingestion, when compared with saline, caused increased acetate concentrations and turnover in overweight insulin-resistant subjects [7,8], accompanied by a decline in lipolysis of −30%. Whether such a decline in lipolysis (decrease of plasma FFA and glycerol) following chronic acetogenic carbohydrate intake improves insulin sensitivity is unknown. The aim of the second step, detailed in the present study, was to investigate the hypothesis that the daily intake of acetogenic carbohydrates for 5 weeks is associated with an improvement of peripheral insulin sensitivity, endogenous glucose turnover, and plasma biomarkers of the metabolic syndrome, in metabolic syndrome patients.

11.2 Materials and Methods

11.2.1 Clinical Study

The volunteers were adult males with symptoms of the metabolic syndrome, as defined by ATPIII guidelines [9]. They had abdominal obesity with waist circumference >102 cm, glycated hemoglobin <7%, and normal liver enzyme, urea, and creatinine concentrations. Subjects that were diabetic or had any medication likely to influence lipid metabolism were excluded. The volunteers were 47 ± 12 years, weighed 101 ± 12 kg, and had a BMI of 33.4 ± 3.0 kg $\cdot$ m^{-2} and a waist circumference of 112 ± 7 cm. At baseline, their systolic and diastolic blood pressures were 149 ± 22 and 89 ± 14 mmHg. Baseline plasma concentrations were insulin 17.1 ± 7.6 mIU $\cdot$ L^{-1}, glucose 5.54 ± 0.85 mmol $\cdot$ L^{-1}, glycated hemoglobin $5.6\% \pm 0.5\%$, FFAs 628 ± 439 µmol $\cdot$ L^{-1}, and triglycerides 2.08 ± 1.16 g $\cdot$ L^{-1}. All subjects gave written informed consent to participate in the study, which was approved by the Human Ethics Committee of the Hospital of Nantes, France.

The study was a double-blind, single-center, crossover, randomized controlled trial. The dietary treatments were 5 weeks long with inclusion of a 6 week washout period between treatments. Anthropometric data and fasting blood samples were collected during all visits. Additionally, after each treatment, the subjects participated in a stable isotope kinetic study combined with a euglycemic-hyperinsulinemic (EH) clamp. The subjects arrived at 8:00 a.m. after a 10 h overnight fasting, and breath gas was collected in air-tight bags. Two catheters were inserted: one into a hand vein and another one into a vein of the contralateral arm. Arterialized blood samples were collected at time T-10 and T0 in the fasting state, after which primed-continuous infusions of the isotope tracers were started and continued for 3 h. The priming doses of [1-^{13}C]acetate, [1,1,2,3,3-^{2}H$_5$]glycerol, and [6,6-^{2}H$_2$]glucose tracers (99% enrichment, Cambridge Isotope Laboratories, Andover, MA) were 19.25, 1.60, and 18.30 μmol·kg^{-1}, with continuous infusions at 0.50, 0.11, and 0.163 μmol·kg^{-1}·min^{-1}, respectively. Further blood samples were collected at 90, 120, 140, 160, and 180 min. The [1-^{13}C] acetate and [^{2}H$_5$]glycerol infusions were stopped at 180 min, while that of [6,6-^{2}H$_2$] glucose was continued for a further 3 h during the EH clamp. The 3 h EH clamp was performed, as described by Molina et al. [10]. Insulin (NovoRapid®, Novo Nordisk, Paris, France) and a 20% glucose solution (Baxter, Maurepas, France) were infused intravenously. The insulin infusion rate was 40 mU·m^{-2}·min^{-1} and reached a steady-state plasma concentration of ~80 mIU·L^{-1}. Insulin-stimulated glucose disposal (glucose infusion rate, GIR) was determined over a steady-state 30 min interval during last hour. Arterialized blood samples were collected at 240, 300, 315, 330, 345, and 360 min. Plasma was aliquoted and stored at −80°C. The subjects were offered a meal before leaving the investigation center.

The acetogenic fibers were defined as fibers producing more acetate in vitro, reported by Titgemeyer et al. [11]. We selected a blend of 20% pectin (90% ± 5% soluble fiber, Herbapekt SF 50 LV, Herbafood Ingredients GmbH, Germany) and 80% acacia gum (>80% dietary fiber, Fibergum P IRX 61410, Colloïdes Naturels International SA, Rouen, France) as acetogenic fibers. The acetogenic fiber drink contained 14.1 g dietary fiber solubilized in 150 mL water, flavored with apple and lemon, colored with Sunset yellow FCF (Bühlmann, Basel, Switzerland), and sweetened with acesulfame K. The placebo drink was of identical composition with no fiber. The subjects consumed 28 g of acetogenic fiber per day (two drinks per day) as a supplement during the 5 week treatment period. The subjects consumed one drink 3–4 h before lunch and the other 3–4 h before dinner in order to synchronize the elevation in plasma acetate from colonic fermentation. The subjects did not consume the test drinks on the day of the clamp study. Volunteer compliance was evaluated by daily recording and gut comfort monitoring. A 3 day diet questionnaire was done during treatments. Total energy intake was 2151 ± 682 and 2199 ± 547 kcal during the fiber and control treatments, respectively; carbohydrate intake was 214 ± 69 and 239 ± 92 g·day^{-1}, protein 87 ± 27 and 85 ± 20 g·day^{-1}, lipid 96 ± 40 and 97 ± 33 g·day^{-1}, and fiber 42 ± 4 and 17 ± 6 g·day^{-1} during the fiber and control treatments, respectively. The subjects maintained their usual dietary habits and normal physical activity.

11.2.2 Biochemistry

Capillary blood glucose was measured using an electrochemical glucose analyzer (Accu-Chek, Roche Diagnostics GmbH, Mannheim, Germany) during the EH clamp. Arterialized blood glucose was assayed enzymatically using a multiparametric analyzer (Hitachi 747; Roche Molecular Biochemicals, Meylan, France). Glycated hemoglobin (HbA1c) was measured using a conventional immunological method.

Plasma concentrations of FFA and triglycerides were measured with commercially available kits (917 Hitachi, Roche, Meylan, France). Total cholesterol, HDL cholesterol, and LDL cholesterol were assessed with enzymatic kits (Modular, Roche, Meylan, France). Plasma glycerol concentrations were determined with an enzymatic method [12]. Plasma concentration of insulin was measured by immunoassay with commercially available kits (Aecsys 2010, Roche, Meylan, France). Hydrogen and methane concentrations in breath samples were analyzed using a gas chromatograph (Quintron Microlyser™, Model DP, Quintron Instruments) and expressed as parts per million (1 ppm ≈ $0.05 \, \mu mol \cdot L^{-1}$ for both gases). Analysis of plasma glycerol isotope enrichments was based on a published method [8]. Plasma acetate concentration and isotope enrichment were analyzed based on a previously published method by a gas chromatograph mass spectrometer (Hewlett Packard, Palo Alto, CA) [7]. Glucose isotope enrichment was determined in $50 \, \mu L$ plasma that was deproteinized. After derivatization with acetic anhydride and pyridine, the penta-acetate glucose derivative was analyzed by a gas chromatograph mass spectrometer. Calibration curves were obtained from solutions with known isotope enrichments which were expressed as mole percent excess (MPE).

11.2.3 Calculations

The HOMA index of IR (in %) was calculated from fasting glucose (in $mmol \cdot L^{-1}$) and fasting insulin (in $\mu UI \cdot mL^{-1}$) concentrations, as previously described [13]. Acetate and glycerol turnovers (rate of appearance, Ra in $\mu mol \cdot kg^{-1} \cdot min^{-1}$) were calculated using the equation for steady-state conditions [14]. Glucose turnover ($Ra_{glucose}$ in $\mu mol \cdot kg^{-1} \cdot min^{-1}$) was calculated using the steady-state equation given earlier during the first 3 h. During the EH clamp, the rate of appearance ($Ra_{glucose}$ in $\mu mol \cdot kg^{-1} \cdot min^{-1}$) and rate of disappearance ($Rd_{glucose}$ in $\mu mol \cdot kg^{-1} \cdot min^{-1}$) of glucose were calculated using Steele's nonsteady-state equations [14]. Insulin sensitivity was determined during the EH clamp from the GIR (GIR expressed in $mg \cdot kg^{-1} \cdot min^{-1}$) necessary to maintain euglycemia during steady-state insulin concentrations. Insulin sensitivity (GIR) was also normalized to the insulin concentration during the clamp and was expressed as $\times 10^{-2} mg \cdot kg^{-1} \cdot min^{-1} / mIU \cdot L^{-1}$ insulin.

11.2.4 Statistics

According to normality distribution, the paired t-test/one-sample t-test or nonparametric Wilcoxon signed-rank test was used for comparison of the primary outcome (insulin sensitivity) and secondary outcomes (endogenous glucose turnover and biomarkers) between both treatments. An ITT (intention-to-treat) analysis was done using SAS software (version 8.2). The rejection level in statistical tests was equal to 5% ($P < 0.05$). The results are presented as the mean ± standard deviation.

11.3 Results

Of the 25 volunteers who were enrolled, randomized, and allocated to treatments, 21 completed the study. The volunteers were nondiabetic, insulin-resistant, obese men diagnosed with the metabolic syndrome. No significant difference in food

Table 11.1 Data after Fiber and Control Treatments in Metabolic Syndrome Men at the Fasting State

	Fiber	Control	P-Value
Insulin ($\mu UI \cdot mL^{-1}$)	14.4 ± 5.4	14.6 ± 7.7	$P = 0.88^a$
Glucose ($mmol \cdot L^{-1}$)	5.86 ± 0.71	5.87 ± 1.08	$P = 0.56^b$
Acetate concentration ($mmol \cdot L^{-1}$)	101 ± 30	88 ± 23	$P = 0.13^a$
Acetate turnover ($\mu mol \cdot kg^{-1} \cdot min^{-1}$)	5.0 ± 1.5	4.9 ± 1.2	$P = 0.38^a$
Glycerol concentration ($mmol \cdot L^{-1}$)	0.08 ± 0.02	0.10 ± 0.03	$P = 0.02^a$
Glycerol turnover ($\mu mol \cdot kg^{-1} \cdot min^{-1}$)	2.2 ± 0.9	2.3 ± 1.0	$P = 0.33^b$
FFA ($\mu mol \cdot L^{-1}$)	664 ± 253	664 ± 222	$P = 0.64^a$
Triglycerides ($g \cdot L^{-1}$)	2.10 ± 1.91	1.65 ± 1.07	$P = 0.25^b$

Note: All values are mean ±SD.
[a] One-sample *t*-test.
[b] Wilcoxon signed-rank test.

intake was observed between treatments except for fiber. Body weight and BMI were not significantly different at the end of the acetogenic fiber and control treatments (100.8 ± 12.5 vs. 100.7 ± 12.4 kg and 33.2 ± 3.1 vs. 33.3 ± 3.1 kg·m⁻², respectively). At the end of the treatments, fasting plasma concentrations of glucose and insulin were not different (Table 11.1). At the end of the fiber treatment, fasting endogenous glucose turnover (7.9 ± 1.3 µmol·kg⁻¹·min⁻¹) was significantly less than after the control treatment (8.6 ± 1.6 µmol·kg⁻¹·min⁻¹, $P = 0.03$, Figure 11.1). The GIR, normalized or not with insulinemia, during the EH clamp was unchanged between treatments (Figure 11.1, Table 11.2). The HOMA-IR index was 3.9 ± 1.7 after the fiber treatment and 4.0 ± 3.2 (NS) after the control treatment. Finally, glycated hemoglobin was unchanged (5.70% ± 0.53% vs. 5.62% ± 0.57%, NS). The methane and hydrogen breath gases of the fasting subjects were 9.1 ± 17.1 and 10.3 ± 11.7 ppm after fiber treatment, respectively, and were not significantly greater than after the control treatment (6.3 ± 15.1 and 7.5 ± 6.0 ppm, respectively, NS). Glycerol concentrations were slightly decreased after the fiber treatments ($P = 0.02$, Table 11.1). The concentration and turnover of acetate, glycerol turnover, and lipid concentrations in fasting subjects were unchanged between treatments, as indicated in Table 11.1. Compliance of subjects was good, as indicated by their records of daily intake of test drinks and records of gut comfort that included flatulence and fecal state. The number of days with flatulence was significantly higher with the fiber (10.6 ± 7.2 days) than with the control treatment (1.8 ± 3.4 days, $P = 0.003$). The proportion of hard stools was significantly lower with the fiber (2% ± 5%) than with control treatment (11% ± 18%, $P = 0.03$).

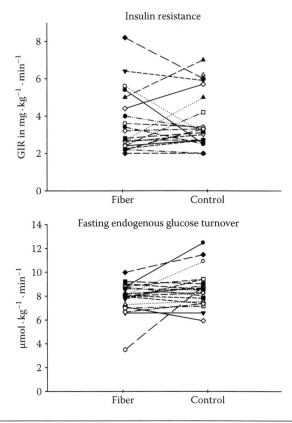

Figure 11.1 Insulin resistance and glucose turnover of subjects. GIR, glucose infusion rate.

Table 11.2 The GIR (GIR, Peripheral IR), the Normalized GIR (Normalized IR with Insulinemia), the Glucose Turnovers, and the Biochemistry after Fiber and Control Treatments in Fasting Metabolic Syndrome Men during the EH Clamps

	Fiber	Control	*P*-value
Insulin (mIU·L^{-1})	81.7 ± 32.7	81.2 ± 13.0	*P* = 0.53[b]
Glucose (mmol·L^{-1})	5.33 ± 0.36	5.24 ± 0.44	*P* = 0.50[a]
GIR (mg·kg^{-1}·min^{-1})	3.7 ± 1.7	3.8 ± 1.5	*P* = 0.50[a]
GIR/insulin (×10^{-2} mg·kg^{-1}·min^{-1}/mIU·L^{-1})	4.4 ± 2.1	4.7 ± 2.1	*P* = 0.78[a]
Glucose Ra (μmol·kg^{-1}·min^{-1})	17.6 ± 8.8	19.5 ± 8.9	*P* = 0.25[a]
Glucose Rd (μmol·kg^{-1}·min^{-1})	17.6 ± 8.9	19.7 ± 9.1	*P* = 0.25[a]

Note: All values are mean ±SD. Ra and Rd for rate of appearance and rate of disappearance, respectively.

[a] One-sample *t*-test.

[b] Wilcoxon signed-rank test.

11.4 Discussion

From previous observations, we hypothesized that acetate, one of the main end products of colonic fermentation, would be antilipolytic and would consequently improve long-term insulin sensitivity and glucose control. We found that 5 week intake of soluble acetogenic fibers (acacia gum and pectin) improved fasting endogenous glucose production but had no effect on fasting glycemia, insulinemia, or peripheral IR in men with the metabolic syndrome.

In the first-step study, overweight men ingested a single dose of 30 g lactulose that caused an acute, large increase in plasma acetate concentrations and acetate turnover (from 11 ± 1 to $16 \pm 2\,\mu mol \cdot kg^{-1} \cdot min^{-1}$) in parallel with a significant reduction in lipolysis (decreased FFA concentrations and glycerol turnover from 4.8 ± 1.9 to $2.8 \pm 1.4\,\mu mol \cdot kg^{-1} \cdot min^{-1}$) [8]. In this second-step study, the chronic intake of acetogenic fibers did not change fasting plasma acetate and FFA concentrations. There are several possible explanations. Volunteer compliance was satisfactory since the ingestion of fibers was accompanied with more flatulence and less hard stools than during the ingestion of the control drinks. Fasting hydrogen and methane breath gases were also higher, but not significantly so, after the fiber treatment. The main reason why plasma acetate and glycerol turnovers were unchanged may be that the hypothesized mechanism only occurs acutely during colonic fermentation and is time limited. Indeed, the subjects did not absorb the test drink on the day of the turnover and clamp studies and did not exhibit a high level of colonic fermentation. In support of our working hypothesis, Weickert et al. recently observed improved peripheral insulin sensitivity, using the EH clamp, in obese women (GIR = 6.9 ± 0.3 vs. $6.1 \pm 0.3\,mg \cdot min^{-1} \cdot kg^{-1}$, $P = 0.003$) who had consumed oat fiber for 3 days and who had enhanced levels of colonic fermentation, as indicated by a high breath hydrogen [15]; however, plasma acetate was not measured. Robertson et al. also observed a 14% increase in GIR after 4 week supplementation with 30 g highly fermentable, but insoluble resistant starch compared with placebo [16]. In sum, although we did not observe a long-term change in plasma lipids after chronic acetogenic fiber ingestion, we cannot exclude that an acute inverse association between colonic acetate and lipolysis exists. Nonetheless, chronic ingestion of acetogenic fibers (acacia gum and pectin) has no effect on whole body insulin sensitivity in men with the metabolic syndrome.

We observed a beneficial reduction in the rate of endogenous glucose production, which almost totally originates in the liver in the fasting state. Short-chain fatty acids produced by colonic fermentation could play a role in hepatic glucose regulation. In vitro studies have shown that hepatocytes exposed to SCFA increase glucose oxidation, decrease fatty acids, and increase insulin clearance [17]. Thorburn et al. observed a significant decrease in hepatic glucose output in healthy men who acutely ingested fiber-rich pearl barley compared with rice [18]. The 3 h decrease in hepatic glucose output, in that study, was further related to a 3 h decrease in plasma FFA, in parallel with a higher breath hydrogen concentration after pearl barley than after rice ingestion, but with no acetate measurement. The liver is one of the first organs exposed to large amounts of portal acetate and propionate produced during colonic fermentation which may subsequently influence hepatic glucose production. Propionate is a precursor of glucose synthesis in ruminants and has been described to modulate glucose production in humans [19]. The ratio of acetate and propionate may regulate hepatic glucose output via an antilipolytic effect of acetate and a gluconeogenic effect of propionate [19]. The reason why acetogenic fibers might modulate liver metabolism rather than that of the peripheral tissues is still uncertain; however, the SCFA gradient in the portal vein may be part of the explanation. Another possible mechanism may involve stimulated secretion of incretins (glucagon-like peptide 1) by short-chain fatty acids in the colon which inhibit hepatic glucose production [20]. The role of short-chain fatty acids on liver metabolism is unclear in humans and deserves further investigation.

Finally, we have shown that chronic 5 week ingestion of acetogenic fibers (acacia gum and pectin) that were a soluble nonviscous and readily fermentable fiber blend does not improve peripheral insulin sensitivity measured with the EH clamp technique in metabolic syndrome patients. However, we showed that chronic acetogenic fiber intake is associated with a reduction in fasting endogenous glucose turnover, which is mainly hepatic in origin. Improving glucose control and especially hepatic glucose output would be relevant for type 2 diabetics.

Acknowledgments

Mme Hivernaud, Mme Seveno, and Mme Pouvreau are acknowledged for the excellent completion of the trial at the Hospital. The personnel from CIC Nantes is acknowledged. A. Rytz, C. Hager, JC. Maire, and B. Decarli are acknowledged for their advices. C. Magliola and I. Perrin are acknowledged for the product release and the safety clearance, respectively. I. Meirim and V. Giller are acknowledged for their analytical support. We also thank M. Kuslys and S. Tan for providing the drinks (Nestlé, PTC Konolfingen). Finally, we thank K. Acheson for reviewing the paper. We sincerely appreciate the participation of all volunteers.

The present work has been accepted for publication in Clinical Nutrition.

References

1. Boden, G., Effects of free fatty acids (FFA) on glucose metabolism: Significance for insulin resistance and type 2 diabetes, *Exp. Clin. Endocrinol. Diabetes,* 111, 121–124, 2003.
2. Santomauro, A.T. et al., Overnight lowering of free fatty acids with Acipimox improves insulin resistance and glucose tolerance in obese diabetic and nondiabetic subjects, *Diabetes,* 48, 1836–1841, 1999.
3. Segerlantz, M. et al., Inhibition of the rise in FFA by Acipimox partially prevents GH-induced insulin resistance in GH-deficient adults, *J. Clin. Endocrinol. Metab,* 86, 5813–5818, 2001.
4. Sierksma, A. et al., Effect of moderate alcohol consumption on adiponectin, tumor necrosis factor-alpha, and insulin sensitivity, *Diabetes Care,* 27, 184–189, 2004.
5. Facchini, F., Chen, Y.D., and Reaven, G.M., Light-to-moderate alcohol intake is associated with enhanced insulin sensitivity, *Diabetes Care,* 17, 115–119, 1994.

6. Abramson, E.A. and Arky, R.A., Acute antilipolytic effects of ethyl alcohol and acetate in man, *J. Lab. Clin. Med.,* 72, 105–117, 1968.
7. Pouteau, E. et al., Production rate of acetate during colonic fermentation of lactulose: A stable-isotope study in humans, *Am. J. Clin. Nutr.,* 68, 1276–1283, 1998.
8. Ferchaud-Roucher, V. et al., Colonic fermentation from lactulose inhibits lipolysis in overweight subjects, *Am. J. Physiol. Endocrinol. Metab.,* 289, E716–E720, 2005.
9. American Heart Association, Third report of the national cholesterol education program (NCEP) expert panel on detection, evaluation, and treatment of high blood cholesterol in adults (adult treatment panel III) final report, *Circulation,* 106, 3143–3421, 2002.
10. Molina, J.M. et al., Use of a variable tracer infusion method to determine glucose turnover in humans, *Am. J. Physiol.,* 258, E16–E23, 1990.
11. Titgemeyer, E.C. et al., Fermentability of various fiber sources by human fecal bacteria in vitro, *Am. J. Clin. Nutr.,* 53, 1418–1424, 1991.
12. Wieland, O.H., UV method, in *Methods in Enzymatic Analysis,* Vol. VI, 3rd edn., Bergmeyer, H.U. (Ed.), Deerfield Beach, FL, Verlag Chemie, 1984, pp. 504–510.
13. Matthews, D.R. et al., Homeostasis model assessment: Insulin resistance and beta-cell function from fasting plasma glucose and insulin concentrations in man, *Diabetologia,* 28, 412–419, 1985.
14. Wolfe, R.R., *Radioactive and Stable Isotope Tracers in Biomedicine—Principles and Practice of Kinetic Analysis,* New York, Wiley-Liss, 1992.
15. Weickert, M.O. et al., Cereal fiber improves whole-body insulin sensitivity in overweight and obese women, *Diabetes Care,* 29, 775–780, 2006.
16. Robertson, M.D. et al., Insulin-sensitizing effects of dietary resistant starch and effects on skeletal muscle and adipose tissue metabolism, *Am. J. Clin. Nutr.,* 82, 559–567, 2005.
17. Venter, C.S., Vorster, H.H., and Cummings, J.H., Effects of dietary propionate on carbohydrate and lipid metabolism in healthy volunteers, *Am. J. Gastroenterol.,* 85, 549–553, 1990.
18. Thorburn, A., Muir, J., and Proietto, J., Carbohydrate fermentation decreases hepatic glucose output in healthy subjects, *Metabolism,* 42, 780–785, 1993.
19. Wolever, T.M., Spadafora, P., and Eshuis, H., Interaction between colonic acetate and propionate in humans, *Am. J. Clin. Nutr.,* 53, 681–687, 1991.
20. Freeland, K.R., Wilson, C., and Wolever, T.M., Adaptation of colonic fermentation and glucagon-like peptide-1 secretion with increased wheat fiber intake for 1 year in hyperinsulinaemic human subjects, *Br. J. Nutr.,* 103, 82–90, 2009.

12

Assessing Immune Health Outcomes Following Dietary Interventions in Healthy Adults

A Model Using Galactooligosaccharides

BOBBI LANGKAMP-HENKEN

Contents

12.1 Introduction

Recently, consumers and consequently the food and dietary supplement industries have become very interested in products that maintain immune health. Probiotics, prebiotics, and nutrients such as vitamin E, zinc, and omega-3 fatty acids are being added to products to modulate immune function. In fact, it was reported that 144 new foods or beverages with structure/function claims related to immune health were introduced in North America during 2009. This is in contrast to only nine new products with similar claims in 2006.[1] Prior to marketing products using immunity claims, substantial supporting evidence must be available. These data can be difficult to obtain because structure/function claims must reflect maintenance of health in *healthy* individuals, where immune function may already be adequate to prevent potential illness. Consequently, human intervention studies examining maintenance of immune health frequently use infants or aged adults. These are times during the life cycle when the immune system may be immature or immune function becomes dysregulated (i.e., immunosenescence).[2-4]

Obtaining scientific evidence to support immunity claims in healthy adults would be an easier task if biomarkers for optimal immune function were available.

Unfortunately, such markers have yet to be identified. Immune responses, which consist of the simultaneous activation and suppression of various immune cells and cytokines, occur locally within the infected tissue and not necessarily within the circulating blood. This makes it difficult to measure and interpret immune responses and almost impossible to find surrogate markers of immune health. Therefore, the best indicators of optimal immune function may be health outcomes, such as fewer days of illness. This chapter will discuss strategies for examining immune health in healthy adults using galactooligosaccharides (GOS) as a model.

12.2 Galactooligosaccharides: Potential Mechanisms in Immune Health

Animal studies and observed health relationships associated with intake of oligosaccharides in humans are helpful for identifying the potential impact of GOS on immune function. Once possible mechanisms of action have been identified, human trials can be designed to examine these mechanisms and their related health outcomes. The primary mechanisms of action of GOS on immune function are likely related to the fact that GOS are not digested in the small intestine. Enzymatically derived from lactose, GOS are chains of galactose units which typically have a terminal glucose and a degree of polymerization between 2 and 10. The enzymes and conditions used to produce GOS determine the type of β-glycosidic linkages within the oligosaccharide.[5] These bonds are resistant to digestion by intestinal enzymes. This allows GOS to arrive intact in the ileum and colon where they may act as antimicrobial agents by mimicking pathogen binding sites on epithelial cells. Microbes, which must adhere to the epithelium to infect the tissue, adhere to GOS instead of the intestinal cells and are displaced from the gastrointestinal tract. These antiadhesive properties were demonstrated in vitro with GOS significantly reducing the adherence of enteropathogenic *Escherichia coli* to HEp-2 and Caco-2 cells.[6]

12.2.1 Reduction of Inflammatory Burden

In addition to potentially changing the intestinal microbial populations through antiadhesive effects, GOS increase the number and proportion of bifidobacteria.[7,8] Bifidobacteria, which are considered beneficial intestinal bacteria, could potentially decrease the inflammatory burden to the host through competition with pathogenic bacteria for residence sites, direct interaction with the intestinal mucosa, or by decreasing lipopolysaccharide (LPS) in the blood.[9–12] Cani and colleagues investigated the latter mechanism by feeding mice with an inflammatory phenotype (*ob/ob*) a control diet or the same diet with added fermentable dietary fiber (oligofructose) or a nonfermentable fiber (microcrystalline cellulose).[12] The mice fed the fermentable oligofructose had higher cecal *Bifidobacterium* spp. and *Lactobacillus* spp. and reduced intestinal permeability to 4000 Da fluorescent dextrans compared to mice fed the control or cellulose diets. The mRNA expression of the intestinal epithelial tight-junction proteins ZO-1 and occludin was negatively correlated with plasma levels of the permeability marker. Additionally, plasma LPS levels, which were positively correlated with plasma levels of the permeability marker, were reduced in mice fed the oligosaccharide compared to mice fed the control or cellulose diets. Oligofructose feeding was also associated with reduced plasma levels of tumor necrosis factor (TNF)-α, interleukin (IL)-1α, IL-1β, IL-6, IL-10, interferon (IFN)-γ, macrophage inflammatory protein (MIP)-1a, and monocyte chemoattractant protein (MCP)-1.[12] These data suggest that fermentable oligofructose may modulate plasma levels of LPS and the associated inflammation by altering the microbiota and intestinal barrier function.

Fermentation products, which also change with diet and bacterial populations within the: play a role in decreasing inflammatory burden. Short-chain fatty acids, which are produced during microbial fermentation of GOS, are trophic to the colon and alter mucosal permeability.[13,14] In vitro studies show that the short-chain fatty acids butyrate, propionate, and acetate induced a concentration-dependent increase in transepithelial resistance (i.e., decreased epithelial permeability) in Caco-2 cells.[15]

The possible mechanisms of action discussed earlier lend themselves to finding a measurable difference in inflammatory processes with dietary GOS, but only in populations where inflammation is likely. For example, one may expect to see a decrease in proinflammatory cytokines and possibly acute phase proteins with dietary GOS supplementation in individuals with a chronic low-grade inflammation but not in individuals with low to normal levels of inflammatory cytokines or acute phase proteins. Low-grade inflammation and/or a leaky intestine is associated with obesity, metabolic syndrome, advanced age, alcohol abuse, and stress.[16–18]

12.2.2 Enhancing Mucosal Immune Function

Dietary GOS may also impact immune health through the gut-associated lymphoid tissue (GALT) or the larger common mucosal lymphoid system. Within the GALT, GOS may directly or indirectly interact with immune cells found within the lymphoid tissues that line the length of the intestine. Peyer's patches, which are organized lymphoid tissues, are inductive sites for immune responses. The Peyer's patches are covered by specialized epithelial cells that allow luminal contents to be sampled. Sampled antigens are presented to T lymphocytes and stimulate B cells. Activated lymphocytes travel to the mesenteric lymph nodes where they begin to proliferate and differentiate. Dendritic cells also appear to sample luminal contents throughout the intestine by transepithelial penetration of the epithelial barrier.[19] A subset of mucosal dendritic cells travel to the mesenteric lymph nodes where they initiate immune responses.[20] Activated and differentiating lymphocytes from the mesenteric lymph nodes travel via the lymphatic system to the thoracic duct where they reenter the bloodstream and home back to the intestine to offer protection. Through the common mucosal immune system, it is proposed that T and B lymphocytes also travel to other mucosal tissues including the respiratory tract (bronchial-associated lymphoid tissue or BALT), tonsils and adenoids (nasal-associated lymphoid tissue or NALT),

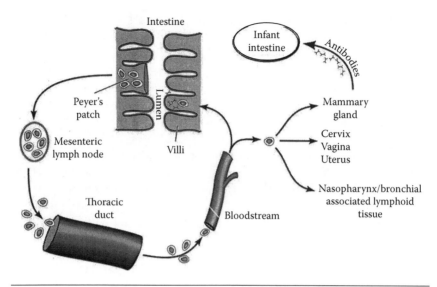

Figure 12.1 Gut-associated lymphoid tissue. (Modified from Langkamp-Henken, B., Glezer, J.A., and Kudsk, K.A., *Nutr. Clin. Pract.*, 7, 100, 1992. With permission of SAGE Publications.)

urogenital tract, and mammary glands (Figure 12.1).[21] Within the lamina propria of the mucosal tissues, activated T lymphocytes may play a number of roles, such as inducing inflammation or tolerance, killing tumor or virus-infected cells, or helping B cells differentiate into immunoglobulin (Ig)A-producing cells. A histological study in mice fed a homologous strain of immunofluorescence-labeled *Bifidobacterium animalis* showed the presence of the bacteria within the Peyer's patches of the intestine and significantly more IgA-secreting cells within the lamina propria of the large intestine after 5 days of feeding 1×10^7 bifidobacteria.[22] Although the study did not examine whether the IgA-secreting cells were specific for *B. animalis*, these data demonstrate that bacteria can be taken up by Peyer's patches and influence mucosal immune function.

B lymphocytes within the mucosal tissue differentiate into plasma cells and produce polymeric IgA (pIgA). The pIgA is typically composed of two IgA monomeric units joined by a J chain. The pIgA binds to the polymeric-Ig receptor (pIgR) on the basolateral surface of epithelial cells. The ligand-bound pIgR is transported across the epithelial cell to the apical surface where the pIgR is cleaved leaving part of the pIgR still bound to the pIgA, thus forming secretory IgA (sIgA). The sIgA, which is resistant to digestion and does not activate complement, prevents the attachment and translocation of bacteria and viruses across the epithelium into the lamina propria. The pIgA also functions to clear antigens on the basolateral side of the epithelial cell (i.e., within the lamina propria), as well as intracellular viruses. If the pIgA is specific for an antigen found within the lamina propria, it can bind to the antigen and the pIgR. This immune complex is then transported across the epithelial cell and released into the mucus lining of the epithelium.[23] Additionally, if an infecting virus is encountered during transcytosis, pIgA specific for that virus can bind to it and neutralize it.[24] The receptor for pIgA also functions as an antimicrobial and anti-inflammatory protein.[25] During the process of transcytosis of the pIgA-pIgR complex, unbound pIgR is also released at the epithelial barrier. The cleaved extracellular portion of the pIgR is called the secretory component. Dallas and Rolfe showed that free secretory component can bind *Clostridium difficile* toxin A and prevent interaction with intestinal receptors.[26] It is of interest that butyrate, a short-chain fatty acid which is produced during fermentation of oligosaccharides, enhances pIgR expression on human colonic cells in vitro, and this effect is potentiated in the presence of proinflammatory cytokines.[13,27]

Although there are no studies examining the effect of GOS on immune cells within GALT and the impact of these changes on tissues within the common mucosal immune system, animal studies demonstrate that diet can impact GALT and clearance of upper respiratory tract infections.[28–30] Mice fed a complete diet parenterally (intravenously) or the same fiber-free elemental diet intragastrically had lower numbers of T and B lymphocytes in the Peyer's patches and intestinal lamina propria than mice fed a standard complex rodent diet. Additionally, intestinal IgA was also reduced compared to that found in mice fed the standard rodent diet.[30] The lack of enteral stimulation with parenteral nutrition is also associated with impaired generation of immune responses to an H1N1 influenza virus infection.[28] To demonstrate this, Johnson and colleagues started mice on a parenteral diet and inoculated the mice with A/PR8 influenza virus on the same day. In the parenterally fed mice, total lymphocyte cell numbers were reduced in the NALT as were the number of IgA-forming cells and virus-specific IgA compared with mice that had free access to a standard rodent diet. By the 8th day postvirus inoculation, the nasal washes were positive for virus in seven of nine parenterally fed mice but only one of the nine fed the standard diet.[28] These data suggest that enteral intake is important for maintaining mucosal-associated immune function and recovery from influenza.

Some of the first evidence in humans showing that GOS may have an effect on GALT and the common mucosal immune system comes from breast-fed infants. Oligosaccharides, which include GOS, are a major component of human milk.[31] Breast-fed infants have a higher proportion of bifidobacteria and higher fecal sIgA levels when compared to infants who are formula fed.[32–34] Additionally, breast-fed infants from developed countries have a reduced risk of nonspecific gastroenteritis, necrotizing enterocolitis, acute otitis media, severe lower respiratory tract infections, and atopic dermatitis.[35] Supplementation of infant formula with GOS and fructooligosaccharide (FOS) in a ratio of 9:1 increases fecal bifidobacteria, produces a fermentation profile that is closer to that of breast-fed infants, and increases fecal sIgA.[32,34,36,37] The data also suggest that healthy infants fed a GOS:FOS supplemented formula have a decreased number of infectious episodes (e.g., upper respiratory, gastrointestinal, and urinary tract infections and otitis media) and incidence of recurrent upper respiratory tract infections compared to infants fed the same formula without oligosaccharides.[2,38]

If GOS modulates mucosal immunity in adults, then one might expect to see outcomes similar to those observed in infants. A number of studies in healthy adults show that GOS intake increases the number of fecal bifidobacteria.[7,8,39–41] Bouhnik and colleagues randomly assigned healthy adults (18–54 years of age) to ingest 0, 2.5, 5.0, 7.5, or 10 g of GOS in addition to their usual diet each day for 7 days. The number of fecal bifidobacteria increased with all doses of GOS, but no linear dose response was observed; however, a low bifidobacteria count at baseline was significantly associated with increased counts with treatment.[7] Future studies need to address whether the increase in bifidobacteria is associated with changes in immune function and improved health.

12.3 Strategies for Examining Immune Health in Healthy Adults

Interventions designed to examine the maintenance of health (e.g., decreased incidence of gastrointestinal or respiratory tract infections) in healthy adults must be administered over a long period. This is to allow sufficient time to accrue the number of days of illness required to detect a measurable difference between the treatment and control groups. To shorten the required time, healthy aged adults or healthy populations engaging in activities known to weaken immune function or increase risk of infection can be used.

12.3.1 Immunosenescence

Aging is associated with a decline in immune function.[42–44] With age there is a shift in T lymphocytes from naive to memory cells. This shift impairs one's ability to respond to novel antigens encountered within the environment or through vaccination. A shift in T-cell subtypes contributes to altered cytokine production (i.e., decreased IL-2, IFN-γ, IL-12, and increased IL-4, IL-6, IL-10). These shifts impair cytotoxic T-lymphocytes, which are important for viral clearance. Altered T-cell activity also impacts B-cell function. Antibody responses and production of high-affinity protective antibodies are reduced.[42,43] Natural killer cells provide a first line of defense against certain malignancies and viral infections. These cells, which are found in the periphery as well as within the mucosal-associated lymphoid tissues, increase in number but decrease in cytotoxic activity with age.[44,45] Neutrophils are part of the initial response to bacterial infection. These cells leave the circulation and migrate through the tissue toward the infected site (chemotaxis). The bacteria are taken up (phagocytosis) and killed by the release of superoxide radicals. Neutrophil chemotaxis, phagocytosis, and oxidative burst decrease with age.[44]

Vulevic and colleagues used a double-blind, placebo-controlled, crossover study to determine whether GOS supplementation could reverse age-related changes in natural killer cells and circulating phagocytic cells.[39] Subjects 64–79 years of age received 2.6 g of GOS or a placebo for 10 weeks. After a 4 week washout period, the subjects were switched to the other treatment. There was a significant increase in the number of Bifidobacterium spp. with placebo and GOS treatment, but the effect was greater with the GOS. Notably, there was a significant positive correlation between the number of *Bifidobacterium* spp. and natural killer cell activity. Total phagocytic activity of leukocytes (i.e., neutrophils and monocytes) was significantly greater with GOS treatment and was again positively correlated with the number of *Bifidobacterium* spp. GOS treatment was also associated with increased IL-10 and decreased IL-1β, TNF-α, and IL-6 production following in vitro LPS stimulation of lymphocytes and monocytes. With placebo treatment, in vitro cytokine levels went in the opposite direction (i.e., IL-10 decreased and IL-1β, TNF-α, and IL-6 increased).[39] The change in cytokine profile suggests that a less inflammatory state was induced with GOS treatment. The increases in fecal bifidobacteria and natural killer and phagocytic cell function with GOS treatment suggest that GOS may confer protection against viral or bacterial infections in aged adults. Future studies need to examine whether these changes result in fewer days of illness.

12.3.2 Immune Challenge

Other populations of healthy adults that may show improved immune function and less naturally occurring illness over a reasonably short period are those who engage in activities that weaken immune function or increase risk of infection. In healthy young adults, immune function is most likely optimal to protect them from gastrointestinal or respiratory tract infections. However, there are occasions when immune function is challenged or immune responses are weakened. These times can be utilized to test interventions on health outcomes in healthy individuals. Drakoularakou and colleagues did this when they examined travelers' diarrhea in healthy adults (mean age 38 years) visiting countries with a high or low risk for travelers' diarrhea.[46] Based on available data regarding the incidence of travelers' diarrhea, the investigators estimated that 50% of the subjects would experience diarrhea within the first 2 weeks of travel. Accordingly, 159 healthy individuals were randomized to receive 2.6 g of GOS or placebo daily for 1 week before traveling and a minimum of 14 days during the travel period. Both the travelers and investigators were blinded to the treatment. The incidence and duration of diarrhea were significantly lower with GOS treatment. A total of 19 out of 81 or 23% of the subjects treated with GOS reported diarrhea that lasted for an average of 2.4 days. In the placebo group, 30 out of 78 or 38% of the subjects reported diarrhea with an average duration of 4.6 days. Although no mechanisms for the treatment difference were examined, it was suggested that GOS may have prevented the adhesion and invasion of pathogens within the small intestine, provided a prebiotic effect within the colon, or enhanced overall immune function of the travelers.[46]

12.3.3 Psychological and Physiological Stress

A time in life that is associated with weakened immune function and increased incidence of illness is during periods of psychological and physiological stress.[47–49] Based on this association, we wondered whether acute psychological stress from academic exams was associated with increased days of naturally occurring cold or flu in healthy undergraduate students. If these young adults experienced illness

during academic exams, then this may be a unique model for testing dietary interventions on health outcomes. Additionally, universities with a large undergraduate
population would provide an ample pool from which to recruit subjects. To test this,
176 undergraduate students were recruited from the University of Florida, which
has an undergraduate population of 32,470 students. The undergraduates were
asked to record their level of stress (0 = no stress to 10 = extremely stressed) and cold
or flu symptoms every day for an 8 week period around the time of fall final exams.
This included the period 3 weeks before exams, 1 week during exams, and 4 weeks
postexams. The probability of getting a cold (defined as two or more cold symptoms
for 2 or more days) increased as the average daily stress level increased (Figure 12.2).
A total of 71 or 40% of the students reported at least one cold over the 8 weeks.[50]

These data suggest that academic stress may provide a good model for examining the effect of dietary interventions on immune outcomes in healthy individuals.
However, the effectiveness of the intervention depends upon the mechanisms by
which academic stress modulates immune function, as well as the mechanisms
by which the intervention boosts immune health. Academic stress is associated
with decreased numbers of lactic acid bacteria, levels of salivary sIgA, and activity of natural killer cells.[51-54] These changes likely contribute to functional gastrointestinal disorders and increased days of cold or flu in academically stressed

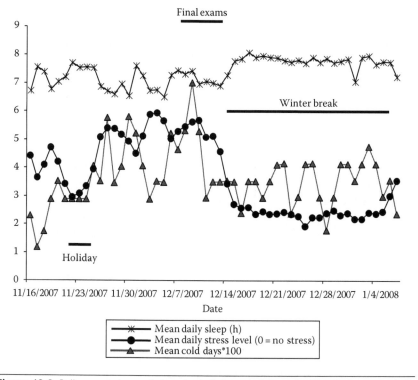

Figure 12.2 Daily average hours of sleep, level of stress, and days of cold or flu for academically
stressed undergraduate students around the time of fall final exams.

university students.[50,55] Dietary interventions designed to maintain health in this population should minimize these stress-induced changes. Based on the previously discussed mechanisms of action, it would be reasonable to test the effect of GOS on maintenance of gastrointestinal and immune health of students undergoing exam stress. Other times when immune function may be weakened resulting in illness in otherwise healthy adults include periods of chronic psychological stress, such as that associated with caring for an individual with Alzheimer's disease, and activities that induce physiological stress, such as endurance exercise competitions and military combat and training.[49,56–58] Although the psychological stress of athletic competitions and military combat and training would affect immune function, the physiological stress also affects immune function. Prolonged, intense exercise is associated with decreased natural killer cell activity, salivary IgA, and measures of T and B cell function.[49] Individuals participating in endurance competitions and combat training are at increased risk for upper respiratory tract infections, and nutritional interventions appear to provide benefits for reducing this risk.[49,58]

12.4 Conclusion

Structure/function claims for food or dietary supplements related to immune health require substantial scientific evidence in support of the claim. This evidence is difficult to obtain because the claim must reflect maintenance of health in *healthy* individuals. Strategies for examining immune health in healthy adults are dependent upon the proposed mechanisms of action of the dietary intervention. However, advanced age, psychological or physiological stress, or immune challenge, such as travelers' diarrhea, may be useful models for examining illness in an otherwise healthy population. Based on the proposed mechanisms of action of GOS, all of the strategies discussed earlier have potential for demonstrating the maintenance of immune health in healthy adults with GOS supplementation.

References

1. Nunes, K., An ounce of prevention—Products promoting immune system support are gaining traction, in FoodBusinessNews.net, May 25, 2010, p. 30, www.foodbusinessnews.net/News/New%20Home/Features/2010/5/An%20ounce%20of%20prevention.aspx
2. Arslanoglu, S., Moro, G. E., and Boehm, G., Early supplementation of prebiotic oligosaccharides protects formula-fed infants against infections during the first 6 months of life, *J. Nutr.*, 137, 2420, 2007.
3. Langkamp-Henken, B. et al., Nutritional formula enhanced immune function and reduced days of symptoms of upper respiratory tract infection in seniors, *J. Am. Geriatr. Soc.*, 52, 3, 2004.
4. Langkamp-Henken, B. et al., Nutritional formula improved immune profiles of seniors living in nursing homes, *J. Am. Geriatr. Soc.*, 54, 1861, 2006.
5. Macfarlane, G. T., Steed, H., and Macfarlane, S., Bacterial metabolism and health-related effects of galacto-oligosaccharides and other prebiotics, *J. Appl. Microbiol.*, 104, 305, 2008.

6. Shoaf, K. et al., Prebiotic galactooligosaccharides reduce adherence of enteropathogenic Escherichia coli to tissue culture cells, *Infect. Immun.*, 74, 6920, 2006.

7. Bouhnik, Y. et al., The capacity of nondigestible carbohydrates to stimulate fecal bifidobacteria in healthy humans: A double-blind, randomized, placebo-controlled, parallel-group, dose-response relation study, *Am. J. Clin. Nutr.*, 80, 1658, 2004.

8. Depeint, F. et al., Prebiotic evaluation of a novel galactooligosaccharide mixture produced by the enzymatic activity of Bifidobacterium bifidum NCIMB 41171, in healthy humans: A randomized, double-blind, crossover, placebo-controlled intervention study, *Am. J. Clin. Nutr.*, 87, 785, 2008.

9. Kankainen, M. et al., Comparative genomic analysis of *Lactobacillus rhamnosus* GG reveals pili containing a human- mucus binding protein, *Proc. Natl. Acad. Sci. USA*, 106, 17193, 2009.

10. Pachikian, B. D. et al., Changes in intestinal bifidobacteria levels are associated with the inflammatory response in magnesium-deficient mice, *J. Nutr.*, 140, 509, 2010.

11. Vijay-Kumar, M. et al., Metabolic syndrome and altered gut microbiota in mice lacking Toll-like receptor 5, *Science*, 328, 228, 2010.

12. Cani, P. D. et al., Changes in gut microbiota control inflammation in obese mice through a mechanism involving GLP-2-driven improvement of gut permeability, *Gut*, 58, 1091, 2009.

13. Hernot, D. C. et al., In vitro fermentation profiles, gas production rates, and microbiota modulation as affected by certain fructans, galactooligosaccharides, and polydextrose, *J. Agric. Food Chem.*, 57, 1354, 2009.

14. Sauer, J., Richter, K. K., and Pool-Zobel, B. L., Products formed during fermentation of the prebiotic inulin with human gut flora enhance expression of biotransformation genes in human primary colon cells, *Br. J. Nutr.*, 97, 928, 2007.

15. Mariadason, J. M., Barkla, D. H., and Gibson, P. R., Effect of short-chain fatty acids on paracellular permeability in Caco-2 intestinal epithelium model, *Am. J. Physiol.*, 272, G705, 1997.

16. Warnberg, J. et al., Physical activity, exercise and low-grade systemic inflammation, *Proc. Nutr. Soc.*, 69, 400, 2010.

17. Rao, R. K., Seth, A., and Sheth, P., Recent advances in alcoholic liver disease I. Role of intestinal permeability and endotoxemia in alcoholic liver disease, *Am. J. Physiol. Gastrointest. Liver Physiol.*, 286, G881, 2004.

18. Rezzi, S. et al., Metabotyping of biofluids reveals stress-based differences in gut permeability in healthy individuals, *J. Proteome Res.*, 8, 4799, 2009.

19. Niess, J. H. et al., CX3CR1-mediated dendritic cell access to the intestinal lumen and bacterial clearance, *Science*, 307, 254, 2005.

20. Schulz, O. et al., Intestinal CD103+, but not CX3CR1+, antigen sampling cells migrate in lymph and serve classical dendritic cell functions, *J. Exp. Med.*, 206, 3101, 2009.

21. Kang, W. and Kudsk, K. A., Is there evidence that the gut contributes to mucosal immunity in humans? *JPEN J. Parenter. Enteral. Nutr.*, 31, 246, 2007.

22. Perdigon, G. et al., Interaction of bifidobacteria with the gut and their influence in the immune function, *Biocell*, 27, 1, 2003.

23. Kaetzel, C. S. et al., The polymeric immunoglobulin receptor (secretory component) mediates transport of immune complexes across epithelial cells: A local defense function for IgA, *Proc. Natl. Acad. Sci. USA*, 88, 8796, 1991.

24. Mazanec, M. B. et al., Intracellular neutralization of virus by immunoglobulin a antibodies, *Proc. Natl. Acad. Sci. USA*, 89, 6901, 1992.

25. Kaetzel, C. S., The polymeric immunoglobulin receptor: Bridging innate and adaptive immune responses at mucosal surfaces, *Immunol. Rev.*, 206, 83, 2005.

26. Dallas, S. D. and Rolfe, R. D., Binding of Clostridium difficile toxin A to human milk secretory component, *J. Med. Microbiol.*, 47, 879, 1998.
27. Kvale, D. and Brandtzaeg, P., Butyrate differentially affects constitutive and cytokine-induced expression of HLA molecules, secretory component (SC), and ICAM-1 in a colonic epithelial cell line (HT-29, clone m3), *Adv. Exp. Med. Biol.*, 371A, 183, 1995.
28. Johnson, C. D. et al., Route of nutrition influences generation of antibody-forming cells and initial defense to an active viral infection in the upper respiratory tract, *Ann. Surg.*, 237, 565, 2003.
29. Kudsk, K. A., Li, J., and Renegar, K. B., Loss of upper respiratory tract immunity with parenteral feeding, *Ann. Surg.*, 223, 629, 1996.
30. Li, J. et al., Effects of parenteral and enteral nutrition on gut-associated lymphoid tissue, *J. Trauma*, 39, 44, 1995.
31. Boehm, G. et al., Prebiotic carbohydrates in human milk and formulas, *Acta Paediatr. Suppl.*, 94, 18, 2005.
32. Bakker-Zierikzee, A. M. et al., Faecal SIgA secretion in infants fed on pre- or probiotic infant formula, *Pediatr. Allergy Immunol.*, 17, 134, 2006.
33. Harmsen, H. J. et al., Analysis of intestinal flora development in breast-fed and formula-fed infants by using molecular identification and detection methods, *J. Pediatr. Gastroenterol. Nutr.*, 30, 61, 2000.
34. Knol, J. et al., Colon microflora in infants fed formula with galacto- and fructo-oligosaccharides: More like breast-fed infants, *J. Pediatr. Gastroenterol. Nutr.*, 40, 36, 2005.
35. Ip, S. et al., Breastfeeding and maternal and infant health outcomes in developed countries, *Evid. Rep. Technol. Assess (Full Rep)*, 1, 2007.
36. Rinne, M. M. et al., Similar bifidogenic effects of prebiotic-supplemented partially hydrolyzed infant formula and breastfeeding on infant gut microbiota, *FEMS Immunol. Med. Microbiol.*, 43, 59, 2005.
37. Moro, G. et al., A mixture of prebiotic oligosaccharides reduces the incidence of atopic dermatitis during the first six months of age, *Arch. Dis. Child*, 91, 814, 2006.
38. Arslanoglu, S. et al., Early dietary intervention with a mixture of prebiotic oligosaccharides reduces the incidence of allergic manifestations and infections during the first two years of life, *J. Nutr.*, 138, 1091, 2008.
39. Vulevic, J. et al., Modulation of the fecal microflora profile and immune function by a novel trans-galactooligosaccharide mixture (B-GOS) in healthy elderly volunteers, *Am. J. Clin. Nutr.*, 88, 1438, 2008.
40. Bouhnik, Y. et al., Administration of transgalacto-oligosaccharides increases fecal bifidobacteria and modifies colonic fermentation metabolism in healthy humans, *J. Nutr.*, 127, 444, 1997.
41. Ito, M. et al., Influence of galactooligosaccharides on the human fecal microflora, *J. Nutr. Sci. Vitaminol. (Tokyo)*, 39, 635, 1993.
42. Gruver, A. L., Hudson, L. L., and Sempowski, G. D., Immunosenescence of ageing, *J. Pathol.*, 211, 144, 2007.
43. Ginaldi, L. et al., Immunosenescence and infectious diseases, *Microbes. Infect.*, 3, 851, 2001.
44. Panda, A. et al., Human innate immunosenescence: Causes and consequences for immunity in old age, *Trends Immunol*, 30, 325, 2009.
45. Cella, M. et al., A human natural killer cell subset provides an innate source of IL-22 for mucosal immunity, *Nature*, 457, 722, 2009.
46. Drakoularakou, A. et al., A double-blind, placebo-controlled, randomized human study assessing the capacity of a novel galacto-oligosaccharide mixture in reducing travellers' diarrhoea, *Eur. J. Clin. Nutr.*, 64, 146, 2010.

47. Cohen, S., Doyle, W. J., and Skoner, D. P., Psychological stress, cytokine production, and severity of upper respiratory illness, *Psychosom. Med.*, 61, 175, 1999.
48. Cohen, S., Tyrrell, D. A., and Smith, A. P., Psychological stress and susceptibility to the common cold, *N. Engl. J. Med.*, 325, 606, 1991.
49. Nieman, D. C. and Bishop, N. C., Nutritional strategies to counter stress to the immune system in athletes, with special reference to football, *J. Sports Sci.*, 24, 763, 2006.
50. Herrlinger-Garcia, K. A. et al., Academic stress in an undergraduate population is associated with increased likelihood of getting a cold, *FASEB J.*, 23, 907.4, 2009.
51. Knowles, S. R., Nelson, E. A., and Palombo, E. A., Investigating the role of perceived stress on bacterial flora activity and salivary cortisol secretion: A possible mechanism underlying susceptibility to illness, *Biol. Psychol.*, 77, 132, 2008.
52. Jemmott, J. B., 3rd and Magloire, K., Academic stress, social support, and secretory immunoglobulin A, *J. Pers. Soc. Psychol.*, 55, 803, 1988.
53. Kiecolt-Glaser, J. K. et al., Psychosocial modifiers of immunocompetence in medical students, *Psychosom. Med.*, 46, 7, 1984.
54. Kiecolt-Glaser, J. K. et al., Modulation of cellular immunity in medical students, *J. Behav. Med.*, 9, 5, 1986.
55. Suarez, K. et al., Psychological stress and self-reported functional gastrointestinal disorders, *J. Nerv. Ment. Dis.*, 198, 226, 2010.
56. Kiecolt-Glaser, J. K. et al., Chronic stress and immunity in family caregivers of Alzheimer's disease victims, *Psychosom. Med.*, 49, 523, 1987.
57. Segerstrom, S. C. and Miller, G. E., Psychological stress and the human immune system: A meta-analytic study of 30 years of inquiry, *Psychol. Bull.*, 130, 601, 2004.
58. Wood, S. M. et al., Novel nutritional immune formula maintains host defense mechanisms, *Mil. Med.*, 170, 975, 2005.

13
Inulin, Gut Microbes, and Health

DIEDERICK MEYER

Contents

13.1 Introduction

Inulins, the β-(2,1)-fructans extracted on industrial scale from chicory roots [1] and present in many other plants [2], are interesting carbohydrates that exhibit a variety of physiological effects and potential health benefits. Being nondigestible—the $\beta(2,1)$-bond cannot be hydrolyzed in our digestive system—these ingredients are dietary fibers with the associated physiological effects. This means that they have a positive effect on bowel habits, as they improve frequency of defecation and stool consistency, and that they may lower serum lipids as other soluble fibers will also do. In addition, they have a low glycemic and insulinemic response and a low caloric value, and may increase feelings of satiety with a possible effect on food and energy intake. Inulin and oligofructose share these important features with many other dietary fibers [3–5]. There is still discussion whether fermentation in the colon is a beneficial physiological effect, but it becomes now accepted that it is important for colonic health and thus should be considered as a beneficial effect of fibers [6,7].

What sets the fructans apart from other fibers is their prebiotic activity: They are able to stimulate specifically the growth of presumably healthy bacteria in our large intestine, thus conferring health benefits to the host [8]. Some of the physiological consequences of these specific changes are already mentioned, as they relate to dietary fibers, but others are more linked to the increase in bifidobacteria:

1. Increased absorption of calcium and magnesium from the colon, with potential benefits for bone health
2. Improved digestion and vitamin status, as a consequence of enzymes and vitamins produced by bifidobacteria

3. Stimulation of the immune system with potential effects for resistance against infections, allergic reactions, and inflammation associated with obesity and metabolic syndrome
4. Increased colonization resistance also leading to a positive effect on resistance against infections
5. Downregulation of risk factors for colon cancer
6. Increased levels of satiety hormones with effects on feelings of satiety, and food and energy intake

Although the last two effects are also dietary fiber effects, the mechanism for inulin is probably different from that of other fibers. As an example, the satiety effects of fibers such as pectins are probably connected with their rheological properties such as an increased viscosity. This may lower the rate of release of nutrients such as glucose from the food matrix and hence affect feelings of satiety.

13.2 Bifidogenic Response

A large number of studies with human volunteers have shown that consumption of inulin and oligofructose leads to an increase in the content of bifidobacteria and when measured often accompanied by a similar effect on lactobacilli, in fecal samples. The first data were shown in 1995 for inulin and oligofructose from chicory [9], and the most recent data show that the same effect is found for inulin from Jerusalem artichoke [10]. For an overview of these data, see [11,12].

The effect is found in infants and in adults of all ages at dosages ranging from about 1.5 g/day in infants to 5 g/day in adults [11]. It is fair to say that inulin is the only prebiotic with proven efficacy in people of all ages [13].

Chain length does not seem to affect the bifidogenic response. If one calculates the yield of bifidobacteria per gram of fructan from the data of human studies, it appears to be independent of chain length (Table 13.1). Literature data show

Table 13.1 Overview of Yield Values of Bifidobacteria on β-(2,1)-Fructans

Prebiotic	Yield of Bifidobacteria	
	Number per g	g/g
Inulin from chicory	1.4×10^{11}	0.14
Oligofructose from chicory	1.5×10^{11}	0.15
sc-FOS from sucrose	1.5×10^{11}	0.15

Note: Yield was calculated with data from human studies for adults (overview in Meyer and Stasse-Wolthuis [11]).

Yield = (number of bifidobacteria per g of feces × fecal output, in g/day)/(inulin consumption, in g/day).

In this calculation, it is assumed that all inulin is only fermented by bifidobacteria and that the fecal output is 150 g/day. To calculate from numbers per gram of inulin to gram of bifidobacteria per gram of inulin, the weight of one Bifidobacterium cell was set at 1 pg ($=10^{-12}$ g).

that the yield of *Bifidobacterium animalis* on oligofructose is about 0.25 g/g [14] and of *B. bifidum* on glucose or galactose ranges from 0.21 to 0.15 g/g [15]. These values are in reasonable agreement with the data in Table 13.1.

The different studies also indicate that the response is more dependent on the starting level of bifidobacteria than of the daily dosage: With lower starting levels, the bifidus increase expressed in log units is higher, and this appears to be the case in adults [16] and in infants [17]. It proves to be more difficult to find a significant increase in people with high starting levels of bifidobacteria. When expressed in numbers of bifidobacteria, the increase is more or less constant as calculated earlier.

These data are based on bacterial enumeration of fecal samples with selective plate counting and with molecular techniques (FISH, RT-PCR). With the introduction of microarrays, it becomes now also possible to look at the effect of inulin or other prebiotics on "all" bacteria present of the colonic microbiota. Such analyses will clearly provide more insight in population changes due to inulin intake (and will also lead to the detection and description of genera and species hitherto unknown) and also in the physiological effects of such changes. As an example, with such techniques, an increase in *Faecalibacterium prausnitzii* has been reported, as well as the fact that not all *Bifidobacterium* spp. may increase after inulin consumption [18]. Kovatcheva-Datchary [19] showed that also members of *Clostridium* cluster XIVa (*Dorrea* spp.) are inulin users. It remains unknown so far what the physiological consequences of a change in these bacterial species are. Another nice example of the potential of the new molecular techniques is provided by Qin et al. [20] who described the metagenomic sequencing, assembly, and characterization of 3.3 million microbial genes from fecal samples of 124 European individuals. They showed that the human gut microbiome gene set is approximately 150 times larger than the human gene complement, and also noted differences in the bacterial species abundance between IBD patients and healthy individuals. They were also able to differentiate between genes necessary for bacteria to survive in the colon and those involved in homeostasis of the whole ecosystem.

13.3 Health Benefits of Bifidobacteria

Bifidobacterium and *Lactobacillus* spp. are used extensively as probiotics, one of the reasons being that there are no known pathogens within these genera. The fermentation patterns of these genera are saccharolytic rather than proteolytic, and it has been accepted that a saccharolytic microbiota consisting mainly of bifidobacteria and lactobacilli is beneficial for gut health [7]. The fermentation products of bifidobacteria and lactobacilli, mainly short-chain fatty acids (SCFA), acetate, propionate, and butyrate, all have benefits. Butyrate is considered a health-promoting metabolite, which functions as the major energy source for epithelial cells of the colon [21], but it may also play a role in the inhibition of colon carcinogenesis and in the regression of colitis [21,22]. Acetate and propionate are used systemically in the body, especially in the liver [21]. Lactate is metabolized by the muscle tissue (and will also be used to a large extent by the colonic microbiota). The branched chain fatty acids are products typical for protein fermentation, e.g., *iso*butyrate and *iso*valerate are formed from the amino acids valine and leucine, respectively [23]. These products may have a negative impact on health and can cause liver problems [21]. Proteolytic fermentation can also lead to other (potentially) toxic components, such as ammonia, phenolic, and sulfur-containing compounds [23]. Ammonia is toxic to the colonic epithelium and promotes colon cancer in rats [24]. In addition, ammonia is a (potential) liver toxin and has been implicated in the onset of neoplastic growth [24,25]. The production of phenolic compounds, such as skatole or indole, by intestinal bacteria has been associated with a variety of disease states in humans, including schizophrenia [23], and sulfur-containing products such as hydrogen sulfide inhibit butyrate metabolism in colon cells [26].

The production of vitamins by bifidobacteria is well documented from in vitro experiments [27], but recent evidence suggests that this may also occur in vivo, when Ramirez-Farias et al. [18] showed that the increased serum folate level in pregnant women was associated with an increased level of fecal bifidobacteria.

The effects described earlier are based on the shift in metabolic activity of the colon flora brought about by the consumption of inulin; other effects probably more related to increased fermentation in the colon include the following:

1. Improved bowel habits, especially in slightly constipated people. As an example, Marteau et al. [28] showed an increase in defecation frequency in such volunteers with 15 g/day of inulin in combination with a bifidogenic effect, and den Hond et al. [29] found similar results with 10 g/day of long-chain inulin.

2. The increased fermentation leads to higher levels of SCFA which lowers the pH of the luminal content and thus improves the solubility of calcium and magnesium salts. This is most likely (part of the) mechanism responsible for the increased absorption of calcium and magnesium as found in studies with adolescents (e.g., [30,31]) and postmenopausal women [32]. In adolescents, this may also lead to an improved bone mineral density with 8 g/day of inulin consumption [31].

3. The lowered pH together with the production of antimicrobial substances by bifidobacteria, such as lactate or bacteriocins [33], may also be responsible for growth inhibition of potential pathogens in the colon. Altogether, this leads to enhanced colonization resistance to infection on the host.

4. More and more evidence becomes available that the increase in bifidobacteria may also lead to effects on the immune system. These effects will be described in more detail later, but they may also contribute to increased resistance to infections in healthy people and to positive effects in people with inflammatory bowel disease (IBD) or with irritable bowel syndrome (IBS).

Table 13.2 Overview of Physiological Effects of Inulin or Oligofructose from Chicory and Lowest Efficacious Dosages Based on Data from Studies with Adult Volunteers

Effect	Dosage (g/Day)
Bifidogenic/prebiotic	5
Improved calcium absorption	8
Enhanced resistance	12
Cholesterol maintenance	9
Enhanced satiety	16
Improved bowel habit	10

5. Emerging evidence shows that in humans, consumption of oligofructose or inulin may lead to enhanced feelings of satiety and less energy intake. Cani et al. [34] reported such data for a daily intake of 16 g/day of oligofructose for 2 weeks, while Parnell and Reimer [35] showed that with 21 g/day for 12 weeks, not only energy intake decreased but also more weight was lost than in the control diet without oligofructose. Long-chain inulin when consumed at breakfast as a fat replacer in sausages also led to an acute decrease of energy intake [36]. These effects are probably due to effects on secretion of satiety hormones [37].

An overview of the lowest efficacious dosage for these effects as reported in human studies is given in Table 13.2.

13.4 Beneficial Effects of Inulin or Oligofructose in Diseased People

In many gastrointestinal diseases or disorders, the microbiota seems to play a role, and in some cases, a beneficial effect has been associated with the consumption of inulin-type prebiotics and increased bifidobacteria content. Table 13.3 summarizes the data with inulin or oligofructose obtained from studies in people with inflammatory bowel conditions.

In people with IBS, Kerckhoffs et al. [42] found a lowered fecal count of bifidobacteria, which could be related to the disorder symptoms. It appears that for IBS, inulin or oligofructose alone does not affect symptom scores. Possibly this lack of effect may be related to the great variety of symptoms connected with IBS (diarrhea vs. constipation). Paineau et al. [43] showed improvements of gastrointestinal discomfort in people with IBS-type symptoms with consumption of 5 g/day of short-chain fructooligosaccharides (sc-FOS) from sucrose.

With IBD patients, a limited number of (small) trials have been published showing promising results (Table 13.3). For patients with Crohn's disease (CD), there is a study with positive results for inulin/oligofructose [39], and a study with ulcerative colitis (UC) patients gave indications for less inflammation (as measured by a lower fecal calprotectin concentration) and perception of abdominal pain [40]. Treatment of patients with an ileal pouch-anal anastomosis seems to

Table 13.3 Effects of Inulin or Oligofructose from Chicory in Humans with Inflammatory Conditions

References	Fructans Used (Dosage)	Study Design, Duration, Number of Subjects	Target Group/ Condition	Results
[37]	OF (6 g/day)	DB, CO, 4 weeks, $n = 21$	Adults/IBS	No effects on symptom scores
[38]	OF (20 g/day)	RCT, DB, parallel, 12 weeks, $n = 98$	Adults/IBS	Greater improvement in placebo group; no difference for symptoms at end of treatment
[39]	OF/inulin (7/3, 15 g/day)	3 weeks, $n = 10$	Adults/ IBD (CD)	Lower disease activity scores
[40]	OF/inulin (1/1, 12 g/day)	RCT, DB, parallel, 2 weeks, $n = 19$	Adults/ IBD (UC)	Lower disease activity; no difference with placebo. Lower fecal calprotectin
[41]	Inulin (24 g/day)	RCT, DB, CO, 3 weeks, $n = 24$	Patients/ pouchitis	No effect on clinical symptoms; lower pouchitis disease index

OF, oligofructose; RCT, randomized controlled trial; DB, double blind; CO, crossover; IBS, irritable bowel syndrome; IBD, inflammatory bowel disease; CD, Crohn's disease; UC: ulcerative colitis.

give mixed results. Welters et al. [41] found some improvement of the conditions with 18 g/day of inulin, whereas a preliminary report of Dahl et al. [44] described no improvement with 10 g/day.

There are also a number of publications in patients with IBD (e.g., [45]) or IBS [46] with inulin-based synbiotics, most, but not all [47], of them showing favorable results. It is not clear whether these effects can be contributed to inulin or the probiotic bacteria or both.

Inflammation also plays a role in atopy, and in studies with infants at risk or with atopy, it has been found that mixtures of prebiotics (9/1 galactooligosaccharides/ inulin, GOS/inulin) gave rise to improved conditions [48], but this effect is not only caused by inulin, and studies with only inulin or oligofructose have not been published so far. Based on the lower abundance of fecal bifidobacteria in infants with eczema [49], it is tempting to suggest that prebiotics, such as inulin, may improve this disorder.

As the microbiota composition of healthy and obese people is different (e.g., [50]), there may be a link between gut microbiota and obesity. Not only satiety hormones may be involved, as described earlier, but also the innate immune system as obesity is also characterized by low-grade inflammation. A high-fat diet induces not only fat storage and obesity but also inflammation. It may be that changing the gut microbiota by prebiotics is also relevant for the control of metabolic diseases connected with obesity. Kalliomäki et al. [51] showed that differences in gut microbiota may precede development of becoming overweight; more specifically these authors showed that bifidobacteria numbers in the first year of life were higher in children that had a normal weight at 7 years than in children being overweight at that age. They also noted the reverse for *Staphylococcus aureus*, and they proposed that this species may trigger low-grade inflammation which contributes to the development of obesity (see also [52]).

In most of these studies, a bifidogenic effect was not measured, but from the dosages applied and the known effective dosages (Table 13.2), a bifidogenic effect is highly likely. It seems therefore fair to conclude that despite some promising results—mainly from studies using pre- or synbiotic mixtures in IBD patients or children at risk for allergy—there are insufficient data to draw firm conclusions on the effect of inulin or oligofructose in people with inflammatory conditions and its connection with the bifidogenic effect. The relationship low-grade inflammation—gut microbiota composition—obesity also offers promising perspectives to establish a link between bifidobacteria/inulin and health.

13.5 Effects of Inulin and Oligofructose on Immune System and Resistance

13.5.1 Effect on Immune Parameters in Humans

Three studies using chicory-derived prebiotics have been published, one of them in elderly people and two in infants (Table 13.4). These studies all measuring antibody response after vaccination, which is a high score marker of systemic immune function, showed mixed results. For instance, Bunout et al. [55] found

Table 13.4 Effects of Inulin and Oligofructose on Immune Parameters in Humans

References	Fructans Used	Study Design, Duration, Number of Subjects	Target Group (Age)	Results
[53]	OF/inulin (7/3, 0.2 g/kg BW/day)	RCT, DB, 10 weeks, $n = 55$	Infants (7–9 months)	Higher **blood IgG levels after measles vaccination**
[54]	OF (0.7 g/day)	RCT, SB, 6 months, $n = 282$	Infants (6–12 months)	No effect on **antibody response after vaccination** with *H. influenzae* type B vaccine
[55]	OF/inulin (7/3, 6 g/d)	RCT, SB, parallel, 28 weeks, $n = 66$	Elderly (>70 years)	Increased **antibody response to influenza and** *S. pneumoniae* **vaccination** in both groups

High score markers in bold letters; see [57].
OF, oligofructose; BW, body weight; RCT, randomized controlled trial; DB, double blind; SB, single blind; CO, crossover.

an increased antibody response in control and prebiotic treated group of elderly subjects, hence no additional effect of the prebiotic treatment, whereas Saavedra and Tschernia [54] reported an increased antibody response after measles vaccination in infants. Another study in infants, however, revealed no effect after influenza vaccination [53]. The prebiotic combination 9/1 GOS/inulin led to higher fecal IgA levels in infants [56].

Although not with chicory-derived fructans, the studies with FOS from sucrose by Langkamp-Henken et al. [58,59] found enhanced immune function, indicated by increased influenza vaccine response and lymphocyte activation, less fever, and fewer newly prescribed antibiotics in seniors living in long-term care facilities.

Schiffrin et al. [60] looked at the effect of the same ingredient on systemic inflammatory markers in elderly people at risk of malnutrition. They found that with consumption of 2–4 g/day of the prebiotic, the level of circulating cytokines was not affected. After 12 weeks of supplementation, less proinflammatory gene activation was found (interleukin-6 (IL-6) and tumor necrosis factor-α (TNF-α)-specific mRNA in blood mononuclear cells was lowered significantly). This confirmed the results of an earlier trial in frail elderly people. Daily consumption of 8 g sc-FOS resulted in a clear bifidogenic effect together with a decreased expression of IL-6 mRNA, suggesting a possible decrease in inflammatory process [61].

A generalized conclusion with respect to immunomodulation in humans by inulin is not possible yet. Limited data suggest that inulin or oligofructose may have a favorable effect on antibody response after vaccination, but the effect may be different depending on age, type of vaccine, and type of fructans. Research data with other prebiotics, such as FOS from sucrose, show promising similar effects.

13.5.2 Effect on Infections in Humans

Table 13.5 provides an overview of human studies on the effect of inulin or oligofructose on the outcome of infections in humans. A division is made in studies with infants and children, and with adults.

Most studies in children and infants show some benefits of inulin/oligofructose or other prebiotic consumption in reducing the duration or severity of common childhood and acute diarrhea. For instance, Waligora-Dupriet et al. [62] showed that with 2 g/day of oligofructose fewer episodes with diarrhea or fever occurred.

Two Indonesian studies with FOS (unknown whether this is chicory derived) show some supportive data. In the first study, duration of diarrhea was found to be reduced with 2.5–5 g/day of prebiotic treatment [63], whereas another trial showed similar but not fully consistent data [64]. Only the group that consumed 3.2% FOS in food showed fewer episodes of diarrhea, while with 4%, no effect was found. Looking at diarrhea episodes of less than 2 days, both FOS percentages were effective. A number of studies using a 9/1 GOS/inulin mixture showed

Table 13.5 Effects of Inulin or Oligofructose on Infections in Humans

References	Fructans Used	Study Design, Duration, Number of Subjects	Target Group/ Condition	Results
[53]	OF (1.1 g/day)	RCT, DB, $n = 123$	Infants 4–24 months/diarrhea prevalence	No effect on diarrhea incidence, less occurrence of fever
[54]	OF (0.55 g/day)	RCT, SB, $n = 282$, 6 months	Infants 6–12 months/diarrhea prevalence	No effect on diarrhea prevalence
[62]	OF (2 g/day)	RCT, DB, $n = 20$; 21 days	Infants 7–19 months/diarrhea prevalence	Less episodes with fever or diarrhea, lower number of infectious disease requiring antibiotic treatment
[68,69]	OF (10 g/day)	RCT, DB, 4 weeks, $n = 244$	Adults/traveler's diarrhea	Trend for less diarrhea, significant decrease of severity of diarrhea
[70]	OF (12 g/day)	RCT, 30 days, $n = 142$	Elderly patients (>65 years) with AAD/*C. difficile*	Less relapse of diarrhea
[71]	OF (12 g/day)	RCT, DB, 2 weeks, $n = 435$	Elderly patients with antibiotic treatment/ *C. difficile*	No protective effect against AAD

OF, oligofructose; RCT, randomized controlled trial; DB, double blind; SB, single blind; CO, crossover; AAD, antibiotic-associated diarrhea.

(a trend toward) significantly less infectious periods, especially for respiratory infections [65–67].

With adults, less data are available (Table 13.5). Cummings et al. [68] reported a trend for shorter duration of travelers' diarrhea, and later analysis showed that severity of diarrhea was decreased significantly [69]. Oligofructose consumption (12 g/day) could not prevent antibiotic-associated diarrhea in elderly patients, despite an increase in fecal bifidobacteria [70], but in another trial, these investigators found that patients taking oligofructose were less likely to develop further diarrhea than those taking the placebo [71].

To conclude, there is some evidence that the incidence and duration of certain infections may be reduced by inulin or oligofructose in infants and children. For adults, much less convincing evidence is available.

13.6 Conclusions

From the data presented earlier, it is clear that inulin and oligofructose do cause a shift in the composition of the colonic microbiota in people of all ages. This shift is associated with a number of physiological effects, such as enhanced calcium absorption, a decrease in blood lipids, a positive effect for energy homeostasis, and a potential effect to increase resistance for infections and decrease of inflammation.

The challenge is to establish a causal link between the microbiota changes and these physiological effects. For some effects, this seems plausible, e.g., the increased production of acid fermentation products by bifidobacteria lowers the colonic pH which increases the solubility of calcium salts and hence improves absorption from the colon.

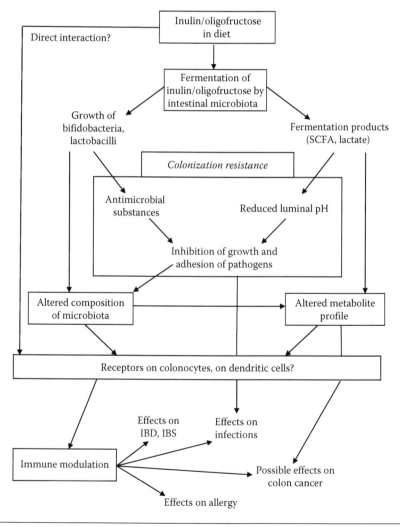

Figure 13.1 Inulin mediated effect on immune health.

For other effects, such links are less clear, but more and more evidence becomes available. Especially the interaction of SCFA with the free fatty acid receptors FFA 2 and FFA 4 (also known as G-protein-coupled receptors GPR 41 and 43, see [72]) on immune cells may explain the effect of fermentation products such as butyrate on immune parameters. It is known that butyrate affects transcription in the colonic mucosa [73]. But also the role of toll-like receptors (TLR) on immune cells of the gut-associated lymphoid tissue, the part of our immune system that constitutes the link between microbiota and immune response, may be important as these receptors may be affected by cell wall components of bifidobacteria (Figure 13.1; [74]).

Continued research will lead to the association between the bifidogenic effect of inulin and oligofructose and beneficial physiological effects becoming ever stronger; in the future, the bifidogenic effect may become a biomarker for gut health.

Further clinical studies in specific patients groups could provide important mechanistic data. For instance, as it has been reported that a reduction of *F. prausnitzii* is associated with a higher risk of recurrent ileal CD (CD; [75]) and as it is also known that *F. prausnitzii* is increased with inulin consumption [18], it would be very interesting to investigate the effect of inulin consumption on the recurrence of ileal CD. It has been suggested that *F. prausnitzii* exhibits anti-inflammatory effects partly due to metabolites blocking NF-κB activation and IL-8 production. Whether this effect is also relevant for healthy people is unknown [75].

Some of the classical dietary fiber effects of inulin and oligofructose (improved defecation, potential to lower serum lipids) can be considered as well established, and for the positive effects on weight management (as a consequence of an effect on satiety hormones) and to lower the risk for diabetes type 2, more and more evidence becomes available. The same holds true for the prebiotic effect and the connection with immune modulation and effects on resistance against infections. The relationship low-grade inflammation—gut microbiota composition—obesity also offers promising perspectives to establish a link between bifidobacteria/inulin and health.

Especially in a time when providing the evidence for health claims becomes more and more important, research on the health benefits of inulin and oligofructose will remain an area of high interest.

References

1. Boeckner, I.S., Schnepf, M.I., and Tungland, B.C., Inulin: A review of nutritional and health implications. *Adv. Food Nutr. Rev.* 43, 1, 2000.
2. Ritsema, T. and Smeekens, S., Fructans: Beneficial for plants and humans. *Curr. Opin. Plant Biol.* 6, 223, 2003.
3. Tungland, B.C. and Meyer, D., Nondigestible oligo- and polysaccharides (dietary fiber): Their physiology and role in human health and food. *Compr. Rev. Food Sci. Food Safety* 1, 73, 2002.
4. IoM (Institute of Medicine), *Dietary Reference Intakes for Energy, Carbohydrate, Fibre, Fat, Fatty Acids, Cholesterol, Protein, and Amino Acids (Macronutrients)*. Food and Nutrition Board, Institute of Medicine. The National Academies Press, Washington, DC, 2005.

5. Health Council of the Netherlands, Guideline for dietary fibre intake. Publication no. 2006/03. In Dutch with a summary in English, 2006.

6. EFSA (European Food Safety Authority), Outcome of the public consultation on the draft opinion of the scientific panel on dietetic products, nutrition, and allergies (NDA) on dietary reference values for carbohydrates and dietary fibre. *EFSA J.* 8, 1508, 2010.

7. Cummings, J.H. et al., PASSCLAIM—Gut health and immunity. *Eur. J. Nutr.* 43(Suppl. 2), 118, 2004.

8. Gibson, G.R. et al., Dietary modulation of the human colonic microbiota: Updating the concept of prebiotics. *Nutr. Res. Rev.* 17, 259, 2004.

9. Gibson, G.R. et al., Selective stimulation of bifidobacteria in the human colon by oligofructose and inulin. *Gastroenterol* 108, 975, 1995.

10. Ramnani, P. et al., Prebiotic effect of fruit and vegetable shots containing Jerusalem artichoke inulin: A human intervention study. *Br. J. Nutr.* 104, 233, 2010.

11. Meyer, D. and Stasse-Wolthuis, M., The bifidogenic effect of inulin and oligofructose and its consequences for gut health. *Eur. J. Clin. Nutr.* 63, 1277, 2009.

12. Roberfroid, M. et al., Prebiotic effects: Metabolic and health benefits. *Br. J. Nutr.* 104(Suppl. 2), S1, 2010.

13. Meyer, D., Native inulin as a prebiotic ingredient in food for infants and young children. *NutraCos* May/June, 49, 2010.

14. Van der Meulen, R., Avonts, L., and De Vuyst, L., Short fractions of oligofructose are preferentially metabolized by *Bifidobacterium animalis* DN-173 010. *Appl. Environ. Microbiol.* 70, 1923, 2004.

15. De Vries, W. and Stouthamer, A., Fermentation of glucose, lactose, galactose, mannitol, and xylose by Bifidobacteria. *J. Bacteriol.* 96, 472, 1968.

16. De Preter, V. et al., Baseline microbiota activity and initial bifidobacteria counts influence responses to prebiotic dosing in healthy subjects. *Aliment. Pharmacol. Therapeut.* 27, 504, 2008.

17. Kim, S.-H., Lee, D.H., and Meyer, D., Supplementation of baby formula with native inulin has a prebiotic effect in formula-fed babies. *Asia Pac. J. Clin. Nutr.* 16, 172, 2007.

18. Ramirez-Farias, C. et al., Effect of inulin on the human gut microbiota: Stimulation of *Bifidobacterium adolescentis* and *Faecalibacterium prausnitzii. Br. J. Nutr.* 101, 541, 2009.

19. Kovatcheva-Datchary, P., Analyzing the functionality of the human intestinal microbiota by stable isotope probing. PhD thesis. Wageningen University, Wageningen, the Netherlands, 2010.

20. Qin, J. et al., A human gut microbial gene catalogue established by metagenomic sequencing. *Nature* 464, 59, 2010.

21. Mortensen, P.B. and Clausen, M.R., Short-chain fatty acids in the human colon: Relation to gastrointestinal health and disease. *Scand. J. Gastroenterol.* 16, 132, 1996.

22. Rowland, I.R., Toxicology of the colon: Role of the intestinal microbiota. In *Human Colonic Bacteria: Role in Nutrition, Physiology and Pathology.* Gibson, G.R. and Macfarlane, G.T., Eds. CRC Press, London, U.K., 1995, p. 155.

23. Macfarlane, S. and Macfarlane, G.T., Proteolysis and amino acid fermentation. In *Human Colonic Bacteria: Role in Nutrition, Physiology and Pathology.* Gibson, G.R. and MacFarlane, G.T., Eds. CRC Press, London, U.K., 1995, p. 75.

24. Hambley, R.J. et al., Effect of high- and low-risk diets on gut microflora-associated biomarkers of colon cancer in human flora-associated rats. *Nutr. Cancer* 27, 250, 1997.

25. Matsui, T. et al., Effect of ammonia on cell-cycle progression of human gastric cancer cells. *Eur. J. Gastroenterol. Hepatol.* 7, S79, 1995.

26. Roediger, W.E. et al., Reducing sulphur compounds of the colon impair colonocytes nutrition: Implications for ulcerative colitis. *Gastroenterol.* 104, 802, 1993.
27. Deguchi, Y., Morishita, T., and Mutai, M., Comparative studies on synthesis of water-soluble vitamins among human species of Bifidobacteria. *Agric. Biol. Chem.* 49, 13, 1985.
28. Marteau, P. et al., Effects of chicory inulin in constipated elderly people: A double-blind controlled trial. *Int. J. Food Sci. Nutr.* 2010. doi:10.3109/09637486.2010.527323.
29. Den Hond, E., Geypens, B., and Ghoos, Y., Effect of high performance chicory inulin on constipation. *Nutr. Res.* 20, 731, 2000.
30. Van den Heuvel, E.G. et al., Oligofructose stimulates calcium absorption in adolescents. *Am. J. Clin. Nutr.* 69, 544, 1999.
31. Abrams, S.A. et al., A combination of prebiotic short- and long-chain inulin-type fructans enhances calcium absorption and bone mineralization in young adolescents. *Am. J. Clin. Nutr.* 82, 471, 2005.
32. Holloway, L. et al., Effects of oligofructose-enriched inulin on intestinal absorption of calcium and magnesium and bone turnover markers in postmenopausal women. *Br. J. Nutr.* 97, 365, 2007.
33. Fooks, L.J. and Gibson, G.R., In vitro investigations of the effect of probiotics and pre-biotics on selected human intestinal pathogens. *FEMS Microbiol. Ecol.* 39, 67, 2009.
34. Cani, P.D., Joly, E., Horsmans, Y., and Delzenne, N.M., Oligofructose promotes satiety in healthy human: A pilot study. *Eur. J. Clin. Nutr.* 60, 567, 2006.
35. Parnell, J.A. and Reimer, R.A., Weight loss during oligofructose supplementation is associated with decreased ghrelin and increased peptide YY in overweight and obese adults. *Am. J. Clin. Nutr.* 89, 1751, 2009.
36. Archer, B.J. et al., Effect of fat replacement by inulin or lupin-kernel fibre on sausage patty acceptability, post-meal perceptions of satiety and food intake in men. *Br. J. Nutr.* 91, 591, 2004.
37. Hunter, J.O., Tuffnell, Q., and Lee, A.J., Controlled trial of oligofructose in the management of irritable bowel syndrome. *J. Nutr.* 129(7 Suppl), 1451S, 1999.
38. Olesen, M. and Gudmand-Hoyer, E., Efficacy, safety, and tolerability of fructooligo-saccharides in the treatment of irritable bowel syndrome. *Am. J. Clin. Nutr.* 72, 1570, 2000.
39. Lindsay, J.O. et al., Clinical, microbiological, and immunological effects of fructo-oligosaccharide in patients with Crohn's disease. *Gut* 55, 348, 2006.
40. Casellas, F. et al., Oral oligofructose-enriched inulin supplementation in acute ulcerative colitis is well tolerated and associated with lowered faecal calprotectin. *Aliment. Pharmacol. Ther.* 25, 106, 2007.
41. Welters, C.F. et al., Effect of dietary inulin supplementation on inflammation of pouch mucosa in patients with an ileal pouch-anal anastomosis. *Dis. Colon. Rectum.* 45, 621, 2002.
42. Kerckhoffs, A.P. et al., Lower Bifidobacteria counts in both duodenal mucosa-associated and fecal microbiota in irritable bowel syndrome patients. *World J. Gastroenterol.* 15, 2997, 2009.
43. Paineau, D. et al., The effects of regular consumption of short-chain fructo- oligo-saccharides on digestive comfort of subjects with minor functional bowel disorders. *Br. J. Nutr.* 99, 311, 2008.
44. Dahl, W.J., Tumback, L.H., and Zello, G.A., Inulin supplementation and quality of life in ileal pouch patients. Abstracts Fourth International Dietary Fibre Conference, Vienna, Austria, July 4–7, 2009, P1/03, 2009, p. 93.
45. Furrie, E. et al., Synbiotic therapy (Bifidobacterium longum/synergy 1) initiates resolution of inflammation in patients with active ulcerative colitis: A randomised controlled pilot trial. *Gut* 54, 242, 2005.

46. Colecchia, A. et al., Symbiotic study group. Effect of a symbiotic preparation on the clinical manifestations of irritable bowel syndrome, constipation-variant. Results of an open, uncontrolled multicenter study. *Minerva. Gastroenterol. Dietol.* 52, 349, 2006.

47. Chermesh, I. et al., Failure of synbiotic 2000 to prevent postoperative recurrence of Crohn's disease. *Dig. Dis. Sci.* 52, 385, 2007.

48. Moro, G. et al., A mixture of prebiotic oligosaccharides reduces the incidence of atopic dermatitis during the first six months of age. *Arch. Dis. Child* 91, 814, 2006.

49. Hong, P.Y. et al., Comparative analysis of fecal microbiota in infants with and without eczema. *PLoS ONE* 5, e9964, 2010. doi:10.1371/journal.pone.0009964.

50. Ley, R. et al., Obesity alters gut microbial ecology. *Proc. Nat. Acad. Sci. USA* 102, 11070, 2005.

51. Kalliomäki, M. et al., Early differences in fecal microbiota composition in children may predict overweight. *Am. J. Clin. Nutr.* 87, 534, 2008.

52. Cani, P.D. and Delzenne, N.M., The role of the gut microbiota in energy metabolism and metabolic disease. *Curr. Pharmaceut. Design* 15, 1546, 2009.

53. Saavedra, J.M. and Tschernia, A., Human studies with probiotics and prebiotics: Clinical implications. *Br. J. Nutr.* 87(Suppl 2), S241, 2002.

54. Duggan, C. et al., Oligofructose-supplemented infant cereal: 2 Randomized, blinded, community-based trials in Peruvian infants. *Am. J. Clin. Nutr.* 77, 937, 2003.

55. Bunout, D. et al., Effects of prebiotics on the immune response to vaccination in the elderly. *J. Parenter. Enteral. Nutr.* 26, 372, 2002.

56. Bakker-Zierikzee, A.M. et al., Faecal SIgA secretion in infants fed on pre- or probiotic infant formula. *Pediatr. Allergy Immunol.* 17, 134, 2006.

57. Albers, R. et al., Markers to measure immunomodulation in human nutrition intervention studies. *Br. J. Nutr.* 94, 452, 2005.

58. Langkamp-Henken, B. et al., Nutritional formula improved immune profiles of seniors living in nursing homes. *J. Am. Geriatr. Soc.* 54, 1861, 2006.

59. Langkamp-Henken, B. et al., Nutritional formula enhanced immune function and reduced days of symptoms of upper respiratory tract infection in seniors. *J. Am. Geriatr. Soc.* 52, 3, 2004.

60. Schiffrin, E.J. et al., Systemic inflammatory markers in older persons: The effect of oral nutritional supplementation with prebiotics. *J. Nutr. Health Aging* 11, 475, 2007.

61. Guigoz, Y., Rochat, F., and Perruisseau-Carrier, G., Effects of oligosaccharide on the faecal flora and non-specific immune system in elderly people. *Nutr. Res.* 22, 13, 2002.

62. Waligora-Dupriet, A.J. et al., Effect of oligofructose supplementation on gut microflora and well-being in young children attending a day care centre. *Int. J. Food. Microbiol.* 113, 108, 2007.

63. Juffrie, M., Fructooligosaccharide and diarrhea. *Biosci. Microflora* 21, 31, 2002.

64. Widjojo, S.R. et al., The effect of FOS supplementation to complementary feeding in diarrhea cases and growth in baby 6–12 months. *Gizi Indonesia* 29, 76, 2006.

65. Arslanoglu, S., Moro, G.E., and Boehm, G., Early supplementation of prebiotic oligosaccharides protects formula-fed infants against infections during the first 6 months of life. *J. Nutr.* 137, 2420, 2007.

66. Arslanoglu, S. et al., Early dietary intervention with a mixture of prebiotic oligosaccharides reduces the incidence of allergic manifestations and infections during the first two years of life. *J. Nutr.* 138, 1091, 2008.

67. Bruzzese, E. et al., A formula containing galacto- and fructo-oligosaccharides prevents intestinal and extra-intestinal infections: An observational study. *Clin. Nutr.* 28, 156, 2009.

68. Cummings, J.H., Christie, S., and Cole, T.J., A study of fructo oligosaccharides in the prevention of travellers' diarrhoea. *Aliment. Pharmacol. Ther.* 15, 1139, 2001.

69. Macfarlane, S., Macfarlane, G.T., and Cummings, J.H., Review article: Prebiotics in the gastrointestinal tract. *Aliment. Pharmacol. Ther.* 24, 701, 2006.
70. Lewis, S., Burmeister, S., and Brazier, J., Effect of the prebiotic oligofructose on relapse of *Clostridium difficile*-associated diarrhea: A randomized, controlled study. *Clin. Gastroenterol. Hepatol.* 3, 442, 2005.
71. Lewis, S. et al., Failure of dietary oligofructose to prevent antibiotic-associated diarrhoea. *Aliment. Pharmacol. Ther.* 21, 469, 2005.
72. Maslowski, K.M. et al., Regulation of inflammatory responses by gut microbiota and chemoattractant receptor GPR43. *Nature* 461, 1282, 2009.
73. Vanhoutvin, S.A. et al., Butyrate-induced transcriptional changes in human colonic mucosa. *PLoS One* 4, e6759, 2009.
74. Abreu, M.T., Toll-like receptor signalling in the intestinal epithelium: How bacterial recognition shapes intestinal function. *Nat. Rev. Immunol.* 10, 131, 2010.
75. Sokol, H. et al., *Faecalibacterium prausnitzii* is an anti-inflammatory commensal bacterium identified by gut microbiota analysis of Crohn disease patients. *Proc. Natl. Acad. Sci. USA* 105, 16731, 2008.

14

Digesta Viscosity and Glucose Behavior in the Small Intestine Lumen

TORU TAKAHASHI, MARI NOBORIKAWA, SEN-ICHI ODA,
SATOMI MARUYAMA, TOMOKO KODA, MIKI TOKUNAGA,
MITSUKO NAOI, and KAZUNARI KITAMORI

Contents

14.1 Introduction

The types of flow behavior of digesta in the intestinal lumen, such as turbulence and laminar flow, can indicate the modes of digestion and absorption. This chapter presents a simulation of flow behavior in the intestinal lumen and considers the behavior of nutrients and enzymes in the intestinal lumen under laminar flow conditions. We then discuss the significance of digesta viscosity in glucose behavior in the intestinal lumen, which is the main modulator of glucose absorption.

14.2 Flow Behavior and Mixing of Digesta

The behavior of glucose in the lumen can be described by the extent of mixing of glucose in digesta on a molecular scale, which is called "micromixing" [1]. Micromixing represents the molecular movement of substrates and enzymes, which directly influences chemical reactions and absorption [1]. The extent of glucose micromixing can be estimated by the flow behavior of digesta in the intestinal lumen, such as turbulence and laminar flow, which can be determined using the Reynolds number for flow of non-Newtonian fluid. Although Reynolds number has been estimated based on a Newtonian model using the viscous properties of non-Newtonian fluids [2], this approach is too simplistic to capture non-Newtonian flow behavior [2]. Our 2005 study was the first to estimate the Reynolds number for the flow of non-Newtonian fluids accurately [3].

The micromixing of digesta in the lumen may occur rapidly through turbulence or slowly through diffusion, which occurs only in the presence of laminar flow [3,4]. In rapid micromixing characterized by turbulence, the influence of the translocation rate of glucose in the lumen on the overall absorption rate can be ignored, as the glucose can be translocated to the epithelial surface at a rate exceeding that of absorption [3,5]. In other words, the overall absorption rate should depend on the transepithelial transport rate (Equation 14.1),

$$\text{(Overall absorption rate)} = a(\text{Transepithelial transport rate}), \qquad (14.1)$$

where a is a constant. This should result in a homogenous concentration of glucose across the intestine. However, in vivo measurement of short-chain fatty acid concentrations and microbiota distributions across the contents of the cecum and colon does not support such homogenous conditions. The short-chain fatty acid concentration of the intestinal contents is higher in the core than at the periphery, and the microbiota at the periphery of the contents differs from that at the core [6,7].

Conversely, glucose can reach the epithelium via diffusion in laminar flow (Figure 14.1) [3]. If the diffusion rate of glucose in the lumen is lower than its transepithelial absorption rate, the overall absorption rate of the glucose should be proportional to either its diffusion rate in the lumen or its membrane transport rate. The slower of these two factors is the rate-limiting factor for the overall absorption process. Considering the mentioned short-chain fatty acid gradient and heterogeneous distribution of microbiota across the intestinal lumen [6,7], the diffusion rate in the lumen should be slower than the membrane transport rate. Therefore, the diffusion rate of glucose in the lumen should correlate with the overall absorption rate in laminar flow (Equation 14.2):

$$\text{(Overall absorption rate)} = b(\text{Diffusion rate in lumen}), \qquad (14.2)$$

where b is a constant.

The flow behavior of digesta in the lumen can be estimated using the Reynolds number, which expresses the ratio of inertial forces to viscous forces in a fluid [8]. The inertial force is the tendency of the fluid to stay in motion or at rest unless acted upon by an outside force [9]. The viscous force is an internal property of a fluid that offers resistance to flow [9]. The Reynolds number is used to determine whether a flow will be dominated by inertial or viscous forces, i.e., whether the flow is turbulent or laminar. A Reynolds number below 2300 indicates that viscous force predominates over inertial force to keep the flow laminar (Figure 14.2a), which results in poor micromixing along the transverse axis. Conversely, a Reynolds number exceeding 2300 indicates that inertial force dominates and that the flow has become turbulent [8] (Figure 14.2b), which completely mixes digesta at the molecular level [4].

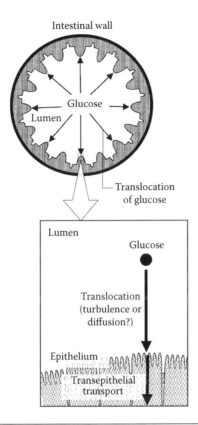

Figure 14.1 Schematic illustration of the possible translocation of glucose to the epithelium in the intestinal lumen.

A vortex can mix a flow moderately by folding the laminar structure of the digesta [4]. Obstructions in the flow can create a Karman vortex (i.e., curl or rotation) in fluids with Reynolds numbers between 40 and 10,000. A Reynolds number below 40 indicates that no Karman vortex is present in the flow downstream from the obstruction [1] (Figure 14.2c). A Reynolds number between 40 and 2300 indicates the existence of a vortex in the laminar flow, suggesting that diffusion is still important for the complete homogenization of the fluid [4]. A vortex is particularly important for macroscopic mixing in laminar flow [3].

To estimate the Reynolds numbers for non-Newtonian fluid, it is necessary to determine the viscosity of the digesta, including particles.

14.3 Viscosity of Digesta Including Particles

The viscosity of digesta has been measured only after removing the particles by centrifugation, under the assumption that particles or insoluble fibers in the diet do not affect the viscosity of the gut contents [10]. However, the complete removal of particles considerably reduces the viscosity of digesta in

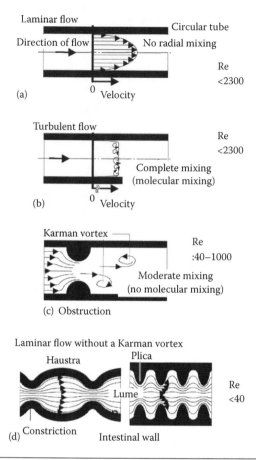

Figure 14.2 Schematic illustration of the flow behavior in a tube. Arrows represent the flow lines for (a) Reynolds number <2300, (b) Reynolds number >2300, (c) Reynolds number 40–9600, and (d) Reynolds number <10.

pigs, chickens, and rats and changes the digesta from a non-Newtonian to a Newtonian fluid [11–14], suggesting that particles are responsible for the basic rheological characteristics of digesta. Furthermore, the addition of particles, such as crystalline cellulose, increases the viscosity of the digesta in vitro [11–14] and in vivo [15]. The viscosity of digesta including particles and that of the digesta supernatant is shown in Figure 14.3 [11–14]. The viscosity of digesta with particles was 500–2800 times greater than the viscosity without particles at a shear rate of $1\,s^{-1}$ ([11–14], Figure 14.3). Larger particles (>1 mm) ($0.35 \pm 0.07\,Pa \cdot s/g$ large particles) have a stronger effect on digesta viscosity than do fine particles ($0.22 \pm 0.03\,Pa \cdot s/g$ large particles) at a shear rate of $1\,s^{-1}$ [4,13]. The water-holding capacity of insoluble fibers increases digesta viscosity [11], which is important for flow behavior in the intestinal lumen and the diffusion of glucose in digesta in the intestinal lumen [16].

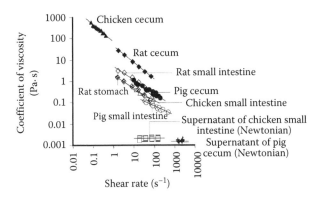

Figure 14.3 Viscosity of digesta with and without particles. The viscosity of digesta with particles was 500–2800 times greater than the viscosity without particles.

14.4 Reynolds Numbers and Flow Behavior Produced by Peristalsis

A mathematical simulation was used to calculate the Reynolds numbers of the flow in the small and large intestines of pigs, chickens, and humans with peristalsis and segmental contraction using the viscosity of digesta including particles [17].

The Reynolds numbers of the flow produced by peristalsis were much lower than 2300 in the small and large intestines of pigs, chickens, rats, and humans (Table 14.1). Reynolds numbers below 10 suggest that the flow of digesta in the intestinal lumen should be laminar and lack a vortex. Therefore, the micromixing of digesta by turbulence was unlikely in the small intestines or ceca examined in this study. The theoretical absence of turbulence implies poor micromixing [4], which supports the validity of Equation 14.2.

At Reynolds numbers below 10 (Table 14.1), a plica, constriction, or haustra should not shed a vortex in the intestine (Figure 14.2d). This suggests that the macroscopic mixing of digesta by a vortex rarely occurs in the small intestine, cecum, or proximal colon. Furthermore, the roughness of the mucosal surface should not alter the frictional drag or disturb the flow of contents in the small and proximal large intestines under laminar flow conditions [18]. Laminar flow without a vortex [18] lacks macroscopic mixing along its transverse axis (Figure 14.2). Glucose should reach the epithelium by diffusion, even with the existence of a plica, constriction, or haustra. In such a situation, the absorption rate should depend on the diffusion rate (Equation 14.2).

14.5 Flow Behavior of the Digesta with Segmentation

Segmental contraction may occur with or without complete constriction. Segmental contraction in the cecum and proximal colon is incomplete, leaving lumen space [19]. Therefore, the calculated Reynolds number of the flow produced by segmental contraction in the cecum and proximal colon of pigs and humans was smaller than 0.5 when the duration exceeded 1 s, given the physiological characteristics of these species [9,20]. Accordingly, this type of segmental contraction should not mix the contents transversally, and the mixture remains incomplete in the intestinal lumen.

Table 14.1 Reynolds Numbers of the Flow Produced by Peristalsis in the Lumen of the Intestine in the Pig, Chicken, and Human

	Radius of the Gastrointestinal Tract (mm)	Velocity of Peristalsis (mm s^{-1})	Shear Rate (s^{-1})	Reynolds Number (Unitless)
Pig				
Small intestine	5.0	18[d]	18	1.0
Cecum	15[b]	11[e]	6.1	0.33
Chicken				
Small intestine	2.5[c]	14[f]	28	0.26
Cecum	4.0[c]	1.0[f]	1.9	0.00010
Human[a]				
Small intestine	7.0[b]	30[d]	29	0.085
Colon	25[b]	10[h]	4.3	0.32

[a] Estimated from the viscosity of pig small intestinal and cecal contents.

[b] Stevens CE, Hume ID (1995) *Comparative Physiology of the Vertebrate Digestive System*, 2nd ed. Cambridge University Press, Cambridge, U.K.

[c] Clark PL (1978) *Br. Poult. Sci.* 19: 595–600.

[d] Hukuhara T (1973) Syoukakan undo no Mekanizumu, pp. 1–16, Tokyo, Japan: Bunkosya.

[e] Cherbut C and Ruckebusch Y (1984) *Br. J. Nutr.* 53: 549–557.

[f] Brummermann M and Braun EJ (1995) *Am. J. Physiol.* 268: R690–R698.

[g] HJ Ehrlein, H Reich and M Schwinger, *Quart. J. Exp. Physiol.* 67: 407–417 (1982).

[h] Crowell MD, Musial F, French W, Kittur D, Anderson D and Whitehead WE (1992) *Physiol. Behav.* 52: 471–474.

Segmental contraction with complete constriction can bring glucose in the center of the lumen into close proximity with the intestinal walls [3]. The laminar flow structure in the lumen should disappear in the area of constriction during a complete segmental contraction. This structure is then reconstructed in the area of constriction upon relaxation. The old laminar structure will be disturbed by this reconstruction in situations characterized by a low Reynolds number, suggesting that moderate mixing occurs in the area of constriction.

There should be no turbulence in complete segmental constriction. As the Reynolds number produced by such constriction should be smaller than 0.5, it is essentially the same as that produced by incomplete constriction. Diffusion in laminar flow is still needed to homogenize the fluid completely [4].

14.6 Behavior of Flow in the Intestinal Lumen and Behavior of Molecules in the Lumen

X-ray computed tomography after a single injection of model digesta containing barium sulfate into the rat ileum or cecum confirmed the poor macroscopic mixing in feces (Takahashi et al. unpublished data). If there is turbulence in the large

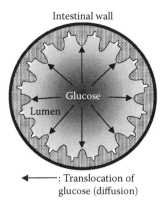

Figure 14.4 Behavior of glucose in the intestinal lumen (cross section). Glucose can reach the epithelium by self-diffusion in laminar flow. The thickness of the black lines represents the glucose concentration.

intestine, then the barium is distributed homogeneously in the feces. Therefore, the heterogeneous distribution of barium in feces suggests the absence of turbulence in the large intestine in vivo (Takahashi et al. unpublished data). Indeed, rapid mixing with turbulence is unlikely to occur in the intestinal lumen [3,7,21–24]. Although folding of digesta is probably induced by segmental contractions of the small intestine and contributes to increased glucose absorption rates [3], the self-diffusion of glucose is an important determinant of the absorption rate because of poor micromixing in the lumen. The diffusion of glucose in the intestinal lumen should depend negatively on the digesta viscosity in laminar flow situations [16]. Therefore, the overall absorption rate is likely to be limited by self-diffusion, rather than by transepithelial transport, because the diffusion rate is slower than the transepithelial transport rate (see Equation 14.2, Figure 14.4) [3].

In laminar flow, greater digesta viscosity should reduce the diffusion rate of glucose in the intestinal lumen and may diminish glucose absorption, decreasing the postprandial blood glucose increment [24]. A greater digesta viscosity may decrease the postprandial blood glucose increment in this way because the digesta viscosity should depend negatively on the diffusion of glucose in the intestinal lumen, as mentioned earlier [24]. Hence, the digesta viscosity is a major modulator of the glucose absorption rate [5,15,24,26].

14.7 Digesta Viscosity and Glucose Absorption

Viscosity is the internal resistance of a fluid to flow [9]. The internal resistance to the flow of digesta is increased by larger water-insoluble fibers, a lower free water content in the digesta, the addition of water-insoluble fibers such as crystalline cellulose, and water-insoluble fibers with greater water-holding capacity; this increase comprises the viscosity of digesta [12,15]. The greater water-holding capacity of fibers can increase the digesta viscosity by decreasing its free water content [15]. Accordingly, the effects of the quantity of water-insoluble fibers, water-holding capacity of fibers, and total and free water contents on the digesta viscosity are not independent [15]. Obviously, water-soluble fibers also increase the digesta viscosity [25], but they should have a synergistic effect in combination with water-insoluble fibers [26]. Furthermore, a synergistic effect on digesta viscosity between water-soluble fibers has also been observed [27]. Therefore, water-insoluble and soluble fibers and the water content of digesta affect digesta viscosity in a complicated manner.

The addition of water-insoluble fibers such as crystalline cellulose to rice or an experimental diet, and of water-soluble fibers such as guar gum or hydro-lyzed guar gum to the experimental diet, decreased the absorption rate of glucose and therefore postprandial blood glucose levels in rats and humans [5,24,26]. We confirmed the depressed diffusion rate of glucose in the intestinal lumen with greater digesta viscosity after the addition of water-soluble fibers [26].

14.8 Depressive Effects of Crystalline Cellulose on the Diffusion in the Intestinal Lumen

Under conditions where (1) laminar flow exists in the intestinal lumen, (2) glucose is translocated by diffusion in the digesta, and (3) the diffusion rate of glucose in the digesta is the rate-limiting factor for the overall glucose absorption (Equation 14.2), as mentioned earlier, a glucose concentration gradient should exist in the intestinal lumen along the radial axis. Glucose in the peripheral lumen should reach the epithelium quicker than that in the center of the lumen because the translocation distance from the center is greater than that at the periphery, and the diffusion rate is slower (Figure 14.5). The existence of a

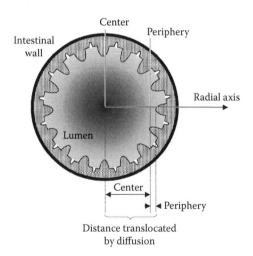

Figure 14.5 Diffusion of glucose in the small intestinal lumen and distance of translocation of glucose (cross section). Glucose in the periphery reaches the epithelium quicker than that in the center. Therefore, the glucose concentration in the periphery is lower than that in the center. Accordingly, a glucose gradient should exist along the radial axis in the small intestinal lumen.

glucose gradient along the radial axis of the small intestinal lumen confirms the validity of the three conditions, i.e., the presence of laminar flow in the lumen, translocation of glucose by diffusion in the lumen, and the predominance of glucose diffusion in the overall glucose absorption. Furthermore, if the three conditions are valid, greater digesta viscosity should make the glucose gradient steeper in the lumen because the diffusion should depend negatively on the viscosity of the digesta [16]. Therefore, we observed the glucose gradient in the intestinal lumen along the radial axis and effect of digesta viscosity on the glucose gradient.

The glucose concentration in the center of the rat small intestinal lumen was higher than that in the periphery in the lumen without crystalline cellulose (Takahashi et al. unpublished data), which supported the validity of (1) the presence of laminar flow in the lumen, (2) the translocation of glucose by diffusion in the lumen, and (3) the predominance of glucose diffusion in the overall glucose absorption.

The glucose gradient in the lumen with high digesta viscosity caused by the addition of crystalline cellulose was steeper than that without crystalline cellulose, which suggested that the digesta viscosity decreased the overall glucose absorption and reduced diffusion of glucose in the digesta in the intestinal lumen. This again supports Equation 14.2 and the earlier three conditions.

14.9 Conclusion

The flow behavior in the intestinal lumen reflects the basal physiological environment in the intestinal lumen. The Reynolds numbers of flow in the intestinal lumen suggest that this flow is laminar. Based on this laminar flow, the luminal environment can explain the mode of glucose absorption. The heterogeneous radial distribution of glucose in the small intestinal lumen can verify the validity of the existence of laminar flow and suggests a way of controlling glucose absorption with high digesta viscosity by decreasing glucose diffusion in the lumen.

Acknowledgment

We thank Prof. T. Sakata of Department of Basic Sciences, Ishinomaki Senshu University for his creative suggestions. This study was supported by a Grant-in-Aid for Scientific Research (No. 22592353).

References

1. Potter, M.C. and Wiggert, D.C., *Mechanics of Fluids*, Prentice Hall, Englewood Cliffs, NJ, 1991. p. 317.
2. Lentle, R.G. and Jansen, P.W., Physical characteristics of digesta and their influence on flow and mixing in the mammalian intestine: A review. *J. Comp. Physiol. B*, 178, 673, 2008.
3. Takahashi, T. and Sakata, T., Insoluble dietary fibers: The major modulator for the viscosity and flow behavior of digesta. *Foods Food Ingredients J. Jpn.*, 210, 944, 2005.

4. Baldyage, J. and Bourne, J.R., Flow phenomena and measurement, In: *Encyclopedia of Fluid Mechanics* (Cheremisinoff NP, eds.), Vol. 1, Gulf Publishing Company, Houston, TX, 1986. p. 148.

5. Takahashi, T., Cellulose, In: *The Handbook of Fiber Ingredients: Health Benefits, Food Applications, and Analysis* (Cho S, ed.), CRC Press, Boca Raton, FL, 2009. p. 263.

6. Yajima, T. and Sakata, T., Core and periphery concentrations of short-chain fatty acids in luminal contents of the rat colon. *Comp. Biochem. Physiol. Comp. Physiol.*, 103, 353, 1992.

7. Takahashi, T., Karita, S., Yahaya, M.S., and Goto, M., Radial and axial variations of bacteria within the cecum and proximal colon of guinea pigs revealed by PCR-DGGE. *Biosci. Biotechnol. Biochem.*, 69, 1790, 2005.

8. Huttula, T., Krogerus, K.Z., and Virtanen, M., Surface and groundwater flow phenomena, In: *Encyclopedia of Fluid Mechanics* (Cheremisinoff NP, ed.), Vol. 10, Gulf Publishing Company, Houston, TX, 1990. p. 212.

9. Sherman, F.S., *Viscous Flow*, McGraw-Hill, Inc., Columbus, OH, 1990. p. 3.

10. Johansen, H., Bach Knudsen, K.E., Sandstrom, B., and Skjoth, F., Effects of varying content of soluble dietary fiber from wheat flour and oat milling fractions on gastric emptying in pigs. *Br. J. Nutr.*, 75, 339, 1996.

11. Takahashi, T. and Sakata, T., Large particles increase viscosity and yield stress of pig cecal contents without changing basic viscoelastic properties. *J. Nutr.*, 132, 1026, 2002.

12. Takahashi, T., Yamanaka, N., Sakata, T., and Ogawa, N., Influences of solid particles on the viscous properties of intestinal contents and intestinal tissue weight in rats. *Nippon Eiyo Shokuryo Gakkaishi (J. Jpn. Soc. Nutr. Food Sci.)*, 56, 199, 2003.

13. Takahashi, T. and Sakata, T., Viscous properties of pig cecal contents and the contribution of solid particles to viscosity. *Nutrition*, 20, 377, 2004.

14. Takahashi, T., Goto, M., and Sakata, T., Viscoelastic properties of the small intestinal and caecal contents of the chicken. *Br. J. Nutr.*, 91, 867, 2004.

15. Takahashi, T. et al., Water-holding capacity of insoluble fibre decreases free water and elevates digesta viscosity in the rat. *J. Sci. Food Agri.*, 89, 245, 2009.

16. Brouwer, A.C. and Kirsch, J.F., Investigation of diffusion-limited rates of chymotrypsin reactions by viscosity variation. *Biochemistry*, 21, 1302, 1982.

17. Borghesani, A.F., Rheology and non-Newtonian flows, in: *Encyclopedia of Fluid Mechanics* (Cheremisinoff NP, ed.), Vol. 7, Gulf Publishing Company, Houston, TX, 1988. p. 89.

18. Cheremisinoff, N.P., Encyclopedia of fluid mechanics, in: *Flow Phenomena and Measurement*, Vol. 1, Gulf Publishing Company, Houston, TX, 1986. p. 285.

19. Berne, R.M. and Levy, M.N., *Physiology*, 3rd edn. Mosby-Year Book, Inc., 1993. p. 615.

20. Ruckebusch, Y. and Fioramonti, J., Motor profile of the ruminant colon: Hard vs soft faeces production. *Experientia*, 36, 1184, 1980.

21. Takahashi, T. and Sakaguchi, E., Behaviors and nutritional importance of coprophagy in captive adult and young nutrias (*Myocastor coypus*). *J. Comp. Physiol. B*, 168, 281, 1998.

22. Takahashi, T. and Sakaguchi, E., Role of the furrow of the proximal colon in the production of soft and hard feces in nutrias, *Myocastor coypus*. *J. Comp. Physiol. B*, 170, 531, 2000.

23. Takahashi, T. and Sakaguchi, E., Transport of bacteria across and along the large intestinal lumen of guinea pigs. *J. Comp. Physiol. B*, 176, 173, 2006.

24. Takahashi, T. et al., Crystalline cellulose decreases blood glucose increment and stimulates water absorption associated with digesta viscosity in the rat. *J. Nutr.*, 135, 245, 2005.
25. Anderson, B.W., Kneip, J.M., Levine, A.S., and Levitt, M.D., Influence of infusate viscosity on intestinal absorption in the rat. An explanation of previous discrepant results. *Gastroenterology*, 97, 938, 1989.
26. Takahashi, T. et al., Hydrolyzed guar gum decreases postprandial blood glucose and glucose absorption in the rat small intestine. *Nutr. Res.*, 29, 419, 2009.
27. Vuksan, V. et al., Viscosity of fiber preloads affects food intake in adolescents. *Nutr. Metab. Cardiovasc. Dis.*, 19, 498, 2009.

15

Manipulating Dietary Intake of Poorly Absorbed and Fermentable Short-Chain Carbohydrates (FODMAPs)

Implications for Laxation and Gastrointestinal Health

JANE G. MUIR, SUSAN J. SHEPHERD, JACQUELINE S. BARRETT,
SHAYLYN B. MITCHELL, DERRICK K. ONG,
ROSEMARY ROSE, OURIANA ROSELLA, CHU K. YAO,
EMMA P. HALMOS, J.R. BIESIEKIERSKI, and PETER R. GIBSON

Contents

15.1 Introduction

Whole grain cereals, legumes, fruit, and vegetables contain a wide range of carbohydrates essential for health. While carbohydrates are a diverse and complex family of compounds, the major classes of importance to human nutrition are sugars (glucose, sucrose, fructose) and sugar polyols (sorbitol and mannitol), oligosaccharides especially galactooligosaccharides (GOS) and fructooligosaccharides (FOS), and the polysaccharides (starch and nonstarch polysaccharides [NSP]) and resistant starch (RS).[1–3]

In relation to the health of the gastrointestinal tract, the long-chain indigestible carbohydrates—NSP (dietary fiber) and RS—have attracted a great deal of worldwide research attention. Over the last decade, the short-chain carbohydrates—FOS and GOS—have also become a major area of research interest.

Many of the physiological properties attributed to the short-chain and long-chain carbohydrates relate to the location and extent of absorption and fermentation.

Carbohydrates can vary greatly in the site and extent to which they are digested and absorbed. Reasons why some carbohydrates are variably absorbed in the small intestine include (i) the absence of certain brush border hydrolase enzymes (e.g., lactase), (ii) the absence of luminal enzymes capable of hydrolyzing the glycosidic linkages in certain short-chain carbohydrate (e.g., GOS), and (iii) the efficiency of various transporter mechanisms (e.g., glucose transporter [GLUT], GLUT-2 and GLUT-5 for fructose) or via passive diffusion (e.g., polyols).[4,5]

15.1.1 FODMAPs: Poorly Absorbed, Rapidly Fermented Short-Chain Carbohydrates

We have recently described a large group of short-chain carbohydrates that can be poorly absorbed by the small intestine and collectively termed these FODMAPs (i.e., fermentable oligo-, di-, and monosaccharides and polyols).[5-7] FODMAPs are found in a wide variety of foods and include lactose (in milk), free fructose (in pears, apples), fructans (polymers of fructose) and FOS (in artichoke, garlic, onions, rye, and wheat), GOS (in legumes), and sugar polyols (e.g., sorbitol, mannitol found in stone fruits and artificial sweeteners).[5-7] FODMAPs may have wide-ranging effects on gastrointestinal health, and this area clearly requires more research attention.

The monosaccharide, fructose, is one of the major FODMAPs present in the Western diet.[4,8] It is present in high levels in fruits, fruit juices, honey, and high fructose corn syrup.[9] The absorption of fructose across the villous epithelium is via a low capacity, carrier-mediated facilitated diffusion GLUT5 (fructose transporter GLUT5).[10,11] This low capacity to absorb fructose can result in its malabsorption. Interestingly, the absorption of free fructose is markedly enhanced in the presence of luminal glucose, and this effect is probably mediated via the low affinity, facultative transporter—GLUT2 (GLUT, GLUT2).[10,11] The capacity of free glucose to enhance the absorption of fructose could be used to minimize the malabsorption of fructose. For this reason, it is important to know the quantity of fructose present in excess of glucose in a food to predict the potential for malabsorption. It should be noted that malabsorption of fructose occurs in healthy people at the same frequency as in people with functional gut disorders (at around 34%) and should not be considered an abnormality.[12]

15.1.1.1 Quantifying Level of FODMAPs in Foods

We have developed the analytical techniques that can be used to quantify levels of these FODMAPs in foods.[13,14] Total fructan levels (i.e., oligo- and polysaccharides consisting of short chains of fructose units with a single D-glucosyl unit at the nonreducing end) are measured using the enzymatic hydrolysis method described and now commercially available in kit form (Megazyme Fructan HK Assay kit).[13] Other short-chain carbohydrates of interest (i.e., fructose, glucose, lactose, sorbitol, mannitol, stachyose, raffinose) are separated and quantified using high-performance liquid chromatography (HPLC) with evaporative light scattering detection (ELSD).[14] These analytical approaches have been used to quantify levels of FODMAPs in common Australian vegetables and fruit and more recently in grains, cereal, and breads.[13-15] The data shown in Table 15.1 provide examples of the major FODMAPs measured in a range of fruit, vegetables, grains, cereal, and breads (Table 15.1).[13-15]

Table 15.1 Short-Chain Carbohydrates Separated via HPLC with ELSD, Total Fructans (via Megazyme Fructan Assay), and Total FODMAPs in Foods (g/Average Serve Size)

Food	Serve (g)	Short-Chain Carbohydrates via HPLC with ELSD[a]								Total Fructan via Megazyme Fructan Assay[c]	Total[d] FODMAP
		Mono- and Disaccharides				Sugar Polyols			GOS		
		Fructose	Glucose	Excess Fructose[b]	Lactose	Sorbitol	Mannitol	Raffinose	Stachyose		
Vegetables											
Artichoke	50	1.04	0.29	0.76	0	0	0	0	0	6.10	6.86
Garlic	3	tr	tr	tr	0	0	0	0	0	0.52	0.52
Onion	16	0.28	0.66	0	0	0	0	0.03	0	0.32	0.35
Broccoli	47	0.13	0.32	0	0	0.18	0	0	0.06	0.07	0.31
Mushroom	74	0	0	0	0	0.08	2.13	0	0	0.20	2.41
Sugar pea	60	1.99	0.35	1.64	0	0	0	tr	0	0.02	1.66
Fruit											
Apple	165	2.64	1.67	0.97	0	1.53	0	0	0	tr	2.50
Pear	165	5.48	1.82	366	0	3.76	0	0	0	nd	7.42
Avocado	60	0.10	0.42	0	0	0.39	0	0	0	0	0.39
Blackberry	100	1.51	2.87	0	0	4.07	0	0	0	nd	4.07
Cherries	84	4.31	3.70	0.61	0	0.45	0	0	0	0	1.06
Nectarine	151	0.94	2.25	0	0	1.54	0	0	0	0.89	2.45

(continued)

Table 15.1 (continued) Short-Chain Carbohydrates Separated via HPLC with ELSD, Total Fructans (via Megazyme Fructan Assay), and Total FODMAPs in Foods (g/Average Serve Size)

| | | Short-Chain Carbohydrates via HPLC with ELSD[a] | | | | | | | | | Total Fructan via Megazyme Fructan Assay[c] | Total[d] FODMAP |
| | | Mono- and Disaccharides | | | | Sugar Polyols | | GOS | | | |
Food	Serve (g)	Fructose	Glucose	Excess Fructose[b]	Lactose	Sorbitol	Mannitol	Raffinose	Stachyose		
Nuts											
Pistachios	23	tr	tr	0	0	0	0	0.81	0	0.21	1.02
Legumes (cooked)											
Borlotti	91	tr	tr	0	nd	nd	nd	0.44	0.47	0.12	1.03
Kidney	95	0.03	0.04	0	nd	nd	nd	0.23	1.10	0.51	1.84
Grains (cooked)											
Couscous	154	0.02	0.05	0	nd	nd	tr	nd	nd	1.12	1.12
Pasta, wheat	148	tr	tr	0	nd	nd	nd	nd	nd	0.50	0.50
Rice, white	190	tr	tr	0	nd	nd	nd	nd	nd	nd	0

Cereals											
All bran	32	0.35	0.19	0.18	nd	nd	nd	0.43	nd	0.76	1.37
Cornflakes	30	0.34	0.40	0	nd	nd	nd	tr	nd	0.32	0.32
Rice bubbles	30	0.34	0.40	0	nd	nd	nd	tr	nd	0.31	0.31
Muesli	55	6.91	8.87	0	nd	0.07	nd	0.19	tr	0.69	0.95
Breads											
Rye	42	0.16	0.05	0.11	tr	nd	nd	0.10	nd	0.44	0.65
White	49	0.13	0.05	0.08	tr	tr	tr	0.10	nd	0.33	0.51
Multigrain	68	0.13	0.15	0	nd	nd	nd	0.26	nd	0.38	0.64
Gluten free	52	0.24	0.11	0.12	nd	tr	tr	0.07	nd	0.10	0.29

Sources: Adapted from Muir, J.G. et al., *J. Agric. Food Chem.,* 55, 6619, 2007; Muir, J.G. et al., *J. Agric. Food Chem.,* 57, 554, 2009; Biesiekierski, J.R. et al., *J. Hum. Nutr. Diet.,* in press, 2010.

nd, not detected; tr, trace amounts detected only.

[a] Fructose, glucose, sorbitol, and mannitol data were obtained from the Sugar Pak Column; data for lactose, GOS (raffinose and stachyose), and FOS (nystose and kestose) were obtained using the high performance column.

[b] Excess fructose = fructose − glucose.

[c] Total fructan levels were determined using the Megazyme Fructan Assay kit.

[d] Total FODMAP = excess fructose + lactose + sorbitol + mannitol + raffinose + stachyose + total fructan.

FODMAPs are clearly found naturally in a wide range of vegetable, fruits, grains, and cereals.[13-15] These short-chain carbohydrates may have important implications for the proper functioning and health of the gastrointestinal tract. Good food composition knowledge will also provide us with the knowledge to design dietary trials to investigate the physiological effects of FODMAP sugars in the diet.

15.1.2 Role of FODMAPs in Health

15.1.2.1 Prebiotic Effects of FODMAPs Fructans and GOS are examples of FODMAPs that have attracted research interest worldwide. Fructans include FOS, with degree of polymerization (DP) of 2–9 units, and inulin (DP ≥ 10) and GOS include stachyose, raffinose, and verbascose. The beneficial effects of FOS/inulin and GOS have been attributed to their malabsorption in the small intestine and delivery of carbohydrate to the large bowel, where they undergo rapid fermentation by bacteria with the subsequent expansion of bacterial population—bifidobacteria and lactobacilli.[16-18] These bacteria are believed to mediate a wide range of responses.

It is important to note, however, that the majority of these studies have been undertaken with pure sources of these FOS and inulin sugars (mostly from chicory and artichoke) and very few studies have been undertaken in this area using fructans—FOS and inulin—that are naturally present in the diet. The information shown in Table 15.1 shows the total fructan and GOS levels in a range of foods. Many foods contain significant amounts of both fructans and GOS, e.g., nuts, legumes, grains, and cereals. The richest sources of fructans (gram/serve) were artichoke > garlic > onion > nectarine > all bran > muesli. For GOS, the legumes and nuts were the richest source. Some foods contain both GOS and fructans (legumes and some cereals).[13-15]

The physiological benefits of prebiotics have been reportedly achieved at around the dose range of 3.5–7 g per day using purified prebiotic FOS/inulin and GOS sugars.[18] The data in Table 15.1 clearly shows that food that will be naturally high in prebiotic fructans and GOS that include dark rye, couscous, pulses, onions, and garlic. A dose of around 7 g per day could be reached easily by ½ cup of couscous (1.1 g), 23 g pistachio nuts (1.02 g), 1 cup of pasta (0.50 g), 2 slices of dark rye bread (1.1 g), and 32 g serve of onion (2.02 g) plus a 6 g serve of garlic (1.04 g).[13-15]

It is also possible that many of the physiological and postulated health effects of fructans/FOS and GOS may also be mimicked by other FODMAPs, and clearly more research is required in this area.

15.1.2.2 Laxation Effects of FODMAPs FODMAPs have a number of physiological effects in the bowel that may contribute to healthy gut functioning and laxation. The relatively small molecular size of FODMAPs has led to the suggestion that FODMAPs as part of the diet are osmotically active and promote the movement of water into the lumen (see Figure 15.1).

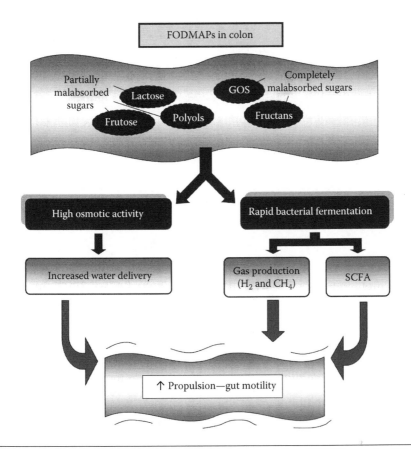

Figure 15.1 Possible consequences of malabsorption and fermentation of FODMAPs on gut motility.

15.1.2.2.1 Effects of Water Movement into the Lumen We have recent evidence for this in a study we conducted in individuals with an ileostomy.[19] In this study, 12 volunteers were randomized to two 4 day dietary periods, comprising diets differing only in FODMAP content (low versus high). The aim of this study was to determine the effect of dietary FODMAPs on the volume of ileal effluent. All food was provided to study participants (an example of the types of foods used during the low and high FODMAP dietary periods is shown in Table 15.2).[19] The macronutrient content, total dietary fiber, and RS content of the two test diets were the same.[19]

The daytime ileal effluent (14 h) was collected hourly and frozen immediately on day 4 of each diet. The FODMAP content of the diet and effluent was measured by enzymatic and HPLC methods. The results showed that of the ingested FODMAPs, 32% were recovered in the high FODMAP diet effluent. In addition, the weight of the effluent collected increased in the high FODMAP dietary period by a mean of 22% ($P = 0.01$), including water volume by 20% ($P = 0.013$) and dry weight by 24% ($P = 0.028$). There was also a significant ($P = 0.018$) positive correlation ($r = 0.72$)

Table 15.2 Example of a Low and High FODMAP Diet

Meal	Low FODMAP Diet	High FODMAP Diet
Breakfast	Rice flakes	Weet-Bix
	Lactose-free milk	Low fat milk
	Corn/rice bread	Rye bread
	Jam	Honey
	Orange cordial	Apple juice
	Tea/coffee with lactose-free milk	Tea/coffee with milk
Morning tea	Orange	Pear
Lunch	Rice/corn pasta with bolognese sauce[a]	Durum wheat pasta with bolognese sauce[a]
	Lemonade sweetened with sucrose	Soda sweetened with high fructose corn syrup
Afternoon tea	Mandarin	Apple
Dinner	Salmon patties	Vegetable patties[b]
	Cheddar cheese	Lettuce leaves
	Lettuce leaves	Spanish onion rings
	Slices tomato	Cottage cheese
	Slices cucumber	
	Sucrose-containing chewing gum	Sorbitol-containing chewing gum

Source: Adapted from a table, see Ong, D.K et al., *J. Gastroenterol. Hepatol.* 25, 1366, 2010.

[a] Low FODMAP bolognese sauce made without using onion, garlic, or mushroom; high FODMAP bolognese sauce made including onion, garlic, and mushroom and also a small quantity of Jerusalem artichokes were added.

[b] High FODMAP vegetable patties contain canned chickpeas, onion, and garlic.

between the output water volume and the total FODMAP content of the output.[19] These data support the hypothetical mechanism that FODMAPs increase delivery of fermentable substrate and water to the proximal colon.

15.1.2.2.2 Effects of Gas Generation and SCFA on Gut Motility   Another consequence of the fermentation of FODMAPs in the gastrointestinal tract relates to the other important by-products of colonic fermentation including short-chain fatty acids (SCFA) (acetate, propionate, and butyrate) and gases (H_2, CO_2, CH_4).[20,21] Gases generated in the lumen can have a wide range of effects on gut motility. Certainly the volume of gas that is generated in the colon will assist in propulsion along the gut—but is becoming clearer that the type of response may in turn depend on the nature of the gas (e.g., H_2 or CH_4) present in the lumen.

We have recently published a study involving 15 healthy individuals and 15 individuals with irritable bowel syndrome (IBS).[22] These volunteers were supplied with two experimental diets that varied only in FODMAP content while leaving the total dietary fiber and RS the same.[22] The two test diets that were either low (9 g/day) or high (50 g/day) in FODMAPs were given for 2 days each, and breath gas samples were collected on day 2. The results demonstrated clearly that a diet high in poorly absorbed short-chain carbohydrates—FODMAP—produced a large and sustained increase in breath hydrogen across the day in both healthy individuals (181 ± 77 ppm.14h vs. 43 ± 18; mean $\pm$ SD $P < 0.0001$) and in patients with IBS (242 ± 79 vs. 62 ± 23; $P < 0.0001$).[22]

Interesting changes in the production of methane gas were also evident from this study. For 10 healthy subjects who were "methane producers," the production of breath methane was lower during the high FODMAP dietary periods compared to the low FODMAP dietary period (47 ± 29 vs. 109 ± 77; $P = 0.043$).[22]

Pimentel and colleagues demonstrated that methane perfusion into the distal small bowel of dogs slowed intestinal transit.[23] They suggested that as with other potent gases (NO, H_2S, CO_2), CH_4 may have major implications in the control of certain physiological processes.[24] Certainly the production of methane gas has been strongly associated with constipation.[25,26] Factors that influence the balance of certain gases in the colonic lumen may in turn impact on the laxation process, and this area requires more investigation.

It is also well known that SCFA (acetate, propionate, and butyrate) can impact on sodium and water movement.[27] SCFA may also influence directly gut motility by acting as chemical stimuli.[28,29] There does appear to be a complex relationship between stimulatory and inhibitory processes that may be reflected by the nature of the SCFA (i.e., acetate, propionate, butyrate) and the location of the SCFA production. The effects of SCFA on gut motility are complex and there is evidence that SCFA produced in one part of the gut can impact on more distant regions. For example, caecal infusion of SCFA has been shown to induce relaxation of the proximal section of the stomach.[28] The more recent observation and investigation of SCFA receptors—G-protein-coupled receptors (GPR41 and GPR43)—may help to unravel the important SCFA-induced effects on gut motility and hence laxation.[29]

The fermentation of unabsorbed carbohydrate can produce a number of by-products (gases—H_2 and CH_4 and SCFA) that may have important implications for the movement of fluid (water) in and out of the lumen. This, in turn, will have important implication for the process of laxation in humans (see Figure 15.1).

15.1.3 Role of FODMAPs in Modifying Symptoms Associated with Irritable Bowel Syndrome

For some individuals, however, the delivery of FODMAPs to the distal small and proximal large bowel and their subsequent rapid fermentation may lead to an exacerbation of symptoms (such as bloating, abdominal discomfort or pain, and altered bowel habits) associated with IBS and other functional gut disorders.[5-7,22] IBS affects one in seven Australians (about 15% of the adult population) and is the most common reason for referral to a specialist gastroenterologist. We have designed a dietary strategy that reduces the quantities of the fermentable FODMAPs in the diet. This approach has been highly successful in reducing gas production and in relieving functional gut symptoms of patients with IBS.[5-7,22]

Consequently, knowledge about the FODMAP composition of foods may have a number of uses in individuals attempting to increase their levels to gain the putative health benefits, or in patients with gastrointestinal disorders who may want to limit their intake of FODMAPs due to undesirable gastrointestinal symptoms.

15.1.4 Implications/Future Research

Clearly more research is required in this area—and indeed, a study is currently underway in our laboratory in which the effect of diets low and high in FODMAPs on transit time is being examined in healthy individuals and in patients with IBS. This work should help to verify the role of FODMAPs in the process of laxation. Finally, future research aimed at investigating the physiological effects of various prebiotic supplements should consider and control the "background levels" of naturally occurring dietary-fermentable short-chain carbohydrates (e.g., FODMAPs).

References

1. Cummings, J.H., Stephen, A.M., Carbohydrate terminology and classification, *Eur. J. Clin. Nutr.*, 61(Suppl 1), S5, 2007.
2. Roberfroid, M., Dietary fibre, inulin and oligofructose: A review comparing their physiological effects, *Crit. Rev. Food. Sci. Nutr.*, 33, 103, 1993.
3. FAO/WHO, Carbohydrates in human nutrition. Report of a Joint FAO/WHO Expert Consultation, Food and Nutrition, Paper 66, Series No. 1, 1998.
4. Gibson, P.R., Newham, E., Barrett, J.S., Shepherd, S.J., Muir, J.G., Review article: Fructose malabsorption and the bigger picture, *Aliment. Pharmacol. Ther.*, 25, 349, 2007.
5. Gibson, P.R., Shepherd, S.J., Personal view: Food for thought—Western lifestyle and susceptibility to Crohn's disease. The FODMAP hypothesis, *Aliment. Pharmacol. Ther.*, 221, 1399, 2005.
6. Shepherd, J.S., Parker, F.C., Muir, J.G., Gibson, P.R., Dietary triggers of abdominal symptoms in patients with irritable bowel syndrome: Randomised placebo-controlled evidence, *Clin. Gastro. Hepatol.*, 6, 765, 2008.
7. Gibson, P.R., Shepherd, S.J., Evidence-based dietary management of functional gastrointestinal symptoms: The FODMAP approach, *J. Gastroenterol. Hepatol.*, 25, 252, 2010.
8. Gibney, M., Sigman-Grant, M., Stanton, J.L., Keast, D.R., Consumption of sugars, *Am. J. Clin. Nutr.*, 62(Suppl 1), 178S, 1995.
9. Park, Y.K., Yetley, E.A., Intakes and food sources of fructose in the United States, *Am. J. Clin. Nutr.*, 58(Suppl), 737S, 1993.
10. Rumessen, J.J., Gudmand-Hoyer, E., Absorption capacity of fructose in healthy adults. Comparison with sucrose and its constituent monosaccharides, *Gut*, 27, 1161, 1986.
11. Thorens, B., Cheng, Z.Q., Brown, D., Lodish, H.F., Liver glucose transporter: A basolateral protein in hepatocytes and intestine and kidney cells, *Am. J. Physiol.*, 259, C279, 1990.
12. Barrett, J.S., Irving, P.M., Shepherd, S.J., Muir, J.G., Gibson, P.R., Comparison of the prevalence of fructose and lactose malabsorption across chronic intestinal disorders, *Aliment. Pharmacol. Therap.*, 30, 165, 2009.

13. Muir, J.G., Shepherd, S.J., Rosella, O., Rose, R., Gibson, P.R., Fructan and free fructose content of common Australian fruit and vegetables, *J. Agric. Food Chem.*, 55, 6619, 2007.

14. Muir, J.G., Rose, R., Rosella, O., Liels, K., Barrett, J.S., Shepherd, S.J., Gibson, P.R., Measurement of short chain carbohydrates in common Australian vegetables and fruit by high performance liquid chromatography, *J. Agric. Food Chem.*, 57, 554, 2009.

15. Biesiekierski, J.R., Rosella, O., Rose, R., Liels, K., Barrett, J.S., Shepherd, S.J., Gibson, P.R., Muir, J.G., Quantification of fructans, galacto-oligosaccharides and other short-chain carbohydrates in processed grains and cereals, *J. Hum. Nutr. Diet.*, 24, 154, 2010.

16. Macfarlane, G.T., Steed, H., Macfarlane, S., Bacterial metabolism and health-related effects of galactooligosaccharides and other prebiotics, *J. Appl. Microbiol.*, 104, 305, 2008.

17. Silk, D.B.A., Davis, A., Vulevic, J., Tzortzis, G., Gibson, G.R., Clinical trial: The effects of a trans-galactooligosaccharide prebiotic on faecal microbiota and symptoms in irritable bowel syndrome, *Aliment. Pharm. Ther.*, 29, 508–518, 2009.

18. Roberfroid, M., Gibson, G.R., Hoyles, L. et al., Prebiotic effects: Metabolic and health benefits, *Br. J. Nutr.*, 104(Suppl 2), S3, 2010.

19. Barrett, J.S., Muir, J.G., Gearry, R.B., Irving, P.M., Rose, R., Rosella, O., Haines, M.L., Shepherd, S.J., Gibson, P.R., Dietary poorly absorbed, short-chain carbohydrates increases delivery of water and fermentable substrates to the proximal colon, *Aliment. Pharmacol. Ther.*, 31, 874, 2010.

20. Macfarlane, G.T., Cummings, J.H., The colonic flora, fermentation and large bowel digestive function. In *The Large Intestine: Physiology, Pathophysiology and Disease*, Phillips, S.F., Pemberton, J.H., Shorter, R.G., Eds., Mayo Foundation, Raven Press Ltd., New York, pp. 51–92, 1991.

21. Topping, D.L., Clifton, P.M., Short-chain fatty acids and human colonic function: Roles of resistant starch and nonstarch polysaccharides, *Physiol. Rev.*, 81, 1031, 2001.

22. Ong, D.K., Mitchell, S.B., Barrett, J.S., Shepherd, S.J., Irving, P.I., Biesiekierski, J.R., Smith, S., Gibson, P.R., Muir, J.G., Manipulation of dietary short chain carbohydrates alters the pattern of gas production and genesis of symptoms in irritable bowel syndrome, *J. Gastroenterol. Hepatol.*, 25, 1366, 2010.

23. Pimentel, M., Lin, H.C., Enayatic, P. et al., Methane, a gas produced by enteric bacteria, slows intestinal transit and augments small intestinal contractile activity, *Am. J. Physiol. Gastrointest. Liver Physiol.*, 290, G1089, 2006.

24. Sahakian, A.B., Jee, S.R., Pimentel, M., Methane and the gastrointestinal tract, *Dig. Dis. Sci.*, 55, 2135, 2010.

25. Soares, A.C., Lederman, H.M., Fagundes-Neto, U. et al., Breath methane associated with slow colonic transit time in children with chronic constipation, *J. Clin. Gastroenterol.*, 39, 512, 2005.

26. Chatterjee, S., Park, S., Low, K. et al., The degree of breath methane production in IBS correlates with the severity of constipation, *Am. J. Gastroenterol.*, 102, 837, 2007.

27. Ruppin, H., Bar-Meir, S., Soergel, K.H., Wood, C.M., Schmitt, M.G., Absorption of short-chain fatty acids by the colon, *Gastroenterology*, 78, 1500, 1980.

28. Cherbut, C., Aubé, A.C., Blottière, H.M., Galmiche, J.P., Effects of short chain fatty acids on gastrointestinal motility, *Scand. J. Gastroenterol. Suppl.*, 222, 58, 1997.

29. Tazoe, H., Otomo, Y., Kaji, I., Tanaka, R., Karaki, S.I., Kuwahara, A., Roles of short-chain fatty acids receptors, GPR41 and GPR43 on colonic functions, *J. Physiol. Pharmacol.*, 59, 251, 2008.

16

Colonic Metabolism of Bioactive Molecules
Potential Impact of Dietary Fiber

CHRISTINE A. EDWARDS, ADA L. GARCIA, and EMILIE COMBET

Contents

16.1 Introduction

The colonic bacterial metabolism of dietary compounds that escape absorption in the small intestine has been studied for many decades in humans. However, most studies have focused on the metabolism of carbohydrates, dietary fiber and proteins, while much less emphasis has been placed on the metabolism of other potentially bioactive molecules such as polyphenolic compounds. It is becoming increasingly reported that the majority of plant food–associated polyphenols enter the human colon either as (i) the parent ingested compound or (ii) as a metabolite produced in the small intestine and/or via the enterohepatic circulation after absorption and cellular metabolism. The subsequent colonic bacterial metabolism of these compounds will determine which bioactive molecules become available to the colonic mucosa and which are absorbed and available in the plasma and tissues of the body.

It may well be that it is the bioactivity of these colonic metabolites that is of more importance in promoting health than that of the parent compounds of which, for many plant polyphenolic rich foods, a much smaller amount enters the body.

There is much individual variability in the metabolism of bioactive molecules in the colon, and this may, in part, be due to the influence of other dietary compounds which can alter small intestinal absorption and colon bacterial activity. An obvious key factor is the intake of dietary fiber, either in the meal along with the polyphenolic compounds (most food sources will also include a rich source of fiber) or as part of the rest of the diet which causes longer-term changes in the properties and metabolic capacity of the colonic microbiota. However, very few studies have investigated the interactions of the food matrix on events in the small intestine and colon and on the final bioactive products that become available to the colonic cells and finally to the tissues of the body.

16.2 Health Benefits of Dietary Fiber

The impact of dietary fiber on human health has been extensively studied. Different types of dietary fiber have been associated with a range of health benefits including reduced rate of absorption of glucose [1] and dietary fat [2] and reabsorption of bile acids [3]. This promotes improved glycemic control, lowering of plasma lipids [4], and reduced risk of diabetes and heart disease (Table 16.1). Dietary fiber also provides the fuel for fermentation by bacteria in the large intestine, resulting in the production of short-chain fatty acids (SCFA). The SCFA have an increasing evidence base for a variety of health effects including promotion of gut mucosal health, increased apoptosis and cell differentiation of cancer cells (mainly associated with butyrate [5]), and possible effects on lipoprotein metabolism and satiety (mainly mediated by propionate [6]). Finally, insoluble fiber and other fiber sources like psyllium, which are less well fermented, dilute colonic contents and speed colonic transit. These play a role in the prevention of constipation and are believed to reduce the risk of colon cancer. However, some effects of dietary fiber on the risk of colonic cancer may be related to their associated phenolic compounds such as ferulic acid and other related hydroxycinnamic acids [7]. The interactions between fiber and phenolic compounds and their combined impact on health need to be explored further.

16.2.1 Physiological Actions of Dietary Fiber in the Gastrointestinal Tract

It has been well established, over the second half of the twentieth century, that dietary fiber, and especially soluble dietary fiber, can influence the absorption of nutrients and nonnutrients in the small intestine. This may be due to increased viscosity, slowing of gastric emptying, reducing the impact of mixing by intestinal contractions, and entrapping or binding of molecules within the fiber structure (Table 16.1; [8]). In recent years, the impact of the food matrix on the absorption of nutrients has been considered as an important influence on their health benefits, with dietary fiber as a major component of the food matrix. Despite the plethora of research on the impact of fiber on the absorption of glucose, amino acids,

Table 16.1 Physiological Action of Dietary Fiber in the GI Tract

Upper gut
Increased viscosity
    Delayed gastric emptying
        Increased satiety
    Reduced impact of intestinal mixing
        Slower absorption of nutrients including glucose
        Possible reduction in rate/extent of absorption of nonnutrient food
          molecules, e.g., polyphenols
        Reduced fat absorption
        Reduced bile acid reabsorption
    Altered mouth to cecal transit time

Large intestine
Production of SCFA
    Increased cell proliferation
    Stimulated apoptosis
    Increased absorption of water
    Energy for colonocytes
    Gut healing
Low colonic pH
    Inhibition of damaging enzymes such as 7 alpha dehydroxylase
    Precipitation of fatty soaps and other harmful compounds
    Inhibition of ammonia production and absorption
    Improved calcium and magnesium absorption
    Decreased cell proliferation
Faster transit
    Reduced exposure to toxins, carcinogens
Dilution of colonic contents
    Dilution of toxins and carcinogens

Systemic effects
Reduced postprandial glycemia
Improved plasma lipids
Lower plasma cholesterol
Increased satiety and reduction in body weight

fats, and bile acids, very little research has considered its impact on the absorption and metabolism of other bioactive plant compounds such as polyphenolics despite most plant food sources being rich in both fiber and phenolics.

16.3 Other Plant-Associated Bioactive Molecules

Plant materials contain a wide range of potentially bioactive molecules, some of which will be digested and absorbed in the upper gastrointestinal (GI) tract, some of which will pass unchanged into the colon, while others may be partially metabolized and returned to the GI lumen (via the enterohepatic circulation). Coingestion of fiber may impact on the small intestinal handling of these compounds, and fermentation of fiber itself may influence what happens when these compounds enter the colon.

The undigested plant materials which reach the colon are then subjected to microbial degradation, yielding a broader variety of small bioactive compounds, including SCFA, phenolic acids, benzene alcohols, equols [9,10], and isothiocyanates [11–13].

16.3.1 Plant-Associated Polyphenolic Compounds

The main flavonoid polyphenolic compounds in the human diet include flavonols, flavones, flavan-3-ols, anthocyanidins, flavanones, and isoflavones with lower amounts of dihydroflavonols, flavan-3,4-diol, coumarins, chalcones, dihydrochalcones, and aurones. The diet also contains nonflavonoid compounds including phenolic acids, hydroxycinnamic acids, and stilbenes [14]. Different combinations of these are found in most fruits, vegetables, and plant-derived beverages (Table 16.2). Research on the bioavailability of plant-associated polyphenols has shown that although a small fraction are readily absorbed in the small intestine and enter the systemic circulation in the form of the parent compounds, substantial metabolism takes place in the small intestine with most metabolites absorbed before reentering the small intestine and passing into the colon (Table16.3). Most polyphenols do not occur in plant food as aglycones, but as glycosides, and the nature of the sugar moiety esterified to the aglycone (e.g., glucose, rhamnose, xylose, rutinose) impacts greatly on subsequent metabolism of the polyphenol molecules and its bioavailability. While glucosides are usually cleaved by the lactase-phlorizin hydrolase (LPH), a β-glucuronidase on the brush border membrane, other glycosides remain intact or only partially degraded and are not absorbed in the small intestine. For example, some compounds such as rutin (quercetin-3-rutinoside) are very poorly absorbed and enter the colon intact (Table 16.3). Thus, in a study by ileostomists who ingested tomato juice supplemented with rutin [23], 86% of the ingested flavonol disaccharide was recovered in ileal fluid collected over a 24h period after ingestion. In subjects with an intact colon, but not those with an ileostomy, the rutin in tomato juice was metabolized by the colonic bacteria, resulting in excretion of 3,4-dihydroxyphenylacetic acid, 3-methoxy-4-hydroxyphenylacetic acid (homovanillic acid), and 3-hydroxyphenylacetic acid in urine. This accounted for 22% of the rutin intake.

For those compounds absorbed in the small intestine, the rate and extent of absorption can be influenced by other components of the food matrix. In subjects who ingested strawberries (containing pelargonidin-3-O-glucoside) with or without cream, the cream delayed gastric emptying and small bowel transit time, as expected [28]. This change in the transit through the upper gut resulted in a delay of over 1h in the peak plasma concentration of the main metabolite pelargonidin-3-O-glucuronide and delayed urinary excretion of metabolites but did not reduce the amount absorbed.

Table 16.2 Principal Polyphenol Classes and Their Food Sources

Class	Subclass	Example[a]	Example of Food Source
Flavonoids	Flavonol	Quercetin, myricetin, rhamnetin	Most fruit and vegetables, including onions, tomatoes, apples, green and black teas, red wine
	Flavone	Apigenin, luteolin (mostly glycosylated)	Parsley, celery, citrus fruits
	Flavan-3-ol	Catechin isomers and their galloylated derivatives, proanthocyanidins (catechin polymers), theflavins	Green tea, cocoa
	Anthocyanidins	Pelargonidin, cyanidin, delphinidin, malvidin	Strawberries, blueberries, blackberries
	Flavanones	Hesperetin, naringenin	Citrus fruits
	Isoflavones	Daidzein, genistein	Soybean
	Coumarins	Umbelliferone, aesculetin	Cinnamon
	Chalcones and dihydrochalcones	Phloretin	Apples
	Aurones	Aureusidin	
	Flavan-3,4-diols	Leucoanthocyanidin, leucopeonidin	
	Dihydroflavonols	Taxifolin	Milk thistle seed extract, red onion (traces)
Non-flavonoids	Phenolic acids	Gallic acids and galloyl esters including ellagic acids, sanguiin H6	Grapes, wine, green and black tea, berries
	Hydroxycinnamic acids	Chlorogenic acid, caffeic acid, ferulic acid	Coffee, apples, artichokes
	Stilbenes	Resveratrol, piceatannol	Grapes, red wine, nuts, peanuts

Source: Crozier, A. et al., *Nat. Prod. Rep.*, 26, 1001, 2009.

[a] Most aglycones occur in plant source esterified to a sugar, which, to a large extent, influences the metabolic fate of the compound.

Table 16.3 Amount and Type of Phenolic Compounds Which Enter the Colon after Ingestion of Plant Foods

	Feed	Main Compounds	Recovered	% Dose in Ileal Fluid	Main Compounds in Ileal Fluid	Not Present in Ileal Fluid	Comments
Hydroxycinnamic acids							
Hagl et al. [15]	Apple smoothie, 0.7 L	58% 5 CQA, 4.8% 4 CQA, 36.7% 3, 4, and 5-p-coumaroylquinic acids	115 ± 28 mg	~61%	~95% Parent compounds (4 and 5 CQAs and 3, 4, and 5-p-coumaroylquinic acids); ~5% metabolites (1 and 3 CQAs) and 0.3% aglycones (p-coumaric acid)	Caffeic acid	Isomerization and esterification of 4 and 5 CQAs to 1 and 3 CQAs; hydrolysis of p-coumaroylquinic acids to p-coumaric acid. Additional liberation of D-(−)-quinic acid
Olthof [16]	Chlorogenic acid supplement	3, 4, and 5 CQAs	27 ± 18 mg	~67%	3, 4, and 5 CQAs		
Olthof et al. [17]	Caffeic acid	Caffeic acid	668 ± 165 mg	~5%	Caffeic acid		

Kahle [18]	Cloudy apple juice, 1 L	~475 µmol	69.6% 5 CQA, 8.7% 4 CQA, 18.3% 3, 4, and 5-p-coumaroylquinic acids	~134 µmol	~28%	44.4% Parent compounds (4 and 5 CQAs and 3, 4, and 5-p-coumaroylquinic acids); 55.6% metabolites (1 and 3 CQAs, methyl coumarate and methyl caffeate)	Caffeic acid	The breakdown of CQAs, FQAs, and p-coumaroylquinic acids contributes to D-(−)-quinic acid formation (14% of parent compound intake)
Stalmach et al. [19]	Instant coffee, 0.2 L	~385 µmol	72.2% 3, 4, and 5 CQAs; 12.5% 3, 4, and 5-FQAs, 10.1% CQA lactones, 1.7% coumaroylquinic acids, 3.6% diCQAs	274 ± 28 µmol	~71%	77.7% Parent compounds (3,4, and 5 CQAs; 3, 4, and 5-FQAs, 3 and 4 CQA lactones, 4 and 5 p-coumaroylquinic acids); 18.8% metabolites (sulfate and glucuronide derivatives of each major category) and 3.6% aglycones (caffeic and ferulic acids)		The specific recovery for each parent compound ingested ranges from ~6% for the CQA lactones >46% for diCQAs and p-coumaroylquinic acids >59% for the CQAs >77% for the FQAs. The specific recoveries from ingested dose for the metabolites ranged from ~4%

(*continued*)

Table 16.3 (continued) Amount and Type of Phenolic Compounds Which Enter the Colon after Ingestion of Plant Foods

	Feed	Main Compounds	Recovered	% Dose in Ileal Fluid	Main Compounds in Ileal Fluid	Not Present in Ileal Fluid	Comments
Dihydrochalcones							
Hagl et al. [15]	Apple smoothie, 0.7 L	~82 mg	61.2% Phloretin glucoside, 38.8% phloretin xyloglucoside	39 ± 8 mg	~48%	45.8% Parent compounds (phloretin xyloglucoside); 50.1% metabolites (three phloretin glucuronides) and 4% aglycones (phloretin)	Phloretin glucoside
Kahle et al. [18]	Cloudy apple juice, 1 L	~81 µmol	79.9% Phloretin glucoside, 21.1% phloretin xyloglucoside	~20 µmol	~25%	63.2% Parent compounds (phloretin xyloglucoside); 27.8% metabolites (phloretin glucuronide) and 9% aglycones (phloretin)	Phloretin glucoside

Reference	Source	Dose	Composition	Amount	%	Metabolites	Comments
Marks et al. [20]	Apple cider, 0.5 L	~46 μmol	67.4% Phloretin glucoside, 30.4% phloretin xylosylglucoside	~18 μmol	~38%	21.8% of parent compounds (phloretin xylosylglucoside and xylohexoside), 64.5% metabolites (three phloretin glucuronides, two phloretin sulfate and one phloretin glucuronide sulfate)	Phloretin glucoside
Flavonols							
Hagl et al. [15]	Apple smoothie, 0.7 L	~31 mg	95.5% Quercetin glycosides (rhamnoside, galactoside, xyloside, and arabinoside) and 4.5% quercetin	~15 ± 3 mg	~46%	89.8% Parent compounds (including all four quercetin glycosides) and 10.1% aglycones (quercetin)	Glycosides are hydrolyzed at different rates depending on the sugar moieties
Hollman et al. [21]	Fried yellow onions	~89 mg aglycone equivalent	Quercetin glucoside	—	~48%		Flavonols quantified postacid hydrolysis, which does not permit to distinguish between parent compounds/aglycones

(continued)

Table 16.3 (continued) Amount and Type of Phenolic Compounds Which Enter the Colon after Ingestion of Plant Foods

		Feed	Main Compounds	Recovered	% Dose in Ileal Fluid	Main Compounds in Ileal Fluid	Not Present in Ileal Fluid	Comments
	Quercetin rutinosides	100 mg	Quercetin rutinoside	—	~83%			
	Quercetin aglycones	100 mg	Quercetin	—	~76%			
Walle et al. [22]	Fried yellow onions	76–150 mg	Quercetin mono- (54.4 ± 8.1%) and diglucosides (45.6 ± 8.1%) and quercetin traces	~29 ± 19 mg	~24%	~100% Aglycone (quercetin)	Glucosides	Quercetin was mostly recovered 0–12 h postingestion
Jaganath et al. [23]	Tomato juice fortified with quercetin rutinoside, 0.3 L	~176 μmol	Quercetin rutinoside	~151 ± 5 μmol	~86%	Quercetin rutinoside		Main excretion 2–5 h postingestion
Kahle et al. [18]	Cloudy apple juice, 1 L	~24 μmol	Only quercetin glycosides (glucoside 16.1%, rhamnoside 24.8%, galactoside 13.2%, xyloside 37.2%, and arabinoside 8.7%)	~0.7 μmol	~3%	95.8% Parent compounds (only quercetin arabinoside and rhamnoside) and 4.2% aglycones (quercetin)	Quercetin glucoside, arabinoside, and xyloside	

Flavan-3-ols

Hagl et al. [15]	Apple smoothie, 0.7 L	~1138 mg	0.3% Monomers (catechins and epicatechins) and 99.7% polymers (procyanidins DPm = 4.8)	~708 ± 198 mg	~62%	99.6% Parent polymer (procyanidins DPm 1.5–3), 0.24% metabolites ((epi)-catechin sulfates) and 0.15% monomer (catechin and epicatechin)		
Auger et al. [24]	Polyphenon E supplement, 200 mg	~452 μmol	Monomers only, including 69% EGCG, 15.7% EC, 7% ECG, 4% EGC, and 4% (+)-epimers	~194 ± 50 μmol	~43%	Parent monomer (82% EGCG, 7.7% EC, 5.7% ECG, 4% GCG)	EGC	Specific recoveries—nongalloylated monomers: ~28% vs. galloylated monomers: ~60%
Kahle et al. [18]	Cloudy apple juice, 1 L	~186 μmol	33.3% Monomers (catechins and epicatechins) and 66.7% polymers (procyanidins DPm = 5.7)	~97 μmol	~52%	90.9% Parent polymer (procyanidins DPm 3.4) and 9.1% monomer (catechin and epicatechin)	(+)-Catechin, dimeric procyanidins	

(*continued*)

Table 16.3 (continued) Amount and Type of Phenolic Compounds Which Enter the Colon after Ingestion of Plant Foods

	Feed	Main Compounds	Recovered	% Dose in Ileal Fluid	Main Compounds in Ileal Fluid	Not Present in Ileal Fluid	Comments
Stalmach et al. [25]	Green tea, 0.3 L	~634 µmol 51.6% Monomers (C, EC, GC, EGC) and 49.3% galloylated monomers (EGCG, GCG, ECG)	439 ± 13 µmol	~69%	47.1% Parent compound (mainly galloylated compounds and EC) and 52.8% metabolites (mainly (E)C and (E)GC metabolites)		Specific recoveries were highest for GCG (89% of the dose ingested) and lowest for C and EC (~7% and 11%, respectively)
Isoflavones							
Walsh et al. [26]	Soy meal (236 mL) fortified with 125 mg isoflavonoid extract	~65 mg 94.7% Isoflavone glucosides (daidzin, genistin, glycitin, malonylgenistin), 5.3% isoflavone aglycones (daidzein, glycitein, genistein)	~24 ± 6 mg	~37%	4.2% Isoflavone glucosides (daidzin, glycitin, genistin, malonylgenistin), 95.8% isoflavone aglycones (daidzein, glycitein, genistein)		

Anthocyanins

Gonzales-Barrio et al. [27]	Homogenized raspberries, 300 g	~204 µmol	Cyanidin and pelargonidin glycosides: 57% sophorosides, 11.2% rutinosides, 13.6% glucosides, 23.2% glucosylrutinosides, 0.6% xylosylrutinosides	81 µmol	~40%	Cyanidin and pelargonidin glycosides: 58% sophorosides, 7.3% rutinosides, 2.7% glucosides, 31.2% glucosylrutinosides, 1.6% xylosylrutinosides	Pelargonidin rutinoside (present in minimal amount in the feed)	The specific recoveries for each compound ranged from 6% for cyanidin glucosides to 40–59% for all other cyanidin and pelargonidin glycosides, but cyanidin xylosylrutinoside (with a recovery of 93% the ingested dose)

Ellagitannins

Gonzales-Barrio et al. [27]	Homogenized raspberries, 300 g	~140 µmol	87.8% Ellagitannins (mainly sanguiin H6) and 12.2% ellagic acid aglycone and pentoside derivative	42 µmol	~30%	54.7% Sanguiin H6 and 45.2% ellagic acid	Ellagic acid pentoside, lambertianin C or sanguiin H10	The specific recovery rate for sanguiin H6 was 23%, while for monomeric ellagic acid recovery was 241%

Abbreviations: CQA, caffeoylquinic acid; FQA, feruoylquinic acid; C, catechin; EC, (–)-epicatechin; CG, (=)-catechin gallate; ECG, (–)-epicatechin gallate; GC, (+)-gallocatechin; EGC, (–)-epigallocatechin; GCG, (+)-gallocatechin gallate; EGCG, (–)-epigallocatechin gallate.

The impact of milk on the bioavailability of the polyphenols in cocoa has been a matter of debate with some studies showing an inhibition of absorption when milk is present [29] but with a greater impact on excretion of urinary metabolites than plasma pharmacokinetics [30]. Other studies, however, showed that, particularly with enriched products, the decrease in bioavailability is negligible [31,32]. This difference in the observed impact of milk on absorption may mean that the inhibitory effect of milk is saturable: If the level of flavan-3-ols in the product is sufficiently high, as in Keogh's and Shroeter's studies [31,32], the impact of the milk may be overcome; however, the reduced amounts of polyphenols found in common milk chocolate products will be less bioavailable [29]. Other researchers have suggested that the sucrose content may be important in determining the pharmacokinetics [33]. Similarly, a recent study by Renouf et al. [34] demonstrated that nondairy creamer and sugar had a significant effect on the T_{max} and C_{max} for hydroxycinnamic acid absorption from coffee (but not the overall dose absorbed), while milk had no effect. The creamer had no overall impact on the dose absorbed, with the area under the curve (AUC) did not differ significantly from the control. Another interesting food matrix interaction was seen when yogurt greatly reduced the urinary phenolic metabolites after ingestion of orange juice containing hesperidin-7-O-rutinoside (hesperidin) and naringenin-7-O-rutinoside (narirutin) [35].

While several studies have focused on the bioavailability of plant polyphenols using supplements, extracts, single meals, and feeding programs spanning several days or weeks, no work yet has investigated the impact of dietary fiber on the bioavailability of such polyphenolic compounds.

16.3.2 Cereals and Polyphenols

Cereals, and in particular whole grains (i.e., oats, wheat, and rye) and pseudocereals (i.e., buckwheat, quinoa, and amaranth), are an important source of dietary polyphenols, but the bioavailability of these in the small intestine is generally very low, either because the molecular structure of cereals prevents liberation of these polyphenols or because of the sugar moiety attached to the polyphenol aglycone.

The amount and range of phenolic compounds in cereals depends on the variety and degree of processing [36]. The main type of polyphenols in cereals is the hydroxycinnamates (ferulic, p-coumaric, caffeic, and sinapic acids). Whole cereal grains, especially the outer layers of wheat grain, contain high concentrations of ferulic acid [37]. Hydroxycinnamates in cereals are commonly present as insoluble esterified forms instead of aglycones (free forms) [38,39], with 90% of the ferulic acid found in wheat being esterified to arabinoxylan and hemicellulose structures in the grain cell walls [40].

The absorption of polyphenols from cereals is very low in the small intestine; 40 g of bran cereal contains ~130 mg of free and ester-linked hydroxycinnamates—with a minor proportion being free phenolic acids—from these, very low concentrations (150–250 nM) can be detected in plasma after a test meal, and just 3% can be recovered in 24 h urine. Among the metabolites recovered, ferulic acid is found in plasma mainly as a glucuronide conjugate. Urinary metabolites of ferulic acid are mainly feruloyl glycine (~70% of total ferulic acid excreted) as well as glucuronide derivatives and a small proportion of sulfate derivatives [41].

The absorption of cereal hydroxycinnamates depends on their level of esterification. Ferulic acid aglycones and a proportion of ester-1 ferulic acids from bran cereals are mainly absorbed within 1–3 h after a test meal in humans, which suggests that absorption occurs in the small intestine and that some deesterification via the small intestine esterases takes place; however, as the majority of hydroxycinnamates are ester bound, and because very low concentrations of hydroxycinnamic acid are found in plasma 6 h after a bran meal, this suggests that there is very little absorption in the large intestine either. The urinary recovery of these compounds is very low, which suggests that extensive action by colonic bacteria in the large intestine may be a major pathway of metabolism for phenolics in cereals.

16.4 Colonic Metabolism of Bioactive Molecules: Possible Interactions with Fiber

The bacteria in the human colon are capable of many different chemical reactions. When colonic metabolism is considered, the focus is usually on a limited number of pathways and substrates, mainly on the fermentation of dietary fiber itself. However, the presence and/or fermentation of dietary fiber and other nondigestible carbohydrates can have major impact on the colonic metabolism of many other important compounds and the release or destruction of related bioactive molecules.

The colonic fermentation of fiber may have significant impact on the colonic metabolism of bioactive molecules by (i) changing the composition and activity of the microbiota; (ii) by reducing colonic pH, which may in turn influence bacterial metabolism and colonic absorption; and also (iii) by influencing colonic motility and residence time (Figure 16.1). These interactions have been very little studied.

16.4.1 Studying Colonic Metabolism of Bioactive Molecules

The major issue for any study of colonic metabolism is the inaccessibility of the proximal colon where most of the fermentation and other bacterial metabolic activities occur. It is not yet possible to effectively measure the colonic metabolism of any compound in vivo without using very invasive techniques such as intubation. Most studies have used, instead, in vitro fermentation with human fecal bacteria as the inoculum [42,43] or animal studies with a variety of species on conventional and test diets [44,45], germ-free animals associated with human gut microbiota [46], or gnotobiotic animals colonized with single or combined bacterial species [47].

While providing essential information on metabolic pathways, capabilities of individual species, and interactions between bacteria in a controlled environment

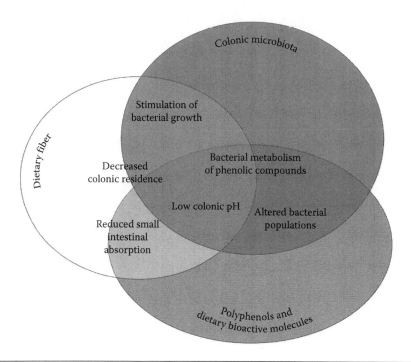

Figure 16.1 Interactions among dietary fiber, colonic microbiota and dietary bioactive molecules (including polyphenols).

or system, these methods have major limitations in terms of translation of results to what happens to humans in vivo. The in vitro cultures used are usually static batch cultures which demonstrate exponential growth of bacteria after an initial lag phase. However, because of the loss of substrate and buildup of inhibitory products and low pH, bacteria enter a stationary and finally a death phase over a short period of 24–48 h. It is difficult to predict the exact timing of the phases and important time points required for the production of intermediate compounds and then final products. Many studies focus on 24 h incubations, while others concentrate on the first few hours when intermediate products may appear. Considering the metabolism of polyphenolic compounds in the presence of fermentable carbohydrate, it may be necessary to take serial samples over several hours to capture the production and degradation of important metabolites, the timing of which may differ substantially between fecal donors [43,48,49].

The animal models assume similarities between the species used and man; however, there are major differences in the bacterial microbiota in both the small and large intestine and differences in the transit time and other metabolic processes. The use of human flora–associated rats/mice may improve on this, but there may be other important differences in gut function that may influence the results. Many of the studies in vitro or in gnotobiotic rats have concentrated on a small number of individual bacterial species in an attempt to unravel particular metabolic pathways, and on single phenolic compounds or individual foods sources. This may not reflect the metabolism seen on a mixed fiber and phenolic-rich diet with the complex microbial ecosystem normally present in the human colon.

In human studies, acute and longer-term feeding experiments can enable monitoring of the products issued from colonic metabolism into the plasma, urine, feces, and breath. The products of colonic fermentation that are absorbed pass to the liver where they may be further metabolized before being distributed to the tissues. The concentrations in plasma, therefore, do not reflect only absorption but also hepatic sequestration and metabolism. The timing of individual peaks may vary between metabolites and individuals and thus require blood sampling over an extended period after the meal, often several hours to capture the full metabolite profile, accounting especially for colonic metabolites. Fecal samples [50,51] provide an end-point sample reflecting the sum of the metabolite production, further metabolism, and then absorption and so may not be representative of the events occurring in the proximal colon, or representative of the production of intermediate metabolites which may have an important influence if produced in high enough amounts for a significant length of time. However, these samples do inform about the compounds that reach the distal colon and which may have an impact there. An alternative approach is to detect colonic metabolites (including phenolic acids and SCFA) in urine collected over 24 h (Table 16.4), although these are further influenced by tissue and renal metabolism of the compounds in plasma. Unfortunately, there are also many similar compounds in urine, which are produced in the body with no contribution from colonic bacteria and therefore interfere with the estimation of colonic products. For example, the liver produces acetate during fasting, and this may be a major source for plasma and urinary acetate. Detoxifying enzymes in the endoplasmic reticulum and microsomes also provide another route for hippuric acid production, independent from colonic microbial action. Meanwhile, 4-hydroxyhippuric acid is a marker of chronic renal failure [52], and homovanillic acid (3-methoxy-4-hydroxyphenylacetic acid) is a product of dopamine metabolism [53]. 4-Hydroxyphenylacetic acid and hippuric acid are found in the urine of people with ileostomies, which indicates that these compounds are not derived solely from microbial metabolism in the colon [54].

Another approach is to compare the urinary output after ingestion of foods or compounds of interest by patients with an ileostomy and those with an intact colon [54]. The difference in metabolites in urine should correspond with those originating from bacterial metabolism in the colon, albeit with possible further metabolism after absorption. The detection of these compounds in urine has focused mainly on measuring the phenolic acid aglycones, although it is increasingly recognized that more focus should be given to the measurement of metabolites such as sulfate derivatives. Examples of urinary phenolic compounds and catabolites derived from colonic bacteria metabolism of plant-associated phenolics are shown in Table 16.4.

Table 16.4 Examples of Products of Colonic Metabolism of Phenolic Compounds Recovered in Urine from Plant Foods and Beverages

Phenolic Acids and Polyphenol Catabolites Significantly Increased in Urine after Supplementation	Grun et al. [55] — Extract of Red Wine and Grape (~800 mg Polyphenols/Day for 4 Weeks)	Roowi et al. [35] — Orange Juice (Single Feed)—Hesperetin-7-O-Rutinoside (168 μmol)	Jaganath et al. [23] — Tomato Juice Fortified with Quercetin-3-O-Rutinoside (176 μmol)	Combet et al. [56] — Flavonol-Rich Diet (>3 Portions Flavonol-Rich Foods/Day for 3 Days)	Olthof et al. [16] — Chlorogenic Acid Supplement (5.5 mmol/Day for 7 Days)	Olthof et al. [16] — Supplement Quercetin-3-Rutinoside (660 μmol/Day for 7 Days)	Rios et al. [57] — 80 g Chocolate (439 mg Proanthocyanidins, 147 mg Catechin Monomers)	Roowi et al. [54] — 300 mL of Green Tea	Ward et al. [58] — Polymeric Proanthocyanidin-Rich Grapeseed Extract (1 g/Day for 6 Weeks)
Pyrocatechol								x	
Pyrogallol								x	
(-)-5-(3,4,5-Trihydroxyphenyl)-γ-valerolactone								x	
Benzoic acid							x		
3-Hydroxybenzoic acid							x		
4-Hydroxybenzoic acid								x	
3,4-Dihydroxy-5-methoxybenzoic acid (4-methylgallic acid)									x
Vanillic acid—4-hydroxy-3-methoxybenzoic acid	x						x		
4-Hydroxy-3,5-dimethoxybenzoic acid (syringic acid)	x				x				
3-Hydroxyphenylacetic acid	x	x		x		x	x		x
4-Hydroxyphenylacetic acid	x								
3,4-Dihydroxyphenylacetic acid			x		x	x	x		

Compound							
3-Methoxy-4-hydroxyphenyl acetic acid (homovanillic acid)	x			x	x		x
3-(3-Hydroxyphenyl)-3-hydroxyphenylacetic acid	x						
4-Hydroxymandelic acid (2-hydroxy-2-(4-hydroxyphenylacetic acid)	x						
3-Hydroxyphenylpropionic acid	x			x	x	x	
3,4-Dihydroxyphenylpropionic acid			x				
3-Hydroxy-cinnamic acid			x				
4-Hydroxy-3-methoxyphenylpropionic acid (dihydroferulic acid)		x					
3-Methoxy-4-hydroxy-cinnamic acid (ferulic acid)			x		x		
3,4-Dihydroxy-cinnamic acid (caffeic acid)			x				
3-(3-Hydroxyphenyl)-3-hydroxypropanoic acid (3-hydroxyphenylhydracrylic acid)		x				x	
3-Methoxy-4-hydroxyphenylhydracrylic acid		x					
Benzoyl amidoacetic acid (hipurric acid)	x						
3-Hydroxyhippuric acid	x	x					
4-Hydroxyhippuric acid	x						

The range of (poly)phenolic and non(poly)phenolic metabolites produced varies between different foods and individuals, with examples being shown in Table 16.4. However, many of the final pathways seem to converge to produce a smaller range of final low-molecular-weight compounds, including benzene alcohols, the phenolic acids benzoic acid, phenylacetic acids, phenylpropionic acid, and their hydroxy and methoxy derivatives.

16.4.2 Intermediates and Final Metabolites

In vitro fermentation studies allow the process of colonic metabolism of phenolic compounds to be studied in detail, with particular emphasis on the production of intermediary compounds and potentially the effect of dietary fiber on the rate and extent of production of compounds that may be, for a short period at least, available to the colonic mucosa, and, if absorbed, to the tissues of the body. These intermediate products are not easily identified in plasma or urine.

16.4.3 Impact of Fermentable Carbohydrate on Bacterial Metabolism of Phenolic Compounds

In a study of the bacterial metabolism of rutin [43], fecal slurries from three individuals were incubated anaerobically in batch culture with either (a) 28 μmol of rutin, (b) 28 μmol of rutin plus 0.5 g glucose, (c) 55 μmol of quercetin, (d) 55 μmol of quercetin plus 0.5 g glucose, and (e) no substrate control. The degradation of rutin was greatly accelerated when the cultures contained fermentable carbohydrate and the appearance/release of quercetin was faster or undetectable compared with cultures without carbohydrate when quercetin was clearly released but much more slowly by the bacteria from all three donors. This suggests that fermentable fiber will influence the speed of colonic metabolism of polyphenols and this is likely to affect the appearance and persistence of metabolic intermediates.

16.5 Bioactivity and Potential Impact on Colonic and Systemic Health

The flavonoids have many potential effects on health and have been associated with antioxidant, anti-inflammatory [59], and other effects which may decrease risk of chronic diseases [60,61], including cardiovascular disease [62], Alzheimer's disease [63], and cancer [64,65]. They may also have specific impact in the colon. Different polyphenolics have been shown to inhibit the growth of some bacteria [66] but not Bifidobacteria and Lactobacilli [67], resulting in a potential probiotic effect. Recently, Tzounis et al. [68] demonstrated the prebiotic effect of a daily flavan-3-ol-rich cocoa drink consumed for 4 weeks, with an increase in Bifidobacteria and Lactobacilli population, together with a modest decrease in plasma triglycerides and CRP levels. Polyphenols and their metabolites may have a beneficial impact on colonic health via reduction of the adhesion of pathogens to gut cells [69] and via a direct anticancer effects such as reduction in carcinogen-induced aberrant crypt foci in rats by hesperitin [70]. However, many of these effects may be associated with the parent compound solely, which may not reach high enough concentrations as it rapidly serves as substrate for the colonic bacteria, which in turn release small molecules of unknown bioactivity. It is therefore important to focus not only on the bioactivity of the parent compounds reaching the colon but also to the dynamic of their metabolism, with particular emphasis on the levels reached, as well as the duration of exposure before further metabolism or excretion takes place.

16.6 Impact of Polyphenols on Colonic Fermentation

Although there are little published data on the effects of fiber on the metabolism and bioavailability of the polyphenolics and their metabolites, some studies have tested the influence of polyphenols on the production of SCFA from the fermentation of nondigestible carbohydrate. Polyphenolic compounds are known to have antibacterial properties [71] and may inhibit certain species in the GI tract. They may also influence the metabolic pathways by changing the populations of bacteria, as they have been shown to have some prebiotic properties [66]. However, recent studies in rats did not identify any impact of polyphenols on the fermentation of chicory root fructans [44], nor any inhibitory effect associated with the ability of rat cecal microflora to ferment pectin after exposure to grape pomaces [67].

16.6.1 Impact of Polyphenol-/Fiber-Rich Foods

Although there have been very few studies properly investigating the interactions between fiber and polyphenolic compounds, there have been several studies investigating the properties and effects of polyphenol- and fiber-rich foods such as blueberry husks [68], grape extract [69], and carob fiber [70]. In these cases, the food extract has been shown to both stimulate colonic production of SCFA and to increase the antioxidant capacity of plasma. However, it is difficult to know from these studies whether the impact of each component has been influenced by the other.

16.6.2 Interindividual Variation in Colonic Metabolism of Bioactive Molecules

In all studies related to the bioavailability and colonic metabolism of polyphenolic compounds, a substantial variability in the individual rate and extent of colonic metabolites has been reported. Some of this variability is likely to be due to physiological differences in the gut function of individuals but more importantly, for the colonic metabolism, differences in the gut microbiota. Gross et al. [48] studied the in vitro metabolism of black tea and red wine/grape juice by fecal samples from 10 human volunteers in batch cultures. They analyzed their fermentation fluid by NMR and GC-MS and measured intermediates and final products from the colonic metabolism of polyphenols at several time points over 72 h and produced detailed profiles for each individual. They showed that major metabolites formed from all food sources were 3-phenylpropionic acid and its hydroxylated derivatives and phenylacetic acid and its hydroxylated derivatives with lower amounts of benzoic acid indicating common final pathways and products for a diverse range of polyphenolic parent compounds. This is in agreement with other in vitro colonic metabolism studies which also show a small range of products from different parent compounds [71]. What is not known is how much of the interindividual variation, in the timing and extent of colonic metabolism, was due to the host physiology, genetics, or previous diet. Indeed, the colonic microbiota is determined by a complex interaction between host, environment, and diet. Past dietary fiber intake occurring in infancy, as the microbiota was colonizing the gut [72], or in the more recent past, is likely to have significant effect on the colonic metabolism of bioactive compounds, even if fiber is not included in the same meal. Gardana et al. [73] studied the microbial transformation of daidzein to equol using in vitro batch cultures and found that equol producers were those that consumed less fiber, vegetable, and cereals and more animal-derived lipids.

16.7 Conclusion

It is now clear that some of the effects of a high-fiber diet may be partly determined by the polyphenolic content of the fiber source. Indeed, the majority of the polyphenolic compounds present in the human diet escape absorption in the small intestine and may be metabolized by colonic bacteria. Moreover, subsequent metabolites may be the most important components to study in relation to bioactivity and health-promoting properties of polyphenols. To fully understand the likely impact of polyphenols, and of dietary fiber in the diet, it is essential to understand the interaction between the fiber, as well as other component of the food matrix, with polyphenolic metabolism and absorption in the small and large intestine. This bears particular relevance to the food industry, when formulating new food products and researchers, when devising and interpreting experimental and epidemiological studies of the impact of diet on health. At the moment, very few studies have explored this new research area, and both carefully designed dietary interventions in humans, as well as the use of elegant in vitro and in vivo animal models, will be required to fully document the complicated pathways involved.

References

1. Jenkins, D.J. and Jenkins, A.L., Dietary fiber and the glycemic response, *Proc. Soc. Exp. Biol. Med.*, 180, 422, 1985.
2. Kritchevsky, D., Dietary fibre and lipid metabolism, *Int. J. Obesity*, 11, 33, 1987.
3. Theuwissen, E. and Mensink, R.P., Water soluble fibers and cardiovascular disease, *Physiol. Behav.*, 94, 285, 2008.
4. Wolever, T.M.S. et al., Physicochemical properties of oat β-glucan influence its ability to reduce serum LDL cholesterol in humans: A randomized clinical trial, *Am. J. Clin. Nutr.*, 92, 723, 2010.
5. Wong, J.M.W. et al., Colonic health: Fermentation and short chain fatty acids, *J. Clin. Gastroenterol.*, 40, 235, 2006.
6. Al-Lahham, A. et al., Biological effects of propionic acid in humans; metabolism, potential applications and underlying mechanisms, *Biochim. Biophys. Acta*, 1801, 1175, 2010.
7. Janicke, B. et al., The anti-proliferative effect of dietary fiber phenolic compounds ferulic acid and p-coumaric acid on the cell cycle of Caco 2 cells, *Nutr. Cancer*, 63, 611, 2011.

8. Edwards, C.A., Mechanisms of action of dietary fibre on small intestinal absorption and motility, *Adv. Exp. Med. Biol.*, 270, 95, 2011.
9. Cavallini, D.C.U. and Rossi, E.A., Equol: Biological activities and clinical importance of an isoflavone metabolite, *Aliment. Nutricao*, 20, 677, 2009.
10. Raimondi, S. et al., Bioconversion of soy isoflavones daidzin and daidzein by Bifidobacterium strains, *Appl. Microbiol. Biotechnol.*, 81, 943, 2009.
11. Fuller, Z. et al., Influence of cabbage processing methods and prebiotic manipulation of colonic microflora on glucosinolate breakdown in man, *Br. J. Nutr.*, 98, 364, 2007.
12. Krul, C. et al., Metabolism of sinigrin (2-propenyl glucosinolate) by the human colonic microflora in a dynamic in vitro large-intestinal model, *Carcinogenesis*, 23, 1009, 2002.
13. Serra, A. et al., Metabolic pathways of the colonic metabolism of procyanidins (monomers and dimers) and alkaloids, *Food Chem.*, 126, 1127, 2010.
14. Crozier, A., Jaganath, I.B., and Clifford, M.N., Dietary phenolics: Chemistry, bioavailability and effects on health, *Nat. Prod. Rep.*, 26, 1001, 2009.
15. Hagl, S. et al., Colonic availability of polyphenols and D-(-)-quinic acid after apple smoothie consumption, *Mol. Nutr. Food Res.*, 55, 368, 2010.
16. Olthof, M.R. et al., Chlorogenic acid, quercetin-3-rutinoside and black tea phenols are extensively metabolized in humans, *J. Nutr.*, 133, 1806, 2003.
17. Olthof, M.R., Hollman, P.C.H., and Katan, M.B., Chlorogenic acid and caffeic acid are absorbed in humans, *J. Nutr.*, 131, 66, 2001.
18. Kahle, K. et al., Polyphenols are intensively metabolized in the human gastrointestinal tract after apple juice consumption, *J. Agric. Food Chem.*, 55, 10605, 2007.
19. Stalmach, A. et al., Bioavailability of chlorogenic acids following acute ingestion of coffee by humans with an ileostomy, *Arch. Biochem. Biophys.*, 501, 98, 2010a.
20. Marks, S.C. et al., Absorption, metabolism, and excretion of cider dihydrochalcones in healthy humans and subjects with an ileostomy, *J. Agric. Food Chem.*, 57, 2009, 2009.
21. Hollman, P.C.H. et al., Bioavailability of the dietary antioxidant flavonol quercetin in man, *Cancer Lett.*, 114, 139, 1997.
22. Walle, T. et al., Quercetin glucosides are completely hydrolyzed in ileostomy patients before absorption, *J. Nutr.*, 130, 2658, 2000.
23. Jaganath, I.B. et al., The relative contribution of the small and large intestine to the absorption and metabolism of rutin in man, *Free Radic. Res.*, 40, 1035, 2006.
24. Auger, C. et al., Bioavailability of polyphenon E flavan-3-ols in humans with an ileostomy, *J. Nutr.*, 138, 1535S, 2008.
25. Stalmach, A. et al., Absorption, metabolism, and excretion of green tea flavan-3-ols in humans with an ileostomy, *Mol. Nutr. Food Res.*, 54, 323, 2010b.
26. Walsh, K.R. et al., Isoflavonoid glucosides are deconjugated and absorbed in the small intestine of human subjects with ileostomies, *Am. J. Clin. Nutr.*, 85, 1050, 2007.
27. Gonzalez-Barrio, R. et al., Bioavailability of anthocyanins and ellagitannins following consumption of raspberries by healthy humans and subjects with an ileostomy, *J. Agric. Food Chem.*, 58, 3933, 2010.
28. Mullen, W. et al., Bioavailability of perlagonidin-3-O-glucoside and its metabolites in humans following the ingestion of strawberries with and without cream, *J. Agric. Food Chem.*, 56, 713, 2008.
29. Serafini, M. et al., Plasma antioxidants from chocolate, *Nature*, 424, 1013, 2003.
30. Mullen, W. et al., Milk decreases urinary excretion but not plasma pharmacokinetics of cocoa flavan-3-ol metabolites in humans, *Am. J. Clin. Nutr.*, 89, 1784, 2009.
31. Keogh, J.B., McInerney, J., and Clifton, P.M., The effect of milk protein on the bioavailability of cocoa polyphenols, *J. Food Sci.*, 72, S230, 2007.
32. Schroeter, H. et al., Nutrition: Milk and absorption of dietary flavanols, *Nature*, 426, 787, 2003.

33. Neilson, A.P. et al., Influence of chocolate matrix composition on cocoa flavan-3-ol bioaccessibility in vitro and bioavailability in humans, *J. Agric. Food Chem.*, 57, 9418, 2009.
34. Renouf, M. et al., Nondairy creamer, but not milk, delays the appearance of coffee phenolic acid equivalents in human plasma, *J. Nutr.*, 140, 259, 2010.
35. Roowi, S. et al., Yoghurt impacts on the excretion of phenolic acids derived from the colonic breakdown of orange juice flavanones in humans, *Mol. Nutr. Food Res.*, 53, S44, 2009.
36. Adom, K.K., Sorrells, M.E., and Liu, R.H., Phytochemicals and antioxidant activity of milled fractions of different wheat varieties, *J. Agric. Food Chem.*, 53, 2297, 2005.
37. Hatcher, D.W. and Kruger, J.E., Simple phenolic acids in flours prepared from Canadian wheat: Relationship to ash content, color, and polyphenol oxidase activity, *Cereal Chem.*, 74, 337, 1997.
38. Adom, K.K. and Liu, R.H., Antioxidant activity of grains, *J. Agric. Food Chem.*, 50, 6182, 2002.
39. Mattila, P., Pihlava, J.M., and Hellstrom, J., Contents of phenolic acids, alkyl- and alkenylresorcinols, and avenanthramides in commercial grain products, *J. Agric. Food Chem.*, 53, 8290, 2005.
40. Lempereur, I., Rouau, X., and Abecassis, J., Genetic and agronomic variation in arabi-noxylan and ferulic acid contents of durum wheat (*Triticum durum* L.) grain and its milling fractions, *J. Cereal Sci.*, 25, 103, 1997.
41. Kern, S.M. et al., Absorption of hydroxycinnamates in humans after high-bran cereal consumption, *J. Agric. Food Chem.*, 51, 6050, 2003.
42. Braune, A. et al., Degradation of neohesperidin dihydrochalone in human intestinal bacteria, *J. Agric. Food Chem.*, 53, 1782, 2005.
43. Jaganath, I.B. et al., In vitro catabolism of rutin by human fecal bacteria and the anti-oxidant capacity of its catabolites, *Free. Rad. Biol. Med.*, 47, 1180, 2009.
44. Juskiewicz, J. et al., Effect of the dietary polyphenolic fraction of chicory root, peel, seed and leaf extracts on caecal fermentation and blood parameters in rats fed diets containing prebiotic fructans, *Br. J. Nutr.*, 105, 710, 2011.
45. Le Gall, M. et al., The role of whole wheat grain and wheat and rye ingredients on the digestion and fermentation processes in the gut—A model experiment with pigs, *Br. J. Nutr.*, 102, 1590, 2009.
46. Lhoste, E.F. et al., The human colonic microflora influences the alterations of xenobiotic-metabolising enzymes by catechins in male F344 rats, *Food Chem. Toxicol.*, 41, 695, 2003.
47. Schnieder, H. et al., Degradation of quercitin-3-glucoside in gnotobiotic rats associated with human intestinal bacteria, *J. Appl. Microbiol.*, 89, 1027, 2000.
48. Gross, G. et al., In vitro bioconversion of polyphenols from black tea and red wine/grape juice by human intestinal microbiota displays strong inter-individual variability, *J. Agric. Food Chem.*, 58, 10236, 2010.
49. Bazzoco, S. et al., Factors affecting the conversion of apple polyphenols to phenolic acids and fruit matrix to short chain fatty acids by human bacteria in vitro, *Eur. J. Nutr.*, 47, 442, 2008.
50. Jenner, A.M. et al., Human fecal water content of phenolics: The extent of colonic exposure to aromatic compounds, *Free Rad. Biol. Med.*, 38, 763, 2005.
51. Gill, C.I.R. et al., Profiling of phenols in human fecal water after raspberry supplementation, *J. Agric. Food Chem.*, 58, 10389, 2010.
52. Gelboin, H.V., Wiebel, F.J., and Kinoshita, N., Microsomal arylhydrocarbon hydroxy-lases: On their role in polycyclic hydrocarbon carcinogenesis and toxicity and the mechanism of enzyme induction. In: Boyd GS, Smellie RMS, editors. *Biological Hydroxylation Mechanisms*. New York: Academic Press, 1972, pp. 103–133.

53. Eisenhofer, G., Kopin, I.J., and Goldstein, D.S., Catecholamine metabolism: A contemporary view with implications for physiology and medicine, *Pharmacol. Rev.*, 56, 331, 2004.
54. Roowi, S. et al., Green tea flavan-3-ols: Colonic degradation and urinary excretion of catabolites by humans, *J. Agric. Food Chem.*, 58, 1296, 2010.
55. Grun, C.H. et al., GC-MS methods for metabolic profiling of microbial fermentation products of dietary polyphenols in human and in vitro intervention studies, *J. Chromatogr. B Anal. Technol. Biomed. Life Sci.*, 871, 212, 2008.
56. Combet, E. et al., Dietary flavonols contribute to false-positive elevation of homovanillic acid, a marker of catecholamine-secreting tumors, *Clin. Chim. Acta*, 412, 165, 2011.
57. Rios, L.Y. et al., Chocolate intake increases urinary excretion of polyphenol-derived phenolic acids in healthy human subjects, *Am. J. Clin. Nutr.*, 77, 912, 2003.
58. Ward, N.C. et al., Supplementation with grape seed polyphenols results in increased urinary excretion of 3-hydroxyphenylpropionic acid, an important metabolite of proanthocyanidins in humans, *J. Agric. Food Chem.*, 52, 5545, 2004.
59. Monagas, M. et al., Dihydroxylated phenolic acids derived from microbial metabolism reduce lipopolysaccharide-stimulated cytokine secretion by human peripheral blood mononuclear cells, *Br. J. Nutr.*, 102, 201, 2009.
60. Arts, I.C.W. and Hollman, P.C.H., Polyphenols and disease risk in epidemiologic studies, *Am. J. Clin. Nutr.*, 81, 317S, 2005.
61. Erlund, I., Review of the flavonoids quercetin, hesperetin naringenin. Dietary sources, bioactivities, and epidemiology, *Nutr. Res.*, 24, 851, 2004.
62. McCullough, M.L. et al., Hypertension, the Kuna, and the epidemiology of flavanols, *J. Cardiovasc. Pharmacol.*, 47, S103, 2007.
63. Dai, Q. et al., Fruit and vegetable juices and Alzheimer's disease: The Kame project, *Am. J. Med.*, 119, 751, 2006.
64. Sing, M.F. et al., Epidemiological studies of the association between tea drinking and primary liver cancer: A meta-analysis, *Eur. J. Cancer Prev.*, 20, 157, 2011.
65. Smith-Warner, S.A., Epidemiology of polyphenols and cancer, *J. Nutr.*, 133, 3846S, 2003.
66. Tzounis, X. et al., Prebiotic evaluation of cocoa-derived flavanols in healthy humans by using a randomized, controlled, double-blind, crossover intervention study, *Am. J. Clin. Nutr.*, 93, 62, 2011.
67. Martin-Carron, N. and Goni, I., Prior exposure of cecal microflora to grape pomaces does not inhibit in vitro fermentation of pectin, *J. Agric. Food Chem.*, 46, 1064, 1998.
68. Branning, C. et al., Blueberry husks and multi-strain probiotics affect colonic fermentation in rats, *Br. J. Nutr.*, 101, 859, 2009.
69. Saura-Calixto, F. et al., Proanthocyanidin metabolites associated with dietary fibre from in vitro colonic fermentation and proanthocyanidin metabolites in human plasma, *Mol. Nutr. Food Res.*, 54, 939, 2010.
70. Gruendel, S. et al., Carob rich preparation rich in insoluble dietary fibre and polyphenols increases plasma glucose load in humans, *Br. J. Nutr.*, 98, 105, 2007.
71. Rechner, A.R. et al., Colonic metabolism of dietary polyphenol: Influence of structure on microbial fermentation products, *Free Rad. Biol. Med.*, 36, 212, 2004.
72. Armstrong, E.F. et al., The effect of weaning diet on the subsequent colonic metabolism of dietary fibre in the adult rat, *J. Nutr.*, 68, 741, 1992.
73. Gardana, C., Canzi, E., and Simenetti, P., The role of diet in the metabolism of daidzein by human faecal microbiota from Italian volunteers, *J. Nutr. Biochem.*, 20, 940, 2009.

17

Impact of Low Viscous Fiber on Postprandial and Fasting Glycemia

GEOFFREY LIVESEY

Contents

17.1 Introduction

Dietary fiber plays an important role in modifying several aspects of health, including the prevention and management of metabolic diseases: metabolic syndrome, diabetes, and coronary heart disease (Liu et al., 2000; Livesey et al., 2008a,b; Salmerón et al., 2001; Schulze et al., 2004a,b; Weickert et al., 2005, 2006). Numerous mechanisms of action have been implicated in how fiber affects digestion and metabolism (Brennan, 2005; Livesey, 2005; Weickert and Pfeiffer, 2008). Of particular relevance for resistant maltodextrin (RMD) are mechanisms leading primarily to a reduction in the glycemic response to carbohydrate foods and in the longer-term mechanisms that involve the metabolism of dietary fiber (Livesey, 2005; Weickert et al., 2005).

17.2 Fiber, Glycemic Index, and Glucose Control: Early Knowledge

Early accounts of dietary treatments exist for diabetes, and these used a cereal product, wheat germ (Egypt: The Ebers Papyrus, 1550 BC), and a low glycemic starchy food, chana dahl (Kapur and Kapur, 2001). A Medical Research Council Special Report "The carbohydrate content of foods" (McCance and Lawrence, 1929) made clear that dietary fiber (or fiber) is a nonglycemic carbohydrate and could replace metabolizable carbohydrate in the diet of diabetics. The fiber content and glycemic response to foods covary, though inexactly (Wolever et al., 1986). This covariance has made it difficult to identify the separate roles of fiber and glycemic response in blood glucose control, and hence, their independent help in the prevention and management of type-2 diabetes and coronary heart disease.

That a lower glycemic response to high-fiber foods was not simply due to a displacement of metabolizable carbohydrate in foods by fiber became evident on feeding foods containing similar amounts of metabolizable carbohydrate but which generated different glycemic responses (Foster-Powell et al., 2002; Jenkins et al., 1981; Wolever et al., 1986). Although this idea had gained pace in years prior to 1981, Jenkin's work was pivotal for acknowledgment by the scientific community and was captured in the concept of glycemic index. Thus, not only was dietary fiber a means to help control blood glucose by the replacement of the metabolizable carbohydrate, but the source of metabolizable carbohydrate also became important.

Among food sources of dietary fiber helpful for the primary and secondary control of type-2 diabetes and coronary heart disease is cereal (Schulze et al., 2007; Wolk et al., 1999). However, in type-2 diabetics, a higher-cereal-fiber diet is reported to be less effective than a lower-glycemic-index diet for diabetes control over 6 months intervention (Jenkins et al., 2008). Also, a low-glycemic-index diet improved insulin sensitivity more than a high-cereal diet in women with polycystic ovary syndrome (Marsh et al., 2010). For dietetic purposes, nevertheless, it is important to recognize that both low-glycemic-index and high-cereal-fiber diets can have important, independent, and additive roles. Our meta-regression analyses confirm cereal fiber to be effective in the cohort studies on risk of type-2 diabetes, with a fall in incidence rate of 5% (SE 1%, $P > |z| < 0.001$) for each 1 g increase in cereal fiber intake. No inconsistency (heterogeneity) among the first eight published cohort studies is evident (author, unpublished). The beneficial effects of cereal fiber and low glycemic index in respect of fasting glycemia and glycated proteins are likely additive—both among published intervention studies on health markers (Livesey et al., 2008a) and among persons within populations studied prospectively, as first shown for heart disease and type-2 diabetes in women (Liu et al., 2000; Salmerón et al., 1997).

17.3 Mechanisms by Which Fiber Affects Glycemia

In addition to a direct role for cereal fiber (and associated substances), dietary fiber has several modes of action by which it can help to maintain a low blood glucose concentration either postprandially or in the fasting state. Mechanisms in general are not discussed here, though two are of particular interest for soluble fibers. As exemplified by guar gum and β-glucan, one important mechanism relates to fiber viscosity, which slows convection mixing and so diffusion of both carbohydrates and hydrolases during digestion (Blackburn et al., 1984; Jenkins et al., 2002) and can encapsulate particles of food so partitioning food starches from the digestive juices containing the starch-degrading enzyme, amylase. When this occurs, the fiber is more effective when incorporated into foods than when taken in a drink (Brennan, 2005; Poppitt et al., 2007). However, this does not always apply or does not apply to all soluble fibers because it does not apply to RMD, which is more effective when taken in a drink than when incorporated into foods (Livesey and Tagami, 2009).

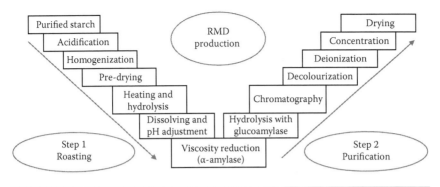

Figure 17.1 The two step production of resistant maltodextrin.

17.4 Resistant Maltodextrin

RMD is a purified fraction from roasted starch. It is produced in two major steps (Figure 17.1). First, starch is heat treated making approximately 50% resistant to digestive enzymes of the gastrointestinal tract (GI) (Ohkuma et al., 1990b; Okuma and Matsuda, 2002, 2003). This process involves partial hydrolysis using moisture already in the starch, eventual drying, and dehydration of reducing ends. During this process, α1-6 anhydroglucose is produced, which initiates reactions and rearrangement of the linkages between glucose units. Hence, the product has linkages other than enzyme-susceptible ones of α1-4 and α1-6. The second major step purifies the resistant fraction (Figure 17.1). Methylation analysis identifies the purified fraction (RMD) to be highly branched. This product is stable in solution, resists depolymerization by acid or heat treatment, and has a dextrose equivalent dispersed across the range DE 10–15. Consequently, RMD has a low viscosity in common with other dextrins of similar size (Ohkuma et al., 1990a).

The RMD is 90% assayable as AOAC fiber (Gordon and Okuma, 2002) and, when ingested with water alone, has negligible acute effect on blood glucose or plasma insulin responses (Kawasaki et al., 2000; Ohkuma et al., 1990b; Okuma and Matsuda, 2002; Shoya et al., 2004; Tokunaga and Matsuoka, 1999; Wakabayashi et al., 1999). The quantitative impact of RMD on carbohydrate metabolism in humans, assessed by indirect calorimetry and breath hydrogen production, is also consistent with the AOAC fiber analysis (Goda et al., 2006). Numerous studies indicate that RMD is well tolerated, for example, (Satouchi et al., 1993). Because RMD resists primary digestion, it becomes a substrate of fermentation in the large bowel, where it is both bifidogenic and butyrogenic (Fastinger et al., 2008). RMD has found use as a means to lower the glycemic response to carbohydrate foods and for such purpose can be found in foods and drinks regulated by FOSHU in Japan. In the United States, RMD has GRAS status (CFR21, 184-1277), and FAO/WHO has rated the product to be "A1 safe" with no limit to ADI (acceptable daily intake).

17.5 Acute Impact of RMD on the Glycemic Response to Meals

Studies have examined the impact of RMD on the glycemic response to rice. Rice is a staple food in many countries and especially in Asia, and increasingly world-wide as Western palates engage with oriental foods. Long-grain rice is commonly found to have a high glycemic index, though different forms have glycemic indices that range from as low as 34 (high amylose rice) to as high as 109 for Jasmine rice (low amylose rice) when compared with glucose. Prospective studies indicate high consumption of rice to make a very significant contribution to the development of diabetes among Orientals (Villegas et al., 2007), so much so that even total carbohydrate intake becomes associated with the development of this condition.

Nine randomized controlled intervention studies investigated 5–8 g RMD consumed in a beverage (e.g., tea) and found this fiber to lower the glycemic response to regular sized portions of boiled rice. In these studies, the beverage was taken with the rice—neither before nor after. Meta-analysis of these studies shows the glycemic response to be reduced by 20% compared with a control beverage without the RMD (Figure 17.2). Among 37 similar studies with varied sources of starches and sugars and varied methods of taking RMD, it has become clear that among Oriental persons, a reduction of the glycemic response due to RMD consumption is a typical finding (Livesey and Tagami, 2009). Variation between studies (inconsistency or heterogeneity) does occur but is likely due to a high variability in the glycemic response within persons from one occasion to another.

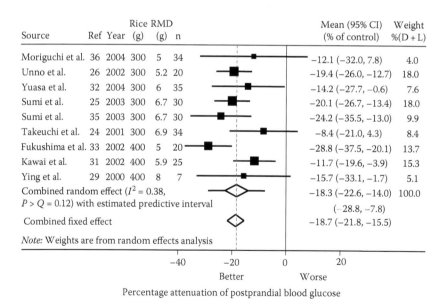

Source	Ref	Year	Rice (g)	RMD (g)	n		Mean (95% CI) (% of control)	Weight %(D + L)
Moriguchi et al.	36	2004	300	5	34		−12.1 (−32.0, 7.8)	4.0
Unno et al.	26	2002	300	5.2	20		−19.4 (−26.0, −12.7)	18.0
Yuasa et al.	32	2004	300	6	35		−14.2 (−27.7, −0.6)	7.6
Sumi et al.	25	2003	300	6.7	30		−20.1 (−26.7, −13.4)	18.0
Sumi et al.	35	2003	300	6.7	30		−24.2 (−35.5, −13.0)	9.9
Takeuchi et al.	24	2001	300	6.9	34		−8.4 (−21.0, 4.3)	8.4
Fukushima et al.	33	2002	400	5	20		−28.8 (−37.5, −20.1)	13.7
Kawai et al.	31	2002	400	5.9	25		−11.7 (−19.6, −3.9)	15.3
Ying et al.	29	2000	400	8	7		−15.7 (−33.1, −1.7)	5.1
Combined random effect ($I^2 = 0.38$, $P > Q = 0.12$) with estimated predictive interval							−18.3 (−22.6, −14.0) (−28.8, −7.8)	100.0
Combined fixed effect							−18.7 (−21.8, −15.5)	

Note: Weights are from random effects analysis

−40   −20   0   20

Better   Worse

Percentage attenuation of postprandial blood glucose

Figure 17.2 Attenuation of the glycemic response to boiled rice in humans by RMD dissolved in a beverage, e.g. tea.

Among a wider range of foods and drinks, the percentage attenuation of the glycemic response was found to be independent of the amount of carbohydrate ingested in the range 30–173 g at one meal (Livesey and Tagami, 2009). This would be consistent with a modification of the glycemic index.

Over the wider range of intakes of RMD, from 4 to 10 g per meal among the totality of studies, there is evidence of dose dependency (Livesey and Tagami, 2009). Such provides stronger evidence of the effectiveness of RMD than can be claimed by a randomized control study alone. Intakes lower than 4 g per meal are not likely to show statistically significant effect.

In addition to attenuating the glycemic response to starchy foods (boiled rice, Figure 17.2), there is attenuation of the glycemic response to refined carbohydrates (maltodextrin, glucose, and sucrose combined) and to an approximately similar extent (Table 17.1). RMD also attenuates the postprandial triglyceride response to a fatty meal in healthy persons (Kishimoto et al., 2007). This lack of substrate specificity suggests that one or more mechanisms operate independently of the nature of the substrate and so independently of the specificity of the digestive enzymes. In the case of the triglyceride response to dietary fat, in burger and chips, 5–10 g RMD per meal reduced the response (incremental area under the 6 h curve) by an average of 23%. Such is similar in magnitude to the attenuation of the glycemic response to carbohydrate foods.

RMD is more effective when taken in drinks than when incorporated into foods (Livesey and Tagami, 2009). Effectiveness is evident with RMD independently of the type of drinks (tea, soft drink, and in one publication with coffee) and several types of tea taken with carbohydrate meals (Table 17.1).

A slowing of stomach emptying by RMD is one possibility that would explain a lower glycemic response to carbohydrate in the presence of RMD, but such would not obviously be due to gel formation in the stomach because RMD does not form a gel. Ileal short-chain fatty acids can inhibit gastric motility via a humoral pathway (Cuche et al., 2000). However, such an effect also seems an unlikely explanation for RMD because it would take perhaps 1 h for such an effect to manifest, whereas the size of the effect is independent of the time course for glucose absorption in humans (Livesey and Tagami, 2009). Similarly, modification of gastric tone via colonic short-chain fatty acid production would not explain attenuation of the glycemic response by RMD (Ropert et al., 1996).

Because RMD impairs the absorption of triglycerides from dietary fat (Kishimoto et al., 2007), it might be thought that RMD could, in some way, act via an interaction with dietary lipids. For example, impaired lipid absorption might enhance the ileal break on stomach emptying, small intestinal motility, and ileal excretion into the colon (Van Citters and Lin, 1999). However, such would not readily explain the attenuation of the glycemic response to fat-free meals such as starch in boiled rice, sucrose, glucose, and maltodextrin taken as the sole source of substrate other than RMD.

Table 17.1 Attenuation of the Glycemic and Insulinemic Responses to Food Carbohydrate by RMD under Various Circumstances

Carbohydrate Source and Mode of RMD Administration	No. of Studies	Attenuation (% per 10 g RMD)		P-Value	Heterogeneity
		Trend[a]	SE		$I^{2\,b}$
Plasma glucose response					
Refined carbohydrates[c]	5	−23[d]	3	<0.001	0.80
Starchy foods	32	−26	3	<0.001	0.80
RMD in foods	16	−18	4	<0.001	0.71
RMD in drinks taken with foods	16	−33	4	<0.001	0.71
Oolong tea	3	−20	8	<0.001	0.41
Green tea	3	−38	6	<0.001	0.48
Other teas	6	−32	7	<0.001	0.75
Soft drinks	3	−33	8	<0.001	0.00
Coffee	1	−63	—	—	—
In tea preadaptation	3	−42	5	<0.001	0.00
In tea postadaptation (4–26 weeks)	3	−36	−8	<0.001	0.00
Plasma insulin response					
Refined and unrefined carbohydrates[e]	6	−25	7	<0.001	0.67

Sources: Based on Livesey, G. and H. Tagami, *Am. J. Clin. Nutr.*, 89, 114, 2009; Livesey, G. and H. Tagami, The significant impact of a low viscous fibre on glycaemic response, in J.W. van der Kamp et al., eds. *Dietary Fibre: New Frontiers for Food and Health*, Wageningen Academic Publishers, Wageningen, the Netherlands, 2010, pp. 475–491.

[a] The trend for the meta-regression dose-response curve is forced through zero effect at zero dose. For consistency in bringing data together from different studies, the trend is expressed as a % per 10 g RMD, whereas in the studies undertaken, the precise values for RMD ingestion may have been lower, between 3 and 10 g RMD per meal.

[b] I^2, the proportion of total variance due to the among-studies variance.

[c] Maltodextrin or glucose or sucrose.

[d] All such values compared with a placebo of identical food and drink intake without RMD.

[e] Starch, maltodextrin, glucose, and sucrose.

A more direct effect of RMD earlier than the terminal ileum, such as a jejunal brake (Lin et al., 1997), remains unexplored. The nondigestible and marginal osmotic effects of RMD may impact on this break (Vu et al., 2000).

Owing to its resistance to digestion, RMD contributes both dry bulk and some bulk water. RMD is also of relatively small size osmotically for fiber (DE 10–15). Each of these characteristics potentially quickens intestinal motility and movement of carbohydrate toward a more distal site in the small intestine where carbohydrate and glucose absorption is least rapid (Livesey et al., 1998).

Carbohydrate metabolism and hydrogen excretion after RMD ingestion together with a low carbohydrate meal are consistent with the amounts of carbohydrate entering the colon being that due to the greater consumption of nondigestible carbohydrate in RMD, and no more than this (Goda et al., 2006). A reduced glycemia due to impaired digestion and so ileal excretion into the colon is therefore unlikely.

The insulinemic response to starchy foods during coingestion of a beverage with RMD if enhanced would explain a lower postprandial blood glucose response. However, this idea is improbable because RMD attenuates the insulin response to an extent similar to that seen for attenuation of the glycemic response (Table 17.1). This similarity also implies no substantially enhanced release of GI peptides that potentiate the insulin response to glucose. Attenuation of the insulin response by RMD is evident for several substrates and meals: glucose, sucrose, maltodextrin (Table 17.1), boiled rice with curry (Livesey and Tagami, 2009), and hamburger and chips (Kishimoto et al., 2007).

Nondigestible polysaccharides have potential to improve glucose tolerance at a second meal (Nilsson et al., 2008). While a second meal effect cannot explain the acute impact of RMD on the glycemic response to dietary carbohydrates in persons without previous ingestion, such cannot be excluded as a contributor to a lower fasting glycemia observed after chronic consumption.

While some mechanisms offer unlikely explanations of how RMD lowers postprandial glycemia, other mechanisms remained to be explored. That RMD in solution appears more potent than RMD in the food matrix may result from some intestinal hurry. Should this be so, the DE equivalent of the RMD could be important to the size of its effect. Possibly also RMD may become entangled in the mucopolysaccharide layer in the GI tract, so increasing the effective "thickness" of the unstirred layer and slowing convection currents and so absorption. Such an effect could explain the wide range of substrates for which RMD affects absorption. Such might also explain why RMD is less effective in a food matrix than in drinks (Table 17.1). However, such a polysaccharide or dextrin effect may not then be unique to RMD and might occur to varying degrees for a range of different dextrins, including maltodextrin. However, the effect with RMD, being nondigestible, would be longer lasting.

17.6 Modification of Fasting Blood Glucose by Chronic Treatment with RMD

Thirty three case-series studies have examined the effects of regular RMD ingestion on fasting plasma glucose consuming RMD daily for 3 months usually divided among three meals a day. The majority of such studies are reported in publications alongside effects on postprandial glycemia [for references see (Livesey and Tagami, 2009)]. Thirteen studied with RMD intakes below 15 g/day were discarded as unduly low powered studies or had group mean plasma glucose below a previously recognized normal mean point of 4.9 mmol/L for which no correction of fasting glucose could be expected.

Seventeen studies of normal healthy persons with fasting plasma glucose in the range 4.9–7.0 mmol/L consumed 15–30 g per day (Figure 17.3). On average

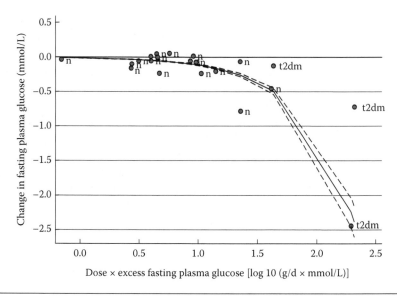

Figure 17.3 Fasting plasma glucose falls during regular RMD consumption over 3 months – dependent on dose and severity of dysglycemia (excess plasma glucose, >4.9 mmol/L).

such treatments, at varied doses, corrected 24% of the plasma glucose in excess of a fasting plasma levels of 4.9 mmol/L, significantly ($P > |kht| = 0.008$). Among these studies, RMD was taken either in drinks or in foods, but not in both. Broadly similar results were observed whether from drinks or from foods, but differences were statistically significant for drinks only ($P > |kht| = 0.044$ for drinks and 0.11 for foods).

Three similar studies have been conducted in persons with a history of type-2 diabetes. Their age range was 55–56 years, body weight range was 55–69 kg, and mean fasting plasma glucose concentration was in the range from 6.3 to 11.1 mmol/L. The dose of RMD was high and in the range 30–60 g RMD daily (Fujiwara and Matsuoka, 1993, 1995; Nomura et al., 1992). Over all three studies, the mean fasting plasma glucose was decreased (−1.15 mmol/L), and the largest effect occurred with the largest dose (Nomura et al., 1992).

Modeling of the results for all studies combined suggested that the reduction in fasting plasma glucose occurred due to an interaction between the dose of RMD and the excess of fasting plasma glucose (Figure 17.3). In other words, larger doses had larger effects, and effects were even larger with increase in severity of dysglycemia above 4.9 mmol/L. Such is consistent with prior observations from randomized controlled studies, which inform us about how dietary fiber in general affects fasting blood glucose in diabetics and nondiabetics combined (Livesey et al., 2008a).

A question arises as to how dysglycemic the normal healthy persons were to begin with. After adjustment of the observations to a constant 30 g RMD ingestion per day—to facilitate comparisons across severity of dysglycemia, a correction of

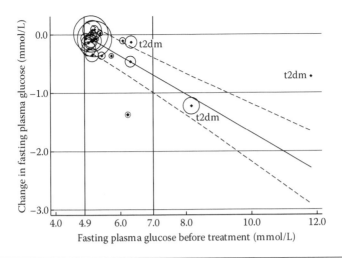

Figure 17.4 Fasting plasma glucose falls during regular RMD consumption over three month's dependent of the severity of dysglycemia (after adjustment for dose to 30 g RMD per day, split between meals).

dysglycemia by RMD is suggested in the range 4.9–7.0 mmol/L fasting glucose, i.e., among nondiabetics as well as in diabetics (Figure 17.4).

17.7 Further and Concluding Discussion

RMD supplies both a source of fermentable carbohydrate and a means to lower the glycemic response to several types of carbohydrates, carbohydrate foods and meals, and is easy to incorporate into drinks and foods. Such incorporation is easy to achieve using RMD as a condiment too because it dissolves readily.

Attenuation of the glycemic response to meals by RMD is more effective when administered simultaneously within drinks than when mixed into a food matrix. In particular, RMD is effective in reducing postprandial glycemia even though in vitro it is a nonviscous source of fiber. Being nonviscous, it can be more palatable than viscous fiber sources and can be consumed with a wide range of foods, optimally by being present in a beverage taken with a meal.

In chronic studies, RMD consumption lowers fasting plasma glucose. Such is evident whenever the fasting plasma glucose is above normal (4.9 mmol/L) in both nondiabetics as well as in type-2 diabetics. Such a result is consistent with similar observations for dietary fiber in general in conventional foods (Livesey et al., 2008a).

That RMD can lower postprandial and fasting blood glucose, and postprandial insulin, implies a potential risk reduction for diabetes and heart disease. Interestingly, such arises without factors associated with cereal fibers which may otherwise be thought important in other circumstances (Institute of Medicine, 2003; Schulze et al., 2007).

Some hypothesized mechanisms of action of RMD on postprandial blood glucose appear unlikely to be involved (as discussed) while several other mechanisms remain to be explored. More than one mechanism might operate so making it difficult to quantify the contribution of each. Although RMD is nonviscous, it may become viscous in vivo, but if not, then its mechanism of action would be largely different to that of viscous fiber sources, such that potential for optimal effects might emerge in some circumstances from combinations of fiber sources.

Although a reduction in postprandial glycemia due to RMD consumption occurs within a timescale that would exclude an involvement of RMD fermentation in the mechanism of effect, fermentation may be implicated in the reduction of fasting blood glucose.

References

Blackburn, N.A., J.S. Redfern, H. Jarjis, A.M. Holgate, I. Hanning, J.H. Scarpello, I.T. Johnson, and N.W. Read. 1984. The mechanism of action of guar gum in improving glucose tolerance in man. *Clin Sci (Lond)* 66:329–336.

Brennan, C.S. 2005. Dietary fibre, glycaemic response, and diabetes. *Mol Nutr Food Res* 49:560–570.

Cuche, G., J.C. Cuber, and C.H. Malbert. 2000. Ileal short-chain fatty acids inhibit gastric motility by a humoral pathway. *Am J Physiol Gastrointest Liver Physiol* 279:G925–G930.

Fastinger, N.D., L.K. Karr-Lilienthal, J.K. Spears, K.S. Swanson, K.E. Zinn, G.M. Nava, K. Ohkuma, S. Kanahori, D.T. Gordon, and G.C. Fahey, Jr. 2008. A novel resistant maltodextrin alters gastrointestinal tolerance factors, fecal characteristics, and fecal microbiota in healthy adult humans. *J Am Coll Nutr* 27:356–366.

Foster-Powell, K., S.H. Holt, and J.C. Brand-Miller. 2002. International table of glycemic index and glycemic load values: 2002. *Am J Clin Nutr* 76:5–56.

Fujiwara, K. and A. Matsuoka. 1993. Continuous administration test of indigestible dextrin; II: Study of the effects of the improvement of fat metabolism in patients with non-insulin-dependent diabetes mellitus. *J Jpn Soc Nutr Food Sci* 83:301–305 (in Japanese).

Fujiwara, K. and A. Matsuoka. 1995. Improvement of glucose tolerance by low-viscosity, water-soluble dietary fiber, indigestible dextrin. *Jpn J Nutr* 53:361–368 (in Japanese).

Goda, T., Y. Kajiya, K. Suruga, H. Tagami, and G. Livesey. 2006. Availability, fermentability, and energy value of resistant maltodextrin: Modeling of short-term indirect calorimetric measurements in healthy adults. *Am J Clin Nutr* 83:1321–1330.

Gordon, D.T. and K. Okuma. 2002. Determination of total dietary fiber in selected foods containing resistant maltodextrin by enzymatic-gravimetric method and liquid chromatography: Collaborative study. *J AOAC Inter.* 85:435–444.

Institute of Medicine. 2003. *Dietary Reference Intakes for Energy, Carbohydrate, Fiber, Fat, Fatty Acids, Cholesterol, Protein, and Amino Acids (Macronutrients)*. Macronutrients and healthful diets. Washington, DC: National Academies Press.

Jenkins, A.L., D.J. Jenkins, U. Zdravkovic, P. Wursch, and V. Vuksan. 2002. Depression of the glycemic index by high levels of beta-glucan fiber in two functional foods tested in type 2 diabetes. *Eur J Clin Nutr* 56:622–628.

Jenkins, D.J., T.M. Wolever, R.H. Taylor, H. Barker, H. Fielden, J.M. Baldwin, A.C. Bowling, H.C. Newman, A.L. Jenkins, and D.V. Goff. 1981. Glycemic index of foods: A physiological basis for carbohydrate exchange. *Am J Clin Nutr* 34:362–366.

Jenkins, D.J., C.W. Kendall, G. McKeown-Eyssen, R.G. Josse, J. Silverberg, G.L. Booth, E. Vidgen, A.R. Josse, T.H. Nguyen, S. Corrigan, M.S. Banach, S. Ares, S. Mitchell, A. Emam, L.S. Augustin, T.L. Parker, and L.A. Leiter. 2008. Effect of a low-glycemic index or a high-cereal fiber diet on type 2 diabetes: A randomized trial. *JAMA* 300:2742–2753.

Kapur, A. and K. Kapur. 2001. Relevance of glycemic index in the management of post-prandial glycemia. *J Assoc Phys India* 49:42–45.

Kawasaki, F., M. Matsuda, T. Hiramatsu, K. Hiroe, K. Kawahara, K. Moriya, and K. Kaku. 2000. Efficacy of tea drink containing indigestible dextrin. *J Nutr Food* 3:65–72 (in Japanese).

Kishimoto, Y., H. Oga, H. Tagami, K. Okuma, and D.T. Gordon. 2007. Suppressive effect of resistant maltodextrin on postprandial blood triacylglycerol elevation. *Eur J Nutr* 46:133–138.

Lin, H.C., X.T. Zhao, and L. Wang. 1997. Intestinal transit is more potently inhibited by fat in the distal (ileal brake) than in the proximal (jejunal brake) gut. *Dig Dis Sci* 42:19–25.

Liu, S., W.C. Willett, M.J. Stampfer, F.B. Hu, M. Franz, L. Sampson, C.H. Hennekens, and J.E. Manson. 2000. A prospective study of dietary glycemic load, carbohydrate intake, and risk of coronary heart disease in US women. *Am J Clin Nutr* 71:1455–1461.

Livesey, G. 2005. Non-digestible carbohydrates and glycaemic control. *In* H. Vorster et al., eds. *Nutrition Safari for Innovative Solutions*, Proceedings of the 18th International Congress of Nutrition. ICC, Durban, South Africa.

Livesey, G. and H. Tagami. 2009. Interventions to lower the glycemic response to carbohydrate foods with a low-viscosity fiber (resistant maltodextrin): Meta-analysis of randomized controlled trials. *Am J Clin Nutr* 89:114–125.

Livesey, G. and H. Tagami. 2010. The significant impact of a low viscous fibre on glycaemic response. In J.W. van der Kamp et al., eds. *Dietary Fibre: New Frontiers for Food and Health*, pp. 475–491. Wageningen Academic Publishers, Wageningen, the Netherlands.

Livesey, G., R. Taylor, T. Hulshof, and J. Howlett. 2008a. Glycemic response and health a systematic review and meta-analysis: Relations between dietary glycemic properties and health outcomes. *Am J Clin Nutr* 87:258S–268S.

Livesey, G., R. Taylor, T. Hulshof, and J. Howlett. 2008b. Glycemic response and health a systematic review and meta-analysis: The database, study characteristics, and macronutrient intakes. *Am J Clin Nutr* 87:223S–236S.

Livesey, G., P.D. Wilson, M.A. Roe, R.M. Faulks, L.M. Oram, J.C. Brown, J. Eagles, R.H. Greenwood, and H. Kennedy. 1998. Splanchnic retention of intraduodenal and intrajejunal glucose in healthy adults. *Am J Physiol* 275:E709–E716.

Marsh, K.A., K.S. Steinbeck, F.S. Atkinson, P. Petocz, and J.C. Brand-Miller. 2010. Effect of a low glycemic index compared with a conventional healthy diet on polycystic ovary syndrome 10.3945/ajcn.2010.29261. *Am J Clin Nutr* 92:83–92.

McCance, R.A. and R.D. Lawrence. 1929. *The Carbohydrate Content of Foods*. Her Majesty's Stationery Office, London, U.K.

Nilsson, A.C., E.M. Ostman, J.J. Holst, and I.M. Bjorck. 2008. Including indigestible carbohydrates in the evening meal of healthy subjects improves glucose tolerance, lowers inflammatory markers, and increases satiety after a subsequent standardized breakfast. *J Nutr* 138:732–739.

Nomura, M., Y. Nakajima, and H. Abe. 1992. Effects of long-term administration of indigestible dextrin as soluble dietary fiber on lipid and glucose metabolism. Nippon Eiyo Shokuryo Gakkaishi. *J Jpn Soc Nutr Food Sci* 45:21–25 (in Japanese).

Ohkuma, K., I. Matsuda, Y. Katta, and Y. Hanno. 1990a. Pyrolysis of starch and its digestibility by enzymes. *Denpun Kagaku* 37:107–114.

Ohkuma, K., I. Matsuda, Y. Katta, and Y. Hanno. 1990b. Pyrolysis of starch and its digestibility by enzymes—Characterization of indigestible dextrins. *Denpun Kagaku* 37:107–114.

Okuma, K. and I. Matsuda. 2002. Indigestible fraction of starch hydrolysates and their determination method. *J Appl Glycosci* 49:479–485.

Okuma, K. and I. Matsuda. 2003. Production of indigestible dextrin from pyrodextrin. *J Appl Glycosci* 50:389–394.

Poppitt, S.D., J.D. van Drunen, A.T. McGill, T.B. Mulvey, and F.E. Leahy. 2007. Supplementation of a high-carbohydrate breakfast with barley beta-glucan improves postprandial glycaemic response for meals but not beverages. *Asia Pac J Clin Nutr* 16:16–24.

Ropert, A., C. Cherbut, C. Roze, A. Le Quellec, J.J. Holst, X. Fu-Cheng, S. Bruley des Varannes, and J.P. Galmiche. 1996. Colonic fermentation and proximal gastric tone in humans. *Gastroenterology* 111:289–296.

Salmerón, J., J.E. Manson, M.J. Stampfer, G.A. Colditz, A.L. Wing, and W.C. Willett. 1997. Dietary fiber, glycemic load, and risk of non-insulin-dependent diabetes mellitus in women. *JAMA* 277:472–477.

Salmerón, J., F.B. Hu, J.E. Manson, M.J. Stampfer, G.A. Colditz, E.B. Rimm, and W.C. Willett. 2001. Dietary fat intake and risk of type 2 diabetes in women. *Am J Clin Nutr* 73:1019–1026.

Satouchi, M., S. Wakabayahi, K. Ohkuma, K. Fujiwara, and A. Matsuoka. 1993. Effects of indigestible dextrin on bowel movement. *Jpn J Nutr* 51:31–37.

Schulze, M.B., S. Liu, E.B. Rimm, J.E. Manson, W.C. Willett, and F.B. Hu. 2004a. Glycemic index, glycemic load, and dietary fiber intake and incidence of type 2 diabetes in younger and middle-aged women. *Am J Clin Nutr* 80:348–356.

Schulze, M.B., M. Schulz, C. Heidemann, A. Schienkiewitz, K. Hoffmann, and H. Boeing. 2007. Fiber and magnesium intake and incidence of type 2 diabetes: A prospective study and meta-analysis. *Arch Intern Med* 167:956–965.

Schulze, M.B., J.E. Manson, D.S. Ludwig, G.A. Colditz, M.J. Stampfer, W.C. Willett, and F.B. Hu. 2004b. Sugar-sweetened beverages, weight gain, and incidence of type 2 diabetes in young and middle-aged women. *JAMA* 292:927–934.

Shoya, H., K. Masuo, T. Shinichiro, Y. Shimada, and K. Shioya. 2004. The inhibitory effect on the postprandial increase in blood glucose exerted by a powdered beverage containing indigestible dextrin, and its safety in over ingestion and long-term ingestion. *J Nutr Food* 7:31–41 (in Japanese).

Tokunaga, K. and A. Matsuoka. 1999. Effects of a FOSHU (food for specified health use) containing indigestible dextrin as a functional component on glucose and fat metabolisms. *J Jpn Diabete Soc* 42:61–63 (in Japanese).

Van Citters, G.W. and H.C. Lin. 1999. The ileal brake: A fifteen-year progress report. *Curr Gastroenterol Rep* 1:404–409.

Villegas, R., S. Liu, Y.T. Gao, G. Yang, H. Li, W. Zheng, and X.O. Shu. 2007. Prospective study of dietary carbohydrates, glycemic index, glycemic load, and incidence of type 2 diabetes mellitus in middle-aged Chinese women. *Arch Intern Med* 167:2310–2316.

Vu, M.K., M.A. Nouwens, I. Biemond, C.B. Lamers, and A.A. Masclee. 2000. The osmotic laxative magnesium sulphate activates the ileal brake. *Aliment Pharmacol Ther* 14:587–595.

Wakabayashi, S., Y. Kishimoto, S. Nanbu, and A. Matsuoka. 1999. Effects of indigestible dextrin on postprandial rise in blood glucose levels in man. *J Jpn Assoc Dietary Fiber Res* 3:13–19 (in Japanese).

Weickert, M.O. and A.F. Pfeiffer. 2008. Metabolic effects of dietary fiber consumption and prevention of diabetes. *J Nutr* 138:439–442.

Weickert, M.O., M. Mohlig, C. Schofl, A.M. Arafat, B. Otto, H. Viehoff, C. Koebnick, A. Kohl, J. Spranger, and A.F. Pfeiffer. 2006. Cereal fiber improves whole-body insulin sensitivity in overweight and obese women. *Diabetes Care* 29:775–780.

Weickert, M.O., M. Mohlig, C. Koebnick, J.J. Holst, P. Namsolleck, M. Ristow, M. Osterhoff, H. Rochlitz, N. Rudovich, J. Spranger, and A.F. Pfeiffer. 2005. Impact of cereal fibre on glucose-regulating factors. *Diabetologia* 48:2343–2353.

Wolever, T.M., Z. Cohen, L.U. Thompson, M.J. Thorne, M.J. Jenkins, E.J. Prokipchuk, and D.J. Jenkins. 1986. Ileal loss of available carbohydrate in man: Comparison of a breath hydrogen method with direct measurement using a human ileostomy model. *Am J Gastroenterol* 81:115–122.

Wolk, A., J.E. Manson, M.J. Stampfer, G.A. Colditz, F.B. Hu, F.E. Speizer, C.H. Hennekens, and W.C. Willett. 1999. Long-term intake of dietary fiber and decreased risk of coronary heart disease among women. *J Am Med Assoc* 281:1998–2004.

18

Essentiality and Beneficial Physiological Effects of Dietary Fiber

Resistant Maltodextrin: A Case Study

DENNIS T. GORDON

Contents

18.1 Introduction

What is dietary fiber (DF)? How much DF intake is needed for its expression of essentiality? What are the minimum DF needs for (1) optimum intestinal regularity (laxation), (2) optimum microbiota composition and mass, and conversely (3) what is the maximum amount of DF that can be tolerated by the intestine? Is there an upper limit (UL) that can be assigned to DF intakes, and what are the consequences of exceeding this UL? What are the health benefits of DF? Are the absolute and/or essential needs of DF versus its health benefits synonymous? Is there one single source of DF that can be considered the most beneficial and/or necessary (possibly essential)? DF is plural and represents a large variety of nondigestible carbohydrates (NDCs) with varying chemical and physical properties, which affect their physiological properties, mainly in and via the intestine. The fact that DF is not digested in the small intestine coupled with its fermentability in the large intestine makes it unique among all carbohydrate food ingredients; these properties contributes to its essentially. It is acknowledged that other nondigestible food components such as plant proteins contribute to intestinal function.

While it has been stated by the Institute of Medicine (IOM), but without evidence, that DF is not an essential nutrient, what are the consequences of absolutely *no* DF? Although possibly a slippery slope, there is justification to discuss the definition and measurement of DF in presenting first its essentiality and then its beneficial physiological effects. Answers and comments, presented in this introduction, are provided using scientific data available on resistant maltodextrin (RMD) (Fibersol-2®). The previous remarks in these proceedings by Buck, Livesey, Baer, and Mai are expanded upon to complement this review. Conventional wisdom on the needs and benefits of DF is challenged. It is further acknowledged that DF is a complex issue literally, legally, scientifically, and from regulatory perspectives. A research scientist wants DF defined to set standards for reproducible research. The nutritionist/food scientist and regulatory agencies want a common identity message to measure consumption, make recommendation on intakes, and provide for a uniform platform for food labeling and related nutrient content and health claims. This chapter is not intended as a definitive review of the literature in defending each point or question presented. While many questions are presented, not all are addressed.

18.2 Defining Dietary Fiber

The active debate as how to define DF has been ongoing for the past decade, first in the United States with an AACC International (AACC) proposed definition that stated as follows:

> Dietary fiber is the edible parts of plants or analogous carbohydrates that are resistant to digestion and absorption in the human small intestine with complete or partial fermentation in the large intestine. Dietary fiber includes polysaccharides, oligosaccharides, lignin, and associated plants substances. Dietary fibers promote beneficial physiological effects including laxation, and/or blood cholesterol attenuation, and/or blood glucose attenuation.

While the first two sentences of the AACC definition clearly and simply state what constitutes DF, the last sentence is an over encompassing health claim. The AACC efforts to provide a comprehensive and international dialogue to define DF were promoted by an FDA inquiry. Since this proposed AACC definition could not be sanctioned by the U.S. Food and Drug Administration (FDA), the FDA was required to contract the U.S. IOM to propose a definition for the purpose of food labeling compliance. The IOM was also in the position to review the benefits of DF that complemented the arduous process of setting Adequate Intake (AI) values, the first step in setting Dietary Reference Intake (DRI) values for DF. The initially presented definition for DF by the IOM was revised, and the IOM further did set values for AIs. The IOM three-tier definition states

> Dietary Fiber consists of nondigestible carbohydrates and lignin that are intrinsic and intact in plants.

Functional Fiber consists of isolated, nondigestible carbohydrates that have beneficial physiological effects in humans.

Total Fiber is the sum of Dietary Fiber and Functional Fiber

The final definition for DF in the United States by the FDA is still pending. However, it is evident that the FDA must consider the IOM definition. This is both interesting and important as how the FDA will finalize its definition to have some reasonable agreement with the recently accepted CODEX definition for DF. While there are many ways to interpret the IOM recommendation to separate the DF in intact plants, *dietary fiber*, from isolated NDCs that have beneficial physiological effects in humans, *functional fiber* (FF), it would appear the emphasis is to retain the original concept of the DF hypothesis and make clear separation between (1) "natural" versus "added," (2) "endogenous" versus "isolated/modified/synthetic," and (3) "whole foods" versus "processed foods" in labeling of foods with sources of NDC or DF. How do the chemical, physical, and physiological properties of the IOM's defined DF differ from those of FF? How does any analytical method differentiate between a DF and an FF? How does the body differentiate between a DF and an FF? Does any source of IOM defined FFs not have some physiological effect, and would not the sum of all ingested DF and FF not contribute to beneficial physiological effects? The original work by Burkitt, Trowell, Walker, and Painter on which the DF hypothesis was developed emphasized that whole plant foods, preferably unprocessed, were the sources of DF in fruits-vegetables-whole grains (F-V-WG) and thus the health-promoting factor(s). While these African populations did not have the processed foods we eat today, their consumption of fruits and vegetables was limited, and they had to cook their starch-based foods. It is not argued that whole plant foods/diets, with more F-V-WG, contribute to a lower-calorie, wholesome, and nutritious diets, but the topic and component being defined, measured, and reported on food labels, on which nutrition/health claims are made, are the NDC, the DF, in or added to foods, but not the foods (i.e., fruits, vegetables, and whole gains).

There is an important nutritional principle or guideline at stake in defining DF. Every set of dietary recommendations implore individuals to eat more F-V-WG. This is sound advice, and possibly the best justification to eat a diet rich in plant foods is to achieve a significant reduction in calorie intake. By allowing sources of isolated, modified, and/or synthesized NDC to be labeled as DF, many traditionalists feel the nutritional importance of F-V-WG will be marginalized. Many opinions are that F-V-WG provides many other important nutrients and components besides DF. Many of these other components, now termed nutraceuticals [1], still require extensive evaluation and proof as to their nutrition/health benefits. While it is true these other components in F-V-WG are important, the issue at hand is the DF in F-V-WG and other NDC (FF) added to foods, but not the foods that contain DF or NDC. The DF hypothesis implies that whole/unprocessed foods are better/healthier than processed foods and that the addition of any isolated/modified/synthesized sources of DF is not the same. Does synthetic/isolated vitamin C differ in its nutritional and physiological properties compared to that ingested with an orange? No. Yes, consumption of the orange might provide other benefits. It would appear the IOM's use of the terms DF and FF would be analogous to characterizing the DF as "natural" and FF as added/isolated/synthetic or "processed." And perhaps this is the one criterion that separates DF from FF; the former exists and can be claimed as a true natural ingredient. The current law in the United States allows for food labels to indicate the amount of total insoluble DF (IDF) and soluble DF (SDF) in a food. Yes, informative but at a cost of label space. Is this information helpful to the consumers? While the FDA saw fit to include the possible inclusion of IDF and SDF information on the food label with the Nutrition Labeling and Education Act of 1990, should the FDA allow for the food labeling of DF that increases viscosity, is fermented, and/or increases levels of bifidobacteria? Will there be space for reporting DF, *functional fiber*, and *total fiber* on all foods labels? Will the consumer benefit from this label information? While it cannot be stated that every processed food contains a FF, many if not most do.

The recently accepted Codex Alimentarius (CODEX) definition is more informative compared to the AACC and IOM definitions, but sets one important caveat,* (footnote 2) that is left to individual countries to decide how to handle this issue. In the long term, continuation of this caveat will only lead to lack of uniformity in nutritional labeling and commerce worldwide. Contrary to CODEX decision to include this caveat mentioned in the following text, nondigestible oligosaccharide (NDO) in the DP range of 3–10 does contribute beneficial physiological effects.

The Codex definition for DF states

> Dietary fibre means carbohydrate polymers[†] with 10 or more monomeric units[‡], which are not hydrolysed by the endogenous enzymes in the small intestine of humans and belong to the following categories:
>
> - Edible carbohydrate polymers naturally occurring in the food as consumed.
> - Carbohydrate polymers, which have been obtained from food raw material by physical, enzymatic or chemical means and which have been

---

[*] Decision on whether to include carbohydrates from 3 to 9 monomeric units should be left to national authorities.

[†] When derived from a plant origin, dietary fibre may include fractions of lignin and/or other compounds when associated with polysaccharides in the plant cell walls and if these compounds are quantified by the Association of Official Analytical Chemists (AOAC) gravimetric analytical method for dietary fibre analysis: Fractions of lignin and the other compounds (proteic fractions, phenolic compounds, waxes, saponins, phytates, cutin, phytosterols, etc.) intimately "associated" with plant polysaccharides are often extracted with the polysaccharides in the AOAC 991.43 method. These substances are included in the definition of fibre insofar as they are actually associated with the poly- or oligo-saccharidic fraction of fibre. However, when extracted or even reintroduced into a food containing non-digestible polysaccharides, they cannot be defined as dietary fibre. When combined with polysaccharides, these associated substances may provide additional beneficial effects (pending adoption of Section on Methods of Analysis and Sampling).

[‡] Decision on whether to include carbohydrates from 3 to 9 monomeric units should be left to national authorities.

shown to have a physiological effect of benefit to health as demonstrated by generally accepted scientific evidence to competent authorities.

• Synthetic carbohydrate polymers that have been shown to have a physiological effect of benefit to health as demonstrated by generally accepted scientific evidence to competent authorities.

It is unfortunate that just a few individuals were able to cause such consternation in championing their idea that DF is a food consisting solely of unprocessed F-V-WG, and not as a majority of people recognize, DF is a food component. While it was anticipated that these few people who suggest the term nonstarch polysaccharides (NSPs) replace the term DF and would provide the significant scientific information to justify their position, their long-promised and then delayed publication just days before a major CODEX meeting left no time for its review and discussion [2]. This publication and its contents can be compared to the belief that DF was a pot of gold at the end of the rainbow. These positions presented by these few individuals have been adequately addressed [3].

The issues that remain unresolved with the CODEX definition of DF have been clearly addressed by Lupton et al. [4]. These remaining unresolved issues are as follows: (issue #1) should NDC polymers with degree of polymerization (DP) three to nine be included as DF; (issue #2) how can the beneficial physiological effect for a DF be proven; (issues #3 and #4) what is the effect of processing on DF chemical, physical, and physiological properties; and what are or what should be considered as animal sources of DF? Regarding issue #3, a case in point is resistant starch (RS) and the difference in RS levels in uncooked and then cooked foods.

And there is an additional issue that appears to be only partly addressed by CODEX, but is an issue of importance in the United States and the FDA. This issue is what AOAC International (AOAC) methods should be accepted to measure all sources of DF, both DF and FF, in foods? While CODEX appears to be accepting all AOAC approved methods, the United States and specifically the FDA currently accepts primarily only AOAC methods 985.29 and 991.43 for purposes of definition (a de facto definition based on methodology) and thus food labeling. There is no method for DF analysis that can differentiate between the DF in plant foods (V-F-WG) and those that are isolated, modified, or synthesized and added to foods. An analogous comment is that once ingested, the body cannot differentiate between the DF in F-V-WG and the NDC (FF) added to foods in their contributing to the quintessential properties of DF. In summation, while the CODEX definition for DF is complete, in an attempt to appease a very few individuals, there appears a lack of harmony in having a worldwide common definition for DF, as endorsed by CODEX.

18.3 Methods of Dietary Fiber Analysis

There are 16 AOAC approved methods for the analysis of NDC or DF. The strengths and limitations of these methods have been reviewed [5]. Often repeated and consistently ignored by the FDA is that while AOAC methods 985.29 and 991.43 can measure IDF and soluble DF components, these methods cannot measure

NDO with DP values of or below 10. There has been a call for a comprehensive method for the analysis of DF that would include the measurement of insoluble and soluble components and individual NDOs. This has recently been accomplished with very high recoveries of insoluble, soluble, resistant starch (RS) and NDO mixtures in bread samples by Nishibata and colleagues [6].

Possibly a second major fault in the CODEX deliberations is their recognizing a non-AOAC-approved method, designed exclusively for the measurement of NSP. However, the recognition of this method appears to be for the sole purpose of appeasing the few people who championed the idea that NSPs are the true heir in defining DF [2,7]. Some wonder why this method is only commercially available in a private laboratory operated by one of the few people supporting the NSP cause; somewhere there is conflict of interest.

Irrespective of the terminology, or the description with limiting caveats used to define DF, ultimately, the method(s) used to measure DF will define its existence in foods and/or clinical experiments that demonstrate beneficial physiological effects. DF is and will always be analyzed as a mixture of NDC, from natural unprocessed foods and processed foods in diets. These diets and the DF they contain will change with regions of a county and regions of the world. While the diversity of DF in foods/diets might appear as a bane to having a unified definition, this diversity in DF components is a benefit to intestinal function and overall health. DF provides beneficial physiological effects because it is so diverse in composition. There can be no method to differentiate between the DF components in F-V-WG from the similar if not identical components extracted, modified, or synthesized (i.e., celluloses, hemicelluloses, pectins). Yes, with modern uses of high-performance liquid chromatography (HPLC), more accurate identification and quantitation of soluble NDO can be possible. For example, the complete chemical profile of RMD can be achieved as described by Buck in these proceedings.

In summary, RMD presents an excellent example as to the current dilemma of having a method be restrictive or limiting in defining a DF. Half of RMD is recovered by AOAC 991.43, and this is defined as DF. The other half of RMD is not detected by this AOAC method and therefore cannot be defined as DF. However, >97% of RMD is fermented, and it all contributes to increased fecal mass and increases levels of bifidobacteria. Further the body does not differentiate between the two factions of RMD in its ability to attenuate blood lipid, glucose, and/or insulin levels.

18.4 Dietary Fiber Hypothesis

While some people would define DF as a collection of NDC to be measured and reported on a food label, to others, it is a hypothesis under constant evaluation. The DF hypothesis is simple, but emphatic and all encompassing: diets high in DF can prevent, and possibly treat, many of the metabolic diseases such as cancer, diabetes, heart disease, hypertension, and obesity and has been reviewed. Furthermore, the hypothesis states that individuals consuming diets low in DF are more susceptible to these diseases, reviewed in reference [3]. Relevant to this review is that most clinical studies providing evidence to support the DF hypothesis have been accomplished with isolated, modified, and/or synthesized sources of NDC or DF; the IOM would describe these as FFs. As will be presented under the heading "Prebiotics and Fermentation: New Next Dietary Fiber Hypothesis," a new hypothesis is suggested that additional health benefits of DF are related to their fermentation in the large intestine, providing energy for the microbiota, resulting in increase in commensal gut microbiota and specific bacteria such as bifidobacteria.

18.5 Dietary Fiber Intakes and Requirements

While there are numerous reports on DF intakes, the medium intakes of DF cited by the IOM range from 16.5 to 17.9 g/day for men and 12.1 to 13.8 g/day for women [8]. Worldwide, DF intakes among different populations do not vary more than 25% of these medium U.S. intakes. The IOM states that food consumption tables only reflect the amount of DF and ingredients added to foods such as pectin and gums which are defined as FFs are not included and are minimal is wrong. What is not included in food consumption tables is the amount of NDO (i.e., polydextrose, RMD, fructans with DP values less than 10, GOS, and others). And while there should be emphasis on eating F-V-WG, examination of the USDA Food Composition Database would indicate that approximately 25% of the reported DF intake comes from isolated and/or modified sources of cellulose in baked products.

The onus placed on DF in setting AI values at 25 and 38 g/day for women and men, respectively, is that it, DF, as a component in diets basically consisting of F-V-WG foods is the principal ingredient that lowers blood cholesterol levels. However contributory increased levels of DF are in lowering blood cholesterol levels, it is the diet modification that helps lower calorie intake and possibly weight loss that really contributes to cholesterol lowering.

If the AI of DF ranges from 25 g/day for women to 38 g/day for men, and mean intakes are only one-half of this amount, three important questions arise: (1) what can be done to fill this DF gap, (2) what types/sources of DF should be added to the diet, and (3) what beneficial physiological effects can be expected/observed with increased consumption of any FF and/or NDO? In attempting to answer these questions, additionally important issues come to our attention. First, it is important to recognize that a diet should contain a mixture of insoluble and soluble components. To what extent should the diet contain, if possible, a distribution of insoluble and soluble components that are not fermented, adding true roughage throughout the intestine and into the feces? Celluloses followed by wheat bran are among possibly the two most common sources of IDF in the diet, yet both can be fermented to vary degrees. Psyllium is a unique DF that exhibits high viscosity in its passage through the entire intestine, but has limited fermentability. While fermented sources of DF contribute to laxation, nonfermentable remnants of insoluble and soluble components certainly add bulk to feces, and, possibly equally important, they help retain fecal water. At present, this distribution is roughly estimated to be 75% and 25% insoluble and soluble components, respectively. While adding more DF to processed foods is continually explored among food scientists and the food industry, the limited palatability of many potential sources of IDF and the limit of how much IDF can be added to a product seemed to be a major limiting factor in closing the DF gap. However, the growing use and acceptability of NDOs that have high functionality and acceptability and especially in the growing beverage market can be considered to be currently filling the DF gap. However significant the consumption of NDOs is currently in foods and beverages, this consumption is not recognized because methods to measure these NDOs in foods and beverages are not recognized.

It is acknowledged that there is no precedent that helps verify that increased fermentation, and thus, increased microbiota mass is a beneficial physiological event. Yes, among Africans upon whom the DF hypothesis was based voided large stool volumes, there is no definitive evidence that this increase was due to increased microbiota. However, there is current scientific belief that increased levels of bifidobacteria, as prebiotics, are important for improved health. Increased levels of bifidobacteria, or other lactic acid bacteria, or any bacteria can only be achieved with increased intakes of more fermentable DF, or just more fermentable NDO. Thus while there is strong evidence to increase DF intakes, the question develops as to from what sources, should there be just be more F-V-WG in the diet, and/or how much more fermentable DF, such as NDO, should be consumed?

In summary, with absolutely no DF being ingested and coming into the intestine, the intestine will fail to function. Yes, a remote possibility, but a real situation among individuals sustained by parental nutrition for long periods. There is no available evidence to suggest the minimum amount of DF for optimum intestinal function. It would appear that an average intake of 13–18 g/day as measured by existing DF methods is adequate for most people, but the question remains how adequate? Yes, it is agreed that DF intakes in the range of 25–38 g/day would be beneficial for a variety of physiological functions. How high a level of DF intake could be tolerated, be beneficial, and without causing any adverse nutritional effects? Again, there is no good evidence to suggest a UL for DF intakes at this time, but the DF hypothesis was based on intakes of 60–90 g/day [3]. While there had been suggestions that DF interferes with mineral absorption/bioavailability, this theory is believed to have been dispelled [9]. The idea that increased fermentation in the large intestine enhances mineral absorption/bioavailability from this organ needs substantial verification.

18.6 Chemical and Physical Properties of Dietary Fiber

The two principal chemical entities (properties) of DF are its monosaccharide units and the glycosidic linkages between units. The common monosaccharide units include glucose, fructose, galactose, mannose, rhamnose, arabinose, ribose, and xylose, and their substituted groups (i.e., carboxyl, methoxy, and others). With one exception, all sources of carbohydrates that exclusively contain only glucose unit with α1-4 and α1-6 glycosidic linkages are digestible, the one exception being RS where the primarily amylose chains are so tightly packed together that they cannot be readily hydrated or gelatinized for digestion. Any other configuration (i.e., β) or numerical designated linkages between monosaccharide units renders the carbohydrate polymer nondigestible. Yes, there are exceptions; lactose contains a β1-4 linkage, but most people have the β-galactosidase to hydrolyze lactose.

While nature has configured many combinations of monosaccharide units and glycosidic linkages to give us the broad complex called DF, there will be continued interest to find and/or synthesize new forms of DF with different combinations of both chemical entities. Why?

One reason will be to give the carbohydrate (i.e., polymer or oligosaccharide) a new or modified physical property to fit a specific food application. In addition, these new combinations might provide a more abundant source of one or more specific monosaccharide units to facilitate more total bacterial mass and/or to stimulate the growth of one or more specific bacterium, a new *prebiotic*. While various fructan products have shown to have *prebiotic* properties and appear to provide the current breath of scientific information on the topic, so do glucose-based NDCs such as RS and RMD.

To expand on the physical properties of DF, the classical insoluble components (i.e., wheat bran and cellulose) provide true bulk particulates in the small intestine, yet are fermented to varying degrees in the large intestine. Viscosity produced by a select group of DF (i.e., β-glucan, psyllium, and pectin) is believed to be the major contributing factor in the attenuation of blood lipid and blood glucose levels. What has been long perceived as an important physiological aspect of DF consumption is its water-holding capacity throughout its movement through the entire intestine. However, this is a difficult parameter to measure and put into quantitative terms for comparison of different DF.

The one important remaining physical property to mention regarding DF is the fact it can be fermented, but to varying degrees. However, while indicting fermentability as a physical property of DF, fermentation is also a physiological property; fermentation is one-half the quintessentiality of DF. Psyllium and β-glucan (from oats and barley) are unique examples of the diversity that can exist between two sources of DF in their physical properties. While both are considered soluble and viscous sources of DF, psyllium is only partially fermented in the large intestine while β-glucan is nearly completely fermented. A looming question that appears to nearing resolution in the near future, are all sources of fermentable DF *prebiotics*?

In summary, the physical properties of DF are its ability to provide insoluble particulate bulk, hold water, provide viscosity, and be fermented. All these properties aid in water retention, and as mentioned, the combined presence of bulk and water, in combination with mucus secretions, helps protect the intestinal surface and helps facilitate nutrient absorption.

18.7 Physiological Properties of Dietary Fiber

The digestion of fats, protein, and carbohydrates in the small intestine is an important and essential physiological event. Conversely, the primary physiological property of DF is that it is not digested in the small intestine, which allows it to transverse the entire small intestine. Ultimately adding bulk as nonfermented insoluble particles or fermented in the large intestine is an important and essential physiological event. The passage of DF exerts its physical properties which in turn influence physiological properties. An IDF provides bulk in a milieu of intestinal liquefaction wherein proper proteolytic, lipolytic, and saccharolytic activities can be achieved. Adequate water in the intestine for the digestion of foods can possibly be compared to the function of bile acids which are necessary for adequate lipid dispersion and subsequent lipolysis. These bulking DFs, and the intestinal motility they produce, enhance nutrient absorption and stimulate goblet cells to produce more mucin. (Beyond the scope of this summary, are mucins the body's endogenous source of DF?) What is the best source of IDF? Is it wheat bran, isolated and/or modified cellulose, or an apple? It appears that some types of IDF in the diet are necessary for laxation, bowel movement. However, this insoluble material need not be of plant origin. Plastic particle has been shown to stimulate laxation. Besides just providing bulk, IDF binds water in the intestine.

The quintessential properties of DF are that it stimulates intestinal motility and provides a source of energy for the intestinal microbiota.

The often repeated rationale for having a definition for DF and its almost universal listing on food labels is that consumers expect DF to offer benefits. Again, possibly a universally accepted health benefit of DF is that it attenuates blood cholesterol levels and/or decreases the incidence of heart disease. In the United States, three of the four FDA approved heath claims that deal with DF specifically refer to the benefits of DF in preventing heart disease. In discussing the endogenous DF in plant foods, the IOM states that since there is a long history on the physiological benefits of "high-fiber foods," there is no justification to re-evaluate these benefits. However strong the intuitive belief that "high-fiber foods" are better for us, it is the past four to five decades of published research on extracted and/or synthesized sources of DF that have shown its physiological benefits. It appears IOM's definition of an FF cannot take advantage of the long history of high-fiber foods as the resulting fiber may be more—or less—beneficial to health than endogenous fiber. The issue remains as to what constitutes a beneficial physiological effect and what requirements should be in place to document such a beneficial effect.

The most commonly cited physiological effects associated with DF are decreased intestinal transit time, increased stool bulk, reduction of blood total and/or LDL cholesterol levels, and reduction of postprandial blood glucose and/or insulin levels, and it is fermentable by the colonic microbiota. In every case suggesting that an isolated, modified, or synthesized source of DF has a beneficial physiology effect, it is now suggested that it will be necessary to conduct a well-designed and well-conducted clinical experiment. Such a study is usually a double-blind, randomized, crossover employing a sufficient number of subjects to see a significant effect between the treatments and the control and, if possible, a study design that would allow observance of a dose effect.

While Health Canada has set some criteria for experiments to evaluate new, novel sources of DF, these standards appear to be over-restrictive [10]. To compare laxation effects of any NDC only to wheat bran presents a difficult standard for comparison; the goal post is too high. As will be presented, the consumption of RMD can increase fecal bulk, but through increased fecal mass. In regard to studies designed to attenuate blood lipid, glucose, and/or insulin levels, test subjects should have been diagnosed as having elevated levels of all or any of these indices. With the increasing prevalence of obesity, many of these individuals will probably have higher than normal blood levels of triglycerides, cholesterol, glucose, or insulin and serve as appropriate subjects, with medical approval, to demonstrate the beneficial physiological effects of a food and/or DF.

The beneficial physiological effects bring us back to the theme of DF essentiality and the question what is the absolute minimum DF needed to initiate intestinal function. It is possible that some degree of peristalsis always occurs due to involuntary intestinal muscle contractions. However, it is known that DF can increase the length of the intestinal villa in the small intestine. This gives rise to more mucosal cells responsible for nutrient absorption and more goblet cells contributing to mucin production. It is well known that animals with a defined cecum will have this organ greatly enlarge with increased levels of fermentable NDC. While these are physiological effects, the current challenge to measure these changes in intestinal morphology as beneficial at least in the human appears realistically unobtainable.

Since the proposed AACC and IOM definitions for DF definitions along with CODEX deliberation, the policy organizations of other countries/regions have presented reviews and opinion of DF. In addition to the most common beneficial physiological effects of DF cited by most committees and organizations, ILSI Europe Concise Monograph on Dietary Fibre [11] expands on the potential effects of the microbiota and the products they might be produced through fermentation. This is not only a positive statement but also one of great challenge in the area of DF research. The ILSI monograph mentions that through increased fermentation, products might be produced that "…. act as immunomodulators (e.g. absorb procarcinogens, promote attack on malignant cells); inhibit growth of harmful yeasts and (peptolytic) bacteria; improve mineral absorption; reduce food intolerances and allergies; stimulate growth of healthy intestinal flora; reduce undesirable compounds (e.g. amines and ammonia, phenols, secondary bile acids); produce nutrients (B group vitamins) and digestive enzymes. These effects are variously linked to health outcomes such as improved bowel function, alleviation of bowel disorders, bone health and improved diabetes management."

18.8 Essentiality of Dietary Fiber

Nutrients are chemicals needed by an organism to live and grow and must be obtained from the organism's environment. Organic nutrients include carbohydrates, proteins, fats, and vitamins. The major inorganic nutrients are minerals or more correctly individual elements.

An *essential nutrient* is a nutrient required for normal bodily function(s) and health that is required in the diet; it cannot be synthesized in the body. Niacin and choline are interesting essential nutrients in that they can be made in the body, in the intestine, but not in adequate amounts. This is interesting in that fermentation must occur in the intestine, and this is dependent on a viable microbiota and the presence of some source of energy that is DF. Essential nutrients exert physiological functions that are diminished when the nutrient is totally lacking in the diet and restored when the essential nutrient is added back to the diet. The time for these deficiency symptoms to develop and corrected can vary among individuals. DF cannot be synthesized in the body. However, the NDC components of mucins and sloughed epithelial cells that are made within the intestine might be considered as endogenous sources of secreted DF. However, to get goblet cells to produce mucin and then have villa expand, function, and then shed, something has to stimulate these events. DF is essential to start and then maintain these events.

The IOM in its 2005 Dietary Reference Intakes for "Dietary, Functional, and Total Fiber" [8] under the heading Clinical Effects of Inadequate Intake states

> Dietary and Functional Fibers are not essential nutrients, so inadequate intakes do not result in biochemical or clinical symptoms of a deficiency. A lack of these fibers in the diet, however, can result in inadequate fecal bulk and may detract from optimal health in a variety of different ways depending on other factors, such as the rest of the diet and the stage of the life cycle.

Among any and all free-living populations, worldwide, it is difficult to image, much less achieve a sustained diet with absolutely no DF. It is impossible to perceive feeding humans for extended periods a purified diet consisting of only essential amino and fatty acids, essential vitamin and minerals, and a totally digestible/absorbable carbohydrate energy source such as glucose, sucrose, or a dextrin. However, there is one realistic exception to this statement, and it is feeding an individual a DF-free diet via parental nutrition. Total parental nutrition is normally used to help a person recover, but in the period of recovery, no food in the intestine leads to intestinal shrinkage and atrophy and lack of an intestinal microbiota. What is known or can be learned from an individual on total parental nutrition? Individuals on parental nutrition have impaired immune function and normally require a steady dose of antibiotics. It is fortunate that the implementation of parental nutrition is normally a short-term experience.

A total review of the physiology (i.e., function), maintenance and health of the intestine of individuals on long-term parental nutrition is beyond the purpose of this chapter, but what is known to occur in these individuals are intestinal atrophy; minimal or complete lack of intestinal peristalsis with no laxation; no intestinal fermentation; near to complete lack of intestinal bacteria, the microbiota; and a severely depressed immune system. It is known that 70% of the body immune system is associated with the intestine.

The question or statement about the essentiality of DF must start with the effects of no DF intake for an extended period and then proceed to determine the minimum amount to observe indirect but positive physiological responses. While DF is clearly not a vitamin or mineral, does not provide essential amino acids or fatty acids, it does stimulate intestinal movement which in turn stimulates goblet cells to produce mucins which can be are fermented. However, DF does provide energy to a unique environment of the human body, the large intestine. What would be the consequence of absolutely no dietary fermentable components reaching the large intestine? Is IDF better than soluble DF? Is fermentation, and especially increased fermentation, good or bad, necessary or unnecessary? Does physical size or molecular size of DF matter?

Is wheat bran the only standard by which all other DF should be compared? While these questions become academic, they do reinforce the idea that the entire topic of DF, the sources of NDC that can constitute DF, and be defined as DF in a diet are varied, and the physiological events influenced by DF are multitude. And finally, our growing knowledge of fermentation and the microbiota, is helping as better understand DF as a complex nutrient. However, with all this complexity, a simple two-sentence definition as proposed by the AACC and recognition of AOAC methods to measure DF might help manage this overcome this complexity.

18.9 Dietary Fiber Requirements

The DF hypothesis was originally presented based upon observations among populations in Africa that were estimated to consume between 60 and 90 g of DF per day [3], amazing amounts compared to today's average DF intakes. One must wonder how this could be possible considering the limited amount of F-V-WG that would have to be consumed each day. Since vegetables and, to a lesser extent, fruits were not principal parts of these African diets, a majority of the NDC among these populations would appear to be in the form of RS. Any person fortunate to see and listen to Dr. Dennis Burkitt will always remember one of his first slides, a photo of a human stool that appeared to be at least 6–8 in. in diameter and about 2–3 in. in depth; the stool occupied the entire slide! Was the bulk of this stool attributed to nonfermentable IDF or increased bacterial mass resulting from the fermentation of DF or more specifically RS? While we really do not know the answer, we do seem to accept that the DF intakes among these African people were extraordinarily high as mentioned. How can modern society achieve these levels, what is the optimum level of DF intake, and can NDOs play a significant part in increasing DF intakes?

Cummings and MacFarlane [12] have suggested that the principal substrates thought to be available for fermentation in the large intestine in g/day are NDOs, 8–18; RS, 8–40; soluble oligosaccharides, 2–8; unabsorbed sugars, 2–8 (mainly as nondigested lactose); dietary protein, 3–9; gut enzymes and secretions, 4–6; mucins, 2–3; and sloughed epithelial cells, unknown amounts. The range of fermentable substrates reaching the large intestine was 29–92 g/day. As previously asked, what is the optimum level of DF intake, and then one asks, what is the optimum level of fermentable DF needed?

It is possible that the current average DF intakes are adequate, but not optimum. But what is needed for an optimum intake, more total DF, or more fermentable DF in the forms of RS and/or a mixture of fermentable NDO?

18.10 Prebiotics and Fermentation: New Next Dietary Fiber Hypothesis

While it appears that "fermentation" is slowly being accepted as a beneficial physiological effect of DF, questions remain as to how or why fermentation in the large intestine contributes to a beneficial physiological effect(s). Is it just the event, or more specific products of fermentation such as the short-chain fatty acids and, as most frequently mentioned, butyric acid; is it the increase in the mass of the microbiota; and/or is it just the great volume of "stuff" and water in the large intestine that just facilitates laxation? Again, no specific answers can be given to these questions, but certainly a topic directly related to fermentation is the concept of *prebiotics*. "A prebiotic is a selectively fermented ingredient that allows specific changes, both in the composition and/or activity in the gastrointestinal microflora that confers benefits upon host well-being and health."

Without specific mention of any product or bacterium, the trend in DF research is to demonstrate that a prebiotic effect is an increase in level of fecal bifidobacteria. While increases and/or decreases in the levels of other bacteria of the commensal microflora could be important, these data are just beginning to be made available.

Again, CODEX has made some interesting comments about NDOs and their fermentation; these comments by CODEX certainly appear to have been influenced by a few people [2,3]:

> Whilst they are fermented this was felt to be part of normal digestive physiology and not something that conferred a specific health benefit. Therefore, inclusion of these water-soluble low molecular weight carbohydrates was potentially misleading for the consumer. Nevertheless the Joint FAO/WHO Scientific Update had acknowledged that NDO were important carbohydrates with unique properties, likely to be shown of importance to other aspects of health after further research. In such case, NDO should be recognized on its own right, but not as dietary fibre.

Irrespective of the limited view of a few people on the importance of intestinal fermentation and the microbiota, these combined topics are the new next hypothesis of DF and its beneficial physiological effects that will lead to better health.

18.11 Resistant Maltodextrin as a Source of Dietary Fiber: The Evidence

Buck in these proceedings has thoroughly reviewed the history of RMD development and its chemical and physical properties. He cites many of the beneficial physiological studies conducted on RMD. Livesey's review in this proceedings and meta-analysis of study [13] dealing with the effects of RMD on attenuation or maintenance of blood glucose and insulin levels appears to have provided the data to substantiate one commonly stated beneficial physiological effect of RMD. The following is a summary of the joint study conducted by Bear and Mai, again presented in these proceedings, to determine the energy value of RMD and its effect on fermentation and the microbiota, respectively. But most importantly, the review of these data presented here is for the purpose of defining RMD as a source of DF with beneficial physiological effects.

Fourteen subjects participated in a randomized, crossover experiment in which they were fed controlled diets of equal energy and nutrient content. The only variable in each of the three 28 day study periods was having the subjects consume three treatments consisting of (1) 50 g of digestible maltodextrin, (2) 25 g of digestible maltodextrin and 25 g of RMD, and (3) 50 g of RMD. All subjects participated in each treatment. During the first 14 days, the subjects were fed the controlled diets and treatments to adapt. The subjects, starting on day 14, then participated in a 7 day balance period in which all feces and urine samples were collected and analyzed. On days 24 and 28, the subjects were placed in a whole body chamber for 24 h to measure net energy gain, and these data are presented elsewhere [13]. On days 1, 13, and 24, a single fecal sample was obtained from each individual for qualitative and quantitative microbiota analyses.

The main objectives of this study relevant to this brief review and only briefly presented were to (1) determine the metabolizable energy (ME) of RMD; (2) determine the extent of RMD fermentation in the large intestine; (3) determine the effects of RMD treatments on (a) number of bowel movements, frequency in 7 day period, (b) changes in daily fecal wet and dry weights, and (c) changes in daily fecal carbohydrate, energy, DF, nitrogen, and ash; (4) determine the qualitative and quantitative changes in the microbiota by DGGE, quantitative polymerase chain reaction (qPCR), and fluorescent in situ hybridization (FISH) analyses; and (5) determine the quantitative changes in bifidobacteria concentrations by qPCR and FISH analyses.

The mean ME values for RMD determined among subjects fed 25 and 50 g RMD/day were 8.3 and 10.4 kJ/g, respectively. These values were not significantly different. Greater than 97% of the ingested RMD was fermented in the large intestine. On initial comment, it can be suggested that about one-half the gross energy in RMD (16.2 kJ/g) is utilized by the host and the other half can be assumed to be used for microbiota growth and maintenance. However, the ME values among subjects fed 25 g RMD/day were unique because of the range in ME values observed, which varied from 0 to 16 kJ/g. This great variability in ME values among subjects consuming 25 g RMD/day is discussed [13]. The ME values among subjects consuming 50 g RMD/day ranged from 6.6 to 14.6 kJ/g.

During the 7 day balance period, there was an increasing trend in the number of bowel movements in subjects consuming 0, 25, and 50 g/day of RMD from 7.0–8.5 to 7.9 per week (SEM = 0.6; $p \leq 0.26$). While there was no significant change in the number of bowel movement, with an average of one bowel movement a day, the subjects did not experience any incidents of intestinal distress.

There were no significant changes in urine weight, urine energy (by bomb calorimetry), urine nitrogen, or fecal fat among subjects consuming the RMD treatments, and these data are not presented here but are available [13].

Significant increases were observed in daily fecal wet weight, fecal dry weight, fecal energy, fecal carbohydrate (measured as IDF + RMD), and fecal nitrogen among subjects consuming RMD. Daily fecal wet weight increased from 118 g in subjects with no RMD by 30.2 g (25.6%) ($p \leq 0.001$) among subjects that consumed 25 g RMD/day and by 42.8 g (36%) ($p \leq 0.001$) among subjects that consumed 50 g/day of RMD. The difference in fecal wet weight between subjects fed 25 and 50 g of RMD was 12.6 g, but this increase was not significant. The daily fecal dry weight increased by 5.5 and 9.3 g in subjects consuming 25 and 50 g/day of RMD, respectively, from the base value of 26.5 g in subjects fed 0 g of RMD/day. Fecal dry weight increased by 3.8 g/day (12%) ($p \leq 0.0001$) in subjects consuming 50 g/day of RMD compared to those consuming 25 g/day. While the total weight of the feces increased with increasing amounts of RMD consumed, the water content of the feces remained constant among all treatments at 78%.

Approximately 0.6 and 1.2 g/day of RMD was recovered in the feces of subjects consuming 25 and 50 g RMD/day, respectively. While these amounts of RMD recovered in the feces were significantly higher compared to the trace amount detected in feces of subjects fed 0 g of RMD and differed between treatments (25 vs. 50), these observations are felt to have no significance in the overall findings. But, these recovered amounts of RMD values in the feces substantiate that >97% of the ingested RMD is fermented. It could have been assumed that as the amount of RMD was increased, the efficiency of RMD fermentation in the large intestine might have declined, but this was not observed.

The carbohydrate measured as IDF and recovered in the feces increased from 10.8 g in subjects with no RMD in their diet by 2.8 and 4.2 g in subjects fed 25 and 50 g of RMD, respectively. These IDF values do not include the small amounts of RMD recovered in the feces. The increase in fecal IDF between subjects consuming 25 and 50 g/day of RMD was 1.4 g, but this was not a significant difference. Daily fecal nitrogen was measured at 1.5 g in subjects with no RMD consumption and significantly increased by 0.3 and 0.6 g in subjects consuming 25 and 50 g/day of RMD, respectively. Since the diets were constant in levels of all macronutrients, micronutrients, and energy fed subjects during the experimental periods, with the exception of the two levels of RMD fed, it is suggested that the increase in carbohydrate and nitrogen measured in the feces is attributed mainly to increased bacterial mass, and this will be verified. However, it is acknowledged that Kjeldahl nitrogen measurements, as employed in this study, are a nonspecific measurement for protein, and part of this nitrogen could be attributed to phenols, indoles, and amines produced by bacteria in the fermentation process.

The initial summary of these data on fecal characteristics is used to substantiate that RMD has important beneficial physiological effects expected of DF, which are (1) increased fecal bulk and (2) is competely fermented and thus promotes fermentation. The consumption of 25 and 50 g for RMD will significantly increase fecal bulk, both wet weight and dry weight. While it is not anticipated that individuals will consume these levels of RMD on a daily basis, extrapolation of these data suggest that every 1 g of RDM would increase fecal wet weight by approximately 1 g and fecal dry weight by 0.2 g. With the dietary habits of most individuals still lacking in DF intakes, a modest intake of a fermentable NDOs could have a significant contributory effect on improved fecal regularity and bulk.

The seemingly appropriate question now to ask after determining that the consumption of RMD can increase fecal bulk and is totally fermented would be, what is contributing to this fecal bulk? What is the beneficial physiological effect of fecal bulk? What is/are the beneficial physiological effects of fermentation? The consumption of inert plastic particles can increase fecal bulk and promote laxation; however, plastic particles are not DF and are not fermented, but do they promote a beneficial physiological effect? A few obvious answers to these questions would be (1) a better definition/description of what constitutes fecal bulk, (2) a better definition/description of what is fermentation, and (3) determine to what extent increased total fecal and/or concentration of fecal bacteria are contributing to fecal bulk.

A multiple set of qualitative and quantitative microbiota assays were used to determine change in the microbiota among individuals consuming RMD. Only a few pertinent observations are reported in this summary, and a full description of the assay techniques and complete listing of results and relevant discussion are presented elsewhere [14].

Briefly reviewing the methodology of the microbiota assays and results, the use of the *denaturing gradient gel electrophoresis* (DGGE) is a simple but efficient method for initial profiling of the fecal microbiota. It was observed that each individual harbored a unique microbiota. However, a distinct band that was consistently present and dose dependent increased after 24 days among 12 of 14 subjects consuming of RMD. This increase was also observed, albeit to a lesser extent, after 13 days of RMD supplementation. The DNA was isolated from the DGGE band, cloned, and conformation was accomplished to insure the correct bands were cloned and the DNA sequenced. The resulting sequences matched closest to sequences in the family Lachnospiraceae in the phylum Firmicutes.

To obtain more targeted quantitative microbiota analyses, the fecal samples were analyzed by FISH and qPCR with probes/primers directed against major groups of Bacteroidetes, Clostridiales, and bifidobacteria. The total bacteria/g of stool increased significantly with RMD consumption among subjects. This association was dose dependent and statistically significant on the linear scale ($p \leq 0.02$). For subjects with no RMD consumption, bacterial counts averaged 8.60E + 09/g of feces and increased to 1.01E + 10 and 1.06E + 10 counts/g in subjects consuming 25 and 50 g/day of RMD, respectively.

While an increase in total bifidobacteria counts/g stool was observed using FISH, this difference could not be verified as significant. However, using the qPCR procedure, a larger and statistically significant increase in bifidobacteria was increased from day 1 to 24 (expressed as genome equivalents/ng DNA) during the period subjects consumed 50 g/day for RMD ($p \leq 0.03$). The mean number of bifidobacteria on day 24 during the period subjects consumed 50 g/day of RMD was 2.7×10^5 compared 5.1×10^4 genome equivalents/ng observed on day 1.

Again, in partial summation as to the beneficial physiological effects of RMD, it is fermented and promotes both fermentation and microbiota growth. These processes lead to increased fecal microbiota concentration and total mass on a daily basis. This observation is supported by the fact that the consumption and then fermentation of RMD lead to increases in fecal NDC, measured as IDF, and nitrogen and suggested to be associated with bacterial cells and possibly to include epithelial remnants. While the fermentation of RMD does not significantly change the unique total microbiota composition of an individual, small but significant changes can occur. The importance of these individual changes does require further investigation. However, one small significant change, the increase in fecal bifidobacteria, does suggest that RMD has similar "prebiotic" potential as reported for other NDO and most notably fructooligosaccharide (FOS).

18.12 Summary

DF is many things to many people. It is a concept, a hypothesis, a marketer's bonanza, a unique complex of NDC, but most importantly an integral necessity of a normal functioning and healthy intestine. DF is universally accepted by the consumer as a healthy and needed ingredient in the diet, and when consumed as a component of foods or beverages, it has no known negative effects. The standard thinking today is that the principal health benefits of DF are to aid laxation and attenuate blood lipid, glucose, and inulin levels. While there is growing interest in the importance of the intestinal microbiota, there is not yet a strong connection of the importance of DF as sources energy for the microbiota in the large intestine. The synergistic relationship between DF and the microbiota for better health is the new DF hypothesis. DF is an essential nutrient for intestinal function and health.

RMD is a synthetic mixture of soluble poly- and oligosaccharides consisting of glucose units with a variety of nonhydrolyzable glycosidic linkages. While a totally soluble source of DF that does not affect the viscosity of a food or beverage, it has been shown to attenuate blood lipid, glucose, and insulin levels. RMD is totally fermentable and increases fecal wet and dry weights, and this increase in fecal mass can be attributed to increased microbiota growth and a significant increase in bifidobacteria. RMD is just one example of DF, and specifically a NDO, that imparts beneficial physiological effects.

CODEX has presented an encompassing definition for DF. The FDA and Health Canada are working to finalize their definitions of DF. Suggestions for both regulatory agencies are as follows:

1. Keep the definition of DF simple (KIS). The first two sentences of the AACC are adequate.
2. Recognize that DF is a complex combination of NDCs naturally occurring in plant foods and those added to foods. This includes the recognition of NDOs in the DP range of 3–10. A single value for the total

amount of all forms of NDC and DF on the Nutrition Facts panel is sufficient. This recommendation is basically an extension of the first recommendation.

3. Acknowledge the importance of exiting AOAC approved methods for the measurement of DF in foods and beverages. Yes, it might take a combination of methods to obtain an accurate measure of the total amount of NDC and DF in a food or beverage.

4. Promote the use of the available AOAC approved methods for DF analyses to expand food composition tables to include information on a food's content of NDOs and RS.

5. Set a reasonable daily value (DV) for DF; the current level of 25 g/day appears acceptable.

6. Enforce current regulations on nutrient content claims and health claims regarding DF.

7. Require the use of well-designed and well-executed clinical experiments to support any health claim regarding DF. The extent of information to substantiate a beneficial physiological effect of a DF should not be as extensive as required for a health claim, but beneficial physiological effects should be supported with good research.

Acknowledgment

While the author acknowledges support from the Matsutani Chemical Industry Co. Ltd., the comments and opinions expressed in this chapter are the sole responsibility of the author.

References

1. Gordon, D.T. and K. Kubomura. 2003. Beverages as delivery systems for nutraceuticals. In: *Beverage Quality and Safety*. Eds. T. Foster and P. Vasavada, CRC Press, Boca Raton, FL, pp. 15–72.
2. Cummings, J.H. and A.M. Stephen. 2007. Carbohydrate classification and terminology. *Eur. J. Clin. Nutr.* 61(Suppl. 1):S5–S18.
3. Gordon, D.T. 2007. Dietary fiber definitions at risk. *Cereal Food World.* 52:112–123.
4. Lupton, J.R., V.A. Betteridge, and T.J. Pijls. 2009. Codex definition of dietary fibre: Issue of implementation. *Quality Assur. Saf. Crop Food* 1:206–212.
5. Gordon, D.T., B. McCleary, and T. Sontag-Srohm. 2006. Summary of dietary fiber methods workshop, Helsinki. In: Dietary fibre components and functions. Eds. H. Salovaara, F. Gates and M. Tenkanen. Wageningen Academic Publishers, the Netherlands, pp. 323–338.
6. Nishibata, N., K. Tashiro, S. Kanahori, C. Hashizume, M. Kitagawa, K. Okuma, and D.T. Gordon. 2009. Comprehensive measurement of total nondigestible carbohydrates in foods by enzymatic-gravimetric method and liquid chromatography. *J Agric Food Chem.* 57:7659–7665.
7. Englyst, K.N., S. Liu, and H.N. Englyst. 2007. Nutritional characterization and measurement of dietary carbohydrates. *Eur. J. Clin. Nutr.* 61(Suppl. 1):S19–S39.
8. IOM. 2001. *Dietary Reference Intakes: Proposed Definition of Dietary Fiber*. National Academies Press, Washington, DC; IOM. 2005. *Dietary Reference Intakes for Energy, Carbohydrate, Fiber, Fat, Fatty Acids, Cholesterol, Protein, and Amino Acids*. National Academies Press, Washington, DC.

9. Gordon, D.T., D. Stoops, and V. Ratliff. 1995. Dietary fiber and mineral nutrition. In: *Fiber in Health and Disease*. Eds. D. Kritchevsky and C. Bonfield, Eagan Press, St. Paul, MN, pp. 267–295.

10. Health Canada. 1997. Guideline concerning the safety and physiological effects of novel fibre sources and food products containing them. Food Directorate Health Protection Branch, Ottawa, ON.

11. Gray, J. 2006. *Dietary Fibre: Definition, Analysis, Physiology & Health*, ILSI Europe, Brussels, Belgium.

12. Cummings, J.H. and G.T. Macfarlane. 1991. The control and consequences of bacterial fermentation in the human colon. *J. Appl. Bacteriol.* 79:443–459.

13. Livesey, G. and H. Tagami. 2009. Interventions to lower the glycemic response to carbohydrate foods with a low-viscosity fiber (resistant maltodextrin): Meta-analysis of randomized controlled trials. *Am. J Clin. Nutr.* 89:114–125.

14. Volker, M., M. Ukhanova, T. Culpepper, X. Wang, S. Kanahori, K. Okuma, H. Tagami, D.T. Gordon, W. Rumpler, and D.J. Baer. 2012. Available energy from resistant maltodextrin varies between individuals and correlates with fecal microbiota composition. *Am. J. Clin Nutr.* (in press).

19

Fecal Microbiota Composition Is Affected by Resistant Maltodextrin, and Bifidobacteria Counts Correlate with Energy Gain

TYLER CULPEPPER, MARIA UKHANOVA,
DAVID J. BAER, SUMIKO KANAHORI, KAZUHIRO OKUMA,
HIROYUKI TAGAMI, DENNIS T. GORDON, and VOLKER MAI

Contents

19.1 Introduction

Resistant maltodextrin (RM) is a low calorie food ingredient that in many ways behaves similar to dietary fiber. RM contains a mixture of oligosaccharides and polysaccharides. Due to the chemical composition of RM, determination of its fiber content requires a specific analytical method.[8] RM is a fine water soluble powder with little taste that has potential utility as a low calorie ingredient in a variety of foods and drinks. Because RM is recalcitrant to digestion by the host enzymes, the energy gain from RM intake depends on the activities of the large intestinal gut microbiota. Although gut microbiota appears unique for each individual, the main metabolic pathways encoded by the gut metagenome appear preserved.[15] Nevertheless, it is feasible that subjects consuming the same amounts of RM derive different amounts of energy from it due to varying efficiencies of their resident microbiota in fermenting this substrate. RM supplementation might have a prebiotic effect by enriching for microbes such as bifidobacteria that are rich in glycohydrolases[21] that can efficiently degrade RM. Indeed, a bifidogenic effect has previously been shown for resistant starch III polymorph B,[17] but only a bifidogenic trend failing to reach significance was reported for RM[6]. *Ruminococcus bromii* numbers were shown to increase upon RS consumption in another study.[1] RM has also been shown to increase fecal bulking[6] and when ingested with fatty meals it suppresses the postprandial elevation of blood triac-ylglycerol levels.[14] The gut microbiota is thought to affect human health, particularly through the generation of beneficial fermentation products, such as butyric acid from the breakdown of nutrients that reach the colon.[9] Although the health effects of some dietary components, including dietary fiber, might depend on the activities of an individual's particular gut microbiota, little is known about interactions between dietary substances and the composition of the microbiota. Directed changes in the intestinal physiology through modification of the gut microbiota by dietary interventions (pre- and probiotics) offer the potential for disease prevention. Many products aiming to promote intestinal health by improving microbiota composition are already commercially available; however, we are only at the beginning of fully understanding the complexity of microbiota composition and activities.

Molecular 16S rRNA-based tools have helped to overcome limitations of conventional microbiological plating methods in studying gut microbiota composition.[23,25] More recently, the developments of high-throughput parallel sequencing methodologies have increased our ability to analyze microbiota at a new level of depth. These tools have already sparked novel microbiota research including studies of potential associations between the proportion of Bacteroidetes and obesity.[5,22,24]

The RM feeding study, from which we now report on fecal microbiota and energy gain, was a double-blinded, randomized, crossover feeding study that investigated the energy gain from RM supplementation in healthy volunteers. We describe here changes that we observed during the RM study in the fecal microbiota composition and associations between microbiota composition and energy gain from RM.

19.2 Material and Methods

19.2.1 Study Design

Volunteers were recruited to participate in a randomized, double-blind, crossover study of 25 g/day of RM (RM25) and 50 g/day of RM (RM50) and compared to a placebo (P, maltodextrin). Fourteen volunteers (subjects A–N) completed the study protocol. Prior to the first fecal collection time point, volunteers were adapted to the diet for 2 weeks. Treatment periods of 28 day duration were separated by at least 2 week washout period. During the three treatment periods, volunteers consumed the same base generic American diet. All foods and beverages were prepared and supplied by the Human Studies Facility at the Beltsville Human Nutrition Research Center (Beltsville, MD). Dinner and breakfast were consumed at the center during the week; carryout lunches and snacks were provided.

Weekend meals and treatments were packaged with instructions for home consumption. The study protocol was reviewed and approved by the Medstar Research Institute Institutional Review Board. All subjects provided written informed consent and were compensated for their participation.

19.2.2 Fecal Collections

Fecal samples were collected on days 1, 13, and 24 of each intervention for a total of nine fecal samples per subject. Subjects obtained a cooler filled with ice for storage of the sample until delivery to the lab. All samples were delivered on ice usually within 4 h of defecation. Samples were processed by kneading in a strong plastic bag immediately upon arrival in the laboratory. A small portion of the sample was fixed for fluorescent in situ hybridization (FISH) analysis as described later, and the remainder was stored at −70°C.

19.2.3 Energy Measurements

Energy gain from RM was determined with bomb calorimetry using residual energy measures and with metabolic data collected in each period during a 24 h stay in a calorimetric room.

19.2.4 Microbiota Analysis

19.2.4.1 DGGE Analysis Bacterial genomic DNA was isolated from the fecal sample by the bead beating method. This method allows for the efficient lysis of most bacterial cells and appears to have little bias.[19] A 457 bp fragment from the V6 to V8 region of the bacterial 16S rDNA was amplified with primers U968-GC (5′ CGC CCG GGG CGC GCC CCG GGC GGG GCG GGG GCA CGG GGG GAA CGC GAA GAA CCT TAC) and L1401 (5′ GCG TGT GTA CAA GAC CC) as described by Zoetendal et al.[27] The GC clamp facilitates separation by denaturing gradient gel electrophoresis (DGGE). DGGE was performed on an 8% [wt/vol] acrylamide gel with a gradient from 40% at the top to 50% at the bottom at a temperature of 60°C. One hundred percent denaturing conditions were defined as 7 M urea and 40% formamide. Gels were run for 16 h at 65 V and stained with Cyber Green. Images of the stained gels were scanned with Quantity One software (Biorad) and analyzed with Diversity Database software (Biorad).

19.2.4.2 FISH Analysis Fecal sample of 0.5 g was added to 4.5 mL of phosphate buffered saline (PBS), and the samples were prepared for FISH analysis as described previously.[7] In short, samples were homogenized by vortexing with a dozen glass beads for 5 min, the fecal debris was removed by centrifuging at low speed, and the bacteria-containing supernatant was fixed in 3% paraformaldehyde in PBS overnight. Aliquots of the samples were stored at −70°C until the time of hybridization. For hybridization, 10 μL of appropriate dilutions of the samples was applied to gelatin-coated microscopic slides and fixed to the slides with 95% ethanol as described previously[13] except that the dilutions were made in PBS and not in 5% Tween solution. The slides were hybridized with the 5 ng/μL of the respective probes using the conditions described previously.[7,11,12] The following probes were used: the EU338 probe detecting almost all bacteria;[2] probe Bac303 for the genera *Bacteroides* and *Prevotella*;[18] the Elgc01 probe detecting *Faecalibacterium*-like species;[26] probe Erec482 for eubacteria, clostridia, and ruminococci belonging to *Clostridium* cluster XIVa;[7] Ato291 for the *Atopobium* group, with *Collinsella aerofaciens* as the predominant fecal species;[12] Rfla730/Rbro729 for ruminococci and clostridia of *Clostridium* cluster IV; the Bif164 probe for all bifidobacteria;[16] and the EC1532 for *Escherichia coli*.[20] Slides were mounted with Vectashield containing DAPI (Vector Laboratories, Burlingame, CA). Fluorescent cells were enumerated by counting at 100× magnification, a minimum of five fields of view per sample. The cells were counted directly with a Zeiss Axioskop-40 epifluorescence-equipped microscope (Zeiss, Germany) or by capturing images and counting cells using ImageJ software (NIH, Bethesda, MD).

19.2.4.3 Quantitative PCR Quantitative PCR (qPCR) analysis was performed in duplicate using a qPCR Core kit (Eurogentec, Cat. No. RT-SN10-05NR, San Diego, CA) on a Stratagene Mx3000P (La Jolla, CA) in 12.5 µL reaction volumes consisting of 1 µL DNA template (containing 25 ng DNA), 1 × reaction buffer, 200 µM dNTP mix, 30 pM forward and reverse primers, 0.025 U/µL HotGoldStar Taq polymerase, 1 × SYBR Green dye, and 30 nM ROX passive reference dye (Stratagene, Cat. No. 600546, La Jolla, CA). The following primers and conditions were used: (1) all eubacteria (V3 F: 5′-CCTACGGGAGGCAGCAG-3′; R: 5′-ATTACCGCGGCTGCTGG-3′, 56°C, 3 mM MgCl2); (2) bifidobacteria (F: 5′-TCGCGTC(C/T)GGTGTGAAAG-3′; R: 5′-CCACATCCAGC(A/G)TCCAC-3′, 58°C, 3 mM MgCl$_2$). *B. adolescentis* DNA was used for generating the standard curve. The amounts of input DNA were converted into genome equivalents by dividing DNA amounts by weight of the genome.

19.2.4.4 454-Based 16S rRNA Pyrosequencing DNA from the fecal samples was isolated as described earlier and amplified using a barcoded pyrosequencing primer set based on universal primers 27F and 338R as described earlier.[10] Sequences of low quality or with a length of less than 150 nucleotides were removed from the analysis. Sequences were analyzed using the RDP pyrosequencing pipeline[4] including features to calculate diversity indices and rarefaction curves.

19.2.5 Statistical Analysis

For the bacterial profiles generated by DGGE, we used imaging software (Quantity One, Biorad) to scan in the gel images. Background was subtracted from each lane, and the profiles were subjected to Gauss modeling. We then calculated a similarity matrix based on Pearson correlation coefficients and generated phylogenetic trees based on various algorithms (Ward, UPMA).

The amounts of bacteria as determined by FISH were analyzed as total counts/g of stool and log$_{10}$ transformed counts/g of stool. The effect of RM on bacterial numbers is defined as the mean during the RM intervention minus the mean during the placebo period subtracted by the mean numbers during the free diet. Subtraction of the amounts during the free diet was done to correct for time trend.

qPCR data were analyzed as genome equivalents/ng of DNA. Changes in amounts of bacterial groups of interest were determined by comparing the change of the genome equivalents/ng DNA between day 1 and day 24 during the RM period with the change between day 1 and day 24 during the placebo period. This approach allowed for consideration of the RM independent effect of the study diet.

The statistical significance of the effects is based on two-sided unpaired t-tests. We did not adjust the p-values for the multiple comparisons that were conducted.

19.3 Results

DGGE, a simple but efficient method for initial profiling of fecal microbiota, revealed that each individual harbored a unique microbiota. We detected a distinct band that was consistently and dose dependently increased after 24 days of RM supplementation in 12 out of 14 subjects (Figure 19.1). This increase was also observed, albeit to a lesser extent, after 13 days of RM supplementation (data not shown). We isolated DNA from two of these bands, cloned the fragments, and after confirmation that we had cloned the correct bands, sequenced them. Both resulting sequences matched closest to sequences in the family Lachnospiraceae, a common commensal in the phylum Firmicutes. The overall microbiota composition in the two samples collected during the two RM periods was in all but one

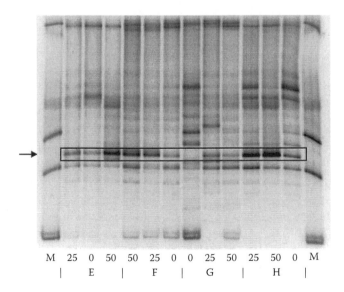

Figure 19.1 DGGE profiles for subjects E, F, G, and H on day 24 during placebo (0), RM 25 (25), and RM 50 (50) intervention periods. M = molecular marker; black arrow indicates position of band increased during RM supplementation (box).

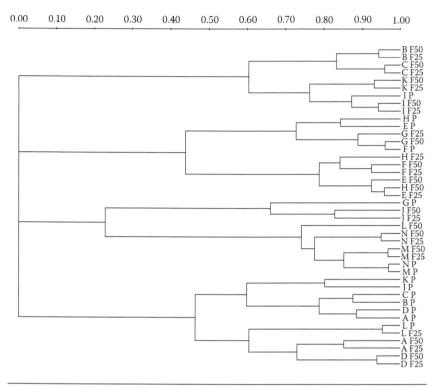

Figure 19.2 Dendogram of DGGE profiles derived for each of the 14 subjects (A–N) during placebo (P), RM25 (F25), and RM50 (F50) intervention periods. Branch length indicates relatedness of the profiles based on Pearson correlation coefficients.

subject closer to each other than either sample was to the sample collected during the placebo period (Figure 19.2). This observation suggests that RM supplementation resulted in a change of overall microbiota diversity in addition to the consistent increase in the single Lachnospiraceae band. Because DGGE is only a crude measure of microbiota diversity, we chose 12 samples from 4 subjects in which we had seen strong effects of RM supplementation on microbiota profiles for an in-depth 16S rRNA analysis using a barcoded 454 pyrosequencing approach. We obtained a total of 283,672 sequence reads with an average read number of 23,639/sample and an average length of 225 nucleotides. Lachnospiraceae sequences were prevalent in all samples (Figure 19.3). However, using 16S rRNA sequencing, we did not detect any increase in the combined operational taxonomic units (OTUs) grouping to the Lachnospiraceae family during RM supplementation. Because there are multiple OTUs that group to the Lachnospiraceae, it is possible that only some OTUs were affected by the intervention, but we detected none among the dominant OTUs. Our DGGE and 16S rRNA sequence analysis varied in the analyzed 16S region (V6–V8 vs. V1–V2), which might have contributed to the divergent results. We detected a variety of other OTUs that appeared affected

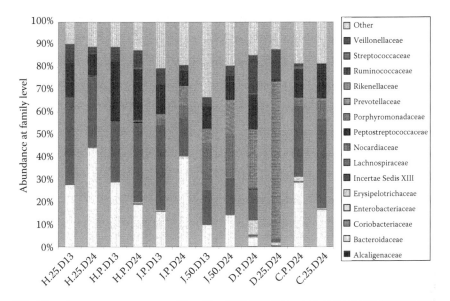

Figure 19.3 Abundance of dominant OTUs on the family level. OTU's grouping to each of the 15 most dominant OTUs, and all other OTUs combined are color coded. Samples from subjects H, J, D, and C were analyzed during placebo (P), RM25 (25), or RM50 (50) on day 13 (D13) and day 24 (D24). Each column shows the bacterial composition of one fecal sample based on 16S rRNA sequencing.

by RM supplementation, including some with closest matches to *Bacteroides*, clostridia, ruminococci, and enterobacteria.

In order to perform a truly quantitative microbiota analysis, we analyzed microbiota by FISH with probes directed against major groups of Bacteroidetes, Clostridiales, and bifidobacteria. Total bacteria/g of stool was increased during RM supplementation (Table 19.1). This association was dose dependent and statistically significant on the linear scale (p = 0.02) during the RM50 period.

A bifidogenic effect has previously been suggested for RM consumption.[6] We initially failed to detect a difference in total bifidobacteria counts/g stool using FISH, partially due to an apparent bifidogenic effect of the control study diet. Mean bifidobacteria counts measured by FISH increased in subjects even during the placebo period. Next, we attempted to confirm the previous qPCR-based report of an RM associated bifidogenic effect with the same method.

Table 19.1 Average FISH Counts by Intervention Period of Total Bacteria and Selected Bacterial Groups to Which the Respective Probes Hybridized

	Placebo	RM25	RM50	p-Value
Total	8.84×10^9	1.01×10^{10}	1.08×10^{10}	0.02
Bacteroidetes	5.16×10^9	5.58×10^9	5.75×10^9	0.5
Clostridia Cl. IVX	4.74×10^9	4.96×10^9	4.63×10^9	0.8
Bifidobacteria	1.69×10^9	2.00×10^9	1.95×10^9	0.3

Using qPCR data, 13/14 subjects showed an increase in bifidobacteria from day 0 to day 24 during the RM50 period, while only 5/14 subjects showed such an increase during the placebo period (p < 0.05). In 12/14 subjects, the increase in bifidobacteria from day 0 to day 24 was larger during the RM50 period compared to the control period. Furthermore, the mean numbers of bifidobacteria tended to be higher on day 24 during RM50 period (2.7×10^5 genome equivalents/ng) compared to the placebo period (1.5×10^5), although not reaching significance (p = 0.29). The increase in bifidobacteria from day 0 to day 24 (expressed as genome equivalents/ng DNA) was larger and statistically significant during the RM50 period (p = 0.03), whereas during the placebo period, the bifidobacteria increase was not significant. This observation suggests that RM had a bifidogenic effect. The fact that results derived from DGGE, 16S rRNA sequencing, FISH, and qPCR differed, although pointing in the same direction, indicates the utility of a multilayered microbiota approach. The various microbiota analysis methods suffer from different biases but when combined allow for a more comprehensive analysis.

The calculated energy value of RM differed in individuals and during the RM50 period, ranging from less than 2 to almost 4 kcal/g (Baer et al. see associated manuscript in this edition). We hypothesized that variations in microbiota composition might have contributed to the observed difference in energy gain from RM. Thus, we analyzed if subjects with an above average energy gain per g of RM harbored a different microbiota. Indeed, using FISH, we detected suggestive increases in total bacteria (p = 0.1) and bifidobacteria (p = 0.07) in the subjects that showed above the mean energy gain from RM; qPCR confirmed the observation that counts of bifidobacteria were increased in subjects gaining above the mean energy from RM (4.1×10^5 vs. 8.3×10^4 bifidobacteria genome equivalents; p = 0.08).

19.4 Discussion

This study of the effects of RM supplementation on microbiota composition in a randomized, placebo-controlled feeding study in 14 male volunteers suggests that RM supplementation increases the total concentration of all fecal bacteria as well as the numbers of bifidobacteria. Microbiota was analyzed in spot stool samples which does not allow us to determine total stool output. It is feasible that increased nutrient availability, due to RM reaching the large intestine, allowed for additional bacterial growth resulting in increased bacterial concentrations in the stool. Using FISH, Bacteroidetes and bifidobacteria also showed slight trends toward increased numbers during RM supplementation, but these associations were small and did not reach significance. Thus, bacteria not targeted by our group-specific FISH probes likely contributed to the observed increase in total bacteria/g stool.

Although we sequenced an average of 23,639 reads/sample, we still did not reach saturation, indicating that even with the current high-throughput sequencing methods, detecting rare bacterial species with high confidence is difficult to achieve in studies with many samples using current longer sequence read technology. Because we performed multiple comparisons in only a few individuals, some of our observations are likely due to chance and need to be confirmed in other studies. The 16S rRNA sequence analysis showed that each of the subjects harbored a unique microbiota. Interestingly, although subjects consumed the same controlled diet each day of the week during the feeding periods, the proportions of dominant bacterial groups changed to some extent.

As increases in bifidobacteria are generally associated with improved immune function and better health, studies of the effects of RM on health outcomes appear warranted. At least over the short-term (28 days) energy gain/g, RM consumed appeared to differ among subjects and correlated with increased numbers of bifidobacteria. A change in microbiota composition and activities over time has previously been implicated to contribute to a change in equol-producing status from long-term soy consumption.[3] Longer-term studies will be needed to determine if over time microbiota composition adapts in subjects deriving less energy from RM intake to become more efficient in deriving additional energy from RM.

Acknowledgments

This study was funded by the U.S. Department of Agriculture and the Matsutani Chemical Industry Co., Ltd. Dr. Mai is funded by a mentored research scholar award from the American Cancer Society (MRSGT CCE-107301). The authors thank the study subjects for their willingness to participate and the BHNRC stuff for all their efforts with running the study.

References

1. Abell, G. C.; Cooke, C. M.; Bennett, C. N.; Conlon, M. A.; McOrist, A. L., *FEMS Microbiol. Ecol.* 2008, 66(3), 505.
2. Amann, R. I.; Krumholz, L.; Stahl, D. A., *J. Bacteriol.* 1990, 172(2), 762.
3. Atkinson, C.; Frankenfeld, C. L.; Lampe, J. W., *Exp. Biol. Med. (Maywood.).* 2005, 230(3), 155.
4. Cole, J. R.; Wang, Q.; Cardenas, E.; Fish, J.; Chai, B.; Farris, R. J.; Kulam-Syed-Mohideen, A. S.; McGarrell, D. M.; Marsh, T.; Garrity, G. M.; Tiedje, J. M., *Nucleic Acids Res.* 2009, 37(Database issue), D141.
5. Duncan, S. H.; Lobley, G. E.; Holtrop, G.; Ince, J.; Johnstone, A. M.; Louis, P.; Flint, H. J., *Int. J. Obes. (Lond.).* 2008, 32(11), 1720.
6. Fastinger, N. D.; Karr-Lilienthal, L. K.; Spears, J. K.; Swanson, K. S.; Zinn, K. E.; Nava, G. M.; Ohkuma, K.; Kanahori, S.; Gordon, D. T.; Fahey, G. C., Jr., *J. Am. Coll. Nutr.* 2008, 27(2), 356.
7. Franks, A. H.; Harmsen, H. J.; Raangs, G. C.; Jansen, G. J.; Schut, F.; Welling, G. W., *Appl. Environ. Microbiol.* 1998, 64(9), 3336.
8. Gordon, D. T.; Okuma, K., *J. AOAC Int.* 2002, 85(2), 435.
9. Guarner, F.; Malagelada, J. R., *Lancet* 2003, 361(9356), 512.
10. Hamady, M.; Walker, J. J.; Harris, J. K.; Gold, N. J.; Knight, R., *Nat. Methods* 2008, 5(3), 235.
11. Harmsen, H. J.; Raangs, G. C.; He, T.; Degener, J. E.; Welling, G. W., *Appl. Environ. Microbiol.* 2002, 68(6), 2982.

12. Harmsen, H. J.; Wildeboer-Veloo, A. C.; Grijpstra, J.; Knol, J.; Degener, J. E.; Welling, G. W., *Appl. Environ. Microbiol.* 2000, 66(10), 4523.
13. Jansen, G. J.; Wildeboer-Veloo, A. C.; Tonk, R. H.; Franks, A. H.; Welling, G. W., *J. Microbiol. Methods* 1999, 37(3), 215.
14. Kishimoto, Y.; Oga, H.; Tagami, H.; Okuma, K.; Gordon, D. T., *Eur. J. Nutr.* 2007, 46(3), 133.
15. Kurokawa, K.; Itoh, T.; Kuwahara, T.; Oshima, K.; Toh, H.; Toyoda, A.; Takami, H.; Morita, H.; Sharma, V. K.; Srivastava, T. P.; Taylor, T. D.; Noguchi, H.; Mori, H.; Ogura, Y.; Ehrlich, D. S.; Itoh, K.; Takagi, T.; Sakaki, Y.; Hayashi, T.; Hattori, M., *DNA Res.* 2007, 14(4), 169.
16. Langendijk, P. S.; Schut, F.; Jansen, G. J.; Raangs, G. C.; Kamphuis, G. R.; Wilkinson, M. H.; Welling, G. W., *Appl. Environ. Microbiol.* 1995, 61(8), 3069.
17. Lesmes, U.; Beards, E. J.; Gibson, G. R.; Tuohy, K. M.; Shimoni, E., *J. Agric. Food Chem.* 2008, 56(13), 5415.
18. Manz, W.; Amann, R.; Ludwig, W.; Vancanneyt, M.; Schleifer, K. H., *Microbiology* 1996, 142(Pt 5), 1097.
19. Miller, D. N.; Bryant, J. E.; Madsen, E. L.; Ghiorse, W. C., *Appl. Environ. Microbiol.* 1999, 65(11), 4715.
20. Poulsen, L. K.; Licht, T. R.; Rang, C.; Krogfelt, K. A.; Molin, S., *J. Bacteriol.* 1995, 177(20), 5840.
21. Schell, M. A.; Karmirantzou, M.; Snel, B.; Vilanova, D.; Berger, B.; Pessi, G.; Zwahlen, M. C.; Desiere, F.; Bork, P.; Delley, M.; Pridmore, R. D.; Arigoni, F., *Proc. Natl. Acad. Sci. USA* 2002, 99(22), 14422.
22. Schwiertz, A.; Taras, D.; Schafer, K.; Beijer, S.; Bos, N. A.; Donus, C.; Hardt, P. D., *Obesity (Silver Spring)* 2010 January, 18(1), 190–195.
23. Tannock, G. W., *Antonie Van Leeuwenhoek* 1999, 76(1–4), 265.
24. Turnbaugh, P. J.; Ley, R. E.; Mahowald, M. A.; Magrini, V.; Mardis, E. R.; Gordon, J. I., *Nature* 2006, 444(7122), 1027.
25. Vaughan, E. E.; Schut, F.; Heilig, H. G.; Zoetendal, E. G.; De Vos, W. M.; Akkermans, A. D., *Curr. Issues Intest. Microbiol.* 2000, 1(1), 1.
26. Wilson, K. H.; Blitchington, R. B., *Appl. Environ. Microbiol.* 1996, 62(7), 2273.
27. Zoetendal, E. G.; Akkermans, A. D.; De Vos, W. M., *Appl. Environ. Microbiol.* 1998, 64(10), 3854.

20

Resistant Maltodextrin Overview

Chemical and Physical Properties

ALLAN W. BUCK

Contents

20.1 Background and History of Development

Furthering the research of Englyst and Cummings on starch [1], Matsutani Chemical Industry scientists can be credited with recognizing the existence of naturally occurring digestion-resistant carbohydrates in common soluble starch hydrolysates such as dextrin, maltodextrin, and corn syrup, investigating their formation and occurrence, and developing optimized production technology for the manufacture of the concentrated soluble dietary fiber known commonly as resistant maltodextrin (RMD) [2–4]. Additionally, they can be credited with advancing clinical research in the areas of intestinal health [5], blood glucose attenuation [6–8], and other physiological effects as applied to RMD [9]. Their research which began in the early 1990s has led to the development and marketing of various forms of RMD, most notably Fibersol®-2 (aka Pinefiber C), a concentrated RMD containing about 90% soluble dietary fiber; Fibersol-2B (aka Pinefiber), containing about 50% fiber and 50% typical maltodextrin; as well as Fibersol-2H or H-Fiber, a hydrogenated form. The product of major commercial importance is Fibersol-2, being freely sold in the United States and around the world. For the most part, unless otherwise specified, this discussion will be around Fibersol-2, the highly concentrated fiber ingredient with characteristics shown in Table 20.1.

With the increasing awareness of the lack of fiber in our diets and increased awareness of the benefits it provides, the development of RMD provides for expanded use and availability of fiber in more food products. This is because RMD properties are very compatible with most food systems, thus providing food product formulators with a highly versatile, easy to formulate, highly concentrated fiber ingredient.

Table 20.1 Typical Characteristics of Fibersol-2 RMD

Appearance	Free-flowing fine white powder
Taste/odor	Bland; odorless
Dispersible	Readily dispersible in water
Solution, 30%	Clear; low viscosity (7 cps)
Total dietary fiber	90+% (dwb) (AOAC 2001.03)
Soluble fiber	90+%
Insoluble fiber	0%
Sugars	2% (dwb)
Dextrose equivalent	8.0–12.0
pH	4–6 in 10% solution
Moisture	5% Max.

It is the purpose of this discussion to review the basic understandings of RMD and relate some of its chemical and physical characteristics compared to other fiber sources to demonstrate that RMD is an invaluable tool for food product developers that can be used to increase the intake of dietary fiber.

20.2 Manufacture and Composition

Figure 20.1 is a graphic illustration for the production of RMD. Various starch sources have been and can be used, but corn starch from the corn wet milling process has been the most widely adopted starting raw material. RMD is made by a combination of hydrolysis and transglucosidation processes. Roasting dry starch at reduced pH conditions results in hydrolysis of the α1-4 and α1-6 glycosidic bonds. The action shortens the starch chain as in hydrolysis reactions but lacking sufficient water, the freed glucose linkages combine within themselves, and transglucosidation occurs creating random glycosidic linkages such as ß1-4, ß1-6, and α and ß1-3 and 1-2 [2–4].

The reaction destroys the granular starch nature of the material, rendering a soluble pyrodextrin. At this point, it contains a mixture of amylase digestible and amylase indigestible material [2–4]. In order to facilitate purification, it is saccharified with alpha-amylase and glucoamylase enzymes.

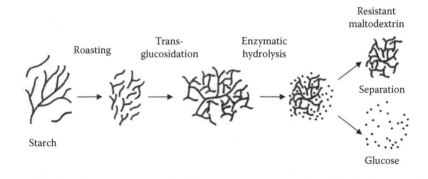

Figure 20.1 Process for manufacturing RMD.

After saccharification, a mixture of readily digestible glucose (depicted as dots on Figure 20.1) and the indigestible maltodextrin units is created. Separating the glucose fraction from the indigestible fraction results in the highly concentrated form of RMD.

Figure 20.2 shows the glycosidic typical linkages and chemical structure as compared to typical maltodextrin [10]. The weight average molecular weight is around 2000 with a polydispersity of about 2. Typical RMD has a reducing sugar content of about 10%–12% (e.g., 10–12 dextrose equivalent).

RMD is essentially all glucose polymers on a dry basis. A typical chromatogram and composition of Fibersol-2 is shown in Figure 20.3. The amount of mono- and disaccharides (DP1 and DP2) can be controlled via the separation process. The intent is generally to have a low amount so that this soluble fiber can be ideal for applications that minimize sugars.

20.3 Digestion and Physiological Properties

The fact that RMD escapes absorption in the small intestine is well known and evidenced by the glycemic response. Although RMD is a polymer of glucose units, there is hardly any postprandial blood glucose response following ingestion [2]. This is illustrated in Figure 20.4. Fifty grams of glucose, Pinefiber, and Fibersol-2 were ingested and blood samples taken every 30 min for over 2 h. The resulting curve shows a significant reduction in the postprandial blood glucose response to Pinefiber, a 50% RMD, and the almost complete absence of either by Fibersol-2, a 90+% RMD [11].

The overall digestive fate of RM has been extensively tested in vitro, in animals and in humans [11–15]. As shown, RMD largely escapes digestion and absorption in the upper gastrointestinal tract. When it reaches the large intestines, it is partly fermented by bacteria, producing short-chain fatty acids. At this point, these studies provide guidance as to how much is absorbed, fermented, and excreted. A review of the three human clinical studies [13–15] concluded that an energy value of 1.4 kcal/g is an appropriate value to assign the fiber fraction in RMD (as supplied, Fibersol-2 is 1.6 kcal/g). This agrees well with values calculated from in vitro and animal studies based on an apparent digestive scheme of 10% absorbed, 50% fermented, and 40% excreted.

Clinical studies show that RMD helps to relieve occasional constipation [16–28]. One example study is a 2 week, placebo-controlled, crossover study with 84 healthy adults. In this particular study, 4.9 g/day of Fibersol-2 was given in a single serving, the control drink contained 2.3 g digestible maltodextrin, and total calories were balanced at 134 kcal. In the subgroup with stool frequencies below 7/week (n = 27) during the run-in phase, there were statistically significant increases in both stool frequency and volume during the treatment period compared to baseline (non-ingestion period), but not different from the control treatment period [22].

Figure 20.5 shows some results from another study demonstrating the effect of RMD on constipation [27]. In this study, 6 g of total Fibersol-2 was consumed in 2–3 g servings. This was a 2 week, placebo-controlled, crossover study with

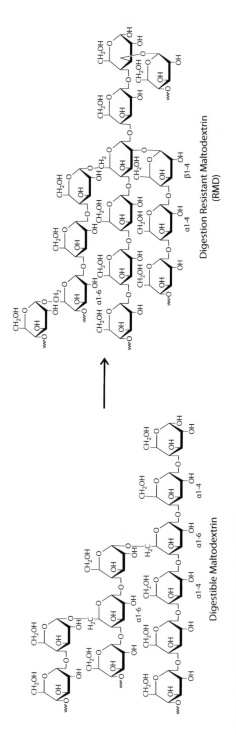

Figure 20.2 Maltodextrin and RMD molecular structure.

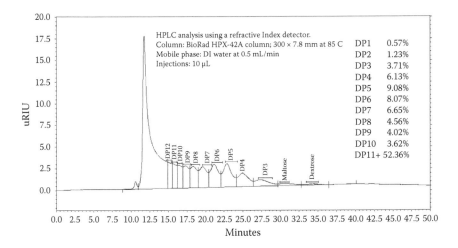

Figure 20.3 DP profile, Fibersol-2 RMD.

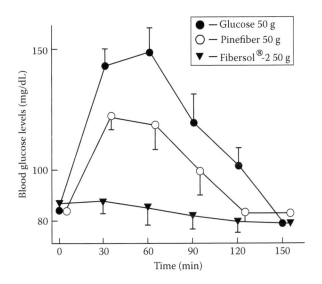

Figure 20.4 Digestibility/glycemic response.

71 healthy adults. In the subjects who were subgrouped as having mild constipation (n = 20), there was a significant increase (p < 0.01) in frequency compared to control and a significant increase in fecal amount compared to control (p < 0.05).

Japan utilizes the FOSHU system for foods demonstrating health benefits. These are foods approved by the Ministry of Health and Welfare as effective for preservation of health by adding certain active ingredients or removing undesirable ones. Further evidence of the utilization of RMD for intestinal benefits is the fact that in Japan 153 of 307 total products formulated for intestinal regularity use RMD.

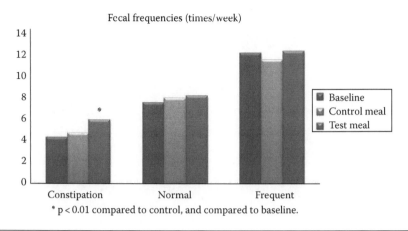

Fecal frequencies (times/week)

* p < 0.01 compared to control, and compared to baseline.

Figure 20.5 Effect of drinks formulated with RMD.

Studies also show that Fibersol-2 when taken with a meal may attenuate the rise in serum glucose following the meal [29–67]. Figure 20.6 is from a study that looked at postprandial blood glucose and insulin after consumption of a cooked rice meal with or without 5 g added Fibersol-2 [39]. A significant decrease in blood glucose levels was noted at 30 and 60 min as well as the area under the curve compared to cooked rice with the placebo food.

The effect on blood glucose is one of the most well studied and used property of RMD. In Japan, 124 of 133 FOSHU products specifically formulated for moderating postprandial blood glucose levels contain RMD.

Certainly many other studies could be illustrated. RMD has been studied, for example, for other gastrointestinal functions, for repeated effects on sugar and fat metabolism, effect on body composition, and others [10]. There are around 100 human clinical studies examining RMD [9,43,57,58,60,64,67,68–72]. Two recent studies demonstrate that foods formulated with Fibersol-2 digestion RMD can provide an increased feeling of satiety, so consumers felt fuller for a longer period of time [73].

20.4 Fiber Definition

As more beneficial effects of fibers are recognized, some regulatory definitions have not caught up with the evolution of current scientific knowledge. Some of the recent authoritative definitions include those generated by American Association of Cereal Chemists [74], Institute of Medicine, National Academy of Sciences [75], and Codex Alimentarius [76]. As definitions evolve, there are some common patterns that can be extracted: Fiber is composed of carbohydrate polymers not hydrolyzed by endemic digestive enzymes, they are derived from food raw materials, and there must be a validated analytical procedure established that measures only the fiber fraction on the ingredient. Also, the material must demonstrate a physiological effect beneficial to humans.

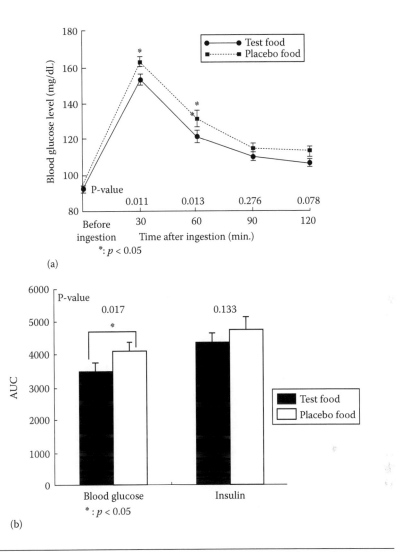

Figure 20.6 Effect of RMD on (a) postprandial blood glucose and (b) insulin in a meal.

RMD meets these criteria. As already discussed, RMD escapes absorption in the small intestine because it is not hydrolyzed by digestive enzymes. RMD is derived from food starch, typically corn, but other food sources would be applicable.

An analytical procedure, AOAC 2001.03, has been developed to measure the fiber fraction in RMD [77]. That method, which was formally adopted in 2005, has recently been expanded, and a new promulgated procedure was developed that universally measures fiber across a wide variety of matrixes and that is AOAC 2009.01 [77]. (These methods are important for detecting RMD in foods. The typical default method for fiber determination commonly referred to as the

Prosky method only determines SDF $\geq$ DP12 or so [78]. In the Prosky test, total dietary fiber is the fraction of ethanol insolubles, precipitated after enzymatic treatment. RMD consists of indigestible components that are lower MW and soluble in ethanol and therefore missed by the Prosky fiber test. In AOAC 2001.03, the water and ethanol insoluble fractions are determined gravimetrically in a single step. The ethanol soluble fraction is collected and analyzed by HPLC with fiber being defined as those polymers DP3 and greater.)

The common physiological effects mentioned by authoritative definitions required for a compound to be identified as fiber include blood glucose attenuation and/or blood cholesterol attenuation and/or laxation and/or intestinal heath and/or others to be determined. RMD has been extensively tested in these areas with examples relating to laxation and blood glucose attenuation provided for the purposes of this discussion to demonstrate its fiber physiological benefits.

20.5 Food Functional Properties

In light of the well-known fact that the population at large is not consuming sufficient dietary fiber, RMD can be easily formulated into foods to boost the fiber content. It is useful in whole-grain foods where it can boost the total dietary fiber to levels attracting the consumer's attention and improve the overall consumer acceptance, as well as to add fiber to foods that normally contain none, enriching the diet and at the same time replacing caloric sugars and carbohydrates with reduced energy fiber. It is quite often referred to as an "invisible fiber." Some of the properties of Fibersol-2 RMD of interest are shown in Table 20.2.

Table 20.2 Characteristics of RMD in Foods

Dietary fiber, 90%
High purity
No inherent or added flavor or odor
Low sweetness
High solubility, 70%
Clear, transparent solution
Rapid dispersion
Very low viscosity
Acid, heat/retort stable
Freeze/thaw stable
Survives culturing
Slow fermentation
Good GI tolerance
Energy control
Low hygroscopicity
Flavor-modifying properties
Moisture control

Table 20.3 Comprehensive Fiber Method: Result of Analysis for Total Nondigestible Carbohydrates (NDC) in Each Test Ingredient Incorporated into Bread for Insoluble Dietary Fiber (IDF), High-Molecular-Weight Soluble Dietary Fiber (HMWSDF), Low-Molecular-Weight Soluble Nondigestible Oligosaccharides (NDO), and Resistant Starch (RS) Contents[a]

Ingredient	IDF + HMWSDF + Part of RS[b]	NDO[c]	−RS[d] (Third Crucible)	RS (AOAC 2002.02)[e]	Total NDC (wt %, Dry Basis)[f]
Cellulose	99.75	0	(0)	0.18	99.33
Wheat bran	39.67	4.86	(0.54)	0.40	44.39
Gum arabic	98.39	0	(0)	0.19	98.58
Polydextrose	0.47	76.54	(0)	0	77.01
RMD	24.69	68.47	(0)	0	93.16
Fructooligosaccharide	0	68.64	(0)	0	68.64
Galactooligosaccharide	0	46.13	(0)	0	46.13
RS	63.44	0.26	(63.22)	43.48	43.96
Bakery flour	4.32	1.66	(0.55)	1.21	6.64

[a] Mean of duplicate measurements, wt %, dry basis.
[b] Determined with AOAC official method 991.43.
[c] Determined by LC with AOAC official method 2001.03.
[d] Subtracted RS value determined from third crucible.
[e] Determined with AOAC official method 2002.02.
[f] Total NDC = (IDF + HMWSDF + part of RS) + NDO − RS (third crucible) + RS (AOAC 2002.02).

Fibersol-2 is a high concentrated source of dietary fiber, being 90% minimum on a dry basis. This allows for minimal addition as a fortifying fiber, so, when used as a bulk ingredient such as when substituting for sugar or corn syrup, makes extremely high fiber contents possible. Table 20.3 is taken from work that led to the development of AOAC 2009.01, the comprehensive method for determining fiber in foods [78]. RMD is among the more concentrated fiber sources available. This work indicates that some soluble fibers such as polydextrose and fructooligosaccharide do not hold up to the enzymatic digestion or are excluded as a result of containing an excess of mono- and disaccharide after digestions and as a result have a lower than expected fiber content.

Low impurities are important in food formulation. The fact that Fibersol is virtually 100% carbohydrate void of residual protein, fat, or ash provides that it is not the limiting factor in shelf life or flavor considerations. For this reason, it is often referred to as an "invisible" fiber but also because it adds no flavor or odor of its own and with minimal viscosity.

Although RMD is composed of glucose polymers, they are low in sweetness, and like common maltodextrin, they are highly soluble. Most forms of RMD are refined by carbon and ion exchange treatments, so solutions are absolutely clear. Typical forms of RMD include spray dried and agglomerated powders. These are readily dispersible, and the agglomerated form, used typically in fiber supplements and powdered beverages, shows rapid dispersibility.

A key benefit to RMD is that it is highly stable to all forms of food processing, withstanding high-acid/high-temperature processing, retort processing, and high-pressure extrusion operations. This property has found favor over many other soluble forms of fiber that do degrade under these conditions, allowing for RMD use in clear, acidified beverages. The high stability of Fibersol has been demonstrated in many applications, and documentation exists to show that there should be no stability issues under typical food processing conditions, including beverage concentrates at pH less than 2, neutral pH retorted soups or extruded cereals.

The highly branched nature of RMD compared to maltodextrin is thought to explain why it prevents retrogradation and hazing during freeze thaw cycles.

While RMD such as Pinefiber contributes a high level of available fermentable carbohydrate via the 50% nonfiber fraction, Fibersol-2 at 90+% is highly resistant to most food cultures. This allows a targeted fiber concentration to be formulated into a product with no need to compensate for fiber that might be utilized as a food source, such as in yeast fermentations or yogurt cultures.

While Fibersol is fermented to some degree in the colon, it is not robustly utilized, generating much less gas production in a given period of time than other soluble fibers, and is quite often a favored selection for its GI tolerance. A study by Flickinger and others published in 2000 is often used to explain why Fibersol has developed such a good reputation from a GI tolerance perspective. While it is utilized by many gut microbes, it is not such a robust fermentation as some highly fermented materials such as fructooligosaccharide [79]. A recent study reports that 20 college age students consuming 20 g of RMD in a beverage 2 h prior to lunch did not experience any adverse gastrointestinal symptoms [73].

It has shown various flavor-modifying properties, improving the metallic aftertaste of aspartame and various nondescript improvements in flavor of other high-intensity sweeteners and whole-grain products.

It is quite common to encounter food product developers who think of fiber as a challenging water-absorbing, bulking agent. RMD is more characteristic of starch hydrolysates such as corn syrups and maltodextrins in terms of their food-formulating properties. Comparing various soluble fibers, some, such as oat beta-glucan show extremely high viscosity at concentrations as lows as 0.3% [80], RMD is a soluble dietary fiber that is not limited in its application by forming gels or excess viscosity.

20.6 Food Applications

As a result of its ease of formulation and functional and other benefits described, RMD has been used in a wide range of applications from beverages to baked goods and snacks. Beverages are well suited to RMD usage. It is stable to thermal processing, even at very low pH, where concentrates can exist below 2.0 pH, and with resulting high clarity. In some applications, it was found to mask off notes associated with high-potency sweeteners, vitamins, and other additives and round out the acidic note in juices and the bitter note on coffee beverages. It has found success in flavored waters, juice and vegetable-based drinks, and functional and nutritional beverages.

Whole-grain bakery items, cereals, and snacks often fall short of expected labeled fiber content, and RMD is useful in bringing them to levels expected by the consumer. It can be incorporated in the base, into coatings, fillings, and other means, often improving shelf life, texture, and overall consumer acceptability. In some cases, it has been found to help mask bitter notes associated with whole grains and bran.

RMD is compatible with all dairy product applications. This includes fluid, frozen, cultured, and fermented dairy foods. Fibersol-2 is stable under all processing and packaging conditions and has been shown to improve flavor, mouthfeel, and sweetness of low-solid dairy foods, acidic products, and dairy foods to which other flavors may be added.

Evidence that RMD is of practical functional benefit in foods is the fact that in Japan it is formulated into many FOSHU products. Not only are a high percentage of products using RMD in foods formulated for intestinal regularity and over 90% of the FOSHU foods for blood glucose control, but also they have been steadily increasing over the last 4 years. It has increased from 99 of 201 products for intestinal regularity in 2005 to 153 of 307 as of June 2009. It has also increased from 61 of 69 products for blood glucose control in 2005 to 124 of 133 also as of June 2009. Both items are easily monitored by the consuming individual.

20.7 Conclusion

There are a growing number of benefits associated with the intake of dietary fiber. It is recognized that no one source of fiber provides all these benefits. Therefore, a diverse range of fiber sources must be consumed. Besides not showing all the physiological benefits associated with fiber, individual fibers show a diversity of functional properties that may limit their suitability in applications. A diversity of fiber-containing foods would help promote increased fiber consumption.

Purified RMD is a highly soluble, bland tasting, nonretrograding dietary fiber prepared from starch. It provides high clarity and low viscosity to aqueous systems and can reduce or replace higher energy sources of carbohydrates. It is highly stable at low pH and elevated temperature and has been shown to be highly versatile in its application to a wide variety of foods.

RMD has been clinically proven to provide physiological benefits associated with fiber. Its physical characteristics and properties provide for its use in foods that normally would not be considered for fiber fortification such as low-viscosity beverages and high-clarity sauces and syrups. RMD also confers functionality that helps increase overall fiber content of foods such as whole-grain formulations where acceptance can be limited as a result of flavor or other functional limitations.

References

1. Okuma, K. and Wakabayashi, S., 44 Fibersol-2: A soluble, non-digestible, starch-derived dietary fibre, in *Advanced Dietary Fibre Technology*, McCleary, B.V. and Prosky, L., Eds., Blackwell Science, Oxford, U.K., 2001, p. 509.
2. Okuma, K. et al., *Denpun Kagaku*, 37, 107, 1990.
3. Okuma, K. and Matsuda, I., *J. Appl. Glycosci.*, 49(4), 479, 2002.
4. Okuma, K. and Matsuda, I., *J. Appl. Glycosci.*, 50, 389, 2003.
5. Wakabayashi, S., *Jpn. J. Nutr.*, 51, 31, 1993.
6. Wakabayashi, S. and Matsuoka, A., *Nippon Naibunpi Gakkai Zasshi (Folia Endrocrinol.)*, 68, 623, 1992.
7. Ueda, Y., Wakabayashi, S., and Matsuoka, A., *J. Jpn. Diab. Soc. (Tohnyobo)*, 36, 715, 1993.
8. Wakabayashi, S. et al., *J. Jpn. Assoc. Dietary Fiber Res.*, 3, 13, 1999.
9. Kishimoto, Y., Wakabayashi, S., and Tokunaga, K., *J. Jpn. Assoc. Dietary Fiber Res.*, 4(2), 59, 2000.
10. Hashizume, C. and Okuma, K., Fibersol®2-resistant maltodextrin: Functional dietary fiber ingredient, in *Fiber Ingredients Food Applications and Health Benefits*, Cho, S. and Samuel, P., Eds., CRC Press, Boca Raton, FL, 2009.
11. Okuma, K. et al., *Tech. J. Food Chem. Chem.*, 6(11), 62, 1990.
12. Tsuji, K. and Gordon, D., *J. Agric. Food Chem.*, 46, 2253, 1998.
13. Nakamura, S. and Oku, T., *J. Jpn. Assoc. Dietary Fiber Res.*, 9(11), 34, 2005.
14. Toshiano et al., *Am. J. Clin. Nutr.*, 83, 1321, 2006.
15. Baer, D. and Rumpler, W. The 9th Vahouny Fiber Symposium, Bethesda, MD, 2010.
16. Satouchi et al., *Jpn. J. Nutr.*, 51, 31, 1993.
17. Kimura et al., *J. Nutr. Food*, 1, 12, 1998.
18. Inaki et al., *J Nutritional Food*, 9(2), 44, 1999.
19. Umekawa et al., *J. Nutr. Food*, 2(2), 52, 1999.
20. Ogiso et al., *J. Jpn. Assoc. Dietary Fiber Res.*, 3(2), 79, 1999.
21. Shi et al., *J. Nutr. Food*, 3(2), 37, 2000.
22. Unno et al., *J. Nutr. Food*, 3(4), 31, 2000.
23. Tanaka et al., *J. Nutr. Food*, 3(4), 39, 2000.
24. Sato et al., *J. Nutr. Food*, 3(4), 47, 2000.
25. Yamamoto et al., *J. Nutr. Food*, 3(2), 29, 2000.
26. Unno et al., *J. Nutr. Food*, 4(4), 21, 2000.
27. Takagaki et al., *J. Nutr. Food*, 4(4), 29, 2001.
28. Furukawa et al., *J. Jpn. Council Advanced Food Ingredients Res.*, 7(1), 55–62, 2004.
29. Fuse et al., *J. Nutr. Food*, 5(1), 69, 2002.
30. Inoue et al., *J. Jpn. Clin. Nutr.*, 26(4), 281, 2005.
31. Mizushima et al., *J. Nutr. Food*, 2(4), 17, 1995.
32. Uno et al., *J. Nutr. Food*, 2(4), 25, 1999.
33. Ito et al., *Jpn. Pharmacol. Ther.*, 34(8), 945, 2006.
34. Kandea et al., *Jpn. Innov. Food Ingredients Res.*, 8(2), 119, 2005.
35. Kawai et al., *Health Sci.*, 21(1), 61, 2005.
36. Kawai et al., *J. Jpn. Council Adv. Food Ingredients Res.*, 8(2), 81, 2005.
37. Suzuki et al., *J. Nutr. Food*, 4(4), 71, 2001.
38. Kawai, *J. Nutr. Food*, 5(4), 33, 2002.
39. Takeyasu, H. et al., *Jpn. Innov. Food Ingredients Res.*, 9(1), 37, 2006.
40. Fukuda et al., *J. Nutr. Food*, 5(2), 21, 2002.
41. Ikeguchi et al., *J. Jpn. Council Adv. Food Ingredients Res.*, 9(1), 57, 2006.
42. Sekizaki, K. and Yonezawa, H., *J. Nutr. Food*, 4(3), 81, 2001.
43. Unno et al., *J. Nutr. Food*, 5(2), 31, 2002.

44. Tamura et al., *J. Nutr. Food,* 6(3), 55, 2003.
45. Shoya et al., *J. Nutr. Food,* 7(4), 31, 2004.
46. Manami et al., *Jpn. Innov. Food Ingredients Res.,* 7(1), 83, 2004.
47. Morita et al., *Jpn. Innov. Food Ingredients Res.,* 8(1), 33, 2004.
48. Fukushima et al., *J. Nutr. Food,* 5(3), 10, 2002.
49. Nakagawa et al., *J. Nutr. Food,* 6(1), 81, 2003.
50. Kawai et al., *J. Nutr. Food,* 6(2), 129, 2003.
51. Sumi et al., *J. Nutr. Food,* 6(1), 89, 2003.
52. Fuse et al., *J. Nutr. Food,* 5(4), 47, 2002.
53. Shinohara et al., *J. Nutr. Food,* 2(1), 52, 1999.
54. Wolf et al., *Nutr. Res.,* 21, 1099, 2001.
55. Wakabayashi et al., *Folia Endocrinol.,* 68, 623, 1992.
56. Fujiwara et al., *J. Nutr. Food,* 53(6), 361, 1995.
57. Kawasaki et al., *J. Nutr. Food,* 3(1), 65, 2000.
58. Kishimoto et al., *Eur. J. Nutr.,* 46, 133, 2007.
59. Takeuchi et al., *J. Nutr. Food,* 4(4), 61, 2001.
60. Kishimoto et al., *J. Nutr. Food,* 3(2), 19, 2000.
61. Moriguchi et al., *Jpn. Innov. Food Ingredients Res.,* 7(1), 63, 2004.
62. In et al., *Eastern Medicinevol.,* 115(2), 19, 1999.
63. Hori et al., *J. Nutr. Food,* 8(2), 27, 2005.
64. Tokunaga, K. and Matsuoka, A., *J. Jpn. Diab. Soc.,* 42(1), 61, 1999.
65. Maeda et al., *J. Nutr. Food,* 4(3), 73, 2001.
66. Shioda et al., *J. Nutr. Food,* 4(2), 7, 2001.
67. Fujiwara et al., *J. Jpn. Clin. Nutr.,* 83, 301, 1993.
68. Nomura et al., *J. Jpn. Soc. Nutr. Food Sci.,* 45, 21, 1992.
69. Kajimoto et al., *J. Nutr. Food,* 3(3), 47, 2000.
70. Matsuoka et al., *J. Jpn. Clin. Nutr.,* 80, 167, 1992.
71. Kajimoto et al., *J. Nutr. Food,* 5(3), 117, 2002.
72. Mizushima et al., *J. Nutr. Food,* 3(3), 75, 2000.
73. Hendrich, S. et al., Higher dose Fibersol-2 increases subjective and biochemical measures of satiety when ingested with a meal compared with control or lower consumption, Presented at the *Ninth Vahauny Fiber Symposium,* Bethesda, MD, June 8–11, 2010.
74. American Association of Cereal Chemists, *Cereal Foods World,* 46, 112, 2001.
75. The National Academies of Science, Institute of Medicine (IOM) Dietary reference intakes for energy, carbohydrate, fiber, fat, fatty acids, cholesterol, protein, and amino acids, Washington, DC: National Academies Press, pp. 339–361, 2002.
76. Codex Alimentarius, FAO, Rome: Joint FAO/WHO Food Standards Programme, Secretariat of the Codex Alimentarius Commission, 2010. Guidelines on nutrition labeling CAC/GL 2-1985 as last amended 2010.
77. *Official Methods of Analysis,* 18th ed. Rev 3, AOAC International, Horwitz and Latimer, 2010.
78. Okuma et al., *J. Agric. Food Chem.,* 57(17), 7659, 2009.
79. Flickinger et al., *J. Nutr.,* 130(5), 1267, 2000.
80. Doublier, J. and Wood, P., *Cereal Chem.,* 72, 335, 1995.

21
Rice Bran Fiber

JIN-HEE PARK, ALBERT W. LEE, STEPHANIE NISHI,
SUSAN S. CHO, and NELSON ALMEIDA

Contents

21.1 Introduction

Rice bran and brown rice (containing rice bran) have been used to produce various types of food products. Examples include breakfast cereals, baked goods, rice cakes, tea, pasta, and noodles. Rice has been cultivated for 2000 years. Historically, rice has constituted an important commercial crop since it was a dietary staple for people in regions around the world. Leading rice-producing countries include the United States, China, and other Asian countries (Lu et al., 1991). Although rice bran is used mostly as animal feed, some is processed for human consumption.

Consumption of rice in developing countries is around 68.5 kg/person/year and 12.8 kg/person/year in developed countries (Kahlon, 2009). Rice is harvested from fields called paddies. In the rice milling process, the hull is first removed to produce brown rice. Brown rice consists of the bran layer, germ, and endosperm (starch). Bran and germ are concentrated sources of vitamins, minerals, flavones, and other phytonutrients present in brown rice. One hundred kilograms of paddy rice on milling yields 10–12 kg rice bran. Rice bran contains the enzyme, lipase, which rapidly degrades the oil and makes the bran rancid and inedible (Kahlon, 2009). To extend shelf life, rice bran is either defatted with hexane or heat-stabilized to deactivate lipase activities.

Each year, between 63 and 76 million tons of rice bran (rice milling byproduct) is produced in the world, and more than 90% of rice bran is sold as animal feed. The remainder is either defatted or stabilized to be used as value-added ingredients. In the United States, rice oil is extracted from 15% to 20% of the rice bran (Kahlon, 2009). Rice bran has been recognized as an excellent source of fiber. The total dietary fiber (TDF) content of full-fat rice bran ranges from 20% to 27% with less than 2% as soluble dietary fiber.

Inadequate intake of dietary fiber increases risk of chronic diseases. Examples include diverticular diseases/constipation, heart disease, cancer, diabetes, metabolic syndrome, and overweight/obesity (IOM, 2002, 2006). Americans consume approximately one-half of the recommended intake levels, the Daily Reference Intakes (DRI). Thus, the IOM (IOM, 2002, 2006) and USDA Dietary Guidelines for Americans (2005, 2010) recommend increased consumption of fiber-rich foods.

The USDA, in partnership with a nonprofit organization, provides a nutritious rice bran drink to preschool children in Latin American countries. Healthy meal replacement drinks made from stabilized rice bran have been introduced in the market.

21.2 Physicochemistry and Structure of Rice Bran Fiber

CJ's rice bran fiber (RBF) is processed from defatted rice bran by a proprietary hydrothermal process. Table 21.1 lists specifications of RBF. Rice bran fiber has >40% TDF (of which >90% is insoluble dietary fiber) and a particle size of <100 μm (Table 21.1). The rice fiber contains no sulfites, added flavors, components from an animal source, BHA, BHT, genetically altered plant material, or irradiated material. Defatted RBF and sugar beet fiber are known to have comparable water-holding capacities (RBF, 4.89 mL/g vs. sugar beet fiber, 4.56 mL/g; Abdul-Hamid and Luan, 2000).

21.3 Functionality

Rice bran fiber consists of mostly insoluble dietary fiber added to food for several purposes. Rice bran fiber can be used as an ingredient in foods and beverages as a food ingredient. Examples include raising TDF content, reducing caloric content, controlling water activity, and modifying the rheological properties of foods and beverages.

Table 21.1 Specifications of RBF

Macronutrient	%	Unit	Analytical Method
TDF (dry wt. basis)[a]	>40	%	AOAC 991.43
Protein	<15	%	AOAC 984.13
Starch	<25	%	AOAC 996.11
Fat	<1.5	%	AOAC 954.02
Moisture	<8.0	%	AOAC 934.01
Ash	<16	%	AOAC 900.02
Lead	<1	ppm	
Arsenic	<1	ppm	
pH, 5% slurry	7.3 ± 0.5	pH	
Microbiological specifications			
Total plate count	<10,000	cfu/g	FDA-BAM2[b] Chap. 3
S. aureus	Negative	cfu/g	FDA-BAM2 Chap. 4
E. coli	Negative	cfu/g	FDA-BAM2 Chap. 4
Salmonella	Negative	cfu/g	FDA-BAM2 Chap. 5
Yeast and mold	<200	cfu/g	FDA-BAM2 Chap. 19

[a] TDF, total dietary fiber; cfu, colony forming units.
[b] BAM, bacteriological analytical manual, January 2001.

21.4 Current Regulatory Status

Rice bran is a GRAS ingredient (GRN 372). FDA has allowed three health claims related to dietary fiber intake and reduced risk of heart disease and cancer: (1) the reduced risk of cancer claim for fiber containing grain products, fruits, and vegetables (21CFR 101.76; FDA 1993a); (2) the reduced risk of coronary heart disease (CHD) claim for fruits, vegetables, and grain products that contain fiber, in particular soluble fiber (21CFR 101.77; FDA, 1993b); and (3) soluble fiber from certain foods and risk of CHD (21CFR 101.81; FDA, 2008). To be eligible for using the health claim, a food product must contain at least 2.5 g of TDF per reference amount customarily consumed (RACC) in food. Foods providing 2.5 g fiber/serving from RBF may be qualified for two health claims (the reduced risk of cancer claim for fiber containing grain products, fruits, and vegetables and the reduced risk of CHD claim for fruits, vegetables, and grain products that contain fiber, in particular soluble fiber), if they meet the jelly bean rules (i.e., as part of low-sodium and low-fat diets).

21.5 Metabolic Fate of Rice Bran Fiber

Rice bran fiber, like most beta-linked fibers, is not digested by human pancreatic or brush border enzymes, and the compounds are not expected to be absorbed intact. Like other dietary fibers, RBF reaches the large intestine without being hydrolyzed by human alimentary enzymes and is fermented by the colonic microflora to SCFAs (e.g., acetate, propionate, and butyrate) that can be utilized as a caloric source by intestinal microflora. Rice bran fiber also has fecal bulking effects to promote intestinal regularity (Miyoshi et al., 1986; Tomlin and Read, 1988). Symptoms caused by fiber deficiency (such as constipation) can be alleviated by RBF.

21.6 Effects of Rice Bran on Growth and Hematology in Animals

21.6.1 Effects of Processing of Rice Bran on Growth and Organ Weights

Sayre et al. (1987) observed that chickens fed with a 60% heat-treated rice bran diet produced weight gains similar to those of chicks fed with a 60% corn diet and that the heat-treated rice bran diet produced significantly greater weight gains than the 60% raw rice bran diet (raw RB, 441 g/3 weeks vs. heat-treated RB, 568 g/3 weeks, $p < 0.05$). The quantity of feed required per unit weight gain was significantly ($p < 0.05$) less for chickens given heat-treated rice bran (1.59) as compared to raw bran (1.86).

Sayre et al. (1988) and Mujajhid et al. (2004) also observed that processing rice bran by extrusion cooking or roasting improved performance of chicks. Extrusion cooking resulted in the best performance, followed by roasting, while nonsignificant differences were observed between raw and pelleted bran (weight gain, g/6 weeks: extrusion 1991[a] ± 249, roasting 1881[b] ± 310, pelleting 1787[c] ± 339, raw rice bran 1788[c] ± 347; lack of a common superscript letter indicates a significant difference, $p < 0.05$; Mujajhid et al., 2004). In this study, raw, extruded, roasted, and pelleted rice brans with three inclusions of antioxidants (0, 125, and 250 ppm) were used at 0%, 10%, 20%, 30%, 40%, and 50% in the diets of broiler chicks. Increasing the amount of rice bran in broiler diets resulted in significantly negative effects on growth performance when rice bran was fed at up to 50% of the diet for 6 weeks (0%: 2296[a] ± 24, 10%: 2172[b] ± 61, 20%: 1949[c] ± 103, 30%: 1738[d] ± 122, 40%: 1575[e] ± 121, 50%: 1442[f] ± 119). No significant differences were observed in mortality or dressing percentage due to different processes or concentrations of rice bran in the diet. Organ weights were significantly higher on raw and pelleted rice bran as compared to extruded and roasted bran (liver, g; extrusion, 2.11[a] ± 0.08; roasting, 2.12[a] ± 0.07; raw, 2.20[b] ± 0.16; pelleted, 2.22[b] ± 0.16). However, these values were within the normal range. Treating rice bran with antioxidants had no significant effect on broiler performance.

The presence of these heat labile antinutritional factors (such as trypsin inhibitors, pepsin inhibitors, and an antithiamine factor) is a reason for poor performance of chicks when the content of raw or pelleted rice bran is increased (Kumar and Chaudhuri, 1976; Lu et al., 1991; Tashiro and Ikegami, 1996; Tashiro and Maki, 1986).

21.6.2 Comparison of Full-Fat and Defatted Rice Bran with Wheat and Corn

Kahlon et al. (1990) studied the influence of stabilized or parboiled rice brans (full-fat or defatted), oat bran, or a cellulose control on weight gain in 4 week old hamsters. All diets contained 10% cellulose and 0.5% cholesterol. Weight gain after 3 weeks was similar in all groups except the parboiled rice bran group that had less ($p < 0.05$) than all other groups (weight gain; control, 2.9; stabilized RB, 2.8;

defatted rice bran, 2.8; parboiled rice bran, 2.3; defatted parboiled RB, 2.7; oat bran, 3.1 g/day). No adverse effects of stabilized full-fat or defatted rice bran were observed.

Other studies also reported that rice bran, corn, and other types of brans (oat or wheat bran) and RBF had comparable weight gains in rats (Ayano et al., 1980; Johnson et al., 1989), mice (Hundemer et al., 1991), geese (Hsu et al., 1996), and chicks (Sayre et al., 1987). Administration of hemicellulose extracted from RBF (10% in diet) had no effect on the body weight and relative tissue weight in rats (Takenaka and Itoyama, 1993).

21.6.3 Hematology

Hemicellulose extracted from RBF increased peripheral blood leukocytes in rats (Takenaka and Itoyama, 1993). Wistar male rats were fed 10% RBF or various proportions of a hemicellulose-containing diet for 2 weeks. The number of peripheral blood leukocytes and lymphocytes was increased by 10% in rats fed with a 10% hemicellulose diet compared with a control diet ($p < 0.01$). The proportion of each lymphocyte subset was not significantly changed.

21.7 Health Benefits of Rice Bran and Rice Bran Fiber in Animals

Rice bran fiber provides several health benefits such as antioxidant, antimutagenic, antigenotoxic, and anticarcinogenic activities. In addition, rice bran enhances the viscosity of the gastrointestinal contents (Dikeman et al., 2006), which attenuates blood glucose and lipid concentrations.

21.7.1 Antioxidant Properties of Rice Bran Fiber

Rice bran fiber (polysaccharides) exhibited good potential for reducing power, chelating ferrous ions, and scavenging effects of 2,2-azino-bis(3-ethylbenzthiazoline-6-sulphonate), 1,1-diphenyl-2-picrylhydrazyl (DPPH), and hydrogen peroxide (Zha et al., 2009). Defatted rice bran extracts and their phytochemical constituents, when assayed by cytochrome c and NBT methods, also showed scavenging effects of superoxide radical and DPPH, largely attributed to flavones, including tricin, phenolics, ferulic acid, and phytic acid (Cai et al., 2004; Renuka Devi and Arumughan, 2007).

21.7.2 Antimutagenic, Antigenotoxic, and Anticarcinogenic Activities of Rice Bran Fiber or Rice Bran

There is no evidence that rice bran or RBF is carcinogenic or mutagenic. Instead, rice bran and its fiber components showed anticarcinogenic and antimutagenic activities in in vitro and in vivo studies (Tables 21.2 and 21.3; Aoe et al., 1993; CIREP, 2006; Hidashi-Okai et al., 2004; Sera et al., 2005; Takenaka et al., 1991; Takenaka, 1992; Takeo et al., 1998; Takeshita et al., 1992; Verschoyle et al., 2007). Inositols and inositol derivatives (Ogawa, 1999), γ-oryzanol (CIREP, 2006), phytic acid (Norazalina et al., 2010), tocols (Sun et al., 2009), phytic acid

Table 21.2 Studies Showing Antimutagenic and/or Anticarcinogenic Activities of RBF

Type of Rice Bran	Test Measure	Tested Mutagens or Carcinogenesis Model	References
RBHs	Chemically induced large-bowel tumors in male rats	DMH	Aoe et al. (1993)
RBF	Binding capacity, in vitro	Various mutagens and carcinogens such as heterocyclic amines,[a] six nitroarenes, 4-nitroquinoline-N-oxide, benzo[a]pyrene, furylfuramide, formaldehyde, and fecal mutagens (glucuronides and sulfates)	Sera et al. (2005)
RBF	Binding capacity, in vitro	Polycyclic biphenyl (PCB)	Takenaka et al. (1991)
RBF	Thymus atrophy in rats as an index of toxicity	Bis(tri-n-butyltin)oxide	Takenaka (1992)

[a] Heterocyclic amines include PCB, polychlorinated dibenzofurans (PCDFs), and polychlorinated-p-dioxins (PCDDs).

(Norazalina et al., 2010), phenols (Rao et al., 2010), and other flavones (Renuka Devi and Arumughan, 2007) are known as active components of rice bran.

21.7.2.1 Antimutagenic Activities of Rice Bran Fiber Rice bran fiber is known to have binding capacity to various mutagens and carcinogens (e.g., heterocyclic amines, six nitroarenes, 4-nitroquinoline-N-oxide, benzo[a]pyrene, furylfuramide, and formaldehyde) and mutagens (e.g., glucuronides and sulfates), as well as metabolites in urine. The binding effects were related to lignin content.

Takenaka et al. (1991) reported that RBF stimulated rat fecal excretion of PCB in rats fed with diets containing RBF, lignin, and cholestyramine. Takenaka (1992) reported that bis(tri-n-butyltin)oxide (TBTO; a biocide, 25 ppm) toxicity (measured as thymus atrophy) in rats was reduced by the administration of 10% RBF diet for 2 weeks (relative thymus weight; TBTO control, 0.08 vs. RBF + TBTO, 0.2 g/kg BW, $p < 0.05$).

21.7.2.2 Anticarcinogenic Activities of Rice Bran Fiber Aoe et al. (1993) reported that water-soluble rice bran hemicellulose (RBH) played a preventive role in 1,2-dimethylhydrazine (DMH)-induced large-bowel carcinogenesis in Fischer 344 rats. Rats were fed with a basal control diet or a diet containing 2% or 4% RBH at 5 weeks of age. At 6 weeks of age, all animals were given an intraperitoneal injection of DMH (20 mg/kg BW) at weekly intervals for 20 weeks and autopsied 7 weeks after the last injection. The incidence of DMH-induced colon tumors was significantly lower in rats fed with the 4% RBH diet than in rats fed

Table 21.3 Studies Showing Antimutagenic and/or Anticarcinogenic Activities of Rice Bran

Type of Rice Bran	Test Measure	Tested Mutagens or Carcinogenesis Model[a]	References
Rice bran saccharide	Chemically induced cancer in Wistar rats	N-ethyl-N′-nitro-N-nitrosoguanidine (ENNG)	Takeshita et al. (1992)
α-Glucan isolated from rice bran saccharide	Inhibition of Meth-A fibrosarcoma tumor in BALB/C mice	Subcutaneous inoculations of Meth-A fibrosarcoma cells (6 × 104 cells/mouse)	Takeo et al. (1998)
Rice bran saccharide	Inhibition of fibrosarcoma tumor in BDF1 mice	Subcutaneous inoculations of Meth-A fibrosarcoma cells (6 × 104 cells/mouse)	Takeo et al. (1998)
α-Glucan isolated from rice bran saccharide	Inhibition of lung carcinogenesis in BALB/C mice	Subcutaneous inoculations of Lewis lung carcinoma cells (105 cells/mouse)	Takeo et al. (1998)
Rice bran saccharide	Inhibition of lung carcinogenesis in BDF1 mice	Subcutaneous inoculations of Lewis lung carcinoma cells (105 cells/mouse)	Takeo et al. (1998)
Rice bran ethanolic extract	umu C gene expression in SOS response associated with DNA damage in S. typhimurium (TA 1535/pSK 1002)	3-Amino-1,4-dimethyl-5H-pyrido[4,3-b]indole (Trp-P-1)	Hidashi-Okai et al. (2004)
Rice bran	Cancer inhibition effects in TAG, TRAMP, or Apc(Min) mice	Genetic mouse models of breast, prostate, and intestinal carcinogenesis	Verschoyle et al. (2007)

[a] Heterocyclic amines include PCB, PCDFs, and PCDDs.

with the basal control diet (adenoma, 7 vs. 3; adenocarcinoma, 32 vs. 19; $p < 0.05$). The number of colon tumors per rat was also significantly lower in rats fed with the 4% RBH diet than in rats fed with the basal control diet (0.9 vs. 1.6; $p < 0.05$).

21.7.2.3 Antimutagenic Activities of Rice Bran Hidashi-Okai et al. (2004) reported antimutagenicity of rice bran extract. When the effect of rice bran extract on umu C gene expression in SOS response associated with DNA damage in *Salmonella typhimurium* (TA 1535/pSK 1002) induced by Trp-P-1 was analyzed, a dose-dependent suppressive activity against Trp-P-1-induced umu C gene expression was observed.

21.7.2.4 Anticarcinogenic Activities of Rice Bran Verschoyle et al. (2007) reported cancer inhibition effects of rice bran in genetic mouse models of breast, prostate, and intestinal carcinogenesis. This study tested the hypothesis that rice bran interferes with the development of tumors in tumor-associated glycoprotein (TAG), transgenic adenocarcinoma of the mouse prostate (TRAMP), or Apc(Min) mice, genetic models of mammary, prostate, and intestinal carcinogenesis, respectively. Mice received rice bran (30%) in an AIN-93G diet throughout their postweaning lifespan. In TAG and TRAMP mice, rice bran did not affect carcinoma development. In TRAMP or wild-type C57Bl6/J mice, dietary rice bran increased kidney weight by 18% and 20%, respectively. Consumption of rice bran reduced numbers of intestinal adenomas in Apc(Min) mice by 51% ($p < 0.01$) compared to mice on the control diet. In parallel, dietary rice bran decreased intestinal hemorrhages in these mice, as reflected by increased hematocrit. At 10% of the diet, rice bran did not significantly retard Apc(Min) adenoma development.

Likewise, low-fiber rice bran (30% of the diet) did not affect intestinal carcinogenesis, suggesting that the fibrous constituents of the bran inhibit carcinogenesis. Other studies also reported anticarcinogenic properties of rice bran (Cai et al., 2004; Fan et al., 2000; Ghoneum and Gollapudi, 2005; Katayama et al., 2003; Kong et al., 2009; Luo et al., 2005; Miyoshi et al., 2001; Nam et al., 2005a,b; Norazalina et al., 2010; Rao et al., 2010).

21.7.3 *Effects of Rice Bran Fiber on Lipid Metabolism in Animals*

Several animal studies (hamster, rat, chick) investigated cholesterol-lowering actions of rice bran or RBF (Tables 21.4 and 21.5; Anderson et al., 1994; Aoe et al., 1989; Ayano et al., 1980; Hundemer et al., 1991; Johnson et al., 1989; Kahlon et al.,

Table 21.4 Animal Studies Reporting Health Benefits of RBF

Animal	Dose, g/Day	Duration	Results	References
Rat	Neutral detergent fiber (NDF) or acid detergent fiber (ADF) isolated from defatted rice bran vs. cellulose control, 5% in diet, with 1% cholesterol and 0.25% cholic acid	3 weeks	NDF—reduced serum ($p < 0.05$) and liver cholesterol (NS) conc.; ADF—no changes in serum and liver lipid profiles	Ayano et al. (1980)
Rat	Hemicellulose fraction from defatted RB vs. high methoxylated pectin, 2% in diet	9 days	Increased fecal excretion of acidic steroids; no changes in serum cholesterol; no histological changes	Aoe et al. (1989)
Rat	RBH	2 weeks	Peripheral blood leukocytes and lymphocytes	Takenaka and Itoyama (1993)
Rat	RBF, 5% in diet	18 months	Reduce toxicity against 5% dye in a diet	Suzuki and Aoyama (1982)

Table 21.5 Animal Studies Related to Rice Bran and Lipid Metabolism

Animal	Dose, g/Day	Duration	References
Studies showing hepatic and/or plasma cholesterol-lowering effects of rice bran			
Hamster	Full-fat RB containing 10% TDF	3 weeks	Kahlon et al. (1989)
Hamster	Defatted RB, defatted parboiled RB, full-fat RB, parboiled RB, OB, or wheat bran vs. cellulose; all diets contained 0.5% cholesterol and 10% TDF	3 weeks	Kahlon et al. (1990)
Hamster	11%, 22%, 33%, or 44% full-fat RB, 35% defatted RB vs. cellulose control containing 10% TDF and 0.3% cholesterol; two additional controls (44% full-fat RB and 10% cellulose) without 0.3% cholesterol	3 weeks	Kahlon et al. (1992a)
Hamster, male	Defatted RB, full-fat RB, or defatted RB + RB oil vs. 10% cellulose; all diets contained 0.3% cholesterol and 10% TDF	3 weeks	Kahlon et al. (1992b)
Hamster	Raw or stabilized RB vs. cellulose, containing 10% TDF and 0.3% cholesterol	3 weeks	Kahlon et al. (1996)
Hamster	RB or wheat bran containing 10% TDF and 0.3% cholesterol	3 weeks	Kahlon et al. (1998)
Hamster	RB diet vs. white or brown rice control containing 10% TDF and 0.5% cholesterol	3 weeks	Kahlon and Chow (2000)
SD rat	6% TDF from RB or cellulose diet containing 1% cholesterol and 0.2% cholic acid	3 weeks	Anderson et al. (1994)
Rat	Heat-stabilized RB vs. unprocessed wheat bran containing 7% TDF and no cholesterol; with or without fish oil	10 days	Topping et al. (1990)
Rat	Raw or parboiled RB vs. wheat bran control; all diets had 10% TDF, 1% cholesterol, and 0.2% cholic acid	3 weeks	Rouanet et al. (1993)
Mice	Five sources of dietary fiber from full-fat RB, soy fiber, OB, barley bran, or mixed bran containing 7% TDF vs. fiber-free diet control; all diets contained 0.06% cholesterol	3 weeks	Hundemer et al. (1991)
Chick	60% defatted (24% TDF) or full-fat RB (20%–21% TDF) vs. corn/soy control (10.5%–18.7% TDF) with 0.5% cholesterol	10 days	Newman et al. (1992)

(continued)

Table 21.5 (continued) Animal Studies Related to Rice Bran and Lipid Metabolism

Animal	Dose, g/Day	Duration	References
Studies showing no significant effects of rice bran on hepatic or plasma cholesterol concentrations			
Hamster	RB or OB vs. cellulose control containing 10% TDF and 0.5% cholesterol. Some diets had an additional 0.1% vitamin E	6 weeks	Kahlon et al. (1999)
Hamster	Stabilized RB, OB, or RB + OB vs. cellulose; all diets contained 0.25% cholesterol and 10% TDF	3 weeks	Kahlon et al. (1993)
Rat	10% stabilized rice bran vs. 10% cellulose or fiber-free control diet	4 weeks	Johnson et al. (1989)

OB, oat bran; RB, rice bran; TDF, total dietary fiber; VFAs, volatile fatty acids.

1989, 1990, 1992a,b, 1993, 1996, 1998, 1999, Kahlon and Chow, 2000; Newman et al., 1992; Rouanet et al., 1993; Suzuki and Aoyama, 1982; Takenaka and Itoyama, 1993; Topping et al., 1990). Except three studies (Johnson et al., 1989; Kahlon et al., 1989, 1999), most of studies demonstrated cholesterol-lowering efficacy of rice bran in various animal models. In these studies, the concentration was up to 60% rice bran or 5% RBF of the diet, and the length of studies was up to 18 months. No studies reported adverse effects of rice bran or RBF. A study investigating the effects of defatted RBF (nonstarch polysaccharides extracted from defatted rice bran, 15% in diet for 7 days) on the nutrient digestibility also reported no adverse effects of RBF (Adrizal and Ohtani, 2002).

21.8 Health Benefits of Rice Bran Fiber in Humans

Numerous human and animal studies examined the health benefits of rice bran (Aoe et al., 1993; Cheng et al., 2009), RBF (Maeda et al., 2004; Miyoshi et al., 1986; Tomlin and Read, 1988), and cereal fiber (Mozaffarian et al., 2003). Cereal fiber intake has been associated with risk reduction of diabetes (Schulze et al., 2007), heart diseases (Pereira et al., 2004), and obesity (Koh-Banerjee et al., 2004). In Western populations, there are no reports of safety concerns related to inherent cereal fibers including RBF.

21.8.1 Human Studies Showing Health Benefits of Rice Bran Fiber

Rice bran fiber has been tested for their hypocholesterolemic, hypoglycemic, gastrointestinal, and immunomodulatory effects in normal human subjects (Table 21.6; Maeda et al., 2004; Miyoshi et al., 1986; Ranhotra et al., 1989; Rodrigues Silva et al., 2005; Sanders and Reddy, 1992; Tomlin and Read, 1988). The maximum dosage of RBF (or total fiber from rice bran) tested was up to 28 g/day, and the duration of the study was up to 6 weeks (Maeda et al., 2004). Rice bran fiber also has fecal bulking effects to promote intestinal regularity (Miyoshi et al., 1986; Tomlin and Read, 1988).

Table 21.6 Human Studies Reporting Health Benefits of RBF

Subjects	Dose, g/Day	Duration	Measurement Endpoints	References
50 elderly, age 70–95 years	0.5 g/day arabinoxylan, RBF, from rice bran hydrolysate	6 weeks	Improved common cold symptoms	Maeda et al. (2004)
5 healthy young men	27.9 vs. 13.7 g/day of RBF (NDF) from brown rice	2 weeks	Increased fecal weight	Miyoshi et al. (1986)
8 normal healthy males	17.1 g RBF (as indigestible residue) from rice	10 days	Increased fecal volume and frequency	Tomlin and Read (1988)
11 subjects with NIDDM	RB diet containing 40 g TDF	1 week	Increased fecal weight	Rodrigues Silva et al. (2005)

21.8.2 Human Studies Showing Health Benefits of Rice Bran

Rice bran has been tested for their hypocholesterolemic and hypoglycemic effects in normal, hypercholesterolemic, or diabetic human subjects (Table 21.7; Cara et al., 1992; Cheng et al., 2010; Gerhardt and Gallo, 1998; Hegsted et al., 1993; Kestin et al., 1990; Ranhotra et al., 1989; Rodrigues Silva et al., 2005; Sanders and Reddy, 1992). Except three studies (Cara et al., 1992; Kestin et al., 1990; Sanders and Reddy, 1992), most of human studies demonstrated cholesterol-lowering efficacy of rice bran. The maximum dosage of rice bran and RBF (or total fiber from rice bran) tested was 100 g/day (Hegsted et al., 1993), and the length of the study was up to 12 weeks (Cheng et al., 2010). Rice bran is known to enhance viscosity of the gastrointestinal contents (Dikeman et al., 2006), which attenuates blood glucose and lipid responses.

Rice bran contains many antioxidants such as phenolic acids (e.g., ferulic acid), vitamin E (alpha-tocopherol, alpha-tocotrienol, gamma-tocopherol, and gamma-tocotrienol), and gamma-oryzanol components (Xu et al., 2001). In addition to fiber, these antioxidants also may contribute to hypoglycemic and hypocholesterolemic effects of rice bran (Jung et al., 2007; Qureshi et al., 2002; Xu et al., 2001). No human clinical studies reported adverse effects of rice bran or its fiber fraction.

21.9 Allergenicity

Unlike wheat and wheat products (containing gliadin), rice bran and RBF were found to be antiallergenic (Choi et al., 2007).

21.10 Summary

Rice bran fiber is an isolate of rice bran and a GRAS ingredient. Numerous human and animal studies examined the health benefits of rice bran, RBF, cereal brans, and cereal fibers. There are no reports of safety concerns in any

Table 21.7 Human Studies Related to Rice Bran and Lipid/Glucose Metabolism

Subjects	Dose, g/day	Duration	Reference
Studies showing cholesterol-lowering effects of rice bran			
11 subjects with moderately elevated blood cholesterol	100 g RB or oat bran vs. wheat flour	3 weeks	Hegsted et al. (1993)
44 moderately hypercholesterolemic adults	84 g heat-stabilized, full-fat RB or oat bran vs. rice starch	6 weeks	Gerhardt and Gallo (1998)
17 moderately hypercholesterolemic and hypertriglyceridemic individuals	Supplementation of 30 g RB and 30 g oat bran vs. usual diet	6 weeks	Ranhotra et al. (1989)
20 healthy young men and women	Supplementation of 30 g defatted RB or 33.3 g full-fat RB vs. low-fiber period	18 days	Tsai and Ting (1992)
28 subjects with NIDDM	20 g stabilized RB	12 weeks	Cheng et al. (2010)
6 normolipidemic males	RB diet containing 2.8 g TDF	Single dose	Cara et al. (1992)
Study showing improved fasting and postprandial glycemic responses			
11 subjects with NIDDM	RB diet containing 40 g TDF	1 week	Rodrigues Silva et al. (2005)
Study reporting no changes in blood lipid and glucose conc. and in glycemic responses			
24 mildly hypercholesterolemic men	60 g/day RB containing 11.8 g TDF vs. baseline	4 weeks	Kestin et al. (1990)
Study reporting no changes in blood lipid conc.			
18 normocholesterolemic subjects	15 or 30 g RB vs. 15 g WB	3 weeks	Sanders and Reddy (1992)
Studies reporting no changes in fasting or postprandial glycemic responses			
6 normolipidemic males	RB diet containing 2.8 g TDF	Single dose	Cara et al. (1992)

of the studies. CJ utilizes an HACCP-controlled manufacturing process and rigorously tests its final production batches to verify adherence to quality control specifications. The literature indicates that rice bran and RBF offer consumers various health benefits such as promoting intestinal regularity and cholesterol-lowering ability, as well as antioxidant, antimutagenic, and anticarcinogenic activities.

References

Abdul-Hamid A and Luan YS. Functional properties of dietary fibre prepared from defatted rice bran. *Food Chem.* 2000;68:15–19.

Adrizal O and Ohtani S. Defatted rice bran nonstarch polysaccharides in broiler diets: Effects of supplements on nutrient digestibilities. *J Poul Sci.* 2002;39:67–76.

Anderson JW, Riddell-Mason S, and Jones AE. Ten different dietary fibers have significantly different effects on serum and liver lipids of cholesterol-fed rats. *J Nutr.* 1994;124:78–83.

Aoe S, Oda T, Tojima T, Tanaka M, Tatsumi K, and Mizutani T. Effects of rice bran hemicellulose on 1,2-dimethylhydrazine-induced intestinal carcinogenesis in Fischer 344 rats. *Nutr Cancer.* 1993;20:41–49.

Aoe S, Ohta F, and Ayano Y. Effect of rice bran hemicellulose on the cholesterol metabolism in rats. *Nippon Eiyoshokuryo Gakkaishi.* 1989;42:55–61.

Ayano Y, Ohta F, Watanabe Y, and Mita K. Dietary fiber fractions in defatted rice bran and their hypocholesterolemic effect in cholesterol-fed rats. *J Nutr Food (Japan).* 1980; 33:283–291.

Cai H, Hudson EA, Mann P, Verschoyle RD, Greaves P, Manson MM, Steward WP, and Gescher AJ. Growth-inhibitory and cell cycle-arresting properties of the rice bran constituent tricin in human-derived breast cancer cells in vitro and in nude mice in vivo. *Br J Cancer.* 2004;91:1364–1371.

Cara L, Dubois C, Borel P, Armand M, Senft M, Portugal H, Pauli AM, Bernard PM, and Lairon D. Effects of oat bran, rice bran, wheat fiber, and wheat germ on postprandial lipemia in healthy adults. *Am J Clin Nutr.* 1992;55:81–88.

Cheng HH, Huang HY, Chen YY, Huang CL, Chang CJ, Chen HL, and Lai MH. Ameliorative effects of stabilized rice bran on type 2 diabetes patients. *Ann Nutr Metab.* 2010;56:45–51. Erratum in: *Ann Nutr Metab.* 2010;56:58.

Choi SP, Kang MY, Koh HJ, Nam SH, and Friedman M. Antiallergic activities of pigmented rice bran extracts in cell assays. *J Food Sci.* 2007;72:S719–S726.

Cosmetic Ingredient Review Expert Panel (CIREP). Amended final report on the safety assessment of oryza sativa (rice) bran oil, oryza sativa (rice) germ oil, rice bran acid, oryza sativa (rice) bran wax, hydrogenated rice bran wax, oryza sativa (rice) bran extract, oryza sativa (rice) extract, oryza sativa (rice) germ powder, oryza sativa (rice) starch, oryza sativa (rice) bran, hydrolyzed rice bran extract, hydrolyzed rice bran protein, hydrolyzed rice extract, and hydrolyzed rice protein. *Int J Toxicol.* 2006;25(Suppl 2):91–120.

Dikeman CL, Murphy MR, and Fahey GC Jr. Dietary fibers affect viscosity of solutions and simulated human gastric and small intestinal digesta. *J Nutr.* 2006;136:913–919.

Fan H, Morioka T, and Ito E. Induction of apoptosis and growth inhibition of cultured human endometrial adenocarcinoma cells (Sawano) by an antitumor lipoprotein fraction of rice bran. *Gynecol Oncol.* 2000;76:170–175.

FDA. § 101.76. Health claims: Fiber-containing grain products, fruits and vegetables and cancer. 58 FR 2639, January 6, 1993a.

FDA. § 101.77. Health claims: Fruits, vegetables, and grain products that contain fiber, particularly soluble fiber, and risk of coronary heart disease. 58 FR 2578, January 6, 1993b.

FDA. § 101.81. Health claims: Soluble fiber from certain food and risk of coronary heart disease. August 15, 2008.

Gerhardt AL and Gallo NB. Full-fat rice bran and oat bran similarly reduce hypercholesterolemia in humans. *J Nutr.* 1998;128:865–869.

Ghoneum M and Gollapudi S. Synergistic role of arabinoxylan rice bran (MGN-3/Biobran) in *S. cerevisiae*-induced apoptosis of monolayer breast cancer MCF-7 cells. *Anticancer Res.* 2005;25:4187–4196.

Harris PJ, Sasidharan VK, Roberton AM, Triggs CM, Blakeney AB, and Ferguson LR. Adsorption of a hydrophobic mutagen to cereal brans and cereal bran dietary fibres. *Mutation Res/Genetic Toxicol Environ Mutagenesis.* 1998;412:323–331.

Hegsted M, Windhauser MM, Morris SK, and Lester SB. Stabilized rice bran and oat bran lower cholesterol in humans. *Nutr Res.* 1993;13:387–398.

Hidashi-Okai K, Kanbara K, Amano K, Hagiwara A, Sugita C, Matsumoto N, and Okai Y. Potent antioxidative and antigenotoxic activity in aqueous extract of Japanese rice bran—Association with peroxidase activity. *Phytother Res.* 2004;18:628–633.

Hsu JC, Lu TW, Chiou PWS, and Bi Yu C. Effects of different sources of dietary fibre on growth performance and apparent digestibility in geese. *Anim Feed Sci Technol.* 1996;60:93–102.

Hundemer JK, Nabar SP, Shriver BJ, and Forman LP. Dietary fiber sources lower blood cholesterol in C57BL/6 mice. *J Nutr.* 1991;121:1360–1365.

Institute of Medicine. *Dietary Reference Intakes for Energy, Carbohydrates, Fiber, Fat, Fatty Acids, Cholesterol, Protein, and Amino Acids.* National Academy Press, Washington, DC. 2002.

Institute of Medicine. *Dietary Reference Intakes.* National Academy Press, Washington, DC. 2006.

Johnson IT, Gee JM, and Brown JC. A comparison of rice bran, wheat bran and cellulose as sources of dietary fibre in the rat. *Food Sci Nutr.* 1989; 42F:153–163.

Jung EH, Ha TY, Hwang IK, and Kim SR. Hypoglycemic effects of a phenolic acid fraction of rice bran and ferulic acid in C57BL/KsJ-db/db mice. *J Agric Food Chem.* 2007; 55:9800–9804.

Kahlon T. Rice bran: Production, composition, functionality, food applications, and physiological benefits. In: *Fiber Ingredients*, Cho SS and Samuel P (eds.). CRC Press, Boca Raton, FL. 2009, pp. 305–321.

Kahlon TS and Chow FI. Lipidemic response of hamsters to rice bran, uncooked or processed white and brown rice, and processed corn starch. *Cereal Chem.* 2000;77:673–678.

Kahlon TS, Chow FI, Chiu MM, Hudson CA, and Sayre RN. Cholesterol-lowering by rice bran and rice bran oil unsaponifiable matter in hamsters. *Cereal Chem.* 1996;73:69–74.

Kahlon TS, Chow FI, Knuckles BE, and Chiu MM. Cholesterol-lowering effects in hamsters of β-glucan-enriched barley fraction, dehulled whole barley, rice bran, and oat bran and their combinations. *Cereal Chem.* 1993;70:435–440.

Kahlon TS, Chow FI, Sayre RN, and Betschart AA. Cholesterol-lowering in hamsters fed rice bran at various levels, defatted rice bran and rice bran oil. *J Nutr.* 1992a;122:513–519.

Kahlon TS, Edwards RH, and Chow FI. Effect of extrusion on hypocholesterolemic properties of rice, oat, corn, and wheat bran diets in hamsters. *Cereal Chem.* 1998;75:897–903.

Kahlon TS, Saunders RM, Chow FI, Chiu MM, and Betschart AA. Effect of rice bran and oat bran on plasma cholesterol in hamsters. *Cereal Food World.* 1989;34: 768–771.

Kahlon TS, Saunders RM, Chow FI, Chiu MM, and Betschart AA. Influence of rice bran, oat bran, and wheat bran on cholesterol and triglycerides in hamsters. *Cereal Chem.* 1990; 67:439–443.

Kahlon TS, Saunders RM, Sayre RN, Chow FI, Chiu MM, and Betschart AA. Cholesterol-lowering effects of rice bran and rice bran oil fractions in hypercholesterolemic hamsters. *Cereal Chem.* 1992b;69:485–489.

Kahlon TS, Wood DF, and Chow FI. Cholesterol response and foam cell formation in hamsters fed rice bran, oat bran, and cellulose + soy protein diets with or without added vitamin E. *Cereal Chem*. 1999;76:772–776.

Katayama M, Sugie S, Yoshimi N, Yamada Y, Sakata K, Qiao Z, Iwasaki T, Kobayashi H, and Mori H. Preventive effect of fermented brown rice and rice bran on diethylnitrosoamine and phenobarbital-induced hepatocarcinogenesis in male F344 rats. *Oncol Rep*. 2003;10:875–880.

Kestin M, Moss R, Clifton PM, and Nestel PJ. Comparative effects of three cereal brans on plasma lipids, blood pressure, and glucose metabolism in mildly hypercholesterolemic men. *Am J Clin Nutr*. 1990;52:661–666.

Kim SM, Rico CW, Lee SC, and Kang MY. Modulatory effect of rice bran and phytic acid on glucose metabolism in high fat-fed C57BL/6N mice. *J Clin Biochem Nutr*. 2010;47:12–17.

Koh-Banerjee P, Franz M, Sampson L, Liu S, Jacobs DR Jr., Spiegelman D, Willett W, and Rimm E. Changes in whole-grain, bran, and cereal fiber consumption in relation to 8-year weight gain among men. *Am J Clin Nutr*. 2004;80:1237–1245.

Kong CK, Lam WS, Chiu LC, Ooi VE, Sun SS, and Wong YS. A rice bran polyphenol, cycloartenyl ferulate, elicits apoptosis in human colorectal adenocarcinoma SW480 and sensitizes metastatic SW620 cells to TRAIL-induced apoptosis. *Biochem Pharmacol*. 2009;77:1487–1496.

Kumar B and Chaudhuri DK. Isolation and partial characterisation of antithiamine factor present in rice-bran and its effect on TPP-transketolase system and *Staphylococcus aureus*. *Int J Vitam Nutr Res*. 1976;46:154–159.

Lu BS, Barber S, and Benedito DBC. Rice bran: Chemistry and technology. In: *Rice Production and Utilization*, Luh BS (ed.). Van Nostrand Reinhold. New York. 1991, Vol. 2, pp. 313–315.

Luo HF, Li Q, Yu S, Badger TM, and Fang N. Cytotoxic hydroxylated triterpene alcohol ferulates from rice bran. *J Nat Prod*. 2005;68:94–97.

Maeda H, Ichihashi K, Fujii T, Omura K, Zhu X, Anazawa M, and Tazawa K. Oral administration of hydrolyzed rice bran prevents the common cold syndrome in the elderly based on its immunomodulatory action. *Biofactors*. 2004;21:185–187.

Miyoshi N, Koyama Y, Katsuno Y, Hayakawa S, Mita T, Ohta T, Kaji K, and Isemura M. Apoptosis induction associated with cell cycle dysregulation by rice bran agglutinin. *J Biochem*. 2001;130:799–805.

Miyoshi H, Okuda T, Oi Y, and Koishi H. Effects of rice fiber on fecal weight, apparent digestibility of energy, nitrogen and fat, and degradation of neutral detergent fiber in young men. *J Nutr Sci Vitaminol*. 1986;32:581–589.

Mozaffarian D, Kumanyika SK, Lemaitre RN, Olson JL, Burke GL, and Siscovick DS. Cereal, fruit, and vegetable fiber intake and the risk of cardiovascular disease in elderly individuals. *JAMA*. 2003;289:1659–1666.

Mujajhid A, Ul Haq I, Asif M, and Gilani AH. Effect of different levels of rice bran processed by various techniques on performance of broiler chicks. *Br Poul Sci*. 2004;45:395–399.

Nam SH, Choi SP, Kang MY, Koh HJ, Kozukue N, and Friedman M. Bran extracts from pigmented rice seeds inhibit tumor promotion in lymphoblastoid B cells by phorbol ester. *Food Chem Toxicol*. 2005a;43:741–745.

Nam SH, Choi SP, Kang MY, Kozukue N, and Friedman M. Antioxidative, antimutagenic, and anticarcinogenic activities of rice bran extracts in chemical and cell assays. *J Agric Food Chem*. 2005b;53:816–822.

Newman RK, Betschart AA, Newman CW, and Hofer PJ. Effect of full-fat or defatted rice bran on serum cholesterol. *Plant Foods Hum Nutr*. 1992;42:37–43.

Norazalina S, Norhaizan ME, Hairuszah I, and Norashareena MS. Anticarcinogenic efficacy of phytic acid extracted from rice bran on azoxymethane-induced colon carcinogenesis in rats. *Exp Toxicol Pathol*. 2010;62:259–268.

Ogawa S. Chemical components of rice bran: Myo-inositol and related compounds: A review. *Anticancer Res.* 1999;19:3635–3644.

Pereira MA, O'Reilly E, Augustsson K, Fraser GE, Goldbourt U, Heitmann BL, Hallmans G, Knekt P, Liu S, Pietinen P, Spiegelman D, Stevens J, Virtamo J, Willett WC, and Ascherio A. Dietary fiber and risk of coronary heart disease: A pooled analysis of cohort studies. *Arch Intern Med.* 2004;164:370–376.

Qureshi AA, Sami SA, Salser WA, and Khan FA. Dose-dependent suppression of serum cholesterol by tocotrienol-rich fraction (TRF25) of rice bran in hypercholesterolemic humans. *Atherosclerosis.* 2002;161:199–207.

Ranhotra GS, Gelroth JA, Reeves RD, Rudd MK, Durkee WR, and Gardner JD. Short-term lipidemic responses in otherwise healthy hypercholesterolemic men consuming foods high in soluble fiber. *Cereal Chem.* 1989;66:94–97.

Rao AS, Reddy SG, Babu PP, and Reddy AR. The antioxidant and antiproliferative activities of methanolic extracts from Njavara rice bran. *BMC Complement Altern Med.* 2010;10:4–12.

Renuka Devi R and Arumughan C. Antiradical efficacy of phytochemical extracts from defatted rice bran. *Food Chem. Toxicol.* 2007;45:2014–2021.

Rodrigues Silva C, Dutra de Oliveira JE, de Souza RA, and Silva HC. Effect of a rice bran fiber diet on serum glucose levels of diabetic patients in Brazil. *Arch Latinoam Nutr.* 2005;55:23–27.

Rouanet J-M, Laurent C, and Besancon P. Rice bran and wheat bran: Selective effect on plasma and liver cholesterol in high-cholesterol fed rats. *Food Chem.* 1993;47:67–71.

Sanders TA and Reddy S. The influence of rice bran on plasma lipids and lipoproteins in human volunteers. *Eur J Clin Nutr.* 1992;46:167–172.

Sayre RN, Earl L, Kratzer FH, and Saunders RM. Nutritional qualities of stabilized and raw rice bran for chicks. *Poultry Sci.* 1987;66:493–499.

Sayre RN, Earl L, Kratzer FH, and Saunders RM. Effects of diets containing raw and extrusion-cooked rice bran on growth and efficiency of food utilization of broilers. *Br Poultry Sci.* 1988;29:815–823.

Schulze MB, Schulz M, Heidemann C, Schienkiewitz A, Hoffmann K, and Boeing H. Fiber and magnesium intake and incidence of type 2 diabetes: A prospective study and meta-analysis. *Arch Intern Med.* 2007;167:956–965.

Sera N, Morita K, Nagasoe M, Tokieda H, Kitaura T, and Tokiwa H. Binding effect of polychlorinated compounds and environmental carcinogens on rice bran fiber. *J Nutr Biochem.* 2005;16:50–58.

Sun W, Xu W, Liu H, Liu J, Wang Q, Zhou J, Dong F, and Chen B. Gamma-Tocotrienol induces mitochondria-mediated apoptosis in human gastric adenocarcinoma SGC-7901 cells. *J Nutr Biochem.* 2009;20:276–284.

Suzuki M and Aoyama H. Preventive effects of fiber against the toxicity of edible tar dyes in rats. *Nippon Eiseigaku Zasshi (Jpn J Hyg).* 1982;37:714–721.

Takenaka S. Hemicellulose in rice bran fibre reduces thymus atrophy in rats treated with bis(tri-n-butyltin)oxide. *Chemosphere.* 1992;25:327–334.

Takenaka S and Itoyama Y. Rice bran hemicellulose increases the peripheral blood lymphocytes in rats. *Life Sci.* 1993;52:9–12.

Takenaka S, Morita K, Tokiwa H, and Takahashi K. Effects of rice bran fiber and cholestyramine on the faecal excretion of Kanechlor 600 (PCB) in rats. *Xenobiotica.* 1991;21:351–357.

Takeo S, Kado H, Yamamoto H, Kamimura M, Watanabe N, Uchida K, and Mori Y. Studies on an antitumor polysaccharide RBS derived from rice bran. II. Preparation and general properties of RON, an active fraction of RBS. *Chem Pharmacol Bull.* 1998;36:3609–3613.

Takeshita M, Nakamura S, Makita F, Ohwada S, Miyamoto Y, and Morishita Y. Antitumor effect of RBS (rice bran saccharide) on ENNG-induced carcinogenesis. *Biotherapy.* 1992;4:139–145.

Tashihiro M and Ikegami S. Changes in activity, antigenicity and molecular size of rice bran trypsin inhibitor by in-vitro digestion. *Nutr Sci Vitamin.* 1996;42:367–376.

Tashiro M and Maki Z. Stability and specificity of rice bran trypsin inhibitor. *J Nutr Sci Vitaminol.* 1986;32:591–599.

Tomlin J and Read NW. Comparison of the effects on colonic function caused by feeding rice bran and wheat bran. *Eur J Clin Nutr.* 1988;42:857–861.

Topping DL, Illman RJ, Roach PD, Trimble RP, Kambouris A, and Nestel PJ. Modulation of the hypolipidemic effect of fish oils by dietary fiber in rats: Studies with rice and wheat bran. *J Nutr.* 1990;120:325–330.

US Department of Agriculture and U.S. Department of Health and Human Services. *Nutrition and Your Health: Dietary Guidelines for Americans,* 6th edn. Government Printing Office, Washington, DC. 2005.

US Department of Agriculture and U.S. Department of Health and Human Services. *Nutrition and Your Health: Dietary Guidelines for Americans,* 7th edn. Government Printing Office, Washington, DC. 2010.

Verschoyle RD, Greaves P, Cai H, Edwards RE, Steward WP, and Gescher AJ. Evaluation of the cancer chemopreventive efficacy of rice bran in genetic mouse models of breast, prostate and intestinal carcinogenesis. *Br J Cancer.* 2007;96:248–254.

Xu Z, Godber JS, and Hua N. Antioxidant activity of tocopherols, tocotrienols, and gamma-oryzanol components from rice bran against cholesterol oxidation accelerated by 2,2′-azobis(2-methylpropionamidine) dihydrochloride. *J Agric Food Chem.* 2001;49:2077–2081.

Zha X-Q, Luo J-P, Zhang L, and Hao J. Antioxidant properties of different polysaccharides extracted with water and sodium hydroxide from rice bran. *Food Sci Biotechnol.* 2009;18:449–455.

22
Hypoglycemic Effects of Oat β-Glucan

BASSAM FARESS, SUSAN S. CHO, ALBERT W. LEE, and NELSON ALMEIDA

Contents

22.1 Glycemic Index of Various Grains

Table 22.1 compares the glycemic index (GI) of common cereal grains. The GI classification system was developed to assess the impact of various foods on postprandial plasma glucose (Jenkins et al., 1978; Truswell, 1992; Wolever, 1990; Wolever et al., 1994, 2003). The GI is the ratio of incremental blood glucose under the curve of a test food to incremental blood glucose under the curve of white wheat bread × 100. Typically, foods with a low degree of starch gelatinization or more compact granules (e.g., spaghetti) and whole grains with high levels of viscous soluble fiber (e.g., barley, oats, and rye) have slower rates of digestion and lower GI values (Liu, 2002). Quick oatmeal, for example, is equivalent to rolled barley. GI is a function of structure, starch type, fiber content, and the interaction of these characteristics (Granfeldt et al., 1994).

Table 22.1 GI of Selected Grains and Grain Products

Whole Grain	GI	Processed Grain	GI
Barley	25	Rolled barley	66
Corn, sweet kernel	55	Corn flakes	84
Oatmeal, old fashioned	49	Oatmeal, quick	66
Rice, brown	55	Krispy, rice	88
Rice, sweet, low amylose	88	Rice, high amylose	59
Rye, whole kernel	34	Rye flour bread	65
Wheat, whole kernel	41	Puffed wheat	74
Bulgur, wheat	48	Wheat flakes	75

Source: From Behall and Hallfrisch (2002).

22.2 Glycemic Index of Various Oat Products

Ten studies determined GI values of various forms of oats (Table 22.2; Alminger and Eklund-Jonsson, 2008; Atkinson et al., 2008; Foster-Powell and Miller, 1995; Foster-Powell et al., 2002; Jenkins et al., 1981, 1983, 2002; Krezowski et al., 1987; Miller et al., 1992; Otto et al., 1980; Tappy et al., 1996; Wolever et al., 1985, 1994).

Table 22.2 GI Values of Various Oats and Oat Brans

Foods Tested	β-Glucan, g	GI	GI Reduction/g β-Glucan	References
High beta-glucan oats				
β-glucan cereal	7.3	52	3.7	Jenkins (2002)
β-glucan bar	6.2	43	5.0	Jenkins (2002)
β-glucan tempe	2.2	63	16.8	Alminger (2008)
Oat bran				
Oat bran	6	72	4.7	Wolever et al. (1994)
Oat bran	6	84	2.7	Jenkins et al. (1985)
Oat bran cereal	4	69	4.0	Tappy et al. (1996)
Oat bran cereal	6	41	7.3	Tappy et al. (1996)
Oat bran cereal	8.4	36.8	5.7	Tappy et al. (1996)
Oat bran breakfast cereal	3.7	86	3.2	Jenkins (2002)
Rolled oats or oat porridge				
Oats, 1 min	4	94	1.5	Wolever et al. (1994)
Oats, quick	4	93	1.8	Wolever et al. (1985)
Oats, porridge	4	70	7.5	Jenkins et al. (1981)
Oats, porridge	4	83	4.3	Brand et al. (1992)
Oats, porridge	4	88	3	Otto et al. (1988)
Oats, porridge	4	98	0.5	Jenkins et al. (1983)
Oats, porridge	4	107	1.8	Krezowski et al. (1987)

Source: Modified from Jenkins, A.L. et al., *Eur. J. Clin. Nutr.*, 56(7), 622, 2002.

A number of these reports evaluated the effect of β-glucan on blood glucose and insulin levels by testing traditional processed products (e.g., bran, porridge, flakes, flour) derived from oat or containing extracted β-glucan fractions. Within the oat category, GI values of oat bran or β-glucan concentrates were much lower than those of thin rolled oats and porridge, which produced postprandial glucose responses similar to the white wheat bread reference (Granfeldt et al., 1995; Liljeberg et al., 1996). These data suggest that the physical form of oats is an important factor in effective glycemic control.

22.3 Oat β-Glucan and Glycemic Responses

Single-dose and longer-term studies show that 3.2 g/day or higher of oat bran and β-glucan isolated from oats consistently reduced postprandial blood glucose and/or insulin concentrations in single-dose or short-term studies (Tables 22.3 through 22.5; Alminger and Eklund-Jonsson, 2008; Battilana et al., 2001; Beck et al., 2009; Behall et al., 2005, 2006; Braaten et al., 1991, 1994; Granfeldt et al., 1994, 1996, 2000, 2008; Hlebowicz et al., 2008; Regand et al., 2009; Tapola et al., 2005; Tappy et al., 1996; Wood et al., 1994, 2000). In long-term studies, consumption of 1–4 g of oat β-glucan produced mixed results. Administration of 3 g/day of β-glucan for 3 weeks improved insulin resistance in subjects with type 2 diabetes (Liatis et al., 2009). In longer-term studies, 6–8 g/day of oat β-glucan for 8–23 weeks lowered fasting blood glucose and insulin levels in healthy volunteers (Table 22.6. Reyna-Villasmil et al., 2007; Rytter et al., 1996).

22.3.1 Acute Tolerance Tests

Single-dose or acute tolerance studies showed that administration of β-glucan from oat bran (tempe) at a dose as low as 2.2 g lowered glycemic and insulinemic responses (Alminger et al., 2008). Healthy subjects as well as those with type 2 diabetes demonstrated improved glycemic or insulinemic responses after consumption of a variety of doses in diverse foods: 2.2 g of oat β-glucan in a form of tempe (Alminger and Eklund-Jonsson, 2008); 4–8.4 g in cereals, including granola and muesli (Beck et al., 2009; Hlebowicz et al., 2008, Tappy et al., 1996); 3.7 g in muffins (Behall et al., 2006); 3.23 g in meals (Behall et al., 2005); or 11.3 g in puddings (Braaten et al., 1991).

However, 4 g of β-glucan administered as oat porridge or crisp did not lower postprandial glucose responses compared to glucose or white wheat reference bread (Liljeberg, 1996; Regand et al., 2009; Tapola et al., 2005). Although studies using low amounts of oat β-glucan, such as 0.5 g oat β-glucan in cereals (Hlebowicz et al., 2007), 2.16 g in cereals (Beck et al., 2009), or 2.7 g in cereals (Ulmius et al., 2009), did not lower glycemic responses, those using 4 g or higher reported lowered glycemic responses. Thus, various single-dose studies suggest that both dosages and food forms have an important influence on glycemic responses. Data indicate that oat β-glucan is effective at 3.23 g or higher and that acceptable food forms include cereals, tempe, muffins, and meal.

Table 22.3 Effects of Oat Beta Glucan on Glycemic Responses in Single Dose Human Clinical Studies

Source	Dose, g/d	Food Form	Duration*	Subject	Results	Reference
High BG oat, 6.6%	2.2 g BG	Tempe	2 h, x	13 healthy men and women	GI: 63; II, 21 (glucose standard, 100; AUC, $p < 0.002$).	Alminger et al., 2008
Oat BG conc. w/ mid or high BG (5.0–21% BG; Oatwell); 52% BG oat bran conc.	2.16–5.65 g/test meal	Corn based cereal	4 h, x	14 healthy overwt. men and women	BG decreased insulin secretion over 2 h (RMANOVA, $p = 0.011$) in a dose responsive manner (Insulin AUC at 2 h: control, 3559; 2.16 g, 3643, NS; 3.8 g BG, 3072, $p < 0.05$; 5.4 g BG, 2952, $p < 0.02$; 5.6 g BG, 2959, $p < 0.05$). Glucose AUC-NS; Insulin AUC at 4 h, NS	Beck et al., 2009
Oat BG conc. (17–33% BG; Oatrim);	0.3, 0.9, and 3.7 g BG (with 3 levels of RS)	Muffin (1 g CHO/kg BW)	4 h, x	10 normal wt and 10 overwt women	3.7 g BG (with low RS) decreased insulin response at 2 h (3.7 g BG, 148, $p < 0.05$; 0.9 g BG, 191, NS; 0.3 g BG, 225; NS; glucose control, 163 pmol/l). BG alone did not decrease glucose response. Synergistic effects between RS and BG were noted.	Behall et al., 2006
Oat flour or oat flakes	3.23 g BG	Meal (1 g CHO/kg BW)	3 h, x	10 overwt and obese women	Oat flour and oat flakes lowered glucose AUC at 2 h (glucose 171; oat flour, 109, $p < 0.05$; oat flakes 122 mmol.min/l, $p < 0.05$). No differences in insulin AUC.	Behall et al., 2005

Oat type	Dose	Food/meal	Duration	Subjects	Results	Reference
Oat gum (78% BG)	11.3 g BG	50 g Glu drink (control), 50 g glu pudding	3 h, x	10 healthy men and women	Compared to glucose control, oat gum lowered postprandial plasma glucose and insulin conc.	Braaten et al., 1991
Rolled oat, thick and thin	N/A	Meals providing 50 g starch, 6.8 g fat, and 12 g protein.	3 h, x	10 healthy men and women	Thick rolled oat (1 mm): GI, 70–78; II, 58–77; thin (0.5 mm) rolled oat, no significant changes in GI and II.	Granfeldt et al., 2000
Oat bran (Oatwell)	4	Muesli (4 g BG) vs. corn flakes meal	90 min, x	12 healthy men and women, aged 22–35 y	Oat BG lowered the postprandial glucose response at 30 min compared to the cornflakes meal (p = 0.045). No differences between the test and control groups were noted at 60 min.	Hlebowicz et al., 2008
Wholemeal oat	0.5	50 g Cereals	120 min, x	12 healthy men and women, aged 23–36 y	No changes in postprandial blood glucose responses.	Hlebowicz et al., 2007
Oat	4.0	porridge	3 h, x	12 healthy men and women, aged 24–46 y	No changes in postprandial blood glucose responses.	Liljeberg et al., 1996
Oat bran (Oatwell 22)	4	Granola, crisp, pasta	3 h, x	12 healthy volunteers mean age 42.3 y	Oat granola and pasta-lower glycemic responses at 30 and 45 min than wheat muffin. Crips-not different from wheat muffin.	Regand et al., 2009

(continued)

Table 22.3 (continued) Effects of Oat Beta Glucan on Glycemic Responses in Single Dose Human Clinical Studies

Source	Dose, g/d	Food Form	Duration*	Subject	Results	Reference
Oat bran flour (Natureal)	Flour, 4.6 or 9.4 Crisp, 3	Flour or crisp	2 h, x	12 healthy volunteers; mean age 66y	The oat bran flour had a lower AUC at 2 h (47+/-45 mmol min/L) than the glucose load (118+/-40 mmol min/L; p < 0.002). No difference between the oat bran crisp (93+/-41 mmol min/L) and the control.	Tapola et al., 2005
Oat bran	4, 6, or 8.4	Breakfast cereal	2 h, x	8 NIDDM aged 34–65y	There was a linear inverse relationship between dose of BG and plasma glucose peak or glucose AUC at 2 h (8, 6, 4, 0 g BG; Maximum increases in plasma glucose, 38, 42, 67, 100; treatment group, (P < 0.05); Glu AUC, 2.5, 2.8, 4.7, 6.8, p < 0.05 for 8 and 6 g BG groups). Postprandial insulin increase was 59–67% (P < 0.01) as high as the continental breakfast after all three levels of BG.	Tappy et al., 1996
Oat bran, oat gum	8.8	porridge meals	3 h	Healthy and NIDDM	Oat bran and wheat farina plus oat gum meals reduced the postprandial plasma glucose excursions and insulin levels when compared with the control wheat farina meal in both control and Type 2 diabetic subjects.	Braaten et al., 1994

Oat powder	2.7–3.0	Breakfast meal	2 h, x	18 healthy volunteers; mean age 66 y	Oat powder –no significant difference in glycemic responses from the control (white bread).	Ulmius et al., 2009
Oat gum	1.45, 2.9, or 5.8; hydrolyzed OG 6.4		3 h, x	20 volunteers	Increasing the dose of OG successively reduced the plasma glucose and insulin responses relative to a control without gum. Reduction of the viscosity of OG by acid hydrolysis reduced or eliminated the capacity to decrease postprandial glucose and insulin levels.	Wood et al., 1994
Oat	4.0 g	Porridge	3 h, x	9 healthy volunteers	No differences in postprandial blood glucose and insulin responses between the test and white wheat bread control.	Liljeberg et al., 1996

BG = beta glucan; GI = glycemic index; II = insulinemic response; AUC = area under the curve; Glu = glucose: OG = oat gum.

Table 22.4 Short Term in Humans

Source	Dose, g/d	Food Form	Duration	Subject	Results	Ref.
Unidentified	8.9 g	Diet as 3 meals a day	3 d; monitor up to 9 h at day 3, x	10 healthy men	26% reduction in plasma insulin concentration during the last 2 h of the 9 h meal ingestion. 12% lower glucose rate of appearance at steady state −21% reduction in the systemic appearance rate of exogenous CHO; unchanged endogenous glucose production.	Battilana et al., 2001
Oat conc	5 g	Polenta meal	2 meals; monitored up to 6 h	12 overwt. men aged 20–60 y	No statistically differences in postprandial glu and insulin responses.	Nazare et al., 2009

Table 22.5 Effects of Oat Beta Glucan on Glycemic Responses in Longer Term Human Clinical Studies

Source	Dose of BG, g/d	Food Form	Duration	Subject	Results	Ref.
Oat (5 or 10% BG) or barley (Ceba foods)	1 or 2 g/d	Beverage containing BG with meal, 2x/d	8 wk, p	89 hyper-cholesterol-emic subjects	Compared to control, intake of 1 g oat BG/d lowered postprandial glu conc. by 19% at 30 min (p = 0.005) and 16% (p – 0.066) at 60 min and insulin conc. by 33 % at 30 min (P = 0.025). No differences in postprandial glucose and insulin responses at 2 h. No changes in fasting blood glucose and insulin conc. by consumption of 1 or 2 g BG/g.	Biörklund et al., 2005
Oat extract	1 or 10% BG	Diet	5 wk, x	23 moderately high cholesterolemic subjects	Glucose responses were reduced by both extracts in both men and women; in women, responses to the 10% extract were lowest. Insulin responses did not differ between men and women, but were lower after oat extracts.	Hallfrisch et al., 1995
Oat bran	4	Soup	5 wk, p	43 healthy men and women	No significant differences in postprandial and fasting blood glucose and/or insulin conc. between test and control groups.	Biörklund et al., 2008

(continued)

Table 22.5 (continued) Effects of Oat Beta Glucan on Glycemic Responses in Longer Term Human Clinical Studies

Source	Dose of BG, g/d	Food Form	Duration	Subject	Results	Ref.
Oat bran	12.8–23.8 g fiber	Diet	2 wk, x	6 healthy males aged 20–27 y	OB delayed the plasma insulin responses insulin peak (at 2–3 h vs. 1 h control) and lowered mean AUC at 7 h. Adding fibers to the test meal induced no change in fasting serum glucose or insulin responses.	Dubois et al., 1995
Oat bran conc.	>9	Bread	12 wk, 8 h profile, x	8 NIDDM men; mean age 45 y	AUC at 4 h: glucose, 810 vs. 470 mmol.min/l, p < 0.01; insulin, 7838 vs. 5916 mU.min/l, 0 < 0.05.	Pick et al., 1996
Oat bran conc	9	Bread	12 wk, x	8 men with NIDDM (mean age = 45 years	Mean glycemic (p < 0.05) and insulin (NS) response areas (AUC) were lower for the oat bran concentrate period than the white bread period. After breakfast, AUC for the oat bran concentrate period was lower for glucose (P < or = .01) and insulin (P < or = .05); insulin peak was reached earlier (P < or = .05) than in the white bread period.	Pick et al., 1996

Table 22.6 Effects of Oat Beta Glucan on Fasting Blood Glucose Concentrations or Insulin Resistance in Longer Term Human Clinical Studies

Source	Dose, g/d	Food Form	Duration*	Subject	Results	Reference
Oat flour	3	Bread	3 wk, x	46 NIDDM	BG improved insulin resistance: test vs. control: fasting plasma insulin changes, −3.23 vs. 3.77 microU/ml (P = 0.03); Homa-IR changes, −2.08 vs 1.33 (P = 0.04).	Liatis et al., 2009
Oat conc. (Ceba foods)	3.5	Soup	8 wk, p	53 NIDDM	No changes in fasting blood glucose and HbA1c conc.	Cugnet-Anceau et al., 2009
Oat bran conc	3 g	Low fat yogurt or milk	8 wk intervention + 4 wk FU, p	62 healthy men and women	No changes in fasting blood glucose and insulin conc.	Longgrove et al., 2000
Oat bran	6, low or high MW	Bread	3 wk, x	22 healthy men and women	No changes in fasting blood glucose and insulin conc.	Frank et al., 2004
Oat bran	6	Bread	8 wk, p	38 men; aged 55–72 y	The BG diet also decreased fasting plasma glucose (82.3 vs. 88.3 mg/dl, P < 0.04), whereas the whole wheat bread diet had no effect (85.6 vs. 83.8, NS).	Reyna-Villasmil et al., 2007
Oats	8 g fiber (BG content, NA)	Soup	23 wk, p	32 volunteers aged 21–57 y	Fasting plasma glucose conc. was decreased significantly from 5.4 to 5.2 mmol/l, and fasting plasma insulin from 122 to 98 pmol/l after 23 weeks.	Rytter et al., 1996

BG = beta glucan; AUC = area under the curve; Glu = glucose: Homa-IR (Homoeostasis model assessment-insulin resistance).

For example, a study in patients with type 2 diabetes (Tappy et al., 1996) incorporated β-glucan into a cooked extruded breakfast cereal. With doses of 4.0, 6.0, or 8.4 g of β-glucan per meal, peak elevations of glucose were reduced by 33%, 59%, and 62%, respectively, compared with control meal values. Likewise, 4 h areas under the curve above basal values were reduced by 29%, 39%, and 65%, respectively, compared with controls. Peak insulin values were reduced by 33%, 38%, and 41%, respectively. Responses were higher compared to those in Braaten et al. (1994). This might be due to differences in the solubility of β-glucan.

22.3.2 Longer-Term Studies (Table 22.5)

In longer-term studies, 1 g/day or higher of oat β-glucan consistently reduced glycemic responses (Biörklund et al., 2005; Dubois et al., 1995; Hallfrisch et al., 1995; Liatis et al., 2009; Pick et al., 1996) except the study of Biörklund et al. (2008) which used 4 g oat beta-glucan in a form of soup. Hallfrisch et al. (1995) found both 1 and 7.6 g/day of an extracted oat β-glucan had comparable effects in lowering glycemic responses. Biörklund et al. (2005) reported that compared to a control, intake of 1 g/day of oat β-glucan lowered postprandial glucose concentration by 19% at 30 min (p = 0.005) and 16% (p = 0.066) at 60 min. Insulin concentration declined by 33% at 30 min (p = 0.025). However, there were no differences in postprandial glucose and insulin responses at 2 h. A dose of 9 g of β-glucan/day for 12 weeks reduced total glucose response area by 46% (p ≤ 0.05) and total insulin response area by 19% (NS) in eight men with type 2 diabetes (Pick et al., 1996). The glucose peak values after breakfast and lunch decreased by 15% and 25%, respectively.

Interest in using the hypoglycemic effect of oat soluble fiber to improve performance in sports is increasing. A comparison of the effects of corn, wheat, and oat cereals on respiratory quotient and blood glucose, insulin, and amino acids at rest and during exercise (Paul et al., 1996) showed that oat cereal produced the lowest glucose and insulin values for 90 min after a meal. After the first 20 min of exercise, the glucose level was higher than with corn or wheat. However, subsequent differences were minimal and performance was the same. The amount of β-glucan from the oat cereal was only approximately 1.1 g, and in view of results from diabetic studies, higher doses could be expected to produce more favorable effects.

Overall, an effective dose for reducing postprandial elevations of glucose and insulin is approximately 3 g/day if the oat β-glucan is administered in a form of cereals, tempe, muffins, or meal. Porridge or soup may not be an acceptable food form to maximize hypoglycemic effects of oat β-glucan.

22.4 Effects of Oat β-Glucan on Fasting Blood Glucose and/or Insulin Levels (Table 22.6)

Oat β-glucan has the potential for use as adjunct therapy for reduction of fasting blood glucose concentrations. In a study with 31 healthy overweight subjects, administration of 8 g/day for 23 weeks decreased fasting plasma glucose concentration from 5.4 to 5.2 mmol/L (p < 0.05) and plasma insulin from

122 to 98 pmol/L ($p < 0.05$; Rytter et al., 1996). Studies using 6 g/day have produced mixed results: consumption of 6 g/day of oat β-glucan bread for 6 weeks decreased fasting blood glucose concentration from 88.3 to 82.3 mg/dL, $p < 0.05$. However, there were no changes with the same amount of bread (6 g/day) for 3 weeks (Frank et al., 2004). It would appear that 3 weeks is not long enough to change fasting blood glucose concentrations.

Consumption of 3–3.5 g/day for 3–8 weeks produced mixed results. Liatis et al. (2009) reported that 3 g/day of β-glucan improved insulin resistance (test vs. control: fasting plasma insulin changes were −3.23 vs. 3.77 microU/mL, $p = 0.03$; homeostasis model of assessment: insulin resistance [Homa-IR] changes were −2.08 vs. 1.33, $p = 0.04$). Conversely, Cugnet-Anceau et al. (2010) and Lovegrove et al. (2000) reported no changes in fasting blood glucose and/or insulin concentrations.

Overall, it appears that oat β-glucan consumption of 6 g/day for over 6 weeks effectively reduces fasting blood glucose and/or insulin concentrations. A number of studies suggest that the more immediate effect of fiber on glucose response requires consumption at every meal. In a review article, Würsch and Pi-Sunyer (1997) reported that foods containing 10% viscous β-glucan soluble fiber from oats and barley can reduce glucose and insulin response in the bloodstream by 50% compared to white bread.

22.5 Factors Influencing Glycemic Responses of Oat β-Glucan

22.5.1 Viscosity

Flattening of postprandial glycemia and viscosity of fiber are positively related (Jenkins et al., 1978; Tappy et al., 1996; Wood et al., 1994). Data show that increasing the dose of oat gum (OG) successively reduced plasma glucose and insulin responses compared to a control. The use of acid hydrolysis to lessen the viscosity of OG reduced or eliminated the capacity to decrease postprandial glucose and insulin levels (Tappy et al., 1996). Wood et al. (2000) related glucose and insulin responses to the concentration and molecular weight of β-glucan in a drink. They found a positive correlation ($R^2 = 0.97$) between viscosity and molecular weight × concentration, which was inversely related to glucose and insulin response.

Wood et al. (1994) reported that the relationship between viscosity and increments in peak plasma glucose and plasma insulin was the same as for guar gum. The author suggested that 79%–96% of the changes in plasma glucose and insulin are attributable to viscosity.

22.5.2 Food Form

The form in which the fiber is ingested is also important. The reduction in GI per gram of beta-glucan in tested foods showed that the effectiveness of β-glucan fiber was similar to minimally processed oat bran (Foster-Powell and Miller, 1995; Foster-Powell et al., 2002; Wolever et al., 1994). For example, Tappy et al. (1996) reported that a cereal containing cooked-extruded oat bran concentrate effectively lowers postprandial glycemia and that oat β-glucan incorporated in the form of crisp or porridge was less effective.

22.5.3 Subjects' Health Status (Type 2 Diabetes)

Effects of β-glucan from OG and oat bran as ingredients in meals have been studied in both healthy and type 2 diabetic subjects (Braaten et al., 1994) with 8.8 g of β-glucan per meal. Subjects with type 2 diabetes have a less sensitive glycemic response to oat β-glucan than healthy individuals. In healthy controls, glucose excursions (differences between the highest and lowest glucose levels) were 43% or 38% lower with OG or oat bran than with a control meal, and the 3 h areas under the curve above baseline were 28.5% or 27.2% lower, respectively, than in controls. In subjects with type 2 diabetes, the levels of excursions were higher and the durations longer than in healthy subjects. With OG and oat bran meals, the glucose excursions were 27.4% or 33.9% lower, respectively, than those in controls. Changes in insulin followed the same pattern.

22.6 Bioequivalency of Barley to Oats in Glycemic Responses

The scientific data indicate that barley and oat β-glucan are bioequivalent in postprandial glycemic control. β-Glucans from both oats and barley were effective in lowering glycemic responses. Hallfrisch et al. (2003) compared glucose and insulinemic responses of barley and oat extract in 9 males and 11 females. Glucose responses to barley and oat extracts were comparable, and the insulinemic response to barley was lower than that of oat extract. However, glycemic and insulinemic responses for both barley and oat extracts were less than for a glucose solution. Like oat β-glucan, barley β-glucan is effective in reducing postprandial glycemic responses at the level of 6 g/serving or above in healthy individuals (Behall et al., 2006; Hallfrisch et al., 2003).

22.7 Comparison of Physicochemical Properties of Barley and Oat Products (Lee et al., 1997)

22.7.1 Viscosity

Newman et al. (1992) reported that oat bran and waxbar barley had an almost identical (7.3 cP) in vitro viscosity that was higher than the barley (2.5 cP) and wheat (1.4 cP).

22.7.2 Solubility

Oat and barley have comparable solubility. Aman and Graham (1987) reported that oat β-glucan solubility was higher than that of barley: oats had an average of 80% soluble β-glucan (65%–90%, 121 cultivars), while barley had an average of 54% (38%–69%, 64 cultivars). The β-glucan solubility of the barley products ranged from 49.9% to 57.4% at 38°C for 2 h and 50.0% to 59.9% at 100°C for 1 h. In comparison, oatmeal had 41.5%–47.6% soluble β-glucan at 38°C and 38.1%–55.9% at 100°C. The correlation between viscosity and β-glucan content is higher for barley than oat, r = 0.98 and 0.84, respectively (Doehlert et al., 1997).

22.7.3 Structure

Barley and oat β-glucan are very similar in structure. In both cases, glucose molecules are linked by two types of β-linkages, about 30% β-(1→3) and 70% β-(1→4). A higher proportion of β-(1–3) linked cellotriosyl units (higher molar ratio) could lead to a greater structural regularity that results in decreased solubility (Wood et al., 2003). Most of the β-(1→4) linkages occur in groups of two (cellotriosyl or DP3) or three (cellotetraosyl or DP4) connected by a single β-(1→3) linkage (Edney et al., 1991).

22.7.4 Molecular Weight

Data suggest that on average, barley β-glucan may have a slightly lower molecular weight than oat β-glucan. The peak molecular weight of barley β-glucan varies from 0.2×10^6 to 2.66×10^6. While oat β-glucan is reported to vary from 1.27×10^6 to 3.03×10^6, most oat cultivars have a β-glucan molecular weight greater than 2×10^6 (Edney et al., 1991). In general, there is significant overlap in the molecular weights of barley and oat β-glucan, which suggests that the difference, if any, is minimal.

References

Alminger M and Eklund-Jonsson C. Whole-grain cereal products based on a high-fiber barley or oat genotype lower post-prandial glucose and insulin responses in healthy humans. *Eur J Nutr.* 2008;47(6):294–300.

Aman P and Graham H. Analysis of total and insoluble mixed-linked (1-3), (1-4) beta-D-glucans in barley and oats. *J AOAC Int.* 1987;35:704–709.

Atkinson FS, Foster-Powell K, and Brand-Miller JC. International tables of glycemic index and glycemic load values: 2008. *Diabetes Care.* 2008;31(12):2281–2283.

Battilana P, Ornstein K, Minehira K, Schwarz JM, Acheson K, Schneiter P, Burri J, Jéquier E, and Tappy L. Mechanisms of action of beta-glucan in postprandial glucose metabolism in healthy men. *Eur J Clin Nutr.* 2001;55(5):327–333.

Beck EJ, Tosh SM, Batterham MJ, Tapsell LC, and Huang XF. Oat beta-glucan increases postprandial cholecystokinin levels, decreases insulin response and extends subjective satiety in overweight subjects. *Mol Nutr Food Res.* 2009;53(10):1343–1351.

Behall KM, Scholfield DJ, and Hallfrisch J. Comparison of hormone and glucose responses of overweight women to barley and oats. *J Am Coll Nutr.* 2005;24(3):182–188.

Behall KM, Scholfield DJ, Hallfrisch JG, and Liljeberg-Elmståhl HG. Consumption of both resistant starch and beta-glucan improves postprandial plasma glucose and insulin in women. *Diabetes Care.* 2006;29(5):976–981.

Biörklund M, Holm J, and Onning G. Serum lipids and postprandial glucose and insulin levels in hyperlipidemic subjects after consumption of an oat beta-glucan-containing ready meal. *Ann Nutr Metab.* 2008;52(2):83–90.

Biörklund M, van Rees A, Mensink RP, and Onning G. Changes in serum lipids and post-prandial glucose and insulin concentrations after consumption of beverages with beta-glucans from oats or barley: A randomised dose-controlled trial. *Eur J Clin Nutr.* 2005;59(11):1272–1281.

Braaten JT, Scott FW, Wood PJ, Riedel KD, Wolynetz MS, Brule D, and Collins MW. High β-glucan oat bran and oat gum reduce postprandial blood glucose and insulin in subjects with and without type 2 diabetes. *Diabetic Med.* 1994;11:312–318.

Braaten JT, Wood PJ, Scott FW, Riedel KD, Poste LM, and Collins MW. Oat gum lowers glucose and insulin after an oral glucose load. *Am J Clin Nutr.* 1991; 53(6):1425–1430.

Brand MJ, Pang E, and Bramall L. Rice: A high or lowglycemic index food? *Am J Clin Nutr.* 1992;56:1034–1036.

Cugnet-Anceau C, Nazare JA, Biorklund M, Le Coquil E, Sassolas A, Sothier M, Holm J, Landin-Olsson M, Onning G, Laville M, and Moulin P. A controlled study of consumption of beta-glucan-enriched soups for 2 months by type 2 diabetic free-living subjects. *Br J Nutr.* 2010;103(3):422–428.

Doehlert DC, Zhang D, and Moore WR. Influence of heat pretreatments of oat grain on the viscosity of flour slurries. *J Sci Food Agric.* 1997;74:125–131.

Dubois C, Armand M, Senft M, Portugal H, Pauli AM, Bernard PM, Lafont H, and Lairon D. Chronic oat bran intake alters postprandial lipemia and lipoproteins in healthy adults. *Am J Clin Nutr.* 1995;61(2):325–333.

Edney MJ, Marchylo BA, and MacGregor AW. Structure of total barley beta-glucan. *J Inst Brew.* 1991;97:39–44.

Foster-Powell K, Holt SH, and Brand-Miller JC. International table of glycemicindex and glycemic load values: 2002. *Am J Clin Nutr.* 2002;76(1):5–56.

Foster-Powell K and Miller JB. International tables of glycemic index. *Am J Clin Nutr.* 1995;62(4):871S–890S.

Frank J, Sundberg B, Kamal-Eldin A, Vessby B, and Aman P. Yeast-leavened oat breads with high or low molecular weight beta-glucan do not differ in their effects on blood concentrations of lipids, insulin, or glucose in humans. *J Nutr.* 2004;134(6):1384–1388.

Granfeldt Y, Eliasson AC, and Björck I. An examination of the possibility of lowering the glycemic index of oat and barley flakes by minimal processing. *J Nutr.* 2000;130(9):2207–2214.

Granfeldt Y, Hagander B, and Björck I. Metabolic responses to starch in oat and wheat products. On the importance of food structure, incomplete gelatinization or presence of viscous dietary fiber. *Eur J Clin Nutr.* 1995;49(3):189–199.

Granfeldt Y, Liljeberg H, Drews A, Newman R, and Björck I. Glucose and insulin responses to barley products: Influence of food structure and amylose-amylopectin ratio. *Am J Clin Nutr.* 1994;59(5):1075–1082.

Granfeldt Y, Nyberg L, and Björck I. Muesli with 4 g oat beta-glucans lowers glucose and insulin responses after a bread meal in healthy subjects. *Eur J Clin Nutr.* 2008;62(5):600–607.

Hallfrisch J, Scholfield DJ, and Behall KM. Diets containing soluble oat extracts improve glucose and insulin responses of moderately hypercholesterolemic men and women. *Am J Clin Nutr.* 1995;61(2):379–384.

Hallfrisch J, Scholfield DJ, and Behall KM. Physiological responses of mean and women to barley and oat extracts (NuTrim X). Comparison of glucose and insulin responses. *Cereal Chem.* 2003;80:80–83.

Hlebowicz J, Darwiche G, Björgell O, and Almér LO. Effect of muesli with 4 g oat beta-glucan on postprandial blood glucose, gastric emptying and satiety in healthy subjects: A randomized crossover trial. *J Am Coll Nutr.* 2008;27(4):470–475.

Hlebowicz J, Wickenberg J, Fahlström R, Björgell O, Almér LO, and Darwiche G. Effect of commercial breakfast fiber cereals compared with corn flakes on postprandial blood glucose, gastric emptying and satiety in healthy subjects: A randomized blinded crossover trial. *Nutr J.* 2007;6:22.

Jenkins AL, Jenkins DJ, Zdravkovic U, Würsch P, and Vuksan V. Depression of the glycemic index by high levels of beta-glucan fiber in two functional foods tested in type 2 diabetes. *Eur J Clin Nutr.* 2002;56(7):622–628.

Jenkins DJ, Wolever TM, Jenkins AL, Thorne MJ, Lee R, Kalmusky J, Reichert R, and Wong GS. The glycaemic index of foods tested in diabetic patients: A new basis for carbohydrate exchange favouring the use of legumes. *Diabetologia.* 1983;24(4):257–264.

Jenkins DJ, Wolever TMS, Kalmusky J, Guidici S, Giordano C, Wong GS, Bird JN, Patten R, Hall M, Buckley G, and Little JA. Low glycaemic index carbohydrate foods in the management of hyperlipidemia. *Am J Clin Nutr.* 1985;42:604–617.

Jenkins DJA, Wolever TMS, Leeds AR, Gasull MA, Haisman P, Dilawari J, Goff DV, Metz GL, and Alberti KGMM. Dietary fibers, fiber analogues, and glucose tolerance: Importance of viscosity. *Br Med J.* 1978;1:1392–1394.

Jenkins DJ, Wolever TM, Taylor RH, Barker H, Fielden H, Baldwin JM, Bowling AC, Newman HC, Jenkins AL, and Goff DV. Glycemic index of foods: A physiological basis for carbohydrate exchange. *Am J Clin Nutr.* 1981;34(3):362–366.

Krezowski PA, Nuttall FQ, Gannon MC, Billington CJ, and Parker S. Insulin and glucose responses to various starch-containing foods in type II diabetic subjects. *Diabetes Care.* 1987;10(2):205–212.

Liatis S, Tsapogas P, Chala E, Dimosthenopoulos C, Kyriakopoulos K, Kapantais E, and Katsilambros N. The consumption of bread enriched with betaglucan reduces LDL-cholesterol and improves insulin resistance in patients with type 2 diabetes. *Diabetes Metab.* 2009;35(2):115–120.

Liljeberg HG, Granfeldt YE, and Björck IM. Products based on a high fiber barley genotype, but not on common barley or oats, lower postprandial glucose and insulin responses in healthy humans. *J Nutr.* 1996;126(2):458–466.

Liu S. Dietary carbohydrates, whole grains, and the risk of type 2 diabetes mellitus. In *Whole-Grain Foods in Health and Disease,* eds. L. Marquart, J. Slavin et al. American Association of Cereal Chemists, St. Paul, MN, 2002, pp. 155–186.

Lovegrove JA, Clohessy A, Milon H, and Williams CM. Modest doses of beta-glucan do not reduce concentrations of potentially atherogenic lipoproteins. *Am J Clin Nutr.* 2000;72(1):49–55.

Miller JB, Pang E, and Bramall L. Rice: A high or low glycemic index food? *Am J Clin Nutr.* 1992;56(6):1034–1036.

Nazare JA, Normand S, Oste Triantafyllou A, Brac de la Perrière A, Desage M, and Laville M. Modulation of the postprandial phase by beta-glucan in overweight subjects: Effects on glucose and insulin kinetics. *Mol Nutr Food Res.* 2009;53(3):361–369.

Newman RK, Klopfenstein CF, Newman CW, Guritno N, and Hofer PJ. Comparison of the cholesterol-lowering properties of whole barley, oat bran, and wheat red dog in chicks and rats. *Cereal Chem.* 1992;69:240–244.

Otto H and Niklas L. Different glycemic responses to carbohydrate-containing foods. Implications for the dietary treatment of diabetes mellitus. *Hyg (Geneve).* 1980;38:3424–3429.

Paul GL, Rokusek JT, Dykstra GL, Boileau RA, and Layman DK. Oat, wheat or corn cereal ingestion before exercise alters metabolism in humans. *J Nutr.* 1996;126:1372–1381.

Pick ME, Hawrysh ZJ, Gee MI, Toth E, Garg ML, and Hardin RT. Oat bran concentrate bread products improve long-term control of diabetes: A pilot study. *J Am Diet Assoc.* 1996;96(12):1254–1261.

Regand A, Tosh SM, Wolever TM, and Wood PJ. Physicochemical properties of beta-glucan in differently processed oat foods influence glycemic response. *J Agric Food Chem.* 2009;57(19):8831–8838.

Reyna-Villasmil N, Bermúdez-Pirela V, Mengual-Moreno E, Arias N, Cano-Ponce C, Leal-Gonzalez E, Souki A, Inglett GE, Israili ZH, Hernández-Hernández R, Valasco M, and Arraiz N. Oat-derived beta-glucan significantly improves HDLC and diminishes LDLC and non-HDL cholesterol in overweight individuals with mild hypercholesterolemia. *Am J Ther.* 2007;14(2):203–212.

Rytter E, Erlanson-Albertsson C, Lindahl L, Lundquist I, Viberg U, Akesson B, and Oste R. Changes in plasma insulin, enterostatin, and lipoprotein levels during an energy-restricted dietary regimen including a new oat-based liquid food. *Ann Nutr Metab.* 1996;40(4):212–220.

Tapola N, Karvonen H, Niskanen L, Mikola M, and Sarkkinen E. Glycemic responses of oat bran products in type 2 diabetic patients. *Nutr Metab Cardiovasc Dis.* 2005;15(4):255–261.

Tappy L, Gügolz E, and Würsch P. Effects of breakfast cereals containing various amounts of beta-glucan fibers on plasma glucose and insulin responses in NIDDM subjects. *Diabetes Care.* 1996;19(8):831–834.

Truswell AS. Glycaemic index of foods. *Eur J Clin Nutr.* 1992;46(Suppl 2):S91–S101.

Ulmius M, Johansson A, and Onning G. The influence of dietary fiber source and gender on the postprandial glucose and lipid response in healthy subjects. *Eur J Nutr.* 2009;48(7):395–402.

Wolever TM. The glycemic index. *World Rev Nutr Diet.* 1990;62:120–185.

Wolever TMS, Katzman-Relle L, Jenkins AL, Vuksan V, Josse RG, and Jenkins DJA. Glycaemic index of 102 complex carbohydrate foods in patients with diabetes. *Nutr Res.* 1994;14:651–659.

Wolever TM, Vorster HH, Bjorck I, Brand-Miller J, Brighenti F, Mann JI, Ramdath DD, Granfeldt Y, Holt S, Perry TL, Venter C, and Xiaomei Wu. Determination of the glycaemic index of foods: Interlaboratory study. *Eur J Clin Nutr.* 2003;57(3):475–482.

Wolever TMS, Wong GS, and Kenshole A. Lactose in the diabetic diet: A comparison with other carbohydrates. *Nutr. Res.* 1985;5:1335–1345.

Wood PJ, Beer MU, and Butler G. Evaluation of role of concentration and molecular weight of oat beta-glucan in determining effect of viscosity on plasma glucose and insulin following an oral glucose load. *Br J Nutr.* 2000;84(1):19–23.

Wood PJ, Braaten JT, Scott FW, Riedel KD, Wolynetz MS, and Collins MW. Effect of dose and modification of viscous properties of oat gum on plasma glucose and insulin following an oral glucose load. *Br J Nutr.* 1994;72(5):731–743.

Würsch P and Pi-Sunyer FX. The role of viscous soluble fiber in the metabolic control of diabetes. A review with special emphasis on cereals rich in beta-glucan. *Diabetes Care.* 1997;20:1774–1780.

23
Oat Fiber

DAN INMAN, ALBERT W. LEE and SUSAN S. CHO

Contents

23.1 Introduction

In Western countries, it is essential to increase fiber intake levels. Fortification of various foods with oat fiber can help improve the fiber intake status of the population. The hull surrounding the bran of an oat seed is one plant fraction that is filled with natural, dietary fiber. Oat fiber, derived from these oat hulls, has in recent years become an important food ingredient that is being added into numerous recipes for their high fiber content (88%–95%) and unique, functional properties. The fiber content is higher than wheat hulls (42%–47%) or corn bran (58%–62%). The hull represents about 30% of the grain's weight and has historically been used as animal feed (Dougherty et al., 1988). Gritty texture and degradation of dough properties are frequently associated with adding native hulls and bran to bakery products. Hull and bran products hydrate superficially. Adding too much water is often attributed to a lower volume index of baked goods, but the right combination of water and fiber can actually improve the volume of bakery items (Gould et al., 1989). Recent advances in the processing of oat hulls to oat fiber have greatly reduced the grittiness and improved the functionality of these fibers.

23.2 Production of Oat Fiber

Processing oat hulls into a more concentrated oat fiber is centered on maximizing consumer acceptability (Yu, 2005). Flavor, color, and texture are improved by physical and chemical treatment, such as hydrogen peroxide with heat and pressure over time. Starch, protein, and fat from the oat hull are removed in minimally processed oat fiber, and the lignin, hemicellulose, cellulose, and silica portions of the oat hull are preserved. As the extraction process is intensified, more of the lignin structure starts to be degraded. Lignin removal is associated with a decrease in the silica content of the oat hulls, reducing the gritty texture of the refined oat fiber. The removal of the lignin allows the fiber bundles to separate into individual fiber strands, a state known as defibrillation.

Changing process parameters allows for varied levels of extraction with different sensory properties. Bulk density and silica content are two factors that affect the end texture of the food. The overall mouthfeel can be classified into two categories: abrasiveness and throat-catch. An abrasive texture is associated with the silica content of a minimally processed oat fiber. Throat-catch has to do with the density of the oat fiber. Density will decrease as fibers become more defibrillated, increasing the likelihood that the fibers will linger in the mouth. The bulk density of the oat fiber increases as the fiber length decreases. Challenging food textures are often overcome by changing the fiber length or degree of extraction (Inglett, 1995).

Aside from changing the color, flavor, mouthfeel, and nutritional profile, processing of oat hulls into oat fiber changes the water-holding capacity (WHC) and mechanics. WHC is defined as the amount of water that is retained by 1 g of dry fiber under specified conditions including temperature, the length and duration of soaking, and speed of centrifugation (Elleuch et al., 2011). Lignin is hydrophobic and lowers overall WHC. Therefore, the more extracted and more defibrillated fibers will have a heightened ability to hold liquids within a given volume (Gould et al., 1989). Fiber length and density also play a key role. Water is loosely held within intermolecular bond sites, and the water holds itself within the fiber matrix via dipole–dipole interaction and capillary action.

These photos show two examples of oat fiber at opposite ends of the extraction spectrum. The minimally extracted oat fiber (Figure 23.1) consists primarily of milled fiber bundles with only a small amount of individual defibrillated fibers. The water absorption properties of this type of fiber would be relatively low. This oat fiber would be useful as an economical source of dietary fiber for items such as cereal, granola bars, cookies, and other low-moisture, high-texture applications. Contrasted with the minimally extracted oat fiber photo, the highly extracted fiber (Figure 23.2) consists almost entirely of small defibrillated strands. This results in a fiber with extremely high water and oil absorption and a low density. This type of fiber would be appropriate for use as a binder/extender in processed meats. It also could be used as carrier for oil-based flavors/colors. Another interesting use for this type of fiber is for structural enhancement of

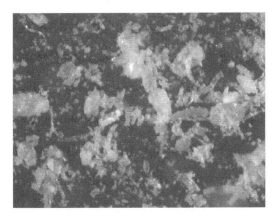

Figure 23.1 Minimally extracted oat fiber.

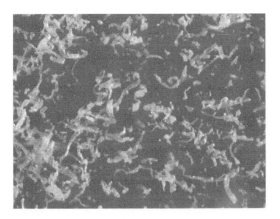

Figure 23.2 Highly extracted oat fiber.

fragile products. When incorporated at low levels (1%–2%), these long-stranded fibers act like reinforcing rods in items like chips, crackers, pretzels, wafers, and ice cream cones to reduce breakage.

23.3 Oat Fiber Characteristics

Oat hull fiber consists of 88%–95% total dietary fiber which has 70% cellulose, 25% hemicellulose, and less than 5% lignin. Oat hull fiber has a high water-binding capacity (300%–800% depending on the extraction level and fiber length).

23.4 Functional Benefits of Oat Fiber as a Fat Replacement

Oat fiber offers numerous functional benefits such as providing structure in food and reduction of calories (Fernandez-Garcia et al., 1988; Hughes et al., 1997; Inglett, 1995). Due to the high WHC of oat fiber, oat fiber and water can increase shelf life and act as a fat mimetic, allowing for a reduction in fat, thus reducing the calories even more. Manufacturers of low-carbohydrate bakery products need to replace flour with fiber ingredients and protein in the formulation. Oat fiber is pH stable and freeze/thaw stable, resulting in a minimization of weeping and product dehydration. This attribute works well in sauces, gravies, and especially frozen entrees.

The following applications demonstrate a minimally extracted oat fiber with a short fiber length for a good source of fiber claim in various foods.

23.4.1 Crispy Cookies

Oat fiber has desirable WHC and mixes easily into dough and does not affect color and flavor. A minimally extracted oat fiber that has lower water-binding capacity would be desirable for manufacturing of cookies and crackers. In these products, too much water binding could damage product integrity since too much water causes structural problems and changes sensory properties. Food products can become bland because the flavor components are diluted with water. Excess water also decreases strength in baked products by reducing the film-forming properties of the dough, resulting in a slow rise or poor volume in the finished product. An appropriate addition of vital wheat gluten will increase the dough strength, allowing the product to maintain the original volume and appearance of the product. The addition of oat fiber makes it possible to produce certain cookies with high fiber without sacrificing sensory properties (Dougherty et al., 1988; Galdeano et al., 2005). In a study of Galdeano et al. (2006), cookies were prepared with the replacement of 20% of wheat flour by physicochemically (extrusion and alkaline hydrogen peroxide) treated oat hulls. Cookies elaborated with the untreated hulls were used as control. Cookies were evaluated for their physical (spread ratio, specific volume, and color) and sensory characteristics, and no difference was detected ($p < 0.05$) among the cookies in relation to the physical properties. Oat fiber cookies contained 9% of added fiber and obtained 91% acceptance when evaluated by potential consumers of the product.

The use of oat fiber providing 5 g fiber per 2 oz. serving of cookies can be prepared as follows (Table 23.1):

1. Scale the following dry ingredients (flour, soda, salt, butter flavor, and oat fiber) into a bowl, dry blend with a wire whisk, and set aside.
2. Add the shortening and brown sugar to the mixing bowl, and cream for 2 min on low speed and 1 min on medium speed.
3. Add eggs and mix on low speed for 1 min and medium speed for 1 min.
4. Add the dry ingredients (flour, soda, salt, butter flavor, and oat fiber) to the mixing bowl and mix on low speed for 1 min.
5. Scrape down the bowl and mix for 15 s on low speed.
6. Add the chopped pecans to the dough and mix on low speed for 15 s.
7. Deposit balls of cookie dough on a baking sheet (spaced out) and flatten and bake in a preheated 350°F oven for 12–14 min.
8. Remove from the pan after 2 min.

Table 23.1 Use of Oat Fiber as a Fat Replacer in Crispy Pecan Cookies (Providing 5 g Fiber per 2 oz Servings [57 g])

Ingredients	Amount Used	Bakers (%)	Finished (%)	Cost per LB	Cost per Usage
All-purpose flour (11% protein, winter wheat)	268	100.00	18.84	$0.1800	$0.1063
Baking soda, sodium bicarbonate	2.7	1.01	0.19	$0.3500	$0.0021
Salt	2.6	0.97	0.18	$0.0762	$0.0004
Butter flavor (natural)	1.4	0.52	0.10	$4.0000	$0.0123
Vitacel oat fiber, HF401-30	128	47.76	9.00	$0.7600	$0.2143
Vegetable shortening, no trans	225	83.96	15.81	$0.5200	$0.2577
Brown sugar, medium	426	158.96	29.94	$0.5000	$0.4692
Eggs, liquid whole eggs	142	52.99	9.98	$0.6000	$0.1877
Pecans, pieces = finely chopped	227	84.70	15.96	$3.2500	$1.6250
Total batch size	1422.7	446.16	100.00		$1.2499
Units	Grams				
Weight per piece	62				
Pieces per batch	22.94677419				
Cost per piece	$0.0545				

23.4.2 Bread

Oat fiber is also used as a fiber source for bread (14.4%–15.5% fiber vs. 1.5% in white bread) and soft cookies (9.8%–12.0% fiber; Dougherty et al., 1988). The bread loaf containing bleached oat fiber had an appealing creamy white interior without any objectionable flavor or aroma. Also addition of oat fiber to pasta shell (2.4% fiber vs. 0.8% in conventional pasta shell) did not affect cooking quality (Dougherty et al., 1988).

For the manufacture of reduced breads providing 5 g of fiber per serving, the following process can be used (Table 23.2):

1. Scale all dry ingredients and set aside (including the oat fiber).
2. Scale the warm water (approximately 95°F) and add to a Hobart 20 quart bowl with a J hook; add the yeast and let it sit for 3 min.
3. Add the rest of the dry ingredients (and oat fiber) and the canola oil on top of the warm water and yeast in the mixing bowl.
4. Begin mixing on low speed (#1) for 3 min, to hydrate and have the dough just come together.
5. Switch the mixer to medium speed (speed #2) and mix to full development (16–18 min). Dough temperature should be 80 ± 2°F.
6. Remove the dough from the mixing bowl, divide, round, mold, pan, and proof for 70–75 min at 95°F at 74% relative humidity (RH).

Table 23.2 Use of Oat Fiber as a Fat Replacer in Bread

White Bread, 1 Slice (28 g)	Control		Test with Oat Fiber	
Ingredients	Amount Used	Finished %	Amount Used	Finished %
Flour (12.5%–13.0% protein from hard red spring wheat)	1000	55.68%	700	28.48%
Water	570	31.74%	1065	43.34%
Sugar	89	4.96%	122	4.96%
Canola oil	55	3.06%	37.6	1.53%
Vitacel oat fiber, HF550-30	0	0.00%	300	12.21%
Yeast, active dry yeast	20	1.11%	27.2	1.11%
Salt	19	1.06%	26	1.06%
Vital wheat gluten	27	1.50%	150	6.10%
Butter flavor	0.6	0.03%	0.8	0.03%
Bakery enhancer/yeast flavor	1.5	0.08%	1.9	0.08%
Dough conditioner/strengthener (DATEM, SSL, Enzymes…)	5	0.28%	12	0.49%
Emulsifier (mono- and diglycerides)	9	0.50%	15	0.61%
Total batch size	1796.1	100.00%	2457.5	100.00%
Units	Grams	510 g dough	Grams	510 g dough
Weight per piece	32		32	
Pieces per batch	56.128125	(Baked)	76.796875	(Baked)
	1 slice = 1.0 g of TDF		1 slice = 5 g of TDF	

7. Bake in a 385°F preheated convection oven for 22–26 min, depending on the oven fan speed.
8. Depan the loaves immediately out of the oven and allow to completely cool on a rack.

23.4.3 Crackers

Long-stranded fibers generally hold more water and reinforce a rod-type structural component. High water absorption, long-stranded fiber with high water aborption also tend to deter susceptibility to breakage. Long-stranded fibers are used to prevent crackers, chips, pretzels, and ice cream cones from deteriorating, reducing breakage and fine dust at the bottom of the package. The following application demonstrates a maximally extracted oat fiber with a long fiber length to increase the strength and structure in a cracker (Table 23.3):

1. Scale and add all of the dry ingredients to the mixing bowl and dry blend for 1 min.
2. Add the canola oil and water; with a dough hook, mix for 2 min on low speed and 10 min at medium speed.

Table 23.3 Use of Oat Fiber as a Fat Replacer in Crackers

Whole Wheat Sesame Crackers	Control		Test with Oat Fiber	
	Grams	(%)	Grams	(%)
Dry ingredients				
Stone-ground whole wheat flour	1000	56.02	930	52.10
Double-acting baking powder	15.5	0.87	15.5	0.87
Salt	25	1.40	25	1.40
Ground toasted sesame seeds	55	3.08	55	3.08
Vitacel oat fiber, HF200	0	0.00	39	2.18
Butter flavor	2	0.11	2	0.11
Bakery enhancer/yeast flavor	2.5	0.14	2.5	0.14
Liquid ingredients				
Canola oil	200	11.20	133	7.45
Warm water (approximately 90°F)	485	27.17	583	32.66
Total batch size	1785	100.00	1785	100.00
Weight per piece	3		3	
Pieces per batch	595		595	

3. Dough should come together and develop into a smooth dough; dough temperature should be around 80°F.
4. Remove the smooth, fully developed dough from the mixer. Let the dough rest for 10–15 min; sheet the dough to the desired thickness. Dock the dough with docking pins for gas release.
5. Mix together an egg wash, combining egg whites with an equal amount of water.
6. Coat the top of the docked sheet with this egg wash.
7. Bake in a preheated conventional oven on an open mesh/screen at 325°F for 13–15 min.
8. Let the baked crackers completely cool before packaging.

23.4.4 Light Bologna, Frankfurters, and Pork Products

Added fiber to the meatball increases the dietary fiber content to 2 g per 91.5 g serving (three meatballs). The fiber in the meatball creates a moister product which could increase the shelf life. Reducing fat in processed meat products can be accomplished by using leaner meats and by dilution of the fat with added water and other nonmeat ingredients (Steenblock et al., 2001). In developing low-fat products, it is essential to find the ingredients which can hold water since adding water to meat products increases cooking losses and purge. Steenblock et al. (2001) reported that addition of both types (bleached and high-absorption oat fibers) of oat fiber at 3% produced greater processing yield for both bologna and frankfurters. Addition of two varieties of oat fiber, bleached and high-absorption oat fibers (each at three levels ranging from 1%–3%), produced greater yields and lighter, less red color in light bologna and fat-free frankfurters. Purge was reduced with oat fiber at 3%. Product hardness

Table 23.4 Use of Oat Fiber as a Fat Replacer in Meatballs

Meatballs, Italian Style	Control		Test with Oat Fiber	
Ingredients	Amount Used	Finished %	Amount Used	Finished %
Ground beef (80:20)	787.95	86.50%	742.95	81.56%
Eggs, whole liquid	57.9	6.36%	57.9	6.36%
Bread crumbs	49.5	5.43%	27	2.96%
Italian seasoning	4.5	0.49%	4.5	0.49%
Garlic salt	4.5	0.49%	4.5	0.49%
Salt	3.15	0.35%	3.15	0.35%
Scallions	2.95	0.32%	2.95	0.32%
Black pepper, fine mesh	0.45	0.05%	0.45	0.05%
Water	0	0.00%	45	4.94%
Vitacel oat fiber, HF251	0	0.00%	22.5	2.47%
Total batch size	910.9	100.00%	910.9	100.00%
Units	Grams		Grams	
Weight per piece (raw)	37		36	
Average cooked weight	30.36	82.1% yield	30.68	85.2% yield
Pieces per batch	24.62		25.30	

increased for bologna with both fiber types as product moistness was reduced when oat fiber was increased. A similar positive effect of oat fiber was reported in processing of pork products (Lee, 1990) and beef patties (Berry, 1997). The USDA has allowed the addition of oat fiber (which must be labeled as isolated oat product) up to 3.5% in meat and poultry products including sausages and franks.

The following application demonstrates a maximally extracted oat fiber with a long fiber length to increase the water- and oil-holding capacity of the meatball (providing 2 g of fiber per 93 g serving of three meatballs) (Table 23.4):

1. Scale all dry ingredients and set aside.
2. Mix oat fiber and water together; set aside.
3. Scale the ground beef and whole eggs and place in a mixing bowl. Mix these together well.
4. Add the dry ingredients and the oat fiber and water mixture to the blended ground beef and whole eggs.
5. Begin mixing on low speed (#1).
6. To mix well and have the meat mixture uniform, bake in a conventional oven preheated for 20 min at 350°F for 2 min.
7. Form into 36–37 g balls and place on a baking sheet pan.

23.5 Health Benefits of Oat Fiber

Numerous scientific studies reported that oat hull fiber promoted glycemic control, weight control, and intestinal health.

23.5.1 Oat Fiber and Glycemic Control

Insoluble fibers can reduce blood glucose levels in normal and diabetic persons. A couple of human studies (Anderson et al., 1991; Weickert et al., 2005) indicated that oat fiber can modulate glycemic responses. Anderson et al. (1991) reported that an oat fiber diet decreased fasting blood glucose levels by 13% ($p < 0.05$), although significant decreases in blood glucose levels were not maintained during the ambulatory phase. In this study, eight lean men with type II diabetes consumed a traditional diabetes diet for 1 week, followed by a control diet plus 30 g/day of insoluble oat fiber for 2 weeks in a hospital metabolic ward. The oat fiber was well accepted and produced no serious side effects. The authors concluded that oat fiber may have beneficial metabolic effects in persons with type II diabetes.

In a study of Weickert et al. (2005), 14 healthy women consumed three matched portions of control or fiber-enriched bread (10.4–10.6 g/portion; wheat fiber, oat fiber). Fiber enrichment accelerated the early insulin response ($p < 0.001$ for oat fiber). It was also associated with an earlier postprandial GIP response after oat fiber (T_{max}, C 83.6 + 7.2). There is a reduced postprandial glucose response on the following day subsequent to ingestion of a control meal (AUC_{C-OF} 2830 + 277 [$p = 0.011$]). No differences in insulin responses were observed after the fiber-enriched diets compared with control ($p > 0.15$). The authors concluded that only 30 g of insoluble dietary fiber from wheat or oats reduces blood sugar levels without raising the insulin response and contributes to a significant improvement in the glucose metabolism.

23.5.2 Oat Fiber and Serum Lipids

Anderson et al. (1991) reported that an oat fiber diet decreased low-density lipoprotein cholesterol by 8.9% ($p < 0.05$) and apolipoprotein B-100 by 17% ($p < 0.01$). Other serum lipid levels did not change significantly, and values returned to pretreatment levels during the ambulatory phase. In this study, eight lean men with type II diabetes consumed a traditional diabetes diet for 1 week, followed by a control diet plus 30 g/day of insoluble oat fiber for 2 weeks in a hospital metabolic ward. Animal studies (Lopez-Guisa et al., 1988; Sunvold et al., 1995) also indicated that oat fiber did not affect serum lipid levels. Oat husk supplementation reduced plasma plasminogen activator inhibitor (PAI) activity in survivors of myocardial infarction with diabetes mellitus type II (Gu et al., 1994). PAN antigen and PAI activity were, though not significantly, reduced by the 10 g/day oat husk supplement.

23.5.3 Oat Fiber and Intestinal Regularity

Animal and human studies reported that oat fiber was effective in improving intestinal regularity and had a role in relieving constipation and/or diarrhea. Table 23.5 summarizes various studies related to the effects of oat fiber on intestinal regularity.

Table 23.5 Oat Fiber and Intestinal Regularity

Positive Effects	No Effect
Broiler chickens—Hetland and Svihus (2001)	Broiler breeders—Hocking et al. (2004)
Rats—Lopez-Guisa et al. (1988)	Human—Kapadia et al. (1995)
Pigs—Mateos et al. (2006)	
Rats—Wang et al. (1994)	
Weaning piglets—Kim et al. (2008)	
Human—Sunvold et al. (1995)	
Human—Stephen et al. (1997)	
Human—Zarling et al. (1994)	

In a pig study of Mateos et al. (2006), oat hull fiber reduced the incidence of diarrhea when oat hulls were used at 2%, 4%, or 4% in the diet ($p < 0.01$). In a young broiler chicken study of Hetland and Svihus (2001), there was a tendency ($p = 0.08$) for faster feed passage with inclusion of coarsely ground oat hulls at the concentration of 0%, 4%, or 10% in the diet. In a rat study of Lopez-Guisa et al. (1988), addition of 5%–15% oat hulls (processed oat hulls, bleached oat hulls, and processed oat hulls coated with starch) in the diet increased fecal weights, and fresh and dry fecal weights increased linearly as the concentration of oat hulls increased.

In a study with 10 healthy males (aged 20–37, who ate, for 2–3 week periods), Stephen et al. (1997) reported that the diet with 25 g providing oat fiber per day (17 g of NSP/day) increased fecal weight from 113 ± 10.4 to 155 ± 10.8 g/day ($p < 0.001$) with no change in transit time. A controlled low-fiber diet contained 13.1 g of non-starch polysaccharide/day. Zarling et al. (1994) reported that supplementation of oat fiber (28.8 g/day of a 50% soy and 50% oat fiber combination for 10 days) significantly increased the number of bowel movements per day (0.9 ± 0.4 vs. 0.5 ± 0.2, $p < 0.05$) and fecal weights (57 ± 31 vs. 32 ± 25 g/day, $p < 0.05$) in medically stable residents of a chronic care facility. Oat fiber also caused a significant increase in fecal nitrogen output (110 ± 65 vs. 75 ± 74 mg/day, $p < 0.05$) and fecal energy (141 ± 73 vs. 76 ± 62 kcal/day, $p < 0.05$). In this study, oat fiber did not affect fecal moisture, gastric emptying, or intestinal transit time. The authors conclude that the addition of a combination of soy and oat fiber to tube feeding material is well tolerated and promotes regular bowel movements without altering the rate of gastric emptying or intestinal transit time. In a healthy human subject study of Sunvold et al. (1995), consumption of diet containing 3.4% oat fiber resulted in slightly firmer stools and provided the greatest amount of fecal output per unit fiber intake.

Kim et al. (2008) reported that addition of 2% oat hulls to an extruded rice-based diet for weaner pigs ameliorates the incidence of diarrhea and reduces indices of protein fermentation in the gastrointestinal tract. The authors concluded that a mostly insoluble oat hull fiber can decrease influenced post-weaning diarrhea in dietary situations where there may be a misbalance of carbohydrate to protein entering the hindgut.

23.5.4 Fermentability of Oat Fiber

It is known that the physicochemical characteristics of fiber modify their fermentation characteristics in the colon. Various studies (Titgemeyer et al., 1991; Bourquin et al., 1993; Roland et al., 1995) indicated that oat fiber does not readily produce short-chain fatty acids (SCFAs) during anaerobic fermentation in the colon. From an in vitro study, Titgemeyer et al. (1991) reported that substrate fermentability based on total SCFA production ranked as follows: citrus pectin > soy fiber > sugar beet fiber > pea fiber > oat fiber. Bourquin et al. (1993) also studied in vitro fermentability of various fiber sources with human colonic bacteria obtained from each of three adult male subjects. In vitro organic matter disappearance during fermentation was less than 20% for the two oat fibers, CMC, and psyllium, intermediate for soy fiber (56.4%), and the greatest for gum arabic (69.5%). Averaged across substrates, acetate, propionate, and butyrate were produced in the molar proportion of 64:24:12. Roland et al. (1995) also confirmed that the lowest amounts of gases and SCFA were found in rats fed on wheat bran, pea, and oat fiber. Cameron et al. (1991) reported that heifers fed larger amounts of treated oat hulls had higher molar percentage acetate and greater acetate:propionate ratios than controls.

23.5.5 Protective Effects of Oat Fiber against Infection and Endotoxemia

Thomsen et al. (2006) reported that both *T. suis* infection and dietary carbohydrates significantly influence the morphological architecture and the production and composition of mucins in the large intestine of pigs. An experiment was performed to study the influence of *Trichuris suis* infection and type of dietary carbohydrates on large intestine morphology, epithelial cell proliferation, and mucin characteristics. Two experimental diets were based on barley flour; oat hull meal was supplemented with oat hull meal, while sugar beet fiber/inulin meal was supplemented with sugar beet fiber and inulin. In this experiment, 32 pigs were allocated randomly into four groups. Two groups were fed oat hull meal and two groups sugar beet fiber/inulin meal. Pigs from one of each diet group were inoculated with a single dose of 2000 infective *T. suis* eggs and the other two groups remained uninfected controls. The pigs were slaughtered 8 weeks post inoculation. Pigs fed oat hull meal had larger crypts both in terms of area and height than pigs fed sugar beet fiber and inulin, and *T. suis*–infected pigs on both diets in Experiment 1 had larger crypts than their respective control groups. The area of the mucin granules in the crypts constituted 22%–53% of the total crypt area and was greatest in the *T. suis*–infected pigs fed oat hull meal. Epithelial cell proliferation was affected neither by diet nor infection in any of the experiments. The study suggests that both diet and infection factors are important in large intestine function and that fibers may play a role in the susceptibility to intestinal helminth infections.

Wan et al. (2010) reported that oat was capable of absorbing intestinal toxins to increase excretion of intestinal toxins in rats. The treatment of taurine (300 mg/kg/day) and oat fiber (15 g/kg/day) induced 21.5% and 18.4% reduction in endotoxin levels, respectively, when compared to the control group ($p < 0.05$). The combination of taurine (300 mg/kg/day) and oat fiber (15 g/kg/day) significantly reduced endotoxin levels in the portal vein by 36.3% when compared to the control group ($p < 0.01$). The authors concluded that the combination of taurine and oat fiber achieved an additive inhibitory effect on intestinal endotoxin release, which might be an effective approach for the treatment of intestinal endotoxemia.

23.6 Summary

In summary, the advances made to the processing of oat hulls for the manufacture of oat fiber have improved the color, flavor, and functionality of the product. As a result of these advances, there are more opportunities for application into a variety of food products with multiple benefits.

References

Anderson JW, Hamilton CC, Horn JL, Spencer DB, Dillon DW, and Zeigler JA. 1991. Metabolic effects of insoluble oat fiber on lean men with type II diabetes. *Cereal Chem.* 68: 291–294.

Berry BW. 1997. Effects of formulation and cooking method on properties of low-fat beef patties. *J Food Service Sys.* 9: 211–228.

Bourquin LD, Titgemeyer EC, Fahey GC Jr., and Garleb KA. 1993. Fermentation of dietary fiber by human colonic bacteria: Disappearance of, short-chain fatty acid production from, and potential water-holding capacity of, various substrates. *Scand J Gastroenterol.* 28: 249–255.

Cameron MG, Cremin JD Jr., Fahey GC Jr., Clark JH, Berger LL, and Merchen NR. 1991. Chemically treated oat hulls in diets for dairy heifers and wethers: Effects on intake and digestion. *J Dairy Sci.* 74: 190–201.

Dougherty M, Sombke R, Irvine J, and Rao CS. 1988. Oat fibers in low calorie breads, soft type cookies, and pasta. *Cereal Food World.* 33: 424–427.

Elleuch M, Bedigian D, Roiseux O, Besbes S, Blecker C, and Attia H. 2011. Dietary fibre and fibre-rich by-products of food processing: Characterisation, technological functionality and commercial applications: A review. *Food Chem.* 124: 411–421.

Fernandez-Garcia E, McGregor JU, and Traylor S. 1988. The addition of oat fiber and natural alternative sweeteners in the manufacture of plain yogurt. *J Dairy Sci.* 81: 655–663.

Galdeano MC and Grossmann MVE. 2005. Effect of treatment with alkaline hydrogen peroxide associated with extrusion on color and hydration properties of oat hulls. *Braz Arch Biol Technol.* 48: 63–72.

Gould JM, Jasberg BK, Dexter LB, Hsu JT, Lewis SM, and Fahey GC Jr. 1989. High-fiber, noncaloric flour substitute for baked foods. Properties of alkaline peroxide-treated lignocellulose. *Cereal Chem.* 66: 201–205.

Gu B, Sundell IB, Keber I, and Keber D. 1994. The effect of oat husk supplementation in diet on plasminogen activator inhibitor type 1 in diabetic survivors of myocardial infarction. *Fibrinolysis.* 8: 44–46.

Hetland H and Svihus B. 2001. Effect of oat hulls on performance, gut capacity and feed passage time in broiler chickens. *Br Poult Sci.* 42: 354–361.

Hocking PM, Zaczek V, Jones EK, and Macleod MG. 2004. Different concentrations and sources of dietary fiber may improve the welfare of female broiler breeders. *Br Poult Sci.* 45: 9–19.

Hughes E, Cofrades S, and Troy DJ. 1997. Effects of fat level, oat fibre and carrageenan on frankfurters formulated with 5, 12 and 30% fat. *Meat Sci.* 45: 273–281.

Inglett GE. 1995. Dietary fiber gels for preparing calorie reduced foods, U.S. Patent application serial number 08/563,834, November 28, 1995.

Kapadia SA, Raimundo AH, Grimble GK, Aimer P, and Silk DB. 1995. Influence of three different fiber-supplemented enteral diets on bowel function and short-chain fatty acid production. *J Parenter Enteral Nutr.* 19: 63–68.

Kim JC, Mullan BP, Hampson DJ, and Pluske JR. 2008. Addition of oat hulls to an extruded rice-based diet for weaner pigs ameliorates the incidence of diarrhoea and reduces indices of protein fermentation in the gastrointestinal tract. *Br J Nutr.* 99: 1217–1225.

Lee S-F. 1990. The utilization of oat fiber and sodium erythorbate for the improvement of PSE pork quality. Dissertation: Thesis (M.S.). Iowa State University, Iowa city, IA.

Lopez-Guisa JM, Harned MC, Dubielzig R, Rao SC, and Marlett JA. 1988. Processed oat hulls as potential dietary fiber sources in rats. *J Nutr.* 118: 953–962.

Mateos GG, Martin F, Latorre MA, Vicente B, and Lazaro R. 2006. Inclusion of oat hulls in diets for young pigs based on cooked maize or cooked rice. *Anim Sci Intl J Fund Appl. Res.* 82: 57–63.

Roland N, Nugon-Baudon L, Andrieux C, and Szylit O. 1995. Comparative study of the fermentative characteristics of inulin and different types of fiber in rats inoculated with a human whole faecal flora. *Br J Nutr.* 74: 239–249.

Steenblock RL, Sebranek JG, Olson DG, and Love JA. 2001. The effects of oat fiber on the properties of light bologna and fat-free frankfurters. *J Food Sci.* 66: 1409–1415.

Stephen AM, Dahl WJ, Johns DM, and Englyst HN. 1997. Effect of oat hull fiber on human colonic function and serum lipids. *Cereal Chem.* 74: 379–383.

Sunvold GD, Titgemeyer EC, Bourquin LD, Fahey GC, and Garleb KA. 1995. Alteration of the fiber and lipid components of a defined-formula diet: Effects on stool characteristics, nutrient digestibility, mineral balance, and energy metabolism in humans. *Am J Clin Nutr.* 62: 1252–1260.

Thomsen LE, Knudsen KE, Hedemann MS, and Roepstorff A. 2006. The effect of dietary carbohydrates and *Trichuris suis* infection on pig large intestine tissue structure, epithelial cell proliferation and mucin characteristics. *Vet Parasitol.* 142: 112–122.

Titgemeyer EC, Bourquin LD, Fahey GC, and Garleb KA. 1991. Fermentability of various fiber sources by human fecal bacteria in vitro. *Am J Clin Nutr.* 53: 1418–1424.

Wan XY, Luo M, Li XD, He P, and Wu MC. 2010. Inhibitory effects of taurine and oat fiber on intestinal endotoxin release in rats. *Chem Biol Interact.* 184: 502–504.

Wang Y, Funk MA, Garleb KA, and Chevreau N. 1994. The effect of fiber source in enteral products on fecal weight, mineral balance, and growth rate in rats. *J Parenter Enteral Nutr.* 18: 340–345.

Weickert MO, Mohlig M, Koebnick C, Holst JJ, Namsolleck P, Ristow M, Osterhoff M, Rochlitz H, Rudovich N, Spranger J, and Pfeiffer AFH. 2005. Impact of cereal fiber on glucose-relating factors. *Diabetologia.* 48: 2343–2353.

Yu P. 2005. Improving the nutritional value of oat hulls for ruminant animals with pretreatment of a multienzyme cocktail: In vitro studies. *J Anim Sci.* 83: 1133–1141.

Zarling EJ, Edison T, Berger S, Leya J, and DeMeo M. 1994. Effect of dietary oat and soy fiber on bowel function and clinical tolerance in a tube feeding dependent population. *J Am Coll Nutr.* 13: 565–568.

24
Sugarcane Fiber

DAN INMAN, ALBERT W. LEE, and SUSAN S. CHO

Contents

24.1 Introduction

Sugarcane is one of the most important crops in the tropics, with global production now estimated at more than 1250 million tons a year (Sangnark and Noomhorm, 2004). Sugarcane contains 73%–76% liquid and 18%–25% fiber. Sugarcane bagasse is the main by-product generated during the processing of granular sugar. Bagasse is a vegetable fiber mainly made up of cellulose in association with lignin (Alonso et al., 2007). A low intake of dietary fiber has been implicated in the etiology of chronic diseases, such as obesity, diabetes, heart disease, diverticular disease, and colon cancer. To increase fiber, healthy-food producers have recently started using bagasse in their products (Fernandez et al., 1996; Pandey et al., 2000).

Based on scientific data, the FDA has allowed several health claims related to dietary fiber. These include reduced risk for (1) cancer (fiber-containing grain products, fruits, and vegetables) (21 CFR 101.76), (2) coronary heart disease (fruits, vegetables, and grain products that contain fiber, particularly soluble fiber) (101.77), and (3) coronary heart disease (soluble fiber from oats and psyllium) (101.81). Increased consumption of dietary fiber also promotes gastrointestinal health and has been linked to lower risk of obesity, overweight, and diabetes (IOM, 2002).

To reduce the risk of chronic diseases, the Institute of Medicine (IOM) and the National Academy of Sciences, United States, have set adequate intake (AI) of total dietary fiber (TDF) for children, adolescents, and adults at 14 g/1000 kcal. But despite these and other guidelines that recommend increased intake, dietary fiber remains a shortfall nutrient in the daily diet of Americans, with more than 90% of the population failing to meet recommended consumption. The total dietary intake for adults is approximately 50% of the recommended amount. This shortfall among most Western people indicates a need for more fiber-rich foods.

Just as health professionals should recommend more consumption of fiber, food developers must formulate more fiber-rich products that appeal to greater numbers of consumers. Several choices of fiber ingredients are already available in the marketplace. Proper use of these ingredients may help improve public health in various countries. This review will focus on the importance of sugarcane fiber in product development and human health.

24.2 Physicochemical Properties of Sugarcane Fiber

Sugarcane bagasse contains cellulose (46.0%), hemicellulose (24.5%), lignin (19.95%), fat and waxes (3.5%), ash (2.4%), silica (2.0%), and other elements (1.7%) (Sangnark and Noomhorm, 2003). Because lignocellulose materials are hydrophobic to some degree, they do not soften or integrate well with dough or batter (Gould et al., 1989). High lignin content contributes to a sandy mouthfeel. To improve texture and functionality of sugarcane fiber, bagasses can be pretreated with hydrogen peroxide or alkaline solutions (Sangnark and Noomhorm, 2003, 2004). This reduces much of the lignin content and opens the fiber structure, making free hydroxyl groups of cellulose available to bind with water. According to Sangnark and Noomhorm, pretreatment can reduce the lignin content of bagasse by approximately 50% and increase the water-holding capacity (WHC) by about the same amount (Sangnark and Noomhorm, 2003).

WHC is defined as the amount of water retained by 1 g of dry fiber under specified conditions of temperature, length of soaking time, and duration and speed of centrifugation. Dietary fibers with high WHC can be used as functional ingredients to avoid syneresis and modify the viscosity and texture of some formulated foods (Elleuch et al., 2011). Fibers with intermediate or low WHC can be used in bakery products that require moisture control to extend shelf life. The relatively low WHC of sugarcane fiber (5.0–9.8 g water/g) improves the shelf life of bakery products.

Oil-holding capacity (OHC) is the amount of oil retained by the fiber after mixing, incubation with oil, and centrifugation. Dietary fiber with high OHC stabilizes high-fat food products and emulsions. Sugarcane has relatively high OHC (3.3–5.1 g oil/g) (Sangnark and Noomhorm, 2003). Thus, it can be used in various emulsion systems.

24.3 Functional Benefits of Sugarcane Fiber

Because sugarcane fiber is insoluble and mostly cellulosic, it is a very stable product for use in food manufacturing. Heat, freeze/thaw, and pH stability enable it to keep its nutritional value throughout harsh processing conditions. The high WHC prevents weeping and product dehydration—features that work well in baked goods, confectionary coatings, beverages, fruit preparations, and frozen and convenience foods. The fiber can be used to replace up to 50% of the fats and oils in bakery products, reducing fat as well as calories. Less expensive than most fats and oils, the combination of sugarcane fiber and water typically cuts costs. Using the product in these ways fortifies fiber and reduces both calories and waste.

24.4 Sugarcane Fiber as a Fat Replacement

A growing body of evidence suggests that high fat intake—more so than other dietary energy sources, such as carbohydrates—may contribute to overeating and obesity. Although fat is energy dense, it has a weak effect on satiety (Gatenby et al., 1995). Also, scientific evidence suggests a relationship between fat intake and weight gain over time in humans (Bes-Rastrollo et al., 2008).

Official recommendations for fat intake are based on the evidence that less fat, particularly the saturated kind, reduces serum cholesterol, a known risk factor for coronary heart disease. The U.S. Surgeon General published a major review on nutrition and health, proposing that dietary energy from fat be cut to 30% of total daily intake (DHHS, 1988).

Reduction in fat intake and/or increased consumption of dietary fiber are associated with decreased risk for heart disease, cancer, and diabetes (Baer et al., 2011; Misra et al., 2010; Vlajinac et al., 2010). If the population followed current dietary recommendations for fat intake, coronary heart disease mortality rates could fall by as much as an estimated 20% (Browner et al., 1991). Replacing fat with substitutes, including oat and sugarcane fibers, could substantially reduce calorie intake.

To succeed as a fat replacement or substitute, a fiber must meet certain criteria in flavor, mouthfeel, texture, structure, process performance, shelf life, and appearance. The sensation of a fatty mouthfeel results from a combination of several inadequately defined and quantified parameters, including viscosity, absorption, cohesiveness, and waxiness. Consumers put product quality before health benefits, even those that they consider important. The major carbohydrate-based fat substitutes include sugarcane and oat fibers, starches, maltodextrins, polydextrose, altered sugars, pectin, gums, and other dietary fibers. By stabilizing substantial quantities of water in a gel-like matrix, this group of fat replacers mimics some of the textural and functional characteristics of fat.

Sugarcane fiber has many functional properties—viscosity, creamy mouthfeel, body, and substance—that make it an ideal fat replacer: Thus, it can be used as a thickener and a binder for stabilization of emulsions, foams, and liquid media.

The low moisture content of carbohydrate replacers has made it difficult to use them in bakery products, especially cookies, biscuits, and crackers. Fat in baked goods is important for tenderness and mechanical handling. Some of the problems that have been encountered—loss of viscosity and moisture, reduced shelf life, and poor aeration, heat transfer, and flavor release—have been improved with the use of sugarcane fiber. Emulsifiers (fatty-acid derived compounds) are usually needed to provide the texture and cohesiveness found in regular fats (Sangnark and Noomhorm, 2003, 2004). By making certain modifications to conventional bakery formulations, a combination of sugarcane fiber and an emulsifier can achieve up to 50% reductions in fat content.

24.5 Food Applications to Bakery Products

Early work by Sangnark and Noomhorm (2003) reported that a 5 g/100 g addition of fiber from alkaline hydrogen peroxide (AHP)-treated bagasse in bread reduced loaf volume and softness. However, a 1.25%–2.0% addition of sucrose ester was effective as a dough strengthener (Barrett et al., 2002; Chung et al., 1981). Grain, crumb color, and aroma of bread made with up to 10% sugarcane bagasse and 1%–1.5% sucrose ester did not differ significantly from bread made with 100% wheat flour (Sangnark and Noomhorm, 2004). Consumers did not accept bread made with a 15% substitution of AHP-treated bagasse and 1%–1.5% sucrose ester addition. At levels of less than 8%, sugarcane fiber does not affect the color and flavor of the finished product. These functional properties make it better suited for the manufacture of sweet bakery goods, such as cookies and muffins. Today, consumers can enjoy fiber fortified foods with a more refined sugarcane fiber that has a finer smoother texture.

24.5.1 Use of Sugarcane Fiber in Cookies

Table 24.1 shows the effect of sugarcane fiber and water by replacing half of the butter in a chocolate chip cookie. The use of sugarcane fiber increased dietary fiber concentration from 0.5 to 1.0 g/cookie while reducing calories and fat levels (total and saturated) by 50%. It also extended shelf life. This cookie can be produced by the following process:

1. Scale all dry ingredients (flour, soda, and salt) into a bowl, blend them with a wire whisk, and set aside.
2. Add butter to the mixing bowl and whip/soften on low speed with a paddle for 2 min on low speed.
3. Add sugar and brown sugar to the whipped/softened butter and mix on medium speed for 2 min.
4. Add eggs and vanilla to the creamed butter and sugar; mix on medium speed for 1 min.
5. Add sugarcane fiber and water to the wet ingredients; rest for 1 min.
6. Add the blended, dry ingredients to the mixing bowl, and mix on low speed for half a minute.

Table 24.1 Use of Sugarcane Fiber in Cookies

Chocolate Chip Cookie		Control			Test with SF601		
Ingredients	Cost/lb	Grams	%	Cost	Grams	%	Cost
Chocolate chips, semisweet	$1.75	340	24.9%	$1.3106	340	24.9%	$1.3106
Flour (11% protein, winter wheat)	$0.20	335	24.5%	$0.1476	335	24.5%	$0.1476
Brown sugar (medium)	$0.65	210	15.4%	$0.3007	210	15.4%	$0.3007
Sugar, granulated	$0.60	140	10.3%	$0.1850	140	10.3%	$0.1850
Butter, lightly salted	$2.00	227	16.6%	$1.0000	113	8.3%	$0.4978
Liquid whole eggs	$0.60	100	7.3%	$0.1322	100	7.3%	$0.1322
Water	$0.00	0	0.0%	$0.0000	89	6.5%	$0.0000
Sugarcane fiber, VITACEL® SF601	$0.90	0	0.0%	$0.0000	25	1.8%	$0.0496
Pure vanilla extract, 2 ×	$7.49	7	0.5%	$0.1155	7	0.5%	$0.1155
Baking soda, sodium bicarbonate	$0.35	4.2	0.3%	$0.0032	4.2	0.3%	$0.0032
Salt	$0.08	3.1	0.2%	$0.0005	3.1	0.2%	$0.0005
Total batch		1366.3	100%	$3.1952	1366.3	100%	$2.7426
Weight per piece		31			31		
Pieces per batch		44			44		
Cost per piece		$0.0725			$0.0622		
Cost reduction		0.00%			14.60%		

7. Fold the chocolate chips into the cookie dough.
8. Deposit balls of cookie dough on a baking sheet and bake in a preheated 375°F oven for 10–12 min.

24.5.2 Use of Sugarcane Fiber in Muffins

Table 24.2 demonstrates the use of sugarcane fiber in muffins to reduce fat/oil and increase total fiber to 3.5 g/95 g serving. Oat fiber muffins can be produced by the following process:

1. Mix the dry ingredients (flour, fiber, baking powder, soda, salt, and preservatives) together in a separate bowl.
2. Add sugar, oil, eggs, and vanilla to a mixing bowl and mix on low speed for 2 min.
3. Add the banana puree and dry ingredients to the liquids, mix on low speed for 1 min, add the water, and mix for 1 min.
4. Scrape down the bowl and paddle, and mix for 1 min on medium speed.
5. Pour 95 g of batter into medium muffin liners in muffin pans (optional); sprinkle a few chopped walnuts on top.
6. Bake in a preheated oven at 375°F for approximately 20–22 min.
7. Let cool for 60 min.

Table 24.2 Use of Sugarcane Fiber in Muffins

Banana Nut Muffin		Control			Test with SF601		
Ingredients	Cost/lb	Grams	%	Cost	Grams	%	Cost
Sugar, granulated	$0.60	460	23.0%	$0.6079	460	23.0%	$0.6079
Flour (11% protein, winter wheat)	$0.20	460	23.0%	$0.2026	430	21.5%	$0.1894
Banana puree	$0.50	300	15.0%	$0.3304	300	15.0%	$0.3304
Water	$0.00	177	8.9%	$0.0001	297	14.9%	$0.0001
Liquid whole eggs	$0.60	200	10.0%	$0.2643	180	9.0%	$0.2379
Vegetable oil, canola	$0.50	240	12.0%	$0.2643	120	6.0%	$0.1322
Walnuts, chopped	$3.25	120	6.0%	$0.8590	120	6.0%	$0.8590
Sugarcane fiber, VITACEL SF601	$0.90	0	0.0%	$0.0000	50	2.5%	$0.0991
Baking powder, double acting	$1.00	19	1.0%	$0.0419	19	1.0%	$0.0419
Pure vanilla extract	$7.49	10	0.5%	$0.1650	10	0.5%	$0.1650
Salt	$0.08	5	0.3%	$0.0008	5	0.3%	$0.0008
Baking soda, sodium bicarbonate	$0.35	3	0.2%	$0.0023	3	0.2%	$0.0023
Sodium propionate	$1.00	3	0.2%	$0.0066	3	0.2%	$0.0066
Potassium sorbate	$1.75	3	0.2%	$0.0116	3	0.2%	$0.0116
Total batch size		2000	100%	$2.7569	2000	100%	$2.6842
Batter weight per piece		107			107		
Pieces per batch		18.69			18.69		
Cost per piece		$0.1475			$0.1436		
Cost reduction		0.00%			2.63%		

24.5.3 Use of Sugarcane Fiber in Bread

Sugarcane fiber can be used as a fiber source in bread. A bread loaf containing sugarcane fiber has an appealing creamy white interior without any objectionable flavor or aroma. Table 24.3 shows that addition of sugarcane fiber increases the fiber content to 4 g/serving. Oat fiber bread can be produced by the following process:

1. Scale warm water, add to a 20 quart mixer with a J hook, add the yeast, and let it sit for 3 min.
2. Scale all dry ingredients and set aside. Add the dry ingredients and canola oil on top of the warm water and yeast in the mixing bowl.
3. Begin mixing on low speed for 3 min. Switch the mixer to medium speed and mix to full development (16–18 min).
4. Remove the dough from the mixing bowl, divide, round, mold, and pan.

Table 24.3 Use of Sugarcane Fiber in Breads

White Bread	Control		Test with SF601	
Ingredients	Grams	%	Grams	%
Water	570	31.7%	975	41.7%
Flour (12.5% protein, hard red spring)	1000	55.7%	800	34.2%
Sugarcane fiber, VITACEL SF601	0	0.0%	200	8.6%
Vital wheat gluten	27	1.5%	130	5.6%
Sugar	89	5.0%	116	5.0%
Canola oil	55	3.1%	35	1.5%
Yeast, active dry yeast	20	1.1%	26	1.1%
Salt	19	1.1%	25	1.1%
Emulsifier (mono- and diglycerides)	9	0.5%	15	0.6%
Dough conditioner/strengthener	5	0.3%	12	0.5%
Fermented yeast flavor	1.5	0.08%	1.9	0.08%
Butter flavor	0.6	0.03%	0.8	0.03%
Total batch size	1796.1	100%	2336.7	100%
Loaf size	510		510	
Loaves per batch	3.52		4.58	
Weight per piece	32		32	
Pieces per batch (baked)	56.13		73.02	
TDF	1		4	

5. Proof for 70–75 min at 95°F at 74% relative humidity (RH). Bake in a 385°F preheated convection oven for 22–26 min depending on the oven fan speed.
6. Depan the loaves immediately out of the oven and allow completely cooling on a rack.

24.5.4 Use of Sugarcane Fiber in Rolls and Yeast-Raised Bakery Products

The addition of sugarcane fiber to rolls and yeast-raised bakery products reduces costs, trans fat (from 0.50 to 0.04 g/roll), and total fat (from 17 to 5 cal/roll). It also increases the level of dietary fiber from 0.71 to 1.24 g/roll (Table 24.4) while extending ambient shelf life. Bakery products containing sugarcane fiber can be produced by the following process:

1. Scale water and add to a 20 quart mixing bowl with a J hook.
2. Scale dry ingredients, mix while dry, and add to the mixing bowl. Scale yeast, fats, oils and/or emulsifiers and add to the mixing bowl, on top of the dry ingredients.
3. Begin mixing on low speed (#1) for 2 min. Switch the mixer to medium speed and mix to full development (control = 13 min, test = 11 min).

Table 24.4 Use of Sugarcane Fiber in Rolls

Dinner Roll		Control			Test with SF601		
Ingredients	Cost/lb	Grams	%	Cost	Grams	%	Cost
Flour (12.5% protein, hard red spring)	$0.20	1500	53.8%	$0.6608	1500	52.0%	$0.6608
Water	$0.00	750	26.9%	$0.0003	922	32.0%	$0.0004
Sugar	$0.60	180	6.5%	$0.2379	180	6.2%	$0.2379
Yeast, fresh compressed crumbled	$0.48	128	4.6%	$0.1353	128	4.4%	$0.1353
Sugarcane fiber, VITACEL SF601	$0.90	0	0.0%	$0.0000	60	2.1%	$0.1189
Salt	$0.08	30	1.1%	$0.0050	30	1.0%	$0.0050
Dough conditioner	$1.85	15	0.5%	$0.0611	15	0.5%	$0.0611
Canola oil	$0.46	0	0.0%	$0.0000	15	0.5%	$0.0152
Emulsifier, 52% mono- and diglycerides	$1.25	5	0.2%	$0.0138	10	0.4%	$0.0275
Malt, nondiastatic	$1.31	9	0.3%	$0.0260	9	0.3%	$0.0260
Vital wheat gluten	$1.10	8	0.3%	$0.0194	8	0.3%	$0.0194
Natural yellow color	$1.00	4	0.1%	$0.0088	4	0.1%	$0.0088
Enzymes (dough strengthener)	$3.75	2	0.1%	$0.0165	2	0.1%	$0.0165
Shortening	$0.52	120	4.3%	$0.1374	0	0.0%	$0.0000
Potato flakes	$0.90	37	1.3%	$0.0733	0	0.0%	$0.0000
Total batch size		2788	100	$1.3957	2883	100%	$1.3329
Weight per piece		32			32		
Pieces per batch		87.13			90.09		
Cost per piece		$0.0160			$0.0148		
Cost savings		0.00%			8.11%		

4. Divide dough into 36 g pieces, round, and pan (full-sheet pan = 8 × 10 pattern, 80 pieces/pan).
5. Panned product is proofed at 98°F at 72% RH for approximately 70–75 min.
6. The top of the proofed product is dusted with cake flour.
7. The pans of proofed dinner rolls are baked in a preheated convection oven at approximately 350°F for 20 min.

24.5.5 *Use of Sugarcane Fiber in Cheesecake*

The use of sugarcane fiber in cheesecake retains moisture, reduces fat by 25%, and provides a good source of fiber (2.5 g of TDF) in a serving. Table 24.5 shows the use of sugarcane fiber in cheesecake.

Table 24.5 Use of Sugarcane Fiber in Cheesecake

Cheesecake, NY Style		Control			Test with SF601		
Shortbread Crust Ingredients	**Cost/lb**	**Grams**	**%**	**Cost**	**Grams**	**%**	**Cost**
Flour (11% protein, winter wheat)	$0.20	200	10.8%	$0.0881	190	10.3%	$0.0837
Water	$0.00	21	1.1%	$0.0000	73	4.0%	$0.0000
Sugar, granulated	$0.60	60	3.2%	$0.0793	60	3.2%	$0.0793
Butter, lightly salted	$2.00	114	6.2%	$0.5022	57	3.1%	$0.2511
Sugarcane fiber, VITACEL SF601	$0.90	0	0.0%	$0.0000	15	0.8%	$0.0297
Pure vanilla extract, 2 ×	$7.49	4	0.2%	$0.0660	4	0.2%	$0.0660
Salt	$0.08	2	0.1%	$0.0003	2	0.1%	$0.0003
Filling ingredients							
Cream cheese	$2.00	908	49.1%	$4.0000	681	36.8%	$3.0000
Sugar, granulated	$0.60	260	14.1%	$0.3436	260	14.1%	$0.3436
Liquid whole eggs	$0.60	200	10.8%	$0.2643	200	10.8%	$0.2643
Water	$0.00	0	0.0%	$0.0000	177	9.6%	$0.0001
Sugarcane fiber, VITACEL SF601	$0.90	0	0.0%	$0.0000	50	2.7%	$0.0991
Amaretto liquor	$8.00	50	2.7%	$0.8811	50	2.7%	$0.8811
Flour (11% protein, winter wheat)	$0.20	30	1.6%	$0.0132	30	1.6%	$0.0132
Total batch size		1849	100%	$6.24	1849	100%	$5.11
Units		Grams			Grams		
Batter weight per piece		95			95		
Pieces per batch		19.46			19.46		
Cost per piece		$0.32			$0.26		
Cost reduction		0.00%			18.06%		

Let all refrigerated ingredients sit at room temperature for 1–2 h.

1. To make the shortbread crust, mix the butter and sugar together well on medium speed for 2 min, as a creaming stage; add the flour, salt, and vanilla (sugarcane fiber and water) and mix for 30 s on low speed until it just comes together.
2. Like a pie crust, roll out the dough on waxed paper and use flour to roll it out slightly larger than the pan.
3. Mold the rolled dough into a spring-form pan and up its sides.
4. Bake the crust in a preheated oven set at 400°F for 15 min.
5. Take the crust out to cool while making the filling.
6. Turn the oven down to 350°F and place a pan of hot water in the oven to keep it moist.

Cheesecake filling:

1. In a large mixing bowl, combine the cream cheese, sugar, flour, eggs, sugarcane fiber, and water.
2. Add eggs one at a time (50 g) and mix each one in well. While mixing on low speed, slowly add Amaretto. Mix only long enough to blend it in.
3. Pour the filling into the baked crust and bake in the preheated oven set at 350°F for 15 min.
4. After this initial bake at 350°F for 15 min, turn the oven down and finish baking at 235°F for 120 min.
5. After this 120 min bake, turn the oven off and leave the cheesecake inside for another 45 min.
6. Remove from oven, let cool at room temperature for another 2 h, and then refrigerate overnight.

24.5.6 Pancake Application

Table 24.6 demonstrates the benefits of adding sugarcane fiber to pancakes. The high WHC and small particle size of the sugarcane fiber retain moisture in pancakes and provide a velvety texture and mouthfeel. The manufacturing process is as follows:

1. Stir all dry ingredients (flour, sugar, baking powder, salt, and fiber) together into a mixing bowl; blend with a wire whisk.
2. Add all liquid ingredients (buttermilk, oil, eggs, water, and fiber) to the dry ingredients.
3. Mix on low speed for 1 min or by hand with a wire whisk until it just comes together as a smooth, thick batter.
4. Pour the batter into a preheated griddle set at 375°F that is sprayed with a pan release coating.
5. Griddle for approximately 140 s on the first side, flip, and griddle for 80 s on the second side.

24.5.7 Use of Sugarcane Fiber in Confectionary Products

Adding sugarcane fiber to confectionary products can reduce calories, increase fiber content to 5 g per serving, and possibly reduce the cost of the formula. Chocolate confectionary coating (Table 24.7) can be processed as follows:

1. Add ingredients to make dark chocolate plus sugarcane fiber and increased fat. Gently melt and mix the slowly melting chocolate to 110°F.
2. Transfer the heated mixture to the conching step or ball-mill mixing tank.
3. Transfer the processed mixture back to a heated mixing tank and heat back up to 110°F while mixing.
4. Hold/temper the mixture at around 85°F–90°F, mix, mold, cool, and package.

Table 24.6 Use of Sugarcane Fiber in Pancakes

Buttermilk Pancakes		Control			Test with SF601		
Ingredients	Cost/lb	Grams	%	Cost	Grams	%	Cost
Water	$0.00	310	34.4%	$0.0001	350	38.9%	$0.0002
Flour (11% protein, winter wheat)	$0.20	300	33.3%	$0.1322	267	29.7%	$0.1176
Liquid buttermilk, reduced fat	$0.35	90	10.0%	$0.0694	90	10.0%	$0.0694
Liquid whole eggs	$0.60	90	10.0%	$0.1189	80	8.9%	$0.1057
Sugar, granulated	$0.60	45	5.0%	$0.0595	50	5.6%	$0.0661
Vegetable oil, canola	$0.52	44	4.9%	$0.0504	22	2.4%	$0.0252
Sugarcane fiber, VITACEL SF601	$0.90	0	0.0%	$0.0000	20	2.2%	$0.0396
Baking powder, double acting	$1.00	12	1.3%	$0.0264	12	1.3%	$0.0264
Salt	$0.08	6	0.7%	$0.0010	6	0.7%	$0.0010
Baking soda, sodium bicarbonate	$0.35	3	0.3%	$0.0023	3	0.3%	$0.0023
Total batch size		900	100.00%	$0.4602	900	100.00%	$0.4536
Units		Grams			Grams		
Batter weight per piece		92			92		
Pieces per batch		9.78			9.78		
Cost per piece		$0.05			$0.05		
Cost reduction		0.00%			1.45%		

Table 24.7 Use of Sugarcane Fiber in Confectionary Products

Dark Chocolate Coating		Control			Test with SF601		
Ingredients	Cost/lb	Grams	%	Cost	Grams	%	Cost
Dark chocolate (8% TDF)	$2.00	454	100.0%	$2.0000	421	92.7%	$1.8546
Sugarcane fiber, VITACEL SF601	$0.90	0	0.0%	$0.0000	22	4.9%	$0.0436
No-trans shortening	$0.60	0	0.0%	$0.0000	11	2.4%	$0.0145
Total batch size		454	100%	$2.0000	454	100%	$1.9128
Units		Grams			Grams		
Grams per serving		38			38		
Servings per batch		11.95			11.95		
Cost per serving		$0.17			$0.16		
Cost reduction		0.00%			4.36%		

Table 24.8 Use of Sugarcane Fiber in Chocolate Coating

Dark Chocolate Coating		Control			Test with SF601		
Ingredients	Cost/lb	Grams	%	Cost	Grams	%	Cost
Dark chocolate (8% TDF)	$2.00	454	100.0%	$2.0000	421	92.7%	$1.8546
Sugarcane fiber, VITACEL SF601	$0.90	0	0.0%	$0.0000	22	4.9%	$0.0436
No-trans shortening	$0.60	0	0.0%	$0.0000	11	2.4%	$0.0145
Total batch size		454	100%	$2.0000	454	100%	$1.9128
Units		Grams			Grams		
Grams per serving		38			38		
Servings per batch		11.95			11.95		
Cost per serving		$0.17			$0.16		
Cost reduction		0.00%			4.36%		

24.5.8 Application of Sugarcane Fiber in Beverages

Sugarcane fiber is an off-white powder that does not dissolve in water. As a result, the addition of an insoluble fiber would require the beverage to be white or opaque. Sugarcane fiber can be used well in chocolate milk, orange juice, fruit smoothies, and thicker (more viscous) protein drinks. A fruit smoothie containing 5 g of fiber per serving can be prepared as follows (Table 24.8):

1. Add all of the ingredients (including the dry ingredients) in a high speed mixer.
2. Mix on high for 5–10 s just long enough to incorporate all of the ingredients well.

Chocolate milk containing 2.5 g of dietary fiber (Table 24.9) can be prepared as follows:

1. Blend the carrageenan, cocoa, and sugar together, dry, and slowly add to the skim milk in a blender.
2. Continue to blend on low speed until well incorporated.

24.5.9 Application of Sugarcane Fiber in Scrambled Eggs

The addition of sugarcane fiber to a typical breakfast product helps retain moistness while reducing costs and fat content. Examples include, but are not limited to, scrambled eggs containing 2.5 g of fiber per serving. These can be manufactured as follows (Table 24.10):

1. Add water to the bottom of the mixing bowl and add the sugarcane fiber to the water; mix well.
2. Add the liquid eggs to the water and fiber, mix well.
3. Pour the batter into a preheated griddle that is set at 350°F and sprayed with a pan release coating. Griddle for approximately 1.5 min.

Table 24.9 Use of Sugarcane Fiber in Chocolate Milk

Chocolate Milk		Control			Test with SF601		
Ingredients	Cost/lb	Grams	%	Cost	Grams	%	Cost
Skim milk (1/2 gal)	$0.19	1771.6	92.3%	$0.7414	1750.6	91.2%	$0.7326
Sugar, granulated	$0.60	116	6.0%	$0.1533	116	6.0%	$0.1533
Cocoa, Hershey's	$1.95	29	1.5%	$0.1246	29	1.5%	$0.1246
Sugarcane fiber, VITACEL SF601	$0.90	0	0.0%	$0.0000	21	1.1%	$0.0416
Salt	$0.08	2.4	0.1%	$0.0004	2.4	0.1%	$0.0004
Carrageenan	$7.49	1	0.05%	$0.0165	1	0.05%	$0.0165
Total batch size		1920	100%	$1.0362	1920	100%	$1.0690
Units		Grams			Grams		
Serving size		240			240		
Servings per batch		8			8		
Cost per serving		$0.1295			$0.1336		

Table 24.10 Use of Sugarcane Fiber in Scrambled Eggs

Scrambled Eggs		Control			Test with SF601		
Ingredients	Cost/lb	Grams	%	Cost	Grams	%	Cost
Liquid eggs	$0.60	100	83.3%	$0.1322	100	72.5%	$0.1322
Milk, whole	$0.20	20	16.7%	$0.0088	20	14.5%	$0.0088
Water	$0.00	0	0.0%	$0.0000	14.2	10.3%	$0.0000
Sugarcane fiber, VITACEL SF601	$0.90	0	0.0%	$0.0000	3.8	2.8%	$0.0075
Total batch size		120	100%	$0.1410	138	100%	$0.1485
Units		Grams			Grams		
Cooked weight per batch		110.76			127.37		
Yield		92.3%			92.3%		
Servings per batch		1			1.15		
Cost per serving		$0.1410			$0.1291		
Cost savings		0.00%			8.39%		

24.6 Effects of Sugarcane Fiber on Gastrointestinal Health

Baird et al. (1977) reported that supplementation of bagasse significantly improved gastrointestinal health in women. In this crossover study, bagasse biscuits contained a supplement of 5.1 g/day of crude fiber. Low-fiber biscuits of similar appearance were given alternatively. Twenty nuns, aged 25–72 years, were divided into two groups of similar age, weight, and plasma cholesterol.

After a preliminary run-in period of 4 months, the supplemental control or bagasse biscuits were given in a randomized order for 2 periods of 12 weeks (dietary periods 2 and 3). Final control observations on a normal diet were made for 1 month. Bagasse has negligible calories and contains 92% fiber, with a high lignin content. Bagasse biscuits (5.1 g of crude fiber daily) were added to the normal diet of 3.7 g of crude fiber daily. The control biscuits had identical ingredients but were low in fiber. The addition on 10.5 g of bagasse containing 5.1 g of crude fiber to a normal diet containing 3.7 g of crude dietary fiber daily raised the mean fecal weight from 88.3 ± 6.4 to 139.7 ± 10.2 g/day (p < 0.005; Baird, 1977). The authors also observed a significant rise in fecal solids and fecal water, although the percentage of water in the stools remained unchanged.

Bagasse supplements accelerated gastrointestinal transit. The overall mean daily stool frequency rose from 0.98 ± 0.05 to 1.35 ± 0.12 when bagasse supplements were added (p < 0.001). The percentage of hard stools dropped from 13.0 ± 3.7 to 8.4 ± 3.6 when bagasse biscuits were consumed. Increased stool frequency is most easily explained by increased fecal weight. The observed improvement may have been related to more fecal bulk and reduced colonic pressure from increased dietary fiber. However, there were no changes in bacteria excreted/g of feces, and the composition of the bacterial flora showed no change.

Excretion of fecal acid sterols on the bagasse supplement increased. The total fecal loss of neutral steroids remained constant on the control and bagasse dietary regimes, but there were dilution and bulking effects from the fiber supplements on the feces. The fecal loss of acid steroids increased significantly (p < 0.01) on the bagasse diet, from 155.6 ± 20.00 to 233.6 ± 16.4 mg. In contrast to bagasse, bran had no effect on the fecal loss of bile acids.

High lignin content makes bagasse more likely to bind bile acids than wheat bran. In the study, individual fecal fat and fecal acid steroid levels were increased in parallel by dietary bagasse, and both returned to their control levels when the dietary supplement ended. Despite the increased fecal loss of acid steroids on the bagasse supplement, no change in plasma cholesterol concentration was observed during the 12 week study.

Sugarcane fiber is a rich source of cellulose. Data indicate that cellulose can relieve constipation. In an observational study (Adamidis et al., 2000), 203 consecutive appendectomized children with histologically proven appendicitis and 1922 controls were studied by the diet history method. Only cellulose and exose were independently correlated to appendicitis, and lower fiber intake was considered the cause in 70% of the cases.

Odes et al. (1986) reported that constipation was treated for 4 weeks in a pilot study with 20–25 g of fiber (cellulose and hemicellulose 89% by weight) daily. Fifteen patients (79%) showed improvement in some or all of five factors, while four patients were largely unresponsive to fiber. Specific symptoms improved as follows: bowel movement frequency in 15 patients (79%), flatulence in 12 (63%), abdominal pain in 10 (53%), stool consistency in 8 (42%), and laxative dependence in 14 (74%). A 4 week posttreatment follow-up showed a return to pre-fiber status in 11 of 13 improved subjects. From a review of 18 human studies,

Stephen et al. (1997) reported that supplementation of 10–24 g of cellulose/day was effective in improving gastrointestinal regularity by reducing mean transit time and increasing stool frequency.

Awais et al. (2011) found that aqueous and ethanolic extracts of sugarcane bagasse had immunotherapeutic efficacy against coccidiosis in industrial broiler chickens. Significantly lower (p < 0.05) oocyst shedding and mortality were observed in chickens administered sugarcane extracts compared to control.

24.7 Summary and Conclusions

Mounting scientific evidence on the role of dietary fats, especially saturated fats, in coronary heart disease will prompt more consumers to choose low-fat foods as a regular part of their diets. Sugarcane fiber may play an important role in the growing low-fat and reduced-fat foods industry. Technological advances in this group of fat mimetics have led to applications previously seen as impossible. With successful marketing and improvements in technology and quality, low-fat products will have a considerable impact upon most sectors of the food industry.

References

Adamidis D, Roma-Giannikou E, Karamolegou K, Tselalidou E, Constantopoulos A. Fiber intake and childhood appendicitis. *Int J Food Sci Nutr*. 2000;51:153–157.

Alonso PW, Garzone P, Cornacchia G. Agro-industry sugarcane residues disposal: The trends of their conversion into energy carriers in Cuba. *Waste Manage*. 2007;27:869–885.

Awais MM, Akhtar M, Muhammad F, Haq AU, Anwar MI. Immunotherapeutic effects of some sugar cane (*Saccharum officinarum* L.) extracts against coccidiosis in industrial broiler chickens. *Exp Parasitol*. February 24, 2011;128:104–110.

Baer HJ, Glynn RJ, Hu FB, Hankinson SE, Willett WC, Colditz GA, Stampfer M, Rosner B. Risk factors for mortality in the nurses' health study: A competing risks analysis. *Am J Epidemiol*. 2011;173:319–329.

Baird IM, Walters RL, Davies PS, Hill MJ, Drasar BS, and Southgate DA. The effects of two dietary fiber supplements on gastrointestinal transit, stool weight and frequency, and bacterial flora, and fecal bile acids in normal subjects, *Metabolism*. 1977;26:117–128.

Barrett A, Cardello A, Maguire P, Richardson M, Kaletunc G, Lesher L. Effects of sucrose ester, dough conditioner and storage temperature on long-term textural stability of shelf-stable bread. *Cereal Chem*. 2002;79:806–811.

Bes-Rastrollo M, van Dam RM, Martinez-Gonzalez MA, Li TY, Sampson LL, Hu FB. Prospective study of dietary energy density and weight gain in women. *Am J Clin Nutr*. 2008;88:769–777.

Browner WS, Westenhouse J, Tice JA. What if Americans ate less fat? A quantitative estimate of the effect on mortality. *JAMA*. 1991;65:3285–3291.

Chung H, Sieb PA, Finney KF, Magoffin CD. Sucrose monoesters and diesters in bread making. *Cereal Chem*. 1981;58:164–167.

Elleuch M, Bedigian D, Roiseux O, Besbes S, Blecker C, Attia H. Dietary fibre and fibre-rich by-products of food processing: Characterisation, technological functionality and commercial applications: A review. *Food Chem*. 2011;124:411–421.

Fernandez M, Borroto B, Rodriguez JL, Beltran G. Dietary fibre from cane bagasse: A new alternative for use of these residues. *Alimentaria*. 1996;277:37–38.

Gatenby SJ, Aaron JI, Morton GM, Mela DJ. Nutritional implications of reduced-fat food use by free-living consumers. *Appetite*. 1995;3:241–252.

Gould JM, Jasberg BK, Dexter LB, Hsu JT, Lewis SM, Fahey GC Jr. High-fiber, noncaloric flour substitute for baked foods. Properties of alkaline peroxide-treated lignocellulose. *Cereal Chem.* 1989;66:201–205.

Institute of Medicine. Dietary reference intakes for energy, carbohydrate, fiber, fat, fatty acids, cholestrol, protein, and amino acids (Macronutrients). National Academy Press, Washington, DC, 2002.

Misra A, Singhal N, Khurana L. Obesity, the metabolic syndrome, and type 2 diabetes in developing countries: Role of dietary fats and oils. *J Am Coll Nutr.* 2010;29:289S–301S.

Odes HS, Madar Z, Trop M, Namir S, Gross J, Cohen T. Pilot study of the efficacy of spent grain dietary fiber in the treatment of constipation. *Isr J Med Sci.* 1986;22:12–15.

Pandey A, Soccol CR, Nigam P, Soccol VT. Biotechnological potential of agroindustrial residues: I. Sugarcane bagasse. *Bioresource Technol.* 2000;74:69–80.

Sangnark A, Noomhorm A. Effect of particle sizes on functional properties of dietary fibre prepared from sugarcane bagasse. *Food Chem.* 2003;80:221–229.

Sangnark A, Noomhorm A. Effect of dietary fiber from sugarcane bagasse and sucrose ester on dough and bread properties. *Lebensmittel-Wissenschaft und-Technologie.* 2004;37:697–704.

Stephen AM, Dahl WJ, Johns DM, Englyst HN. Effect of oat hull fiber on human colonic function and serum lipids. *Cereal Chem.* 1997;74:379–383.

U.S. Department of Health and Human Services (DHHS), Public Health Service (PHS), The Surgeon General's Report on Nutrition and Health, DHHS (PHS) Publication No. 88-50210, U.S. Government Printing Office, Washington, DC, 1988.

Vlajinac H, Ilic M, Marinkovic J, Sipetic S. Nutrition and prostate cancer. *J Buon.* 2010;15:698–703.

25

Galactooligosaccharides
Next Generation Prebiotics

ANNE M. BIRKETT

Contents

25.1 Introduction

Oligosaccharides are a class of carbohydrates that are well known to the food and nutrition industry, and today, various types are commercially available. As a group, they are defined by their chain length, having a degree of polymerization (DP) between 3 and 9 (Food and Agriculture Organization/World Health Organization, FAO/WHO, 1997) or 3 and 10 (American Association of Cereal Chemists, AACC, 2001). Chemically, there is substantial diversity between different types of oligosaccharides, including monomeric composition, polymer architecture, DP range, and average DP.

Nondigestible oligosaccharides (NDOs) have been at the forefront of nutrition science research for more than 20 years. In particular, NDOs have been linked through substantial clinical, animal, and *in vitro* research to an ability to modulate the colonic microflora via stimulating the growth of selected beneficial bacteria (i.e., prebiotic action) and inhibiting colonization of others. Changes in the colonic microflora, and their metabolic products and interaction with the immune system, are now seen as biomarkers of intestinal health. These changes have been linked to a variety of digestive and immune health benefits such as improved stool quality, reduced risk of infection, reduced allergic symptoms, and improved symptoms of irritable bowel syndrome and intestinal discomfort (Roberfroid et al., 2010). Research has revealed that different NDOs have different metabolic and physiological effects, including digestibility, bacterial selectivity (between and within species), bacterial utilization rate, by-products of fermentation, gas production (volume and type), and pathogen antiadhesive activity.

Galactooligosaccharides (GOS) are oligosaccharides in which galactose is the principal monomer. Other monomers may be present to a lesser extent, such as glucose. Commercial interest in GOS largely originated from their structural similarity to oligosaccharides found in human milk (human milk oligosaccharides, HMOs). HMOs represent the third largest solid component in human milk, following lactose and fat, and are present at 15–23 g/L in colostrum and 8–12 g/L in transitional and mature milk (Agostoni et al., 2004; Boehm et al., 2005). It is thought that HMOs are present in human milk primarily to support the growth and development of the infant's microflora and immune system, and as such HMOs are known as the "Bifidus Factor." Commercial GOS ingredients share some structural similarities with selected HMOs, and supplementing infant formula with GOS affords additional immune protection to formula-fed infants (Bruzzese et al., 2006). Consequently, commercial application of GOS ingredients today is primarily in the infant formula market. However, recent formulation and nutrition research has demonstrated the potential for a broader role for GOS— delivering pH and process stable soluble fiber and contributing to digestive and immune health across the life stages, from infants to adults.

This chapter introduces GOS from a commercial, technical, and nutritional perspective.

25.2 Commercial Ingredients

Commercial GOS ingredients are currently available from companies based in Asia, Europe, and the United States. The Japanese market was an early adopter of GOS ingredients, leading the way in areas of development, production, and application. In Japan, GOS has FOSHU (Food for Specified Health Uses) approval.

Tzortzis and Vulevic (2009) have extensively reviewed and compared selected commercial GOS ingredients, including their composition and production processes. GOS ingredients are typically manufactured from lactose by the enzyme β-galactosidase. The primary source of β-galactosidase is bacterial, such as the genus Bifidobacteria or Bacillus; however, other microbial sources have been employed. The resulting ingredients are a heterogeneous mixture of different polymers, so GOS is in fact an ingredient class rather than a specific chemical entity. Most of the polymers have a terminal glucose unit; however, some of the disaccharides do have a terminal galactose unit. Overall, commercial ingredients differ in a number of ways, including polymer composition and architecture, purity (i.e., an amount of residual lactose and monomer sugars), and quality and quantity of supporting nutrition science evidence.

Purimune® is a commercial GOS ingredient which is differentiated by its high purity. Purimune is made from lactose using the enzyme β-galactosidase and is available in powder form from GTC Nutrition in the United States. The high-purity claim is based on a minimum specification of 90% GOS, with a maximum of 10% residual sugars (i.e., lactose, galactose, glucose) on a dry basis. This equates to more than 85% GOS on an as-is basis. Purimune has a DP range of 2–6, and more than 70% of the polymers have DP ≥3. Chain linkages include β 1-3, 1-4, and 1-6 (Figure 25.1). Purimune has GRAS status in the United States (for foods and beverages, and for infant formula and follow-on formula) and is considered "not novel" in Europe. Other certifications include kosher dairy, halal, and non-GMO.

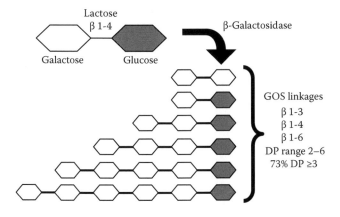

Figure 25.1 Common polymers in Purimune GOS.

25.3 Technical Features

GOS ingredients share some common technical features with the broader oligosaccharide family. Overall, oligosaccharides are typically soluble and nonviscous, making them easy to formulate with, particularly for beverages. GOS does have additional benefits over other oligosaccharides, particularly its stability over a wide pH range. Further, GOS has minimal organoleptic (taste, color, texture) impact, making it suitable for foods, beverages, supplements, and infant products.

Technical features of GOS ingredients may be product specific due to the polymeric differences between ingredients. Therefore, this section will deal specifically with the features of Purimune high-purity GOS:

- It is available as a white powder with a small particle size. Average particle size is 125 μm.
- The caloric value is approximately 2 kcal/g (Macfarlane et al., 2008; Sako et al., 1999). Energy is derived from the bacterial fermentation products.
- It is completely soluble in both hot and cold water. Solution mixing times are dependent upon the liquid temperature—for example, a 10% solution at 4°C–5°C, 23°C–25°C, 40°C–45°C, or 71°C–73°C would require mixing times of 6 min, 2.5, 2.5, and 1 min, respectively.
- It is colorless, forming a clear solution.
- It does not contribute to viscosity. For example, a 60% solution measures less than 500 cps at temperatures ranging 25°C–80°C.
- It has good stability under both high heat and acid conditions (Figure 25.2).
- It has a clean, slightly sweet taste, which is 30% as sweet as sucrose, allowing for partial sugar replacement and masking of off-flavors.

Figure 25.2 highlights the stability of GOS in Purimune, with stability indicated by the analytically measured retention of GOS. In this study, solutions

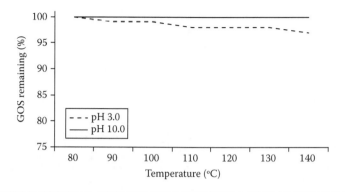

Figure 25.2 Stability of Purimune GOS to heat and temperature.

containing Purimune were subjected to a wide temperature range (80°C–140°C) and pH range (3–10) and held at these conditions for 90 min. There was no loss of GOS at pH 10 across all temperatures, and less than 5% of the GOS was lost at pH 3. This demonstrates the exceptional stability of GOS under extreme pH and temperature conditions.

25.4 Nutritional Benefit Overview

GOS is largely not digested within the upper gastrointestinal tract, so it passes to the large intestine where the health benefits are primarily exhibited. GOS is recognized as a fiber by the AACC (AACC, 2001), and this is supported by nutrition science evidence:

- GOS is not hydrolyzed *in vitro*, under simulated gastric conditions, or by salivary or pancreatic amylase (Chonan et al., 2004; Ohtsuka et al., 1990).
- Some smaller GOS polymers are partially hydrolyzed *in vitro* by rat small intestinal mucosal enzymes (Chonan et al., 2004); however, it is expected that only a relatively low amount is hydrolyzed *in vivo*, since GOS does not increase blood glucose when consumed by human subjects (van Dokkum et al., 1999).
- GOS is fermented, as demonstrated by increased breath hydrogen in clinical studies. Fermentation appears to be rapid, with increases in breath hydrogen appearing 1.5 h after consumption (Chonan et al., 2004) and peaking 3.5 h after consumption (Sako et al., 1999).
- GOS utilization is complete in the adult human and rat gastrointestinal tract, shown by an absence of GOS in fecal material (Alles et al., 1999; Ohtsuka et al., 1991).
- GOS is measured by AOAC Official Method 2001.02 (Association of Official Analytical Chemists, AOAC, 2004). In this method, GOS and lactose are extracted from foods using hot phosphate buffer, and GOS is calculated as the difference in galactose content between portions treated or not treated with β-galactosidase.

In preparing for this chapter, a thorough review of the GOS nutrition science literature was conducted across various databases and reference lists, and 60 references were found that reported on clinical effects of GOS. Twenty-three papers (38%) reported on effects in adult subjects, and 37 papers (62%) reported on effects in infants and children, with many using a combination of GOS and fructooligosaccharide. The higher proportion of studies in infants reflects a general interest in GOS due to its structural similarity to HMOs in human milk and the proposed association between HMOs and intestinal microflora and immune development. The majority of the clinical studies reported benefits relating to digestive and immune health (Table 25.1).

GOS consistently showed prebiotic effects, in particular increasing the counts and/or percentage of Bifidobacteria in more than 30 infant and adult studies (e.g., Scholtens et al., 2008; Vulevic et al., 2008). Indeed, one review by Gibson et al. (2004) suggested that GOS is one of only three carbohydrates that have sufficient evidence to fulfill the criteria for prebiotic classification. The minimum dose reported to obtain bifidogenic effects was 2.5 g/d, when consumed by healthy males with low Bifidobacteria counts (Ito et al., 1993a). Clinical studies have also reported reductions in fecal pathogens such as Candida, *E. coli*, and Clostridia (Ito et al., 1993b; Magne et al., 2008; Scholtens et al., 2008; Vulevic et al., 2008), and animal studies have reported decreased colonization of pathogens such as *Salmonella typhimurium* and *Listeria monocytogenes* after an oral challenge

Table 25.1 Summary of Digestive and Immune Health Benefits Associated with GOS

Evidence Type	Detail
Clinical endpoints—digestive health	Good tolerance[a,i]
	Decreased constipation[a]; increased fecal frequency[a,i]; softer stools[i]
	Decreased travelers diarrhea[a]; decreased diarrhea[i]
	Improved abdominal pain/IBS score[a]
Clinical endpoints—immune and inflammation	Improved eczema/atopic dermatitis/allergic urticaria[i]
	Decreased infections/fever/need for antibiotics[i]
	Decreased recurrent wheezing[i]
Biomarkers—digestive health	Decreased pH[a,i]; increased short-chain fatty acids[a,i]
	Decreased ammonia/p-cresol/indole[a]
Biomarkers—immune and inflammation	Increased Bifidobacteria/Lactobacilli[a,i]
	Decreased Candida,[a] decreased *E. coli*/Clostridia[a,i]
	Immune cell response: increased phagocytosis/natural killer cell activity[a]
	Cytokines: decreased TNF-α/IL-6/IL-1β[a]; increased IL-10[a]
	Immunoglobulins: increased IgA[i]; decreased IgE sensitization[i]

a, adults; i, infants.

(Ebersbach et al., 2010; Searle et al., 2009). GOS is thought to influence the intestinal microflora by multiple mechanisms: (1) selective growth of Bifidobacteria and Lactobacilli, (2) reduced attachment of pathogens on intestinal cells via a decoy mechanism based on the similarity between GOS and receptor oligosaccharides, and (3) short-chain fatty acids produced during fermentation lower the luminal pH and make the environment less hospitable for pathogens.

The International Scientific Association of Probiotics and Prebiotics (ISAPP) recently proposed a definition for dietary prebiotics as "a selectively fermented ingredient that results in specific changes in the composition and/or activity of the gastrointestinal microbiota, thus conferring benefits(s) upon host health" (Gibson et al., 2010). This definition clearly emphasizes that prebiotics should contribute a health benefit. Across the 60 references reviewed for this chapter, various clinical endpoints and biomarkers collectively suggested a benefit of GOS for digestive and immune health. Specifically, in infant studies, GOS was reported to effectively improve skin inflammation, infections, fever, and wheezing (van der Aa et al, 2010; Arslanoglu et al., 2007, 2008; Bruzzese et al., 2009; Kuitunen et al., 2009; Kukkonen et al., 2007; Moro et al., 2006). In adult studies, GOS effectively improved constipation, diarrhea, abdominal pain, and symptoms of irritable bowel syndrome (Drakoularako et al., 2010; Shimoyama et al., 1984; Silk et al., 2009; Teuri and Korpela, 1998). Further, clinical and animal studies combined demonstrated improvements in a number of biomarkers, such as cytokines, immune cell response, antibody response, and intestinal barrier protection and function. Future studies are expected to elaborate on mechanisms whereby GOS plays an important role in digestive and immune health.

25.5 Commercial Uses

A review of global new product introductions (NPIs) across a given time period is useful for market trend analysis, particularly to identify leading market segments for ingredient application. To prepare for this chapter, we reviewed global NPIs containing GOS in the food, beverage, and supplement segments, using the Mintel Global New Products Database. The first mention of products with GOS in this database was found in 1997. Consequently for this chapter, we scanned global NPIs across the period 1997 to March 2010. Key commercial developments for GOS-containing products are as follows:

- Across the entire period, most (57%) of the NPIs were located in the Asian region. Europe was the second most active region, accounting for 39% of the NPIs. Product development with GOS has been slower in other regions of the world, including North America (Figure 25.3).
- From 1997 to 2002, NPI activity recorded each year was low, with less than 10 global NPIs each year. From 2003, the number of NPIs each year has steadily risen, peaking to date in 2008 and 2009, with more than 70 NPIs per year (Figure 25.4). This time line is consistent with trends in clinical research, observed from the PubMed scientific

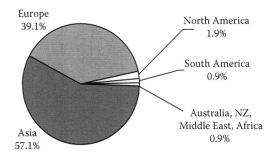

Figure 25.3 Global NPIs containing GOS, 1997–2010.

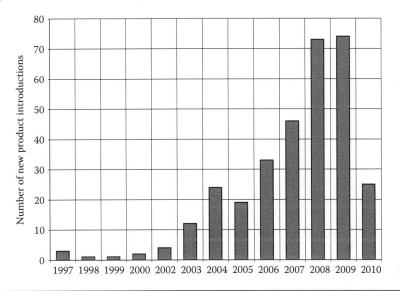

Figure 25.4 Global NPIs containing GOS, 1997–2010, by year.

database, which is managed by the U.S. National Library of Medicine and the National Institutes of Health. A search for clinical studies in this database using the search terms "GOS," "galacto-oligosaccharide," and "galactooligosaccharide" found 183 citations in PubMed across the 1997–2010 period—31 of the citations were relevant to GOS ingredients—and the majority of those (i.e., 8 of 31, representing 26%) were published in 2008 (Figure 25.5).

• The primary market segment for NPIs varied over time. Between 1998 and 2000, beverages were the primary category using GOS. In 2002, NPIs were recorded for infant formula and baby food, and these products have remained the primary category using GOS ingredients through to 2010. The second most dominant category for GOS use today is the dairy segment. NPIs for this category began in 2003 and have continued through to 2010. The three categories mentioned feature the

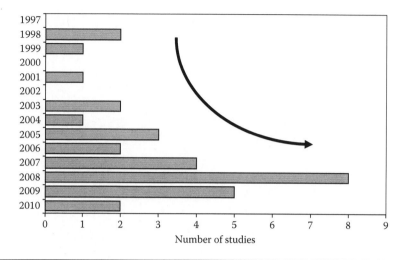

Figure 25.5 Number of clinical studies using GOS, 1997–2010.

core attributes of GOS: (1) soluble and nonviscous, (2) lactose based, and (3) structural similarity with HMOs and relevance to infant health.

- Asia was the first region to have NPIs containing GOS listed in the Mintel database. Asia continued to be the dominant region for NPIs until 2003. Since 2004, the majority of NPIs recorded containing GOS have been shared between Asia and Europe. This progression also reflects trends in clinical research: much of the clinical science has been authored by Asian and European researchers.

25.6 Conclusion

GOS is a relatively new NDO ingredient in the United States but is well established as a functional and nutritional ingredient in other parts of the world, particularly Asia and Europe. GOS provides excellent stability, making it ideal for formulating into a variety of applications that include foods, beverages, supplements, and infant products. GOS is supported by an extensive and growing scientific literature base: current research supports GOS as a prebiotic, and clinical studies link GOS to benefits for digestive and immune health. Ongoing research will contribute to our mechanistic understanding of the role of GOS for health, for both infants and adults.

References

van der Aa, L.B. et al., Synbiotics prevent asthma-like symptoms in infants with atopic dermatitis, *Allergy*, June 17, 2010, 66, 170–177.

Agostoni, C. et al., Prebiotic oligosaccharides in dietetic products for infants: A commentary by the ESPGHAN Committee on nutrition, *J. Pediatr. Gastroenterol. Nutr.*, 2004, 39, 465.

Alles, M.S. et al., Effect of transgalactooligosaccharides on the composition of the human intestinal microflora and on putative risk markers for colon cancer, *Am. J. Clin. Nutr.*, 1999, 69, 980.

American Association of Cereal Chemists (AACC), The definition of dietary fiber. Report of the Dietary Fiber Definition Committee to the Board of Directors of the American Association of Cereal Chemists, *Cereal Foods World*, 2001, 46, 112.

Arslanoglu, S. et al., Early supplementation of prebiotic oligosaccharides protects formula-fed infants against infections during the first 6 months of life, *J. Nutr.*, 2007, 137, 2420.

Arslanoglu, S. et al., Early dietary intervention with a mixture of prebiotic oligosaccharides reduces the incidence of allergic manifestations and infections during the first two years of life, *J. Nutr.*, 2008, 138, 1091.

Association of Official Analytical Chemists (AOAC), AOAC Official Method 2001.02. Trans-galactooligosaccharides (TGOS) in selected food products. First action 2001. Final action 2004. 45.4.12.

Boehm, G. et al., Prebiotic carbohydrates in human milk and formulas, *Acta Paediatrica*, 2005, 94(Suppl 449), 18.

Bruzzese, E. et al., Impact of prebiotics on human health, *Dig. Liver Dis.*, 2006, 38(Suppl 2), S283.

Bruzzese, E. et al., A formula containing galacto- and fructo-oligosaccharides prevents intestinal and extra-intestinal infections: An observational study, *Clin. Nutr.*, 2009, 28, 156.

Chonan, O. et al., Undigestibility of galactooligosaccharides, *Nippon Shokuhin Kagaku Kogaku Kaishi*, 2004, 51, 28.

van Dokkum, W. et al., Effect of nondigestible oligosaccharides on large-bowel functions, blood lipid concentrations and glucose absorption in young healthy male subjects, *Eur. J. Clin. Nutr.*, 1999, 53, 1.

Drakoularakou, A. et al., A double-blind, placebo-controlled, randomized human study assessing the capacity of a novel galacto-oligosaccharide mixture in reducing travellers' diarrhoea, *Eur. J. Clin. Nutr.*, 2010, 64, 146.

Ebersbach, T. et al., Certain dietary carbohydrates promote Listeria infection in a guinea pig model, while others prevent it, *Int. J. Food Microbiol.*, 2010, 140, 218.

Food and Agriculture Organization, World Health Organization (FAO/WHO), Carbohydrates in human nutrition. FAO Food and Nutrition Paper—66. Report of a Joint FAO/WHO Expert Consultation, Rome, Italy, April 14–18, 1997. Chapter 1. The role of carbohydrates in nutrition. http://www.fao.org/docrep/w8079e/w8079e07.htm#description, sourced October 7, 2010.

Gibson, G.R. et al., Dietary modulation of the human colonic microbiota: Updating the concept of prebiotics, *Nutr. Res. Rev.*, 2004, 17, 259.

Gibson, G.R. et al., Dietary prebiotics: Current status and new definition, *Food Sci. Technol. Bull. Funct. Foods*, 2010, 7, 1.

Ito, M. et al., Influence of galactooligosaccharides on the human fecal microflora, *J. Nutr. Sci. Vitaminol.*, 1993a, 39, 635.

Ito, M. et al., Effects of transgalactosylated disaccharides on the human intestinal microflora and their metabolism, *J. Nutr. Sci. Vitaminol.*, 1993b, 39, 279.

Kuitunen, M. et al., Probiotics prevent IgE-associated allergy until age 5 years in cesarean-delivered children but not in the total cohort, *J. Allergy Clin. Immunol.*, 2009, 123, 335.

Kukkonen, K. et al., Probiotics and prebiotic galacto-oligosaccharides in the prevention of allergic diseases: A randomized, double-blind, placebo-controlled trial, *J. Allergy Clin. Immunol.*, 2007, 119, 192.

Macfarlane, G.T. et al., Bacterial metabolism and health-related effects of galacto-oligosaccharides and other prebiotics, *J. Appl. Microbiol.*, 2008, 104, 305.

Magne, F. et al., Effects on faecal microbiota of dietary and acidic oligosaccharides in children during partial formula feeding, *J. Pediatr. Gastroenterol. Nutr.*, 2008, 46, 580.

Moro, G. et al., A mixture of prebiotic oligosaccharides reduces the incidence of atopic dermatitis during the first six months of age, *Arch. Dis. Child.*, 2006, 91, 814.

Ohtsuka, K. et al., Availability of 4' galactosyllactose (O-β-D-galactopyranosyl-(1-4)-O-β-D-galactopyranosyl-(1-4)-D-glucopyranose) in rat, *J. Nutr. Sci. Vitaminol.*, 1990, 36, 265.

Ohtsuka, K. et al., Utilization and metabolism of [U-^{14}C]4'galactosyllactose (O-β-D-galactopyranosyl-(1→4)-O-β-D-galactopyranosyl-(1→4)-D-glucopyranose) in rats, *J. Nutr. Sci. Vitaminol.*, 1991, 37, 173.

Roberfroid, M. et al., Prebiotic effects: Metabolic and health benefits, *Br. J. Nutr.*, 2010, 104(Suppl 2), S1.

Sako, T. et al., Recent progress on research and applications of non-digestible galacto-oligosaccharides, *Int. Dairy J.*, 1999, 9, 69.

Scholtens, P.A.M.J. et al., Fecal secretory immunoglobulin A is increased in healthy infants who receive a formula with short-chain galacto-oligosaccharides and long-chain fructo-oligosaccharides, *J. Nutr.*, 2008, 138, 1141.

Searle, L.E. et al., A mixture containing galactooligosaccharide, produced by the enzymic activity of *Bifidobacterium bifidum*, reduces *Salmonella enterica* serovar Typhimurium infection in mice, *J. Med. Microbiol.*, 2009, 58, 37.

Shimoyama, T. et al., Microflora of patients with stool abnormality, *Bifidobacteria Microflora*, 1984, 3, 35.

Silk, D.B.A. et al., Clinical trial: The effects of a trans-galactooligosaccharide prebiotic on faecal microbiota and symptoms in irritable bowel syndrome, *Aliment. Pharmacol. Ther.*, 2009, 29, 508.

Teuri, U. and Korpela, R., Galacto-oligosaccharides relieve constipation in elderly people, *Ann. Nutr. Metab.*, 1998, 42, 319–327.

Tzortzis, G. and Vulevic, J., Galacto-oligosaccharide prebiotics, in *Prebiotics and Probiotics Science and Technology*, Charalampopoulos, D., Rastall, R.A., Eds., Springer Science+Business Media, New York, 2009, Chapter 7.

Vulevic, J. et al., Modulation of the fecal microflora profile and immune function by a novel trans-galactooligosaccharide mixture (B-GOS) in healthy elderly volunteers, *Am. J. Clin. Nutr.*, 2008, 88, 1438.

Physiochemical Properties of Wheat Bran and Related Application Challenges

DEIRDRE E. ORTIZ and DAVID W. LAFOND

Contents

26.1 Wheat: Types and Processing

The major grains consumed in the world are wheat (~33%) and rice (~25%) (Slavin et al., 1999). In the United States, consumption is mainly from wheat, corn, and oats. These grains have very different amounts of fiber depending on the specific grain. Table 26.1 illustrates the fiber content in each of these grains as well as the relative proportion of the components. The fiber content varies based on growing region, environmental conditions, and specific grain variety, but typically rye, barley, wheat, and oats have the highest levels of fiber from the whole grain, although the fiber chemical structure is different. Wheat is high in arabinoxylans, whereas oats are high in β-glucans.

Wheat is grown widely throughout the world and is consumed in many forms, most commonly bread, biscuits, breakfast cereals, pasta, noodles, and beer. There is significant evidence that the earliest cultivation of wheat took place in the "Fertile Crescent" in today's southern Turkey and northern Syria. Of the wild types that were domesticated and cultivated, two major cultivars of wheat still exist: tetraploid hard wheats (a.k.a. durum wheats, *Triticum turgidum*) and hexaploid wheats (a.k.a. bread wheats, *Triticum aestivum*). In North America, wheat is divided into several major classes. These classes are divided by milling quality (hard vs. soft), color of the bran (red vs. white), and whether the wheat requires vernalization (overwintering) to grow. There are other classes for durum and club wheat, and other "boutique" wheats like purple wheat are kept separate.

The majority of wheat cultivated is hull-less and is relatively easily threshed from the stalk. Wheat kernels have three major components in the caryopsis

Table 26.1 Compositional Differences of the Major Grains

Component (%)	Wheat	Rice	Corn	Barley	Rye	Oats[a]
Endosperm	83.0	90.0	82.0	81.1	83.0	67.0
Germ	3.0	2.5	11.0	3.3	3.0	—
Bran	14.0	7.5	7.0	15.6	14.0	33.0
Total fiber	12.2	2.8	7.3	17.3	15.1	10.6

Sources: From Hoseney, R.C., *Principles of Cereal Science and Technology,* AACC, St. Paul, MN, 1994; USDA Nutrient Database, 2010, http://www.nal.usda.gov.

[a] There is no commercial mill fraction for oat germ. The germ is not present as a discrete layer that can be removed through milling.

(the kernel): endosperm, bran, and germ. The proteins in wheat endosperm give wheat some of its uniqueness. Wheat endosperm contains a complex set of proteins which have viscoelastic properties when hydrated and mixed and are capable of trapping gas, giving wheat products textures unlike products made with other grain flours. Wheat germ has high levels of proteins, lipids, and phytonutrients like vitamin E. Most wheat is cleaned, tempered, and milled into flour. Wheat flour can be milled into a wholemeal or easily separated into its anatomical parts. Generally, the bran and germ are larger particle sizes and can be separated by sifting.

26.1.1 Wheat Bran Definition

For the purposes of this chapter, we will define wheat bran as the millers do (see Figure 26.1), recognizing that the millers' bran has four distinct sections— pericarp, testa, aleurone, and the remnants of endosperm. This chapter will cover the physiochemical properties of the four sections of wheat bran, with our focus being on the pericarp and aleurone sections.

26.1.2 Physical Properties of Wheat Bran

Examination of wheat bran under a microscope reveals outer bran layers (pericarp), the seed coat (testa), and the thick cell-walled aleurone layer (see Figure 26.2). Wheat bran also has bits of the endosperm layer attached. The physical properties of these layers differ significantly. The pericarp layers, which include the epidermis, hypodermis, and cross and tube cells, are functionally a mechanism to protect the germ and storage energy (endosperm) that the germ uses to reproduce. These cells are stacked and aligned in a way to shield the embryonic plant from insects and disease while providing access to water and other nutrients the plant needs. These layers also can be rather rigid unless well hydrated. Wheat millers have referred to the tempering process of hydrating the outer bran layers as "toughening" the bran. In actuality, the bran layers become more flexible, extensible, and rubbery during the hydration process prior to milling, allowing the bran to come off the milling rolls in larger pieces which are more easily separated from the smaller pieces of endosperm.

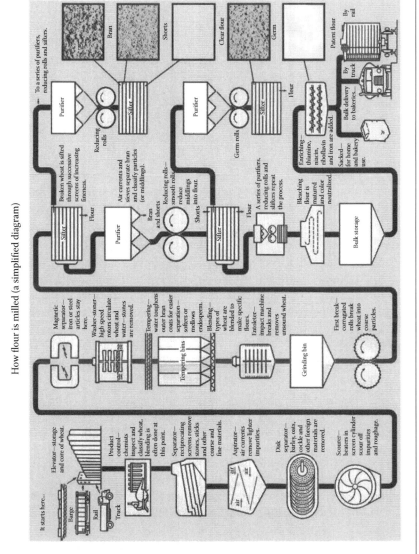

Figure 26.1 Simplified willing process taken from North American Millers Association (NAMA) image library.

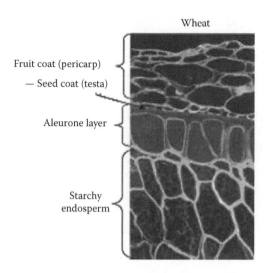

Wheat

Fruit coat (pericarp)

— Seed coat (testa)

Aleurone layer

Starchy endosperm

Figure 26.2 Microstructure of parts of intact grains of wheat. The sections have been stained with Acid Fuchsin and Calcofluor: protein appears red, cell walls rich in β-glucan appear light blue, and lignified cell walls of the fruit coat appear yellowish-brown. (From Kamal-Eldin, A. et al., *Food Nutr. Res.*, 53, 2009.)

In 1992, Glenn and Johnson cut small (2 mm) disks of wheat kernels from the brush end (radial cuts) and the dorsal end (longitudinal cuts) of wheat kernels. They then incubated the disks in a humidity chamber and peeled the bran from the surface of the wheat disks. After mounting the wheat strips and rehumidifying them, they found that the tensile strength, percent deformation to fracture, and initial tangent modulus of elasticity were similar for radial and longitudinal cuts. There were no consistent differences by wheat class (soft vs. hard). Also, the maximum tensile strain to rupture for fully hydrated wheat bran strips (100% RH) was three times greater than for wheat bran strips at 45% RH. They also found that the bran tensile strength was nearly isotropic. This effect of hydration was also linked to tensile strength by Evers and Reed (1988). They found that there was a phase change within cell walls during hydration. The cell wall sections that are most hydrophobic and rich in cutin (a waxy, polyester polymer found on the surface of plant cuticles) are most affected.

The aleurone section of the wheat bran is distinctly different in its physical properties from the outer pericarp layer. Antoine et al. (2003) manually dissected the bran into three sections: the outer pericarp; a mid layer made up of the inner pericarp, testa, and nucellar tissues; and lastly the aleurone layer. They performed tensile strength tests on the isolated strips in both directions (longitudinal and radial orientation). They found that the plastic properties of the bran are nearly exclusively controlled by the middle layers and the aleurone layer. This is likely because the compounds making up the middle layers and the aleurone are biochemically different from the outer layers.

The factors contributing to the mechanical properties of wheat bran are not entirely elucidated. But likely, the biochemical composition and the organization of the

Table 26.2 Phenolic Acid Contents (mg/g wb) in Wheat Kernel Fractions

Bran Fraction	Ferulic Acid	Dehydrodimers of Ferulic Acid	Dehydrotriferulic Acid	Sinapic Acid	*p*-Coumaric Acid
Pericarp	8.18	5.12	1.21	0.01	0.04
Intermediate layer	5.92	0.91	0.07	0.08	0.07
Aleurone	8.17	1.07	0.11	0.44	0.21
Bran	5.26	1.01	0.24	0.25	0.09

Sources: Adapted from Antoine, C. et al., *J. Agric. Food Sci.*, 51, 2026, 2003; Antoine, C. et al., *J. Cereal Sci.*, 39, 387, 2004.

structures are the major contributing factors. Early work by Fincher and Stone have shown that wheat bran cell walls are mainly composed of arabinoxylans, β-glucans, and small amounts of cellulose and lignin (Fincher and Stone, 1986). Later work by Khan and Shewry (see Table 26.3) represent data compiled from multiple studies and thus a slightly different composition. The wheat bran arabinoxylans are esterified with ferulic acid side chains which contribute to cross-linking of the polymers in the bran layers (see Table 26.2). Peyton et al. (2002) found that degree of ferulic acid cross-linking affected the extensibility of the aleurone. The outer structures of the bran (pericarp and testa) have distinct structures with differing shapes, densities, and adhesive interactions. These structures and their properties all contribute to the mechanical properties of the bran.

26.2 Cereal Fibers Are Located in the Cell Walls of the Caryopsis

Plants have two types of cell walls that differ in both chemical composition and physiological function. Primary cell walls surround growing and dividing plant cells. In addition to providing strength to the cells, they must also be able to be flexible and allow the cell to grow and divide. Secondary walls are much thicker and more rigid. They are deposited once the cell has stopped growing and account for most of the fiber in plants.

Cell wall polysaccharides account for about 10% of the dry weight of the mature wheat (*T. aestivum*) grain and about 2%–3% dry weight of the white flour fraction. Primary and secondary cell walls of wheat are composed of hemicellulose (mainly arabinoxylan), β-glucan, cellulose, and lignin, in different proportions. Most of the analytical research in this area is focused on mill fractions of wheat as opposed to cell wall type so the amount of data represented in Table 26.3 is limited.

Table 26.3 shows the principal fibers of wheat cell walls. They also contain smaller amounts of glycoproteins and phenolic esters (ferulic and coumaric acids). Cellulose fibrils are embedded within a network of hemicellulose and lignin (see Figure 26.3). Cellulose is composed of only 1,4-linked β-D-glucose units in long linear polymers. Lignin is composed of highly cross-linked phenolic molecules and is also a component of secondary walls. Lignin serves to form links between the cellulose fibrils and the hemicellulose polymers to form the cell wall structure.

Table 26.3 Distribution (% Dry Weight) of Fiber Types within Various Wheat Cell Wall Components

Component[a]	Arabinoxylan	β-Glucan	Cellulose	Lignin
Endosperm	70	20	2	ND[b]
Aleurone	65	29	2	ND
Bran	64	6	29	8.3

Source: From Khan, K. and Shewry, P.R., *Wheat Chemistry and Technology*, 4th edn., K. Khan and P.R. Shewry, eds., AACC International Inc., St. Paul, MN, 2009.

[a] Numbers in this table were compiled from multiple studies, and totals do not add up to 100%.

[b] None detected.

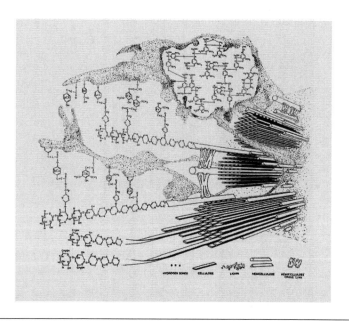

Figure 26.3 Secondary cell wall structure (CW). Components are arranged so that the cellulose microfibrils and hemicellulosic chains are embedded in lignin. Specific linkages and components of non-core lignin are shown for a generalized grass secondary CW. Non-core lignin components include *p*-coumaric (pCA), ferulic (FA), *p*-hydroxybenzoic (BA), sinapic (SA), and cinnamic (CA) acids. (From Oklahoma State University Digital Library, Stillwater, Oklahoma, n.d.)

26.2.1 Chemistry of Plant Fibers

Hemicelluloses are branched polysaccharides that have some structural similarity to cellulose because their backbone is composed of 1,4-linked β-D sugar monomers. Hemicelluloses however, contain a variety of sugar monomers, pentoses, and hexoses and their corresponding uronic acids as opposed to only glucose in the backbone of cellulose. Hemicelluloses are typically highly branched as opposed to the linear cellulose structure. Hemicelluloses are found in both primary and secondary cell walls and include arabinoxylan, glucuronoxylan, glucomannan, and galactomannan. They are present in grain hulls, plant stems, and fruit and represent a major source of plant-based dietary fiber. The complete cell wall structure model has yet to be completely elucidated and is still evolving although the composition is fairly well known.

26.2.2 Chemistry of Wheat Bran

There are a number of nutritionally important compounds within wheat bran. Wheat bran is a critical source of fiber and phenolic compounds. Wheat bran and germ are good sources of the B vitamins (thiamin, riboflavin, niacin, B6, biotin, folate, and pantothenic acid) (see Table 26.5).

Fiber is not a group of structurally similar compounds (see Figure 26.4). The only common factor is that they are all nondigestible by humans. Humans can digest α 1→4 and 1→6 linked hexose and pentose rings; however, the α 1→2, 1→3, and 1→5 as well as the β linkage forms are nondigestible by endogenous enzymes of humans. The fiber in wheat bran includes cellulose, lignin, and a small group of hemicelluloses of which arabinoxylan is the most common (16%–25%). Wheat arabinoxylans are a backbone of β-1,4 linked xyloses with branches of α-L-arabinose attached at either C(O)-2 or C(O)-3.

During wheat milling, millers attempt to separate the outer layers which make up the bran from the starchy endosperm, which becomes the flour. Wheat bran is a combination of many distinct layers of specialized cells (see Figure 26.5). The outermost layers or pericarp is composed of epidermis, hypodermis, and cross and tube cells. The innermost layers include the nucellar and aleurone layers. The aleurone layer is composed of a single layer of cells whose cell walls are high in arabinoxylans linked to ferulic acid. Thus, wheat bran is composed of cell walls from pericarp, seed coats, and aleurone layers with some attached remnants of endosperm. The proportion and structure of arabinoxylans vary in wheat bran by tissue layer (Beaugrand et al., 2004). The majority of the arabinoxylans is found in the pericarp (38%), nucellar epidermis (25%), and aleurone layer (25%) (Swennen et al., 2006).

There is significant chemical variation across the bran tissues. The ratio of arabinose to xylose varies significantly across the bran tissues. The aleurone layers have arabinose (A) to xylose (X) ratio of 0.3–0.5 (Table 26.4) while the epidermis layers have an A/X ratio of ≥1.0. (Antoine et al., 2003). Also, the outer pericarp has significant levels of glucuronic acid and the aleurone has none of this moiety in it.

Arabinoxylans are pentosans (made from pentose sugar monomers) found in the bran of grains such as wheat, rye, and barley. They consist of a xylan backbone (see Figure 26.6) with L-arabinofuranose (L-arabinose) attached randomly by α 1→2 and/or 1→3 linkages to the xylose units throughout the chain (Ring and Selvendran, 1980).

Arabinoxylans are present in the cross-linked form to cellulose, other arabinoxylan chains, ferulic acid and p-coumaric acid at some arabinofuranosyl units,

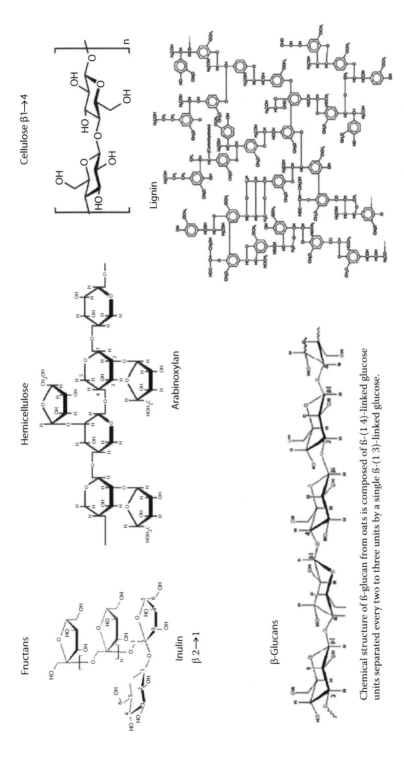

Figure 26.4 Fiber is not a group of structurally similar compounds. Each of these types of carbohydrates is fiber based on the current definition in the United States. Their structures and hence their physical properties are very different from each other.

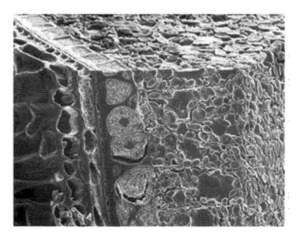

Figure 26.5 Scanning electron micrograph of a portion of the outer surface of a wheat grain showing starchy endosperm, aleurone and overlying nucellar remnants, seed coat, and inner pericarp. The outer pericarp was lost in preparation. (From Joyner, Master's thesis. La Trobe University, Melbourne, Victoria, Australia, 1985.)

Table 26.4 Properties of Wheat Arabinoxylans

	Total Arabinoxylan (g/100 g Flour)	Water Extractable (g/100 g Flour)	A/X Ratio	Intrinsic Viscosity
Whole grain wheat	4.0–9.0	0.3–0.9	0.7	0.8–5.5
Flour	1.4–2.1	0.54–0.68		—
Bran	19.4	0.88		—

Sources: From Fincher, G.B. and Stone, B.A., Cell walls and their components in cereal grains technology, in: *Advances in Cereal Science and Technology*, Y. Pomeranz, ed., AACC International, St. Paul, MN, pp. 207–295, 1986; Fincher, G.B. and Stone, B.A., Chemistry of nonstarch polysaccharides, in: *Encyclopedia of Grain Science*, C. Wrigley, H. Corke, and C.E. Walker, eds., Elsevier, Oxford, U.K., pp. 206–223, 2004.

and to lignins. The fermentation in the gut of wheat bran is greatly impacted by the degree of cross-linking of the ferulic acid molecules. Arabinoxylans have physicochemical properties important to the baking industry. They influence processing and product characteristics because of their water-binding properties which affect the viscosity of dough, the retention of gas bubbles from fermentation, and the final texture of baked products.

Cereal brans, including wheat bran, have large amounts of lignin in them. Marlett and Navis (1988) found that about 5% of the dry weight of wheat bran is lignin. Other nonpolysaccharide components (suberin and cutin) can be found in different parts of the bran. Selvandran et al. (1980) and Ring and Selvendran (1980) found 9.2% protein (including cellular and glycol-proteins) in bran fractions.

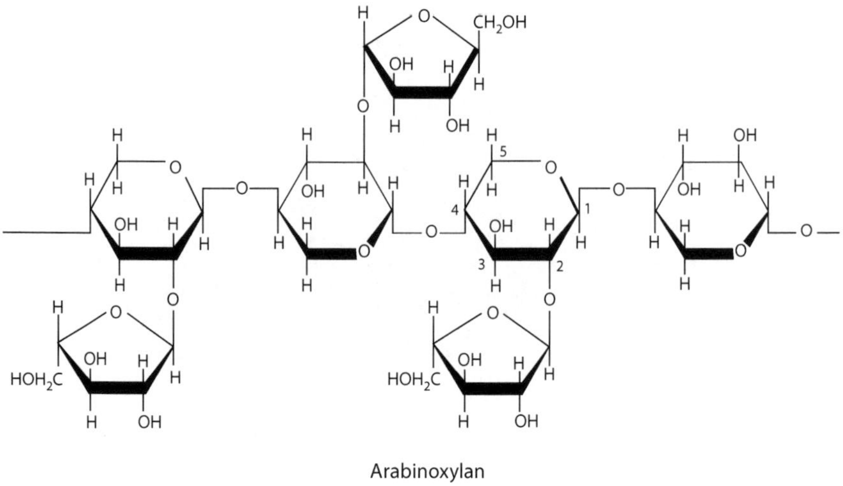

Arabinoxylan

Figure 26.6 Arabinoxylan structural unit.

There is a great diversity of micronutrients and copassengers in wheat bran (see Table 26.5). Morrison et al. (1982) found that 85% of the tocotrienols in wheat were in the testa, pericarp, and aleurone fraction. Bran fractions are also a source of tocopherols but at a significantly lower level than the germ fraction. There are some data that indicate that whole grain flours are higher in carotenoids than flours without the bran and germ component, indicating that there is the possibility of some of the carotenoids in the bran fraction. The bran fraction also contains a significantly higher sterol content (see Table 26.6). Many of the trace minerals like iron, manganese, silicon, and copper are largely present in the bran fraction. This is likely because many of the functional side groups of the fibers in bran can bind cations.

26.3 Issues in Adding Whole Grain Wheat as a Source of Fiber to Food

If used as an ingredient intended to significantly raise fiber levels in a finished product, whole grains are limited in the amount of fiber that they can add, and they bring other calorie-contributing components with them. For example, if you were to make a breakfast cereal using only whole grain wheat, the highest level of fiber you could attain is 12.2 g/100 g (this number could be increased slightly through extensive drying to 13.5 g/100 g). In a typical 30 g serving, this would equate to 3.6 g of fiber, much less than the level required for an excellent fiber source claim (5 g/30 g serving), but sufficient for a good source claim (3 g/30 g serving). Most of the wheat kernel is starch coming from the endosperm which provides considerable energy to the growing plant and calories to the food it is added to. In order to increase the amount of fiber that can be added without raising calories, a more concentrated fiber source is required. Grains are milled to remove the seed coat from the kernel, and to separate

Table 26.5 Fiber and B Vitamin Content of Wheat Fractions

Wheat Part	Fiber Content (%)	Thiamin (µg/g)	Riboflavin (µg/g)	Niacin (µg/g)	Vitamin B$_6$ (µg/g)	Pantothenic Acid (µg/g)	Biotin (µg/g)	Folate (µg/g)
Bran	42.8	5.2–8.9	3.2–5.8	136–296	7.3–16	22–25	0.2–0.5	0.8–2.6
Germ	13.2	4.2–4.4	5.0–10	38–68	4.9–33	10–23	0.2–0.3	1.9–5.2
Endosperm	1.7–2.8	0.8–2.6	0.3–0.6	7.0–15	0.4–2.8	3.0–6.3	0.01–0.03	0.2–0.3

Sources: From USDA Nutrient Database, 2010, http://www.nal.usda.gov; Souci, S.W. et al., *Food Composition and Nutrition Tables,* 6th edn., Medpharm Scientific Publishers, Stuttgart, Germany, 2000; Food Standards Agency, *McClance and Widdowson's the Composition of Foods,* 6th edn., Royal Society of Chemistry, Cambridge, U.K., 2002; National Food Administration (Sweden), 2004, www.slv.se.; National Public Health Institute of Finland, 2004, www.fineli.fi.; Danish Institute for Food and Veterinary Research, 2005, www.foodcomp.dk

Table 26.6 Sterol Content of Finnish Wheat Flour and Bran Fractions (mg/100 g wb)

Wheat Fraction	Total Plant Sterol Content	Sitosterol	Sitostanol	Campesterol	Campestanol	Stigmasterol
1997 wheat sample						
Whole grain	72.6 ± 1.3	40.6 ± 0.4	9.1 ± 1.3	12.1 ± 0.1	6.0 ± 0.4	1.9 ± 0.4
Flour (0.6% ash)	43.0 ± 1.0	26.8 ± 0.5	3.6 ± 0.2	7.6 ± 0.2	2.3 ± 0.1	0.5 ± 0.2
Flour (1.2% ash)	60.7 ± 0.4	36.8 ± 0.2	4.8 ± 0.1	11.1 ± 0.3	4.0 ± 0.0	0.9 ± 0.2
Bran (4% ash)	167.8 ± 1.5	70.4 ± 0.5	31.5 ± 0.1	24.3 ± 0.6	25.6 ± 0.2	7.4 ± 0.1
Bran (4.5% ash)	184.7 ± 1.5	93.8 ± 1.2	20.9 ± 1.2	35.4 ± 0.8	17.6 ± 0.1	5.9 ± 0.1
1998 wheat sample						
Whole grain	83.0 ± 3.2	48.6 ± 1.9	9.8 ± 0.2	15.0 ± 0.7	7.3 ± 0.1	1.5 ± 0.2
Flour (0.6% ash)	39.8 ± 0.2	26.6 ± 0.3	4.1 ± 0.2	7.1 ± 0.1	2.0 ± 0.1	—
Flour (1.2% ash)	70.4 ± 0.8	45.2 ± 0.3	6.5 ± 0.2	15.3 ± 0.2	2.8 ± 0.0	Trace
Bran (4% ash)	177.3 ± 9.4	81.8 ± 4.1	28.3 ± 1.2	28.9 ± 1.9	24.0 ± 1.7	6.1 ± 0.6
Bran (4.5% ash)	177.6 ± 12.2	92.5 ± 6.0	20.7 ± 1.5	34.7 ± 3.0	16.5 ± 0.7	6.3 ± 0.5

Source: From Piironnen, V. et al., *Cereal Chem.*, 79(1), 148, 2002.

Table 26.7 Typical Analysis of Mill Fractions

Analysis	Whole Wheat	Patent Flour	Germ	Bran
Protein (%)	12.0	11.0	30.0	14.5
Ash (%)	1.8	0.4	4.0	6.0
Fiber (%)	2.5	ND[a]	2.0	10.0
Fat (%)	2.9	0.88	10.0	3.3
Digestible carbohydrate (by difference) (%)	80	87	54	66
Calories/100 g	397	402	426	352
Calories/g fiber	158	—	213	35

Source: From Ziegler, E. and Greer, E.N., *Wheat: Chemistry and Terminology,* Y. Pomeranz, ed., American Association of Cereal Chemists, St. Paul, MN, 1971.

[a] Not detected.

out the endosperm from the bran and germ layers, to provide commercially available fractions of the grain. In the case of wheat kernels, the bran fraction provides a higher level of fiber than the whole grain and with fewer calories (see Table 26.7).

26.4 Properties of Wheat Bran in Foods

Fiber can impart textural, flavor, and color properties to foods; these properties become more noticeable and typically less desirable as the fiber concentration increases. Adding wheat bran and other fibers to foods can affect the food texture by making it harder, more brittle, or rougher depending on the application. Wheat bran may change the appearance of the food, making it darker and browner or speckled, particularly in a bland-flavored food or a lightly colored product like a cracker or a rice cake. In dough products where water is added to the mix, fiber may increase the water needed to hydrate the dough, making stickier dough with more water to remove in baking or drying in later unit operations.

Fibers provide solubility, viscosity, and water-binding capacity properties for use in food product development. They can be added to a food product either as part of an ingredient or as an isolated fiber. When fiber is added as an ingredient such as bran, it is part of an existing matrix that can impact the fiber's accessibility to water. The physical structure of the matrix can limit water reaching the fiber, and other components in the ingredient can compete for water. As a result, wheat bran is relatively insoluble even though it contains a large amount of arabinoxylans which are soluble in isolated form. As mentioned earlier, other components in the ingredient can contribute additional calories to the finished product. In the case of wheat bran, this would include starch and protein from the endosperm included in the bran mill fraction.

Isolated fibers are generally classified as soluble or insoluble in water, although when considered soluble, they are present as a colloidal suspension as opposed to a true solution. Solubility is influenced in part by the chemical structure of the fiber. Generally, the more branching a fiber has, the greater its solubility in water, as this structural feature limits the amount of interchain interactions and allows water to interact with the fiber. A high-molecular-weight linear fiber such as cellulose with its repeating structure of β 1-4 linkages is insoluble because of strong interchain interactions, allowing it to form an ordered crystalline structure of polysaccharide chains held together by hydrogen bonding. Guar gum or pectin fibers have a high-molecular-weight highly branched structure and are very soluble because the branching limits crystalline structure formation. Arabinoxylans also have branched structures and thus are soluble as well. The presence of ionizing groups and heterogeneous sugar positional bonding (e.g., β-glucans in oats with mixed β 1-3 and β 1-4 linkages) impact solubility because they too can affect interchain interactions (Tungland and Meyer, 2002).

Solubility has a large impact on food processing and finished product attributes. Insoluble fibers like wheat bran can hydrate and physically entrap water but are still present in the food matrix as discrete particles. The more coarse ground fibers can be abrasive in processing equipment such as extruders. Insoluble fibers often require more water in the dough system to hydrate the particles. Once in a food system, the insoluble fiber particles may interrupt the food macro structure, causing potential weak points in the three-dimensional food matrix. Particles may also impart a gritty mouthfeel if the size has not been reduced low enough.

The viscosity of a fiber ingredient refers to its ability to thicken or form gels in fluids due to entanglement of the polysaccharide chains within the fluid. It is generally related to molecular weight or chain length, and viscosity increases as these properties increase. There is a positive nonlinear relationship between molecular weight and solution viscosity (Dikeman and Fahey, 2006). Long-chain polysaccharides bind or entrap significant amounts of water and thus exhibit high viscosities in solution. Highly soluble fibers that are either short polymer chains or highly branched polymers have low solution viscosities. These fibers can be added to foods and used to affect moisture migration or modify food texture with less effect on viscosity.

The interaction between water and fiber in a food system has been described as water binding or water holding. Water binding of a fiber refers to retention of water after physical stress, whereas water holding refers to water retained within a fiber's structure without stress (Tungland and Meyer, 2002).

Many of the unit operations used to make food products exert physical stresses on the food system (e.g., processes such as extrusion, mixing, pumping). These processes can affect the amount of water retained by the fiber, possibly due to changes in the fiber's molecular structure. Processing can impact the stickiness of insoluble fibers in the dough of cereals due to its water-binding properties. Adding wheat bran to a cereal formula will increase the amount of water held by the ingredient vs. the remainder of the dough ingredients due to insoluble fiber present in the bran. This could require more water to be added in the cooking stage. More water at this stage can make the dough difficult to handle and physically move from the cooker to the next processing stage. The stickier dough can affect remaining unit operations. Hydrolyzed arabinoxylans are much more soluble than wheat bran and require less water at the dough stage, resulting in drier dough and more efficient processing downstream. Thus the properties of wheat bran and fibers may require processing and equipment modifications to achieve desired product attributes.

References

Antoine, C., Peyron, S., Lullien-Pellerin, V., Abecassis, J., and Rouau, X. 2004. Wheat bran tissue fraction using biochemical markers. *J. Cereal Sci.* 39: 387–393.

Antoine, C., Peyron, S., Mabille, F., Lapierre, C., Bouchet, B., Abecassis, J., and Rouau, X. 2003. Individual contribution of grain outer layers and their cell wall structure to the mechanical properties of wheat bran. *J. Agric. Food Sci.* 51: 2026-2033.

Beaugrand, J., Reis, D., Debeire, F., Guillon, P., and Chabbert, B. 2004. Xylanase mediated hydrolysis of wheat bran evidence for subcellular heterogeneity of cell walls. *Int. J. Plant Sci.* 165(4): 553–563.

Danish Institute for Food and Veterinary Research. 2005. www.foodcomp.dk.

Dikeman, C.L. and Fahey, G.C. 2006. Viscosity as related to dietary fiber: A review. *Crit. Rev. Food Sci. Nutr.* 46: 649–663.

Evers, A.D. and Reed, M. 1988. Some novel observations by scanning electron microscopy on the seed coat and nucellus of the mature wheat grain. *Cereal Chem.* 65: 81–85.

Fincher, G.B. and Stone, B.A. 1986. Cell walls and their components in cereal grains technology. In: *Advances in Cereal Science and Technology.* Y. Pomeranz, ed. AACC International, St. Paul, MN, pp. 207–295.

Fincher, G.B. and Stone, B.A. 2004. Chemistry of nonstarch polysaccharides. In: *Encyclopedia of Grain Science.* C. Wrigley, H. Corke, and C.E. Walker, eds. Elsevier, Oxford, U.K., pp. 206–223.

Food Standards Agency. 2002. *McClance and Widdowson's the Composition of Foods,* 6th edn. Royal Society of Chemistry, Cambridge, U.K.

Glenn, G.M. and Johnson, R.K. 1992. Moisture-dependent changes in mechanical properties of isolated wheat bran. *J. Cereal Sci.* 13: 223–236.

Hoseney, R.C. 1994. *Principles of Cereal Science and Technology.* AACC, St. Paul, MN.

Joyner, S.L. 1985. The histochemistry and ultrastructure of wheat aleurone cell wall. Master's thesis. La Trobe University, Melbourne, Victoria, Australia.

Kamal-Eldin, A., Lærke, H.N., Bach Knudsen, K.E., Lampi, A.M., Piironen, V., Adlercreutz, H., Katina, K., Poutanen, K., and Åman, P. 2009. Physical, microscopic and chemical characterisation of industrial rye and wheat brans from the Nordic countries. *Food Nutr. Res.* 53: 10.3402.

Khan, K. and Shewry, P.R. 2009. *Wheat Chemistry and Technology,* 4th edn. K. Khan and P.R. Shewry, eds. AACC International Inc., St. Paul, MN.

Marlett, J.A. and Navis, D. 1988. Comparison of gravimetric and chemical analyses of total dietary fiber in human foods. *J. Agric. Food Chem.* 36: 311–313.

National Food Administration (Sweden) 2004. www.slv.se.

National Public Health Institute of Finland. 2004. www.fineli.fi.

Oklahoma State University Digital Library. http://digital.library.okstate.edu/OAS/oas_image_files/v72/p51_56Fig1.jpg (accessed August 16, 2009).

Peyton, S. et al. 2002. Relationship between bran mechanical properties and the milling behavior of durum wheat (*Triticum durum* Desf.). Influence of tissue thickness and cell wall structure. *J. Cereal Sci.* 36: 377–386.

Piironnen, V. et al. 2002. Plant sterols in cereals and cereal products. *Cereal Chem.* 79(1): 148–154.

Ring, S. and Selvendran, R. 1980. Isolation and analysis of cell wall material from beeswing wheat bran. *Phytochemistry* 19: 1723–1730.

Ring, S.G. and Selvendran, R.R. 1980. Isolation and analysis of cell wall material from beeswing bran (*Triticum aestivum*). *Phytochemistry* 19: 1723–1730.

Selvendran, R.R., Ring, S.G., O'Neill, M.A., and Du Pont, M.S. 1980. Composition of cell wall material from wheat bran using in clinical feeding trials. *Chem. Ind.*, 22: 885–888.

Slavin, J.L., Martini, M.C., Jacobs, D.R., Jr., and Marquart, L. 1999. Plausible mechanisms for the protectiveness of whole grain. *Am. J. Clin. Nutr.* 70: 459S–463S.

Souci, S.W., Fachmann, W., and Kraut, H. 2000. *Food Composition and Nutrition Tables*, 6th edn. Medpharm Scientific Publishers, Stuttgart, Germany.

Swennen, K., Courtin, C., Lindemans, G., and Delcour, J. 2006. Large-scale production and characterization of wheat bran arabinoxylooligosaccharides. *J. Sci. Food Agric.* 86: 1722–1731.

Tungland, B.C. and Meyer, D. 2002. Nondigestible oligo- and polysaccharides (dietary fiber): Their physiology and role in human health and food. *Comp. Rev. Food Sci. Food Safety* 1: 73–92.

USDA Nutrient Database. 2010. http://www.nal.usda.gov

Ziegler, E. and Greer, E.N. 1971. *Wheat: Chemistry and Terminology*. Y. Pomeranz, ed. American Association of Cereal Chemists, St. Paul, MN.

27
Pectin

HANS ULRICH ENDRESS and FRANK MATTES

Contents

27.1 Technological Aspects

27.1.1 Introduction

Pectin is a well-known ingredient used to form gels and to stabilize acidified milk beverages, or it simply acts as a viscosifier in beverages. Pectin is classified as a dietary fiber since pectin is not digested by the human body and can be determined by the AOAC methods 985.29 and 991.43 [1]. The term protopectin is used to describe the native pectin in plant tissues that cannot be purified without using destructive methods. With cellulose, hemicelluloses, glycoproteins, and lignin, pectins form the cell walls of all higher plants. The concentration of pectin is highest in the middle lamella, which is a tissue that connects cells. In plant physiology, pectin takes part in water retention and ion transport and, therefore, is involved in the growth, size, and shape of cells. Pectin content is less concentrated in primary cell walls and almost absent in secondary cell walls [2].

27.1.2 Chemical Structure

Pectin is a polysaccharide consisting of galacturonic acid, which forms a linear chain by α-(1,4)-D glycosidic links. In the polygalacturonic acid chain, α-(1,2)-L-rhamnopyranose units are inserted, which form kinks interrupting the linear chain, resulting in a zigzag-shaped molecule. D-Galacturonic acid units are partially esterified with methanol so that a degree of esterification (DE) or degree of methylation (DM) can be defined. The DE is plant specific and is also influenced by pectin-degrading enzymes during the ripening process of fruits and vegetables by the action of pectinesterases. The DE can also be influenced during the extraction process of commercial pectin types. Per definition, pectins with a DE of higher than 50% are called high-methylester (HM) pectins and pectins with a lower DE than 50% are called low-methylester (LM) pectins. Unesterified pectin is called pectic acid and its salts, pectates. In most plants, HM pectin is found; pectins isolated from apples have a DE of up to 80%. In lemon fruits or sugar beets, pectin with lower DE is found: 75% and 60%, respectively. Sunflower heads contain pectin with a lower DE than 50%.

Also, the distribution of methylester is plant specific as plant pectinesterases de-esterify pectin blockwise during maturation. Pectin, which is de-esterified during the extraction process, has randomly distributed methylester groups. Pectins are rarely esterified with ethanol. Pectins in sugar beet plants have a high content of acetyl groups. Acetic acid is esterified mainly with C-2 and C-3 of the galacturonic acid units (Figure 27.1).

Bound to rhamnose units are so-called neutral sugar side chains consisting mainly of L-arabinose and D-galactose, which form complex structures. Pectins containing arabinan side chains can be isolated from many fruits and vegetables, such as apples, apricots, cabbage, carrots, onions, pears, and sugar beet. Arabinans are polysaccharides consisting of α-(1,5)-linked arabinofuranosyl units to which α-(1,2)- and α-(1,3)-linked arabinofuranosyl units are attached as side chains. In other plants, such as citrus fruits, grapes, onions, potatoes, soy beans, tomatoes,

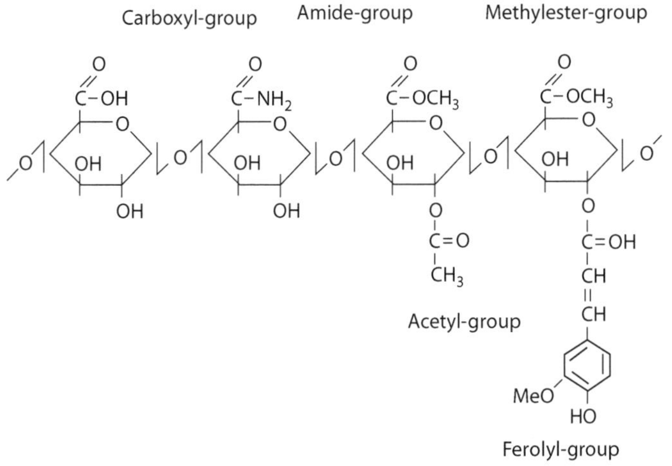
Carboxyl-group
Amide-group
Methylester-group
C-OH
C-NH2
C-OCH3
C-OCH3
OH
OH
OH
OH
OH
OH
C=O
CH3
C=OH
CH
CH
Acetyl-group
MeO
HO
Ferolyl-group

Figure 27.1 Substituents at the galacturonic acid main chain.

and apples, arabinogalactans containing heteropolysaccharide side chains with L-arabinose and L-galactose can be found. There are two structurally different arabinogalactans. Type 1 consists of an α-(1,4)-linked linear chain of D-galactopyranosyl residues with short chains of linear α-(1,5)-arabinans. Type 2 is a highly branched polysaccharide with ramified chains of α-(1,3)- and α-(1,6)-linked D-galactopyranosyl residues terminated by L-arabinofuranosyl and to a small extent by L-arabinopyranosyl residues. Other neutral sugars, such as D-xylose, D-glucose, D-mannose, and/or D-apiose, form single-unit side chains or short side chains. D-fucose can be found at the terminal end of sugar side chains. The distribution of rhamnose units is uneven. Areas having low rhamnose content are called homogalacturonan or smooth regions. Areas of high rhamnose content are named rhamnogalacturonan, and, because of being highly branched, these areas are also called hairy regions [3].

The molecular weight of pectin molecules depends on the type of plant and the maturation stage. It is influenced by pectin-degrading enzymes, such as polygalacturonase, which splits linkages between the galacturonosyl residues of the pectin main chain. Pectin with very high molecular weight is found in apples and in citrus fruits. Commercial pectin types that are used as gelling agent and thickener have a molecular weight of about 100,000 g/mol. For dietary fiber enhancement, pectin types with low molecular weight, such as 30,000 g/mol, are produced.

Not all galacturonic acid–containing polysaccharides can be called pectin. As food additive, the term pectin (INS No. 440; EEC No. E440 pectins with (i) pectin, (ii) amidated pectin; CAS number 9000-69-5; EINECS number 232-553-0) may only be used for polysaccharides containing at least 65% galacturonic acid [4–6]. According to the U.S. Pharmacopeia, pectin has to have a minimum content of galacturonic acid of at least 74% [7].

27.1.3 Physical Properties

Pectin is soluble in water but not soluble in organic solvents. By having carboxylic acid groups, pectin is a polyelectrolyte and a weak organic acid. Added to water, carboxylic acid groups dissociate and the pectin molecule becomes negatively charged. Pectin is very stable at acidic pHs ranging from pH 2.0 to 4.5. The stability of pectin also depends on the DE. At pH below 2, pectin is de-esterified and HM pectins turn into LM pectins. At pH higher than 4.5, pectin degrades by a process called β-elimination. In this reaction, the pectin chain is split next to methylester containing galacturonic acid units. β-elimination is a process driven by hydroxide ions leading to a stronger reaction at neutral pH value. LM pectins are more stable at higher pH than HM pectins. At very high pH, additional saponification occurs. Having no methylester groups, pectic acid and its salts show the highest stability.

Because of its molecular weight and molecular structure, pectin is capable of binding water. Pectin molecules also form convolutions due to the linear characteristic of the molecules and interactions between pectin molecules. This causes increased friction, leading to shear thinning flow behavior of pectin solutions when pectins with high molecular weight are used at high concentration. Diluted pectin solutions or pectin solutions made with low molecular weight pectin show Newtonian flow behavior. Divalent metal ions increase cross-linking of pectin molecules by interacting with carboxylic acid groups of the pectin molecules, leading to increase of viscosity. Interactions with divalent metal ions are also possible when HM pectins with a block-wise distribution of nonesterified carboxylic acid groups are used.

The most important commercial application of pectin is gelation. Under certain conditions, pectin forms a three-dimensional network that is stabilized by interactions between pectin molecules. A minimum concentration of the pectin is necessary for initiating the gelation process. Molecular structure, concentration and type of total soluble solids, pH value, ionic strength, valency and kind of ions, and temperature of the manufacturing process are important factors influencing the gelation process and pectin concentration needed to set [8–10]. The gel structure is formed during cooling down from high temperature in which the product is in a sol status. Gel formation is turning a liquid sol into a solid structure. The point at which a structure is formed is characteristic to a certain temperature, which can be defined as setting temperature. The setting temperature of pectin gels is highly influenced by the pectin type, pH value, content of total soluble solids, and divalent metal ions and is partly influenced by ionic strength, type of total soluble solids, pectin dosage, etc.

A reason for commercially distinguishing HM pectin from LM pectin is their different ability to form gels for different application areas. HM pectins form gels at total soluble solids higher than 55% and pH below 3.5. Junction zones stabilizing the gel structure are formed by hydrophobic interactions between methylester groups and hydrogen bonds between hydroxyl groups. Therefore,

HM pectins are used as gelling agent for traditional jams, jellies, and marmalades. The addition of total soluble solids reduces the water activity for making a shelf-stable product but also reduces the firm hydrate cover surrounding pectin molecules. Acidic conditions are required to reduce the dissociation of the carboxylic acid groups, reducing the negative charge density of pectin molecules. By reducing negative charge density, repulsion of pectin molecules is reduced, and once attracting forces grow stronger than repelling forces, junction zones are formed. In the food industry, this is achieved by adding acidifying ingredients, such as citric acid or lemon juice.

LM pectin is able to form gels relatively independent from the content of total soluble solids content and pH by forming junction zones under the influence of divalent metal ions. LM pectins may find enough ions to establish firm junction zones already present or ions, such as calcium ions, are added separately to the system. Due to the glycosidic bonds of the galacturonic acid units, a folded structure of the pectin molecules forms. As a result, two galacturonic acid units form a hollow body. A positively charged calcium ion can be imbedded into the hollow body which reduces the negative charge density. Sterically seen, only 50% of the size of the calcium ion is imbedded, allowing another pectin molecule to attach to the calcium ion. In these hollow spaces, calcium ions are bound as metal complexes. The calcium content and the affinity of the pectin molecules to divalent metal ions influence the gel strength. The affinity of pectin to divalent metal ions depends on the amount of free carboxylic acid groups, so that typically low methylester shows interactions with calcium ions. HM pectins can also interact with calcium ions if they have areas that have several consecutive free carboxylic acid groups, such as HM citrus pectin. The amount of calcium needed to form gels increases with reduced content of total soluble solids, increasing pH, and increasing ionic strength. Higher concentration of calcium ions is also needed when products are made with sugar alcohols than with sucrose as total soluble solids.

A gel is formed during the cooling process at a certain temperature called the setting temperature. The setting temperature can be measured by an oscillating rheometer, and it is influenced besides by the pectin type especially by pH value, content of total soluble solids, and calcium content. The setting temperature depends on the DE, and it is reduced from high DE to 60% DE, and setting temperature increases again when the DE is further decreased. Due to their different setting temperatures and therefore different setting speeds, respectively, setting time of HM pectins can be classified as rapid set, medium rapid set, to extra slow set pectin. The setting temperature is increased by decreasing the pH and/or increasing total soluble solids and/or the calcium content (LM pectins) in the final product. Filling temperature has to be higher than setting temperature. If products are deposited below setting temperature, an irregular, softer gel is formed with a rough gel structure, usually unwanted besides for bake-stable fruit preparations.

27.1.4 Commercial Pectin

Pectin is produced by extraction from plant sources, and despite the wide occurrence of pectin in nature, only a few materials are used as sources for manufacturing of commercial pectin. Citrus peels, apple pomace, and sugar beet pulp are commercially used for the pectin production. These materials are occurring after juice or sugar production. To get storable and transportable conditions, citrus peels, apple pomace, and sugar beet pulp are immediately dried after processing. Citrus peels are additionally washed to prevent browning and to separate citrus oil. Citrus pectin is also produced from fresh processed citrus peels in citrus growing areas. The yield of citrus pectin from dried peels and apple pomace are approximately 30% and 15% pectin, respectively.

In the manufacturing process, a pectin-containing extract is produced by treating the raw material with inorganic acid at elevated temperature. Under these conditions, the bonds of the neutral sugar side chains that bind the pectin molecule to the cell wall network are clinched, releasing the molecule into the aqueous solution. In the next steps, the pectin-containing extract is separated from the insoluble raw material, which mainly contains cellulose, followed by clarification and concentration. Pectin is isolated by alcoholic precipitation. The alcohol–water mixture is separated from the precipitated pectin, which is then dried, ground, and sieved to defined particle size. Pectin with different degrees of esterification (DEs) can be obtained by adjusting the extraction conditions accordingly. Another possibility is to use extracted HM pectin, which is in a second step de-esterified under acidic conditions. A de-esterification process under alkaline condition with ammonia is used to introduce amide groups.

Pectin extracted from apple pomace or citrus peel typically has high molecular weight and high water-binding capacity. Pectin in sugar beet pulp naturally has a lower molecular weight than pectin made from apple pomace or citrus peels. Pectins with reduced molecular weight, hence reduced viscosity, can be produced besides from poorer raw material by ball milling or treating pectin with oxidizing agents. By treating pectin with pectin esterase (PE; EC 3.1.1.11) and/or endopolygalacturonase (endo-PG; EC 3.2.1.15), pectins with reduced DE and/or reduced molecular weight are obtained.

27.2 Nutritional Aspects

27.2.1 Metabolism of Pectin

Pectin is not digested by the human body; there are no enzymes excreted that are able to degrade the molecule. However, certain bacteria of the gut flora are able to use pectin as substrate. Without the fermentation process (see also Sections 27.2.2 and 27.2.3), pectin would pass almost unchanged through the digestive system. Pectin is quite stable under the acidic conditions of the stomach, although a slight de-esterification process occurs. In patients with an ileum syrinx, applied pectins were recovered from 100% to only 70%. But studies have also excluded fermentation at this early stage of digestion.

Pectins reduce amylase activity by 10%–40%, lipase activity by 40%–80%, and trypsin activity by 15%–80% [12–16]. The activity of pancreatic enzymes is reduced by an increase of viscosity of the digestive fluids, which reduces the contacts between enzymes and substrates. Pectin may also inhibit enzyme activity, such as lipase [17,18], by interacting with substrates inhibiting the adsorption of enzyme to the substrate. The inhibitory activity of the high-molecular-weight fraction (>300.000 g/mol) was strongest and much stronger than that of commercial citrus pectin [19].

There are reports that pectins influence the bioavailability of nutrients; the bioavailability of quercetin was increased in rats consuming the diet containing apple pectin for 6 weeks. The increase in quercetin absorption might be attributed to alteration of the absorptive capacity of the small intestine through apple pectin–induced improvement of its morphological and physiological properties [20].

27.2.2 Fermentation of Pectin

Fermentation of pectin mainly occurs in the cecum, colon ascendens, and colon. Microorganisms such as *Bacteroides*, *E. coli*, *Lactobacillus*, and *Bifidobacterium* are able to use pectin as substrate, and these organisms are able to degrade pectin by 90%–95% [21,22]. When grown on a mixture of polysaccharides, *Bacteroides ovatus* preferred to utilize starch and pectin, which showed that these carbohydrates are important substrates for the bacterium located in the large intestine [23]. Pectin degradation increases with decreasing DE [24] and duration of adaptation time [25].

Products of the fermentation process in the human body are the short-chain fatty acids (SCFA)—acetate, propionate, and butyrate (a molar proportion of 84:14:2 was reported [26,27])—and gases like methane, carbon dioxide, and hydrogen. The pectin concentration seems to have an influence on the molar proportion of SCFA. At low pectin concentration (2.5 mg/mL), the molar proportion of SCFA of 81:10:9 was formed. At high pectin concentrations (30 mg/mL), a molar proportion of 74:7:20 was formed [28]. Homogenates of human feces were incubated anaerobically with pectin, resulting in an increase of SCFA by 6.5 mmol/g pectin or 1.05 mol/mol hexose equivalents [29]. Pectin might be partially fermented to oligogalacturonic acid with different degrees of polycondensation (degree of polymerization, DP). Nonreducing ends of these oligomers can bear Δ-4, 5-double bonds due to β-elimination or by action of pectin and pectate lyases. By incubating pectic acid with human feces galacturonic acid, Δ-4, 5-unsaturated di- and trigalacturonic acids were formed with digalacturonic acid as the main product [30]. The respective enzymes were also found in animal feces [31–33]. Products obtained by further degradation of galacturonic acid were furan-2,5-dicarbonic acid and galactaric acid, which further are transformed into acetoacetic acid. Pectin with lower DE showed increased formation of SCFA [34]. The pectin-fed rats showed increased ileum, cecum, and colon weights. Also during in vitro fermentation of pectin with fecal flora obtained from rats, unsaturated oligogalacturonic acids were formed, and pectin with lower DE was fermented faster than pectin with higher DE. Pectin-fed rats also showed increased total bacterial population in the cecum as well as increased weight of cecal wall and its contents [35].

27.2.3 Prebiotic Nature

Strains of bifidobacteria are able to ferment pectin by 10% [36]. However, not all bifidobacteria are able to utilize pectin [37]. *Bifidobacterium pseudolongum* P6, which was isolated from rabbit cecum, fermented pectin via a modified Entner–Doudoroff pathway. Pectin was degraded by extracellular endopolygalacturonase. The enzyme 2-keto-3-deoxy-6-phosphogluconate (KDPG) aldolase (EC 4.1.2.14) has an important role in the fermentation process of pectin. KPDG aldolase activity has been seen in pectin-fermenting organisms, such as *Treponema saccharophilum* [38], *Butyrivibrio fibrosolvens*, *Prevotella ruminicola* [39], and *Lachnospira multiparus* [40], while no KPDG activity was seen in cell extracts obtained from Bifidobacterium species or *Streptococcus bovis* [37] that are not able to utilize pectin. *Bifidobacterium pseudolongum* P6 fermented pectin to acetate, lactate, succinate, and ethanol (3.22 ± 0.23; 6.01 ± 0.64; 1.58 ± 0.25; 0.66 ± 0.10; 0.32 ± 0.10; mmol/g pectin). In the fermentation process, no carbon dioxide was formed. *Bifidobacterium lactis* showed good growth rates with HM pectin as substrate. LM pectins were better growing media than HM pectin for *Bifidobacterium pseudolongum*, *B. bifidum* Bb12, *Lactobacillus plantarum* 0207, *L. casei shirota*, and *L. acidophilus*. *Bifidobacterium angulatum* and *B. infantis* were not able to utilize HM pectin but were able to ferment LM pectin. Comparing different pectin types, greater fermentation selectivity was seen with decreasing DE as well as reduced molecular weight [41].

27.2.4 Role of Pectin in Weight Management

It has been reported that consuming 36 g pectin per day increased excretion of fatty acids by 80% [42]. Pectins decrease bile acid concentration in the small intestine. If the bile acid concentration is too low, fat absorption is significantly reduced, so that pectin is recommended as a useful adjuvant in the treatment of disorders related to overeating [43]. With results of other studies conducted with the U.S. Army using HM apple pectin, it was concluded that pectin may have an important adjunct role in human nutrition and especially in obese persons [44].

Another hint for the role of pectin in weight management might come from studies with HIV-positive patients [45]. Lipodystrophy has been described with increasing frequency in patients infected with HIV. Differences in the diets of HIV-positive men who developed fat deposition and those who did not were studied. The patients who did not develop fat deposition had overall greater energy intake and greater consumption of total protein, total dietary fiber, soluble fiber, insoluble fiber, and pectin than patients who developed fat deposition. Also, the addition of low-viscosity pectin to low-calorie beverages reduced energy intakes at next meal, presenting a possible tool for intake regulation. A short time interval between consumption of a low-calorie beverage and a meal also increased satiety and decreased food intake, reflecting the short-lived effect of volume [46].

Pectin may play a role in weight management by promoting delayed gastric emptying [47–50], increased mouth–cecum transit time, binding high amounts of water into a gel matrix, prolonging the feeling of satiety, reduction of food consumption, delayed/reduced resorption of nutrients [51], reduced formation of enzyme–nutrient complexes [52–55], reduced degradation and digestion of macromolecules [55], and increasing of unstirred water layer [56]. Pectin and pectin containing systems can partially replace sugar or fat as bulking agent for developing calorie-reduced food.

27.2.5 Affinity to Metal Ions and Excretion of Toxic Metals

As a polyelectrolyte, pectin is able to bind and exchange cations. The stability of the respective complexes is significant for the type of cation [57–63]. Sodium pectinate has different affinity to metal ions and forms strongest complexes with lead [56]. Metal ions can be bound intermolecularly between two pectin molecules as well as intramolecularly. The affinity of pectin to metal ions is influenced by the DE [60,62,63], distribution of free carboxylic acid groups [64], pH [65–67], ionic strength and concentration, and affinity of other present cations.

Supplemented pectin had no negative effect in short-term studies with humans [68–71] on Fe, Cu, and Zn balances. Similar results were seen in studies lasting 5–6 weeks on Ca and Mg levels [42,72]. Also in studies with workers who were exposed to high levels of lead showed no significant change of Cu, Fe, Mg, and Zn when they took 8 g/day pectin over a period of 6 weeks in order to increase excretion of lead by binding to pectin [73]. Excretion of other toxic metal ions was also increased by pectins [74–80].

27.2.6 Influence of Pectin on Jejunal and Ileal Morphology

Pectin influences morphology and ultrastructure of the intestines [81–83]. The effects of pectin on jejunal and ileal morphology were studied with adult male mice fed a semisynthetic diet containing 8% cellulose or pectin for 30 days. No significant differences in the jejunal villus height between the two groups were found, but the jejunal crypt depth and both the ileal villus height and crypt depth of the mice fed the pectin diet were significantly greater than those of the mice fed the cellulose diet. Numerous intercellular spaces were observed in the jejunal absorptive cells of the mice fed the pectin diet, but not the cellulose diet. Moreover, the ileal absorptive cells of mice fed the pectin diet contained numerous peroxisomes, whereas there were few in these cells of mice fed the cellulose diet [81].

27.3 Medical Aspects

27.3.1 Reduction of Symptoms of Dumping, Short Bowel Syndrome, and Short Gut Syndrome

There are reports that individuals with severe dumping syndrome may respond to agents such as pectin, which increase the viscosity of intraluminal contents [84–89]. Pectin significantly increased stool solidity and improved colonic water absorption following resection without significantly altering mucosal structure [90]. Patients with reduced length of remaining small bowel after bowel surgery due to mesenteric thrombosis or Crohn's disease responded well to the approach of a pectin-supported diet program instead of total parenteral nutrition [91]. Pectin supplementation to the enteral feed also increased nitrogen absorption and prolonged stomach-to-anus transit time in a 3-year-old boy with short gut syndrome [92].

27.3.2 Effects on Acute Intestinal Infections

Patients who receive tube-feeding formulas very often show diarrhea. By adding pectin to these formulas, getting liquid stools is significantly reduced, and a normalization of colonic fluid composition can be achieved [93]. This was also achieved when tube-fed patients receiving antibiotics additionally were fed with pectin [94]. Clinical studies showed that pectin has the potential to reduce acute intestinal infections by inhibiting the growth of *Shigella*, *Salmonella*, *Klebsiella*, *Enterobacter*, *Proteus*, and *Citrobacter*. A rapid suppression of diarrhea and other symptoms of acute infections was observed in pectin-supplemented infants and children [95–97].

27.3.3 Effects on Atherosclerosis

An important risk factor for atherosclerosis, stroke, and coronary heart disease is fibrinogen, not only its concentration; it is also believed that the quality of fibrin networks may be an important risk factor for the development of coronary heart disease. The risk is increased with high serum cholesterol level. Coronary heart disease and stroke caused by atherosclerosis and its related problems of hyperinsulinemia, hyperlipidemia, and hypertension are strongly related to the diet [98]. In a study with two groups of 10 male hyperlipidemic volunteers, the effect of pectin on fibrinogen and fibrinogen network was studied. For 4 weeks, each volunteer of one group received a pectin supplement of 15 g pectin per day and the effects compared to the group that received a placebo were studied. The group that received pectin supplementation showed significant decrease in total cholesterol, LDL, and apolipoproteins A and B. Also, the fibrin network became more permeable, and it had lower tensile strength, which is believed to be less atherogenic. In this study, it was suspected that pectin modified network characteristics by a combination of its effects on metabolism and altered fibrin conversion. An in vivo study comparing the effect of pectin with acetate showed that acetate, which is also formed in the fermentation of pectin, may be responsible in part for the pectin supplementation. Fibrinogen levels in the acetate group remained almost unchanged, and like the pectin group, fibrin networks were more permeable, had lower tensile strength, and were more lyseable [99].

In the Los Angeles Atherosclerosis Study [100], the intima-media thickness (IMT) of the common carotid arteries in humans (aged 40–60 years, $n = 573$) in 47% of women was measured ultrasonographically. A significant inverse association was observed between IMT progression and the intakes of viscous fiber ($P = 0.05$) and pectin ($P = 0.01$). The ratio of total to HDL cholesterol was inversely related to the intakes of total dietary fiber ($P = 0.01$), viscous fiber ($P = 0.05$), and pectin ($P = 0.01$). The intake of viscous fiber, especially pectin, appears to protect against IMT progression. Serum lipids may act as a mediator between dietary fiber intake and IMT progression.

Frequent and long-lasting high insulin concentrations promote vascular lesions, which are the primary stadium of atherosclerosis. Suppression of postprandial insulin levels by pectins may therefore have an antiatherogenic effect [101]. Dietary fibers like pectin may also increase peripheral insulin sensitivity in young and old adults [102].

27.3.4 Effects on Cholesterol and Lipid Metabolism

Pectin increases the viscosity of the chymus, leading to a reduced turnover of large molecules, such as fat molecules, bile acid, cholesterol, etc. With low-density lipoproteins (LDL), pectin forms complexes, which leads to a reduction of lipid resorption and an increased excretion of lipid with the pectin molecules. It has been seen that the interaction is electrostatic [103] and the binding of LDL is depending on the DE of pectin. HM pectin can bind LDL by the ratio of 1:4, whereas LM pectin is able to bind less LDL [104]. The positive influence of pectin was already described in 1961. It has been shown that consuming food containing pectin leads to serum LDL cholesterol reduction [105]. Most studies carried out with a wide variety of subjects and experimental conditions showed the potential of cholesterol reduction by consuming 6–15 g pectin per day [104–120]. Pectins have almost no influence on the level of high-density lipoproteins (HDL), leading to a healthier LDL:HDL ratio.

DE of pectin can impact cholesterol-lowering ability of pectin. Studies [121] indicating that a minimum DE of 10% is needed for a pectin to have cholesterol-reducing properties were not able to be reproduced [116]. Studies published since 1985 are summarized in Table 27.1.

Table 27.1 Influence of Pectins on Lipid Metabolism

References	Subjects	Time	Pectin g/Day +a, b, c	Cholesterol, mg/dL			
				Total	LDL	HDL	TG
Schuderer [122]	30 c	3 weeks	20	−17	−21	+4	n.d.
	15 s	3 weeks	20	−12	−14	+12	n.d.
Cerda et al. [123]	27?	4 weeks	15	−15	n.d.	n.d.	n.d.
Grudeva [124]	54	90 days	15 + a	−34.4	n.d.	+24.6	−24.6
	55			−34.5	n.d.	+34.0	−26.2
Grudeva et al. [125]	47	90 days	15 + b	−36	−23.5	+36.3	−18.8
Veldman et al. [98,99]	10	4 weeks	15	−11,6	−11.5	+21.3	n.d.
Bartz et al. [126]	40	4 weeks	10 + c	−44	−45.5	+14	−55

c, controlled; s, self-served; n.d., not determined.
a = +sorbitol 1:1 b = +sorbitol 2:1 c = 1,5 g omega-3 fatty acid.

Synergistic effects on reducing cholesterol with other substances were found; by combining the dose of 15 g pectin with 20 g fish oil per day, the cholesterol ester fraction of plasma lipids was reduced further by 44% [127]. Another beneficial effect was a 30% decline in the fatty acid fraction. Studies with rats showed an increased reduction of plasma cholesterol and plasma triglycerides by combining apple pectin with polyphenols from apples [128].

A meta-analysis also showed that increasing the pectin dosage to more than 10 g per day did not further improve the effects [129]. Pectin was more efficacious than other soluble fibers, such as psyllium, oat products, and guar, in the reduction of cholesterol (Table 27.2; [99,130,131]).

Regarding the effectiveness of pectin, it appears that high molecular weight or high viscosity has a minor influence on the cholesterol-reducing properties of pectin. The ability to form hydrophobic interaction seems to be more important. In a study with several sugar beet pectins, the beet pectin, which was deacetylated and had a low molecular weight, showed highest cholesterol reduction. Sugar beet pectin with reduced neutral sugar content showed lowest cholesterol reduction.

Table 27.2 Effect of Various Soluble Fibers on Blood Lipid Profiles

Soluble Dietary Fibers	Number of Studies	Participants	Change per g Fiber (mg/dL)
Cholesterol			
Oat products	26	1600	−1.43
Psyllium	17	757	−1.08
Pectin	7	277	−2.71
Guar	17	341	−1,00
LDL cholesterol			
Oat products	22	1439	−1.23
Psyllium	17	757	−1.12
Pectin	4	117	−2.13
Guar	12	218	−1.28
HDL cholesterol			
Oat products	24	1542	−0.07
Psyllium	17	757	−0.07
Pectin	7	277	0.14
Guar	15	302	−0.11
Triglycerides			
Oat products	20	1374	+0.7
Psyllium	16	720	+0.3
Pectin	6	247	−1.8
Guar	17	338	−0.9

Source: Brown, et al., *Am. J. Clin. Nutr.,* 69, 30, 1999.

However, apple pectin with high methylester content and high viscosity showed strongest cholesterol reduction in this study [132]. Other studies showed that molecular weights and the fermentability of pectin to SCFA are important factors for cholesterol reduction [133]. The addition of pectin also increased the activity of cholesterol-7-α-hydroxylase in rats. This enzyme activates bile acid synthesis from cholesterol and might also lead to a reduction of the level of LDL [134].

27.3.5 Effects on Glucose Metabolism

Blood glucose level is strongly affected by carbohydrate-rich food and causes a peaking glycemic response. Because of gel formation and increasing chymus viscosity, pectin delays the absorption of glucose and other monosaccharides, as well as reduction of degradation of complex carbohydrates. Pure pectin has a glycemic index of almost zero. Sugar, which is added to standardize commercial food grade pectin, increases the glycemic index, respectively. This also means that pectin and other soluble fibers reduce the glycemic index in case of combined consumption. Studies showed that pectin lowers blood glucose and insulin levels after consuming carbohydrate-rich food. A summary is shown in Table 27.3 [135–146].

In a test with diabetics and nondiabetic consumers, pectin flattened the glycemic response and reduced the insulin demand for both groups. That led to less urinary glucose loss and improved control of diabetes [147].

Several studies suggested that the addition of pectin as a gel and viscosity providing soluble fiber has an influence on the unstirred water layer, which reduced the absorption of large molecules such as fatty acids or glucose. With increasing pectin dosage, the unstirred water expanded, resulting in reduced absorption of glucose and fatty acids [148,149].

Gastric inhibitory polypeptide, which reduces gastric motility and insulin secretion, is reduced by pectin [150,151]. There are indications that gastric motility has an influence on gastric emptying half-time. Insulin reduction could result in reduced activity of α-hydroxy-α-methylglutaryl (HMG)-CoA-reductase. HMG-CoA-reductase is involved in an early step of the endogenous cholesterol synthesis. Since its activity also depends on insulin concentration, cholesterol level could be reduced.

27.3.6 Anticarcinogenic Effects of Pectin

Studies investigating the effects of pectin on carcinogenesis show benefits of pectin. The diet supplemented with 20% apple pectin and 20% citrus pectin significantly reduced azoxymethane-induced colon carcinogenesis [152,153]. Diet supplemented by 20% apple pectin also decreased the number of tumors in 1, 2 dimethylhydrazine-induced colon carcinogenesis [154,155]. These studies showed that pectin significantly lowered fecal glucuronidase activities at the initiation stage group and prostaglandin E2 (PGE2) level in distal colonic mucosa. Glucuronidase is considered a key enzyme in the metabolism and carcinogenic activation of 1, 2 dimethylhydrazine in the colonic lumen. The ability of apple pectin to decrease PGE2 was dose dependent [153]. Studies concluded that pectin and its fermentation products,

Table 27.3 Effects of Pectins on Serum Glucose and Serum Insulin

References	Subjects	Amount Pectin Added in g	Time Interval (min) of Significant Decrease of Serum Glucose	Serum Insulin
Jenkins et al. [135]	8 d	10	30–90	30–120
	3 i	10	30–120	—
Jenkins et al. [136]	13 n	10	At 15 min n.s. 30–90	15–45
Leeds et al. [84]	5 g dumping syndrome	10,5	At 30 min improved retention of load in stomach	—
Jenkins et al. [137]	6 d	14,5	n.s.	n.s.
Monnier et al. [138]	6 d	9/sq. m[a]	30–60	n.s.
Holt et al. [47]	6 n	14,5	30–45	—
Labayle et al. [139]	23 g	10–20	At 30 min	—
Labayle et al. [139]	3 h	5	Hypoglycemia Overted	—
Vaaler et al. [140]	8 i	15	15–90	—
Poynard et al. [141]	7 i	7	60–90	>180 min
Gold et al. [142]	6 n	10	n.s.	n.s.
Gold et al. [142]	6 n	10	60–90	n.s.
Williams et al. [143]	13 d	10	At 60 min	n.s.
Kanter et al. [144]	5 n, 6 o, 5 d	10 + guar	Significant decrease in all but greatest change in obese and diabetic subjects	
Schwartz et al. [48]	7 n	20	n.s.	—

d, diabetics; n, normal subjects; g, gastric surgery; h, hypoglycemic; o, obese; i, insulin-dependent diabetics; n.s., not significant.

[a] Square meter body surface.

such as butyrate, are important contributing factors to the protective effects of fruits against colon cancer [157]. Increased apoptosis frequency or increased apoptotic indexes are also identified as protective factors [156,157]. A pectin-enriched diet induced upregulation of active caspase-1 (20 kDa) and caspase-3 precursor in rats that have been treated with DMH [157]. Inhibition of galectin expression is known to be an antiproliferative factor of citrus pectin [158].

The application and production of modified citrus pectin are also described in several patents. Patent EP 0 716 605 B1 (WO 95/07084), a carrot soup, describes using α-1, 4-galacturonic acid units derived from pectin with a DE of 20%–80% [159]. Other patents are WO 01/60378 A2 [160] and WO 02/42484 [161] and claim different activity mechanisms. However, in common are a rather low DP and a content of unsaturated galacturonides.

27.4 Application of Pectin in Food Products

27.4.1 Fruit Spreads

Fruit spreads are a traditional application for pectin as commercial pectin is used to supplement naturally occurring pectin in fruit. In these products, typically HM pectin is used with a dosage of 0.1%–0.4%. Pectin dosage depends on the used type of fruit product and the fruit type itself. Gel-forming properties of pectin depend on the amount of total soluble solids present in the finished product and the pH of the fruit spread. HM pectin forms gels at a total soluble solids content of at least 60°Brix and a pH value of below pH 3.4. Fruit spreads that have a reduced content of sugar are manufactured with LM conventional or LM amidated pectins. The pectin dosage lies in a range of 0.6%–1.2% and depends highly on the amount of sugar that is used. By using commercial pectin, it is possible to create a variety of different textures. Apple pectin will provide a smooth gelled texture, whereas gels with a brittle texture are obtained once citrus pectin is used.

27.4.2 Industrial Fruit Preparations

Pectin provides the desired texture of the fruit preparation and thermal stability once the product passes through the baking process. Depending on firmness and required baking stability in bakery fillings up to 1.5%, pectin is used. In dairy fruit preparations, typically LM pectin is used. Such a pectin forms shear thinning gel textures, which is an important quality aspect as shear thinning ensures maintaining fruit integrity without the tendency to form syneresis. Additionally, good mixing behavior with the dairy product is seen to maintain mouthfeel and stability. The usage level is between 0.5% and 1.5% and depends mostly on the content of total soluble solids in the fruit preparation. Molecular-weight-reduced pectin can be added to fruit preparations to increase the respective product with soluble dietary fiber.

27.4.3 Confectionery Articles

Pectin is used as a gelling agent for a variety of confectionery products. It is possible to produce acidic fruit jellies with firm and brittle texture and also products with a gummy texture. Also, aerated products can be manufactured using pectin as gelling agent. Typically, HM pectins are used that have been standardized to constant setting temperature in order to prevent pregelling. In order to standardize the production of confectionery products, buffer salts that have retarding properties, such as sodium citrate, are added to the manufacturing process. For manufacturing fruit jellies, 1.3%–1.7% pectin is used, and, with a dosage of about 2.5%, products with a gummy texture are obtained.

27.4.4 Dairy Products

Low-fat or fat-free fermented dairy products, such as yogurt, fresh cheese, etc., might lack mouthfeel and viscosity. LM pectin or LM amidated pectin is used to enhance firmness, mouthfeel, and transport stability with a dosage of 0.2%.

In the manufacturing process, pectin is added to nonfermented milk before homogenizing. Low methylester can be used as gelling agent for dairy dessert products. HM pectin has the ability to stabilize protein at acidic conditions. It is now widely used to stabilize acidified milk drinks, yogurt smoothies, and soy beverages. The amount of pectin that is used depends on the amount of protein that has to be stabilized and the pH of the finished product. Within the pH range of 4.0–4.2, a strong stabilization is seen, so that it is possible to run the beverage through heat treatment for producing a product with long shelf life.

27.4.5 Beverages and Sorbet

Low-calorie soft drinks or juice drinks show a lack of mouthfeel because of the use of nonnutritive high-intensity sweeteners. By adding HM pectin, the viscosity and mouthfeel of low-calorie beverages will be enhanced. The enhanced aroma transfer will create a better impression of the intensive flavor. To create a juicy mouthfeel, a pectin dosage of 0.1% is used. HM pectin also stabilizes pulp particles of juices and juice drinks. The addition of a large amount of pectin with high molecular weight results in full-bodied products, thus limiting the amount of pectin for this application. Low-molecular-weight pectin can be used in beverages that contain 3% soluble fiber. In sorbets, HM pectin is used to provide mouthfeel, and, with strong water binding, pectin controls the growth of large ice crystals. Typically, 0.5% pectin is used in sorbet products.

27.4.6 Condiments and Spreads

Tomato sauces often need to be thickened, and pectin is a suitable ingredient. Medium-methylester and LM pectins give similar textures as the natural tomato pectin. Between 0.6% and 1.0% pectin is used to thicken tomato-based sauces. Condiments, like mint sauce or other fruit condiments, can also be textured with pectin. Fat-reduced spreads have relative high water content. Pectin is able to thicken the water phase of fat-reduced spreads in order to obtain a stable emulsion. Depending on the fat content, either HM pectin or LM pectin is used.

27.4.7 Bakery Products and Cereal Products

With its high water-binding property, pectin is suitable to be used in bakery products to control moisture content. By using about 0.1% high-molecular-weight pectin, stalling is reduced, which increases the shelf life of bakery items, such as rolls. The properties of high-molecular-weight pectin limit the amount of pectin that can be added to dough, but molecular-weight-reduced pectin offers possibilities to enhance items with soluble fiber or be part of a dietary fiber blend. With its water-binding properties, pectin can play a distinctive role in obtaining the desired dough rheology. Pectin can also be used to enhance the soluble fiber content of pasta and cereal products.

References

1. AOAC, Methods 985.29 and 991.43, *Official Methods of Analysis,* 17th edn., Horwith, W., AOAC International, Gaithersburg, MD, 2000.
2. Northcote DH, Control of pectin synthesis and deposition during plant cell wall growth. In: Fishman, M.L. and J.J. Jen, Eds. *Chemistry and Function of Pectins,* ACS Symposium Series 310, American Chemical Society, Washington, DC, 1986, p. 134.
3. Schols HA and Voragen AGJ, The chemical structure of pectins. In: Seymour, G.B. and J.P. Knox, Eds. *Pectins and Their Manipulation,* Blackwell Publishing, Oxford, U.K., 2002, pp. 1–29.
4. Commission Directive 98/86/EC from 11. November 1998; *Official Journal of the European Communities,* 09.12.1998 Pectin (E 440i), Amidated Pectins (E 440ii); pp. L 334/24-L334/25.
5. Compendium on Food Additive Specifications, Joint FAO/WHO Expert Committee on Food Additives, 71st Meeting 2009, FAO JECFA Monographs 7, ISSN 1817-7077, Pectins, Food and Agricultural Organization of the United Nations, Rome, Italy, 2009, pp. 75–80.
6. FCC, *Committee on Food Chemicals Codex,* 5th edn., National Academy Press Washington, DC, 2003.
7. United States Pharmacopeial Convention, *United States Pharmacopeia 34—National Formulary 29 (USP 34-NF29),* ISBN: 9783769253900, 2010, pp. 3831–3833.
8. Kratz E, Factors influencing the behavior of apple pectin as gelling agent, thickening agent and stabilizer in dairy products. *Food Ingredients Europe Conference Proceedings—1989.* Expoconsult Publishers, Maarson, NL, 1989, pp. 118–123.
9. Garnier C, Axelos MAV, and Thibault JF, Phase diagrams of pectin calcium systems: Influence of pH, ionic strength, and temperature on the gelation of pectins with different degree of methylation, *Carbohydrate Res.* 1993, 240, 219.
10. Endress HU, Mattes F, Norz K, Pectins. In: Hui, Y.H., Ed. *Handbook of Food Science, Technology, and Engineering—Volume 3,* CRC Press, Boca Raton, FL, 2006, pp. 140-1–140-30.
11. Walzel E, Einfluss ausgewählter Ballaststoffe auf den Mineralstoffwechsel. In: Schulze, J., and W. Bock, Eds. *Aktuelle Aspekte der Ballaststofforschung,* Behr's Verlag, Hambur, Germany, 1993, pp. 239–275.
12. Isaksson G, Lundquist I, Akesson B, and Ihse I, Influence of dietary fiber on intestinal activities of pancreatic enzymes and on fat absorption in man, Digestion 1982b, 25, 39.
13. Isaksson G, Lundquist I, and Ihse I, Effect of dietary fiber on pancreatic enzyme activity in vitro, *Gastroenterology* 1982a, 82, 918–924.
14. Dutta S and Hlasko J, Dietary fiber in pancreatic disease: Effect of high fiber on fat malabsorption in pancreatic insufficiency and in vitro study on the interaction of dietary fiber and pancreatic enzymes, *Am. J. Clin. Nutr.* 1985, 41, 517–525.
15. Hansen WE, Effect of dietary fiber on pancreatic lipase activity in vitro, *Pancreas* 1987, 2(2), 195–98.
16. Hansen WE, Effect of dietary fiber on proteolytic pancreatic enzymes in vitro, *Int. J. Pancreatol.* 1986, 1(5–6), 341–351.
17. Tsujita T, Sumiyosh M, Han LK, Fujiwara T, Tsujita J, and Okuda H, Inhibition of lipase activities by citrus pectin, *J. Nutr. Sci. Vitaminol.* 2003, 49(5), 340–345.
18. Tsujita J, Tsujita T, Fujiwara T, Okamoto A, Hamada S, Kikuchi S, Fujii Y, and Nomura A, Health food containing pectins, inhibiting lipase activity, JP Patent 2002, 199534.
19. Edashige Y, Murakami N, and Tsujita T, Inhibitory effect of pectin from the segment membrane of citrus fruits on lipase activity, *J. Nutr. Sci. Vitaminol. (Tokyo)* 2008, 54(5), 409–415.
20. Nishijima T, Iwai K, Saito Y, Takida Y, and Matsue H, Chronic ingestion of apple pectin can enhance the absorption of quercetin, *J. Agric. Food Chem.* 2009, 57(6), 2583–2587.

21. Werch, SC and Ivy AC, On the fate of ingested pectin, *Am. J. Dig. Dis.* 1941, 8, 101.

22. Cummings JH and Macfarlane GT, The Control and consequences of bacterial fermentation in the human colon, *J. Appl. Bacteriol.* 1991, 70, 443.

23. Degnan BA, Macfarlane S, and Macfarlane GT, Utilization of starch and synthesis of a combined amylase/alpha-glucosidase by the human colonic anaerobe Bacteroides ovatus, *J. Appl. Microbiol.* 1997, 83(3), 359–366.

24. Nyman M and Asp NG, Fermentation of dietary fibre components in the rat intestinal tract, *Brit. J. Nutr.* 1982, 47, 357.

25. Nyman M and Asp NG, Dietary fibre fermentation in the rat intestinal tract: Effect of adaptation period, protein and fibre levels, and particle size, *Brit. J. Nutr.* 1985, 54, 635.

26. Viola S, Zimmermann G, and Mokady S, Effect of pectin and algin upon protein utilization, digestibility of nutrients and energy in young rats, *Nutr. Rep. Int.* 1970, 1, 367.

27. Englyst HN, Hay S, and Macfarlane GT, Polysaccharide breakdown by mixed populations of human faecal bacteria, *FEMS Microbiol. Ecol.* 1987, 95, 163.

28. Mortensen PB, Hove H, Clausen MR, and Holtug K, Fermentation to short-chain fatty acids and lactate in human faecal batch cultures. Intra- and inter-individual variations versus variations caused by changes in fermented saccharides, *Scand. J. Gastroenterol.* 1991, 26(12), 1285–1294.

29. Vince AJ, McNeil NI, Wager JD, and Wrong OM, The effect of lactulose, pectin, arabinogalactan and cellulose on the production of organic acids and metabolism of ammonia by intestinal bacteria in a faecal incubation system, *Br. J. Nutr.* 1990, 63(1), 17–26.

30. Matsuura Y, Pectic acid degrading enzymes from human feces, *Agric. Biol. Chem.* 1991, 55(3), 885–886.

31. Wojciechovicz M, Partial characterization of pectinolytic enzymes of Bacteroides ruminicola isolated from the rumen of a sheep, *Acta Microbiol. Pol. Ser. A.* 1971, 3, 45.

32. Wojciechovicz M and Ziolecki A, Pectinolytic enzymes of large rumen treponemes, *Appl. Environ. Microbiol.* 1979, 37, 136.

33. Wojciechowicz M and Ziolecki A, A note on the pectinolytic enzyme of *Streptococcus bovis*, *J. Appl. bact.* 1984, 56, 515.

34. Dongowski G, Lorenz A, and Proll J, The degree of methylation influences the degradation of pectin in the intestinal tract of rats and in vitro, *J. Nutr.* 2002, 132(7), 1935–1944.

35. Mallett AK, Wise A, and Rowland IR, Hydrocolloid food additives and rat caecal microbial enzyme activities, *Food Chem. Toxicol.* 1984, 22(6), 415–418.

36. Crociani F, Alessandrini A, Mucci MM, and Biavati B, Degradation of complex carbohydrates by Bifidobacterium spp., *Int. J. Food Microbiol.* 1994, 24, 199–210.

37. Slováková L, Dušková D, and Marounek M, Fermentation of pectin and glucose, and activity of pectin-degrading enzymes in the rabbit caecal bacterium Bifidobacterium pseudolongum, *Lett. Appl. Microbiol.* 2002, 35, 126–130.

38. Paster BJ and Canale-Parola E, *Treponema saccharophilum* sp. nov., a large pectinolytic spirochete from the bovine rumen, *Appl. Environ. Microbiol.* 1985, 50, 212–219.

39. Marounek M and Dušková D, Metabolism of pectin in rumen bacteria *Butyrivibrio fibrisolvens* and *Prevotella ruminicola*, *Lett. Appl. Microbiol.* 1999, 29, 429–433.

40. Dušková D and Marounek M, Fermentation of pectin and glucose, and activity of pectin-degrading enzymes in the rumen bacterium *Lachnospira multiparus*, *Lett. Appl. Microbiol.* 2001, 3, 159–163.

41. Olano-Martin E, Gibson GR, and Rastall RA, Comparison of the in vitro bifidogenic properties of pectins and pectic-oligosaccharides, *J. Appl. Microbiol.* 2002, 93, 505–511.

42. Cummings JH, Southgate DAT, Branch WJ, Wiggins HS, Houston H, Jenkins DJA, Jivraj T, and Hill MJ, The digestion of pectin in the human gut and its effect on Ca absorption and large bowel function, *Br. J. Nutr.* 1979, 41, 477.

43. DiLorenzo C, Williams CM, Hajnal F, and Valenzuela JE, Pectin delays gastric emptying and increases in obese subjects, *Gastroenterology* 1988, 95, 1211–1215.

44. Tiwary CM, Ward JA, and Jackson BA, Effect of pectin on satiety in healthy US Army adults, *J. Am. Coll. Nutr.* 1997, 16(5), 423–428.

45. Hendricks KM, Dong KR, Tang AM, Ding B, Spiegelman D, Woods MN, and Wanke CA, High-fiber diet in HIV-positive men is associated with lower risk of developing fat deposition, *Am. J. Clin. Nutr.* 2003, 78(4), 790–795.

46. Perrigue M, Carter B, Roberts SA, and Drewnowski A, A low-calorie beverage supplemented with low-viscosity pectin reduces energy intake at a subsequent meal, *J. Food Sci.* 2010, 75(9), 300–305.

47. Holt S, Heading RC, Carter DC, Prescott LF, and Tothill P, Effect of gel fiber on gastric emptying and absorption of glucose and paracetamol, *Lancet* 1979, 24, 637–639.

48. Schwartz SE, Levine RA, Singh A, Scheidecker JR, and Track NS, Sustained pectin delays gastric emptying, *Gastroenterology* 1983, 83, 812–817.

49. Schwartz SE, Levine RA, Weinstock RS, Petokas RS, Mills CA, and Thomas FD, Sustained pectin ingestion: Effect on gastric emptying and glucose tolerance in non-insulin-dependent diabetic patients, *Am. J. Clin. Nutr.* 1988, 48, 1413–1417.

50. Sandhu KS, el Samahi MM, Mena I, Dooley CP, and Valenzuela JE, Effect of pectin on gastric emptying and gastroduodenal motility in normal subjects, *Gastroenterology* 1987, 92(2), 486–492.

51. Flourie B, Vidon N, Florent CH, and Bernier JJ, Effect of pectin on jejunal glucose absorption and unstirred water layer thickness in normal man, *Gut* 1984, 25(9), 936–941.

52. Gatfield IL and Stute R, Enzymatic reactions in the presence of polymers, *FEBS Lett.* 1972, 28, 29–31.

53. Wilson F and Dietschy J, The intestinal unstirred water layer: Its surface area and effect on active transport kinetics, *Biochim. Biophys. Acta* 1974, 363, 112–126.

54. Dunaif G and Schneeman BO, The effect of dietary fiber on human pancreatic enzyme activity in vitro, *Am. J. Clin. Nutr.* 1981, 34, 1034–1035.

55. Hansen WE and Schulz G, Pflanzenfasern—Neue Wege in der Stoffwechseltherapie. In: Huth, K., Ed. *Lösliche und Fixierte Inhibitoren der Amylase in Guar und Anderen Ballaststoffen*, Karger S, Basel, Switzerland, 1983, pp. 144–150.

56. Gerencser GA, Cerda J, Burgin C, Baig MM, and Guild R, Unstirred water layers in rabbit intestine: Effects of pectin, *Proc. Soc. Exp. Biol. Med.* 1984, 176(2), 183–186.

57. Harland BF, Dietary fibre and mineral bioavailability, *Nutr. Res. Rev.* 1989, 2, 133.

58. Jellinek HHG and Chen PYA, Polygalacturonic acid—Bivalent metal complexes, *J. Polymer Sci.* 1972, 10, 287–293.

59. Paskins-Hurlburt AJ, Tanaka Y, Skoryna SC, Moore W, Stara JF, and Stara JR, The binding of lead by a pectic polyelectrolyte, *Environ. Res.* 1977, 14, 128–140.

60. Kohn R, Malovikova A, Bock W, and Dongowski G, Bindung von Blei-Ionen an Nahrungspektine in Gemüse und Obst, *Nahrung* 1981, 25, 853.

61. Malovikova A and Kohn R, Binding of cadmium cations to pectin, *Collect. Czech. Chem. Commun.* 1982, 47, 702.

62. Malovikova A and Kohn R, Binding of lead and chromium(III)cations to pectin, *Collect. Czech. Chem. Commun.* 1979, 44, 2915.

63. Kohn R, Ion binding on polyuronates—Alginate and pectin, *Pure appl. Chem.* 1975, 42, 371–397.

64. Markovic O, Kohn R, Mode of pectin deesterification by *Trichoderma reesei* pectinesterase, *Experiencia* 1984, 40, 842.

65. Schlemmer U, Die Bindung von Fe und Zn an Pektin und Alginat, *Ernährungs-Umschau* 1983, 30, 232.
66. Schlemmer U, In vitro-Untersuchungen über die Bindung von Nährstoffen an Pektin und Alginat. Jahresbericht der Bundesforschunganstalt für Ernährung 1982, A 6.
67. Schlemmer U, Studies of the binding of Cu, Zn and Ca to pectin, alginate, carrageenan and guar gum in HCO_3^--CO2 buffer, *Food Chem.* 1989, 32, 223.
68. Lei KY, Davis MW, Fang MM, and Young LC, Effect of pectin on Zn, Cu and Fe balances in humans, *Nutr. Rep. Int.* 1980, 22, 459.
69. Plant A, Kies C, and Fox HM, The effect of Cu and fiber supplementation on Cu utilization in humans, *Fed. Proc.* 1979, 38, 549.
70. Grudeva-Popova J and Sirakova I, Effect of pectin on some electrolytes and trace elements in patients with hyperlipoproteinemia, *Folia Med. (Plovdiv.)* 1998, 40(1), 41–45.
71. Drews LM, Kies C, and Fox HM, Effect of dietary fiber on Cu, Zn, and Mg utilization by adolescent boys, *Am. J. Clin. Nutr.* 1979, 32, 1893.
72. Stasse-Wolthuis M, Albers HFF, van Jeveren JGG, de Jong JW, Hautvast JGAJ, Hermus RJJ, Katan MB, Brydon WG, and Eastwood MA, Influence of dietary fiber from vegetables and fruits, bran, or citrus pectin on serum lipids, fecal lipids, and colonic function, *Am. J. Clin. Nutr.* 1980, 33, 1745–1756.
73. Walzel E, Bock W, Kujawa M, Macholz R, Raab M, and Woggon H, Einfluss von Pektin auf die Bleieliminierung und ausgewählte essentielle Mineralstoffe bei bleiexponierten Personen, in Mengen- und Spurenelemente, Arbeitstagung Leipzig 1987, p. 149.
74. Monnier L, Colette C, Aguirre L, and Mirouze J, Evidence and mechanism for pectin-reduced intestinal inorganic Fe absorption in idiopathic hemochromatosis, *Am. J. Clin. Nutr.* 1980, 33, 1225.
75. Bezzubov AD, Vasilieva OG, and Khatina AI, The influence of pectin on the elimination of lead from the body, *Gig. Truda Prof. Zabol. 4* 1960, 3, 32–37.
76. Bondarev GI, Anisova AA, Alekseeva TE, and Syzrancev JK, Beurteilung von niederverestertem Pektin als prophylaktisches Mittel bei Bleivergiftung, *Vopr. Pitanija* 1979, 2, 65.
77. Livshic OD, Prophylactic role of lead pectin containing food products in lead-poisoning, *Vopr. Pitanija* 1969, 4, 76.
78. Niculescu T, Rafaila E, Eremia R, and Balasa E, Untersuchungen zur Pektinwirkung bei experimenteller Bleivergiftung, *Igiena* 1968, 17, 421–427.
79. Trakhtenberg IM, Lukovenko VP, Korolenko TK, Ostroukhova VA, Demchenko PI, Rabotiaga TE, and Krotenko VV, The prophylactic use of pectin in chronic lead exposure in industry (Russ.), *Lik. Sprava.* 1995, (1–2), 132–136.
80. Stantschev S, Kratschanov C, Popova M, and Kirtschev N, Prevention of chronic satunism by the use of foodstuffs enriched with pectin: 2. Mitt. Application of granulated pectin, *Letopisi Chig. Epidemiol. Sofija* 1980, 12(7), 95.
81. Tamura M and Suzuki H, Effects of pectin on jejunal and ileal morphology and ultrastructure in adult mice, *Ann. Nutr. Metab.* 1997, 41(4), 255–259.
82. Andoh A, Bamba T, and Sasaki M, Physiological and anti-inflammatory roles of dietary fiber and butyrate in intestinal functions, *J. Parenter. Enteral Nutr.* 1999, 23(5 Suppl.), 70–73.
83. Fukunaga T, Sasaki M, Araki Y, Okamoto T, Yasuoka T, Tsujikawa T, Fujiyama Y, and Bamba T, Effects of the soluble fibre pectin on intestinal cell proliferation, fecal short chain fatty acid production and microbial population, *Digestion* 2003, 67(1–2), 42–49.
84. Leeds AR, Ralphs DN, Boulos P, Ebied F, Metz G, Dilawari JB, Elliott A, and Jenkins DJA, Pectin and gastric emptying in the dumping syndrome, *Proc. Nutr. Soc.* 1977, 37, 23A.

85. Leeds AR, Ralphs DN, Ebied F, Metz G, and Dilawari JB, Pectin in the dumping syndrome: Reduction of symptoms and plasma volume changes, *Lancet* 1981, 1(8229), 1075–1078.
86. Lawaetz O, Blackburn AM, Bloom SR, Aritas Y, and Ralphs DNL, Effect of pectin on gastric emptying and gut hormone release in the dumping syndrome, *Scand. J. Gastroenterol.* 1983, 18, 327–336.
87. Harju E, Metabolic problems after gastric surgery, *Int. Surg.* 1990, 75(1), 27–35.
88. Samuk I, Afriat R, Horne T, Bistritzer T, Barr J, and Vinograd I, Dumping syndrome following Nissen fundoplication, diagnosis, and treatment, *J. Pediatr. Gastroenterol. Nutr.* 1996, 23(3), 235–240.
89. Hasler WL, Dumping syndrome, *Curr. Treat. Options Gastroenterol.* 2002, 5(2), 139–145.
90. Roth JA, Frankel WL, Zhang W, Klurfeld DM, and Rombeau JL, Pectin improves colonic function in rat short bowel syndrome, *J. Surg. Res.* 1995, 58(2), 240–246.
91. Sales TR, Torres HO, Couto CM, and Carvalho EB, Intestinal adaptation in short bowel syndrome without tube feeding or home parenteral nutrition: Report of four consecutive cases, *Nutrition* 1998, 14(6), 508–512.
92. Finkel Y, Brown G, Smith HL, Buchanan E, and Booth IW, The effects of a pectin-supplemented elemental diet in a boy with short gut syndrome, *Acta Paediatr. Scand.* 1990, 79(10), 983–986.
93. Zimmaro DM, Rolandelli RH, Koruda MJ, Settle RG, Stein TP, and Rombeau JL, Isotonic tube feeding formula induces liquid stool in normal subjects: Reversal by pectin, *JPEN. J. Parenter. Enteral Nutr.* 1989, 13(2), 117–123.
94. Schultz AA, Ashby-Hughes B, Taylor R, Gillis DE, and Wilkins M, Effects of pectin on diarrhea in critically ill tube-fed patients receiving antibiotics, *Am. J. Crit. Care* 2000, 9(6), 403–411.
95. Potievskii EG, Shavakhabov Sh Sh, Bondarenko VM, and Ashubaeva ZD, Experimental and clinical studies of the effect of pectin on the causative agents of acute intestinal infections (Russian), *Zh. Mikrobiol. Epidemiol. Immunobiol.* 1994, (Suppl. 1), 106–109.
96. de la Motte S, Bose-O'Reilly S, Heinisch M, and Harrison F, Double-blind comparison of an apple pectin-chamomile extract preparation with placebo in children with diarrhea (German), *Arzneimittelforschung* 1997, 47(11), 1247–1249.
97. Triplehorn C and Millard PS, A rice-based diet with green banana or pectin reduced diarrhea in infants better than a rice-alone diet, *ACP. J. Club.* 2002, 136(2), 67.
98. Veldman FJ, Nair CH, Vorster HH, Vermaak WJ, Jerling JC, Oosthuizen W, and Venter CS, Dietary pectin influences fibrin network structure in hypercholesterolaemic subjects, *Throm. Res.* 1997, 86(3), 183–196.
99. Veldman FJ, Nair CH, Vorster HH, Vermaak WJ, Jerling JC, Oosthuizen W, and Venter CS, Possible mechanisms through which dietary pectin influences fibrin network architecture in hypercholesterolaemic subjects, *Throm. Res.* 1999, 93(6), 253–264.
100. Wu H, Dwyer KM, Fan Z, Shircore A, Fan J, and Dwyer JH, Dietary fiber and progression of atherosclerosis: The Los Angeles Atherosclerosis Study, *Am. J. Clin. Nutr.* 2003, 78(6), 1085–1091.
101. Flodin NW, Atherosclerosis: An insulin-dependent disease? *J. Am. Coll. Nutr.* 1986, 5, 417.
102. Fukagawa NK, Anderson JW, Hageman G, Young VR, and Minaker KL, High-carbohydrate, high fiber diets increase peripheral insulin sensitivity in healthy young and old adults, *Am. J. Clin. Nutr.* 1990, 52, 524.
103. Baig MM, Cerda JJ, Pectin: Its interaction with serum lipoproteins, *Am. J. Clin. Nutr.* 1981, 34, 50–53.

104. Falk JD and Nagyvary JJ, Exploratory studies of lipid-pectin interactions, *J. Nutr.* 1982, 112, 182–188.

105. Keys A, Grande F, and Anderson JT, Fiber and pectin in the diet and serum cholesterol concentration in man, *Proc. Soc. Exp. Biol. Med.* 1961, 106, 555–558.

106. Fahrenbach MJ, Riccardi BA, Saunders JC, Lourie IN, and Heider JG, Comparative effects of guar gum and pectin on human serum cholesterol levels, *Circulation* 1965, 31/32 (Suppl. II), 11–14.

107. Palmer GH and Dixon DG, Effect of pectin dose on serum cholesterol levels, *Am. J. Clin. Nutr.* 1966, 18, 437–442.

108. Jenkins DJA, Leeds AR, Gassull A, Houston H, Goff D, and Hill M, The cholesterol-lowering properties of guar and pectin, *Clin. Sci. Mol. Med.* 1976a, 51, 8–9.

109. Durrington PN Bolton CH, Manning AP, and Hartog M, Effect of pectin on serum lipids and lipoproteins, whole-gut transit time and stool-weight, *Lancet* 1976, 21, 394–396.

110. Kay RM and Truswell AS, Effect of citrus pectin on blood lipids and fecal steroid excretion in man, *Am. J. Clin. Nutr.* 1977, 30, 171–175.

111. Raymond TL, Connor WE, Lin DS, Warner S, Fry MM, and Connor SL, The interaction of dietary fibers and cholesterol upon the plasma lipids and lipoproteins, sterol balance, and bowel function in human subjects, *J. Clin. Invest.* 1977, 60, 1429–1437.

112. Delbarre F, Rondier J, and deGéry A, Lack of effect of two pectins in idiopathic or gout-associated hyperdyslipidemia hypercholesterolemia, *Am. J. Clin. Nutr.* 1977, 30, 463.

113. Jenkins DJA, Reynolds D, Leed AR, Walker AL, and Cummings JH, Hypocholesterolemic action of dietary fiber unrelated to fecal bulking effect, *Am. J. Clin. Nutr.* 1979, 32, 2430–2435.

114. Ginter E, Kubec EJ, Vozár J, and Bobek P, Natural hypocholesterolemic agent: Pectin plus ascorbic acid, *Intl. J. Vit. Nutr. Res.* 1979, 49, 406.

115. Nakamura H, Islukawa T, Tada N, Kagami A, Koudo K, Miyazami E, and Takeyama S, Effect of several kinds of dietary fibres on serum and lipoprotein lipids, *Nutr. Rep. Int.* 1982, 26, 215–221.

116. Judd PA and Truswell AS, Comparison of the effects of high and low methoxyl pectins on blood and faecal lipids in man, *Br. J. Nutr.* 1982, 48, 451–458.

117. Challen AD, Branch WJ, and Cummings JH, The effect of pectin and wheat bran on platelet function and haemostatis in man, *Human Nutr. Clin. Nutr.* 1983, 37, 209–217.

118. Miettinen TA and Tarpila S, Effect of pectin on serum cholesterol fecal bile acids and biliary lipids in normolipidemic and hyperlipidemic individuals, *Clin. Chim. Acta* 1977, 79, 471–477.

119. Schwandt P, Richter WO, Weisweiler P, and Neureuther G, Cholestyramine plus pectin in treatment of patients with familial hypercholesterolemia, *Atherosclerosis* 1982, 44, 379–383.

120. Hundhammer K and Marshall M, Wirkung niedriger Dosen Apfelpektin auf die Blutlipide, ihre Verträglichkeit und Akzeptanz bei ambulanten hypercholesterinämischen Patienten, *Akt. Ernähr.* 1983, 8, 222–225.

121. Ershoff BH and Wells AF, Effects of methoxyl content on anti-cholesterol activity of pectic substances in the rat, *Exp. Med. Surg.* 1962, 20, 272–276.

122. Schuderer U, Wirkung von Apfelpektin auf die Cholesterin-und Lipoproteinkonzentration bei Hypercholesterinämie, Dissertation 1986, University of Giessen, Giessen, Germany.

123. Cerda JJ, Studies on the role of citrus pectin in nutrition, Oral version of the lecture held at the X. International Fruit Juice Convention, February 23–24, 1988, in Orlando, FL.

124. Groudeva-Popova J, Application of granulated apple pectin in the treatment of hyperlipoproteinaemia, *Z. Lebensm. Unters. Forsch.* 1996, A 204, 374–378.

125. Groudeva-Popova J, Krachanova M, Djurdjev A, and Krachanov C, Application of soluble dietary fibres in treatment of hyperlipoproteinemias, *Folia Med.* 1996, 39, 39–43.
126. Bartz VP, Blutfette auf natürliche Weise senken: Eine Kombination aus Omega-3-Fettsäuren und Pektin zeigt viel versprechende Ergebnisse, *Ernährung Medizin* 2002, 17, 149–150.
127. Sheehan JP, Wei IW, Ulchaker M, and Tserng KY, Effect of high fiber intake in fish oil-treated patients with non-insulin-dependent diabetes mellitus, *Am. J. Clin. Nutr.* 1997, 66(5), 1183–1187.
128. Aprikian O, Duclos V, Guyot S, Besson C, Manach C, Bernalier A, Morand C, Remesy C, and Demigne C, Apple pectin and a polyphenol-rich apple concentrate are more effective together than separately on cecal fermentations and plasma lipids in rats, *J. Nutr.* 2003, 133(6), 1860–1865.
129. Brown L, Rosner B, Willett WW, and Sacks FM, Cholesterol-lowering effects of dietary fiber: A meta-analysis, *Am. J. Clin. Nutr.* 1999, 69, 30–42.
130. Ullrich IH, Evaluation of a high-fiber diet in hyperlipidemia: A review, *J. Am. Coll. Nutr.* 1987, 6, 19–25.
131. Aroch MG, Hypercholesteremic compositions containing ascorbic acid and pectin, Slovak Patent 1986, CODON: CZXXA9 CS 228809 B 0101.
132. Pfeiffer R, *Wirkung Unterschiedlich Strukturierter Ballaststoffe auf Ausgewählte Merkmale des Lipidstoffwechsels bei der Ratte*, Fachverlag Köhler, Gießen, Germany, 2000.
133. Yamaguchi F, Uchida S, Watabe S, Kojima H, Shimizu N, and Hatanaka C, Relationship between molecular weights of pectin and hypocholesterolemic effects in rats, *Biosci. Biotechnol. Biochem.* 1995, 59(11), 2130–2131.
134. Matheson HB, Colon IS, and Story JA, Cholesterol 7 alpha-hydroxylase activity is increased by dietary modification with psyllium hydrocolloid, pectin, cholesterol and cholestyramine in rats, *J. Nutr.* 1995, 125(3), 454–458.
135. Jenkins DJA, Goff DV, Leeds AR, Alberti KGMM, Wolever TMS, Gassull MA, and Hockaday TDR, Unabsorbable carbohydrates and diabetes: Decreased post-prandial hyperglycaemia, *Lancet* 1976, 2, 172.
136. Jenkins DJA, Leeds AR, Gassull MA, Cochet B, and Alberti KGMM, Decrease in postprandial insulin and glucose concentrations by guar and pectin, *Ann. Intern. Med.* 1977, 86, 20.
137. Jenkins DJA, Wolever TMS, Leeds AR, Gassull MA, Haisman P, Dilawari J, Goff DV, Metz GL, and Alberti KGMM, Dietary fibres, fibre analogues, and glucose tolerance: Importance of viscosity, *Brit. Med. J.* 1978, 1, 1392.
138. Monnier L, Pham TC, Aguirre L, Orsetti A, and Mirouze J, Influence of indigestible fibers on glucose tolerance, *Diabetes Care* 1978, 1, 83.
139. Labayle D, Chaput JC, Buffet C, Rousseau C, Francois P, and Etienne JP, Action du son de blé et de la pectine sur l'hyperglycémie provoquée par voie orale chez les opérés de l'estomac, *Nouv. Presse Med.* 1980, 9, 223.
140. Vaaler S, Hanssen KF, and Aagenaes Ø, Effect of different kinds of fibre on postprandial blood glucose in insulin-dependent diabetics, *Acta Med. Scand.* 1980, 208, 389.
141. Poynard T, Slama G, Delage A, and Tchobroutsky G, Pectin efficacy in insulin-treated diabetics assessed by the artificial pancreas, *Lancet* 1980, 1, 158.
142. Gold LA, McCourt JP, and Merimee TJ, Pectin: An examination in normal subjects, *Diabetes Care* 1980, 3, 50.
143. Williams DRR, James WPT, and Evans IE, Dietary fibre supplementation of a 'normal' breakfast administered to diabetics, *Diabetologia* 1980, 18, 379.
144. Kanter Y, Eitan N, Brook G, and Barzilai D, Improved glucose tolerance and insulin response in obese and diabetic patients on a fiber-enriched diet, *Israel J. Med. Sci.* 1980, 16, 1.

145. Sahi A, Bijlami RL, Karmarkar MG, and Nayar U, Modulation of glycemic response by protein, fat, and dietary fiber, *Nutr. Res.* 1985, 5, 1431.
146. Siddhu A, Sud S, Bijlani RL, Karmarkar MG, and Nayar U, Modulation of postprandial glycaemia and insulinaemia by dietary fat, *Indian J. Physiol. Pharmacol.* 1991, 35(2), 99–105.
147. Tunali G, Stetten D, Schuderer U, and Hofmann H, Wirkung von Pektin—In Form von Apfelpektinextrakt—auf die postprandiale Serumglucose- und Serum-Insulin-Konzentration bei Probanden mit Diabetes Mellitus Type II, 27. Wiss. DGE-Kongress 1990, München Ernährungs-Umschau aus Forschung und Praxis 37, 141
148. Jenkins DJ and Jenkins AL, Dietary fiber and the glycemic response, *Proc. Soc. Exp. Biol. Med.* 1985, 180(3), 422–431.
149. Fuse K, Bamba T, and Hosoda S, Effects of pectin on fatty acid and glucose absorption and on thickness of unstirred water layer in rat and human intestine, *Dig. Dis. Sci.* 1989, 34(7), 1109–1116.
150. Morgan LM, Goulder TJ, Tsiolakis D, Marks V, and Alberti K, The effect of unabsorbable carbohydrates on gut hormones, *Diabetologia* 1979, 17, 85–89.
151. Levitt NS, Vinik AI, Sive AA, Child PT, and Jackson WPU, The effect of dietary fiber on glucose and hormone responses to a mixed meal in normal subjects and in diabetic subjects with and without autonomic neuropathy, *Diabetes Care* 1980, 3, 515–519.
152. Ohkami H, Tazawa K, Yamashita I, Shimizu T, Murai K, Kobashi K, and Fujimake M, Effects of apple pectin on fecal bacterial enzymes in azoxymethane-induced rat colon carcinogenesis, *Jpn. Cancer Res.* 1995, 86(6), 523–529.
153. Tazawa K, Yatuzuka K, Yatuzuka M, Koike J, Ohkami H, Saito T, Ohnishi Y, and Saito M, Dietary fiber inhibits the incidence of hepatic metastasis with the anti-oxidant activity and portal scavenging functions (Japanese), *Hum. Cell.* 1999, 12(4), 189–196.
154. Tazawa K, Okami H, Yamashita I, Ohnishi Y, Kobashi K, and Fujimaki M, Anticarcinogenic action of apple pectin on fecal enzyme activities and mucosal or portal prostaglandin E2 levels in experimental rat colon carcinogenesis, *J. Exp. Clin. Cancer Res.* 1997, 16(1), 33–38.
155. Ohno K, Narushima S, Takeuchi S, Itoh K, Mitsuoka T, Nakayama H, Itoh T, Hioki K, and Nomura T, Inhibitory effect of apple pectin and culture condensate of Bifidobacterium longum on colorectal tumors induced by 1,2-dimethylhydrazine in transgenic mice harbouring human prototype c-Ha-ras genes, *Exp. Anim.* 2000, 49(4), 305–307.
156. Olano-Martin E, Rimbach GH, Gibson GR, Rastall RA, Pectin and pectic-oligosaccharides induce apoptosis in in vitro human colonic adenocarcinoma cells, *Anticancer Res.* 2003, 23(1A), 341–346.
157. Avivi-Green C, Madar Z, and Schwartz B, Pectin-enriched diet affects distribution and expression of apoptosis-cascade proteins in colonic crypts of dimethylhydrazine-treated rats, *Int. J. Mol. Med.* 2000, 6(6), 689–698.
158. Bergman M, Djaldetti M, Salman H, and Bessler H, Effect of citrus pectin on malignant cell proliferation, *Biomed. Pharmacother.* 2010, 64(1), 44–47.
159. Guggenbichler JP, Blockierung der Anlagerung von Keimen an menschlichen Zellen, European Patent 1998, 0 716 605 B1.
160. Stahl B and Boehm G, Antiadhesive carbohydrates, International Patent 2001, WO 01/60378 A2.
161. Kunz M, Munir M, and Vogel M, Method for producing pectin hydrolysis products, International Patent 2000, WO 02/42484 A2.

28

Fruit Fibers

JÜRGEN FISCHER

Contents

28.1 Definition and Origin of Fruit Fibers

The term dietary fiber [1] has been coined for organic components of plants that cannot be degraded by human alimentary enzymes and thus remain unabsorbed in the small intestine. Following the studies of Trowell and coworkers [2] on the connection between dietary fiber intake and occurrence of diseases in modern civilization, fibers are no longer regarded as superfluous for nutrition, and attempts are being made to increase their amount in the food. Traditionally, parts of plants (roots, tubers, leaves, fruits, and seeds) rich in protein, carbohydrate, and fat have been chosen for human consumption. In addition, fiber-depleted raw materials have been selected due to sensory reasons [3]. The main part of dietary fibers in our diet comes from cell walls of fruits, vegetables, pulses, and cereals [4]. The cell wall is a very complex network of different nonstarch polymers, structural proteins, and phenolic substances [5–7]. Nearly all components of the cell wall belong to the group of dietary fibers. The most abundant nonstarch polymers of the plant cell walls are cellulose, hemicellulose, pectin, and lignin. According to the solubility in water, we distinguish soluble from insoluble dietary fiber. The complex, native cell wall material is primarily insoluble in water and has a fibrous structure.

The composition of this intrinsic cell wall material can vary among different plants and depends on the biological function of the plant organs and tissues. The composition undergoes changes during the plant's life. Even within the same cell, changes occur during maturation [7]. In general, the content of cellulose and lignin strongly depends on the maturation of a plant and increases with the need of a tissue for structural stabilization [8]. The highest dietary fiber content in edible parts of plants is located in the outer regions of grains, fruits, or vegetables due to their excellent protective function. In fruits, the reproductive organs of plants that contain one or more seeds (including the embryo), the parenchyma tissue is the main cell type. These cells have comparably thin walls but are highly vacuolated [5,6] and can stabilize a tissue with very high water content. Two facts are responsible for this high functionality: the morphological structure and the higher ratio of pectin and

Table 28.1 Composition of Edible Parts of Fruits

Fruit	Water (%)	Available Carbohydrate	Protein	Fat	Dietary Fiber	Water Binding of Dietary Fiber
Apple	85.3	12.4	0.3	0.4	2.3	31.5
Apricot	85.3	9.4	0.9	0.1	2.0	37.5
Mango	82.0	12.8	0.6	0.5	1.7	40.3
Strawberry	89.5	6.5	0.8	0.4	2.0	41.1
Pineapple	85.3	13.1	0.5	0.2	1.4	51.2
Orange	86.7	9.2	1.0	0.2	2.2	34.7
Plum	83.7	11.4	0.6	0.2	1.7	42.2
Peach	87.5	9.4	0.8	0.1	1.7	45.5

Source: Souci-Fachmann-Kraut, Food Composition and Nutrition Tables 1989/90, and theoretical water binding of dietary fiber.

hemicellulose versus cellulose. For example, in quince [9], the same cellulose content was found in flesh and core tissue but a three times higher pectin content in flesh.

Table 28.1 gives an overview on the composition of some fruits. The fat and protein contents are in general lower than 1%, and sugar is in the range of 6%–13%. Because the cell wall material (=dietary fiber) is responsible for moisture control (and texture), a theoretical water-binding capacity can be determined for dietary fiber. A value of 1 has been considered for sugar and protein.

Raw material to produce fruit fiber is available in large quantities and is more or less a by-product of the processing of fruits to juice or puree [9–14]. The industrial residue is dried, to some extent purified or processed, and milled to a defined grain size [15].

For example, the production of apple juice is accompanied by the accumulation of about 20% pomace [16]. Usually, the pomace is dried immediately after processing of the fruit. The resulting apple fiber consists of skin, seeds, core, and mainly the cell wall material of flesh (parenchymal tissue). It has an average content of about 60% dietary fiber and 12% available sugars. The soluble fiber content is approximately 20%, being mainly pectin.

In case of citrus processing [11], 40%–60% of the total fruit remains after juice and essential oils extraction. The remaining peels and pulp can be used to produce secondary products such as candied peels, pectin, or citrus fiber. Depending on the tissue, commercial dietary fiber with different properties can be produced out of the same raw material. For example, the total dietary fiber content is 9.6% in orange peels, 9.7% in the membranes, and 11% in juice sacs and the water content is 69%, 81%, and 84%, respectively [17]. Hence, the total dietary fiber content of seeds is 14.6%, but their water content is only 48%. This is caused by their different biological needs. Protection versus moisture control is reflected by the high cellulose/lignin fraction of 68% in contrast to only 42% in the other tissues.

Although by-products of fruit processing exist in large amounts [18], the commercial production of fruit fibers is limited to small amounts due to several reasons. By-products are widely used in the feed industry. Fresh fruit tissue after squeezing is not stable against enzymatic degradation and is very sensitive to microbiological spoilage. In addition, fruit ripening is governed by cell wall degradation, which is responsible for softening. With oversoftening, the production of fiber is economically not of interest. Therefore, a drying process soon after fruit processing is necessary (this happens naturally in case of cereal bran or legume hulls during ripening). However, the drying process is expensive due to the high and stable water binding of fruit-derived cell wall material and, in addition, difficult if the aim is to preserve the beneficial native functionality, the high water-binding capacity [19]. This property strongly depends on the maintenance of the cell wall architecture [19–21]. The term *material with cellular structure* (MCS) was chosen for powdered products that can be rehydrated to suspensions that have nearly equal properties as fresh cell wall material [22,23]. Disintegration of the cell clusters is helpful to remove water-soluble substances during preparation but must not destroy the cell wall structure. This is accompanied by lower water-binding properties [24]. In this respect, powdered cell wall material from apples was described with water-binding capacities of more than 30 g/g. Such values are in the range of the theoretical values shown in Table 28.1. The way of rehydration plays an important role in the water-binding properties of fruit fibers. Intensive stirring or shear forces lead to enhanced binding properties [25,26].

In the recent years, fruit fiber–producing companies have focused on obtaining products with a high water-binding property, closer to those in fresh fruits. A comparison of this key property of commercially available fruit fibers can be seen in Figure 28.1. All values are determined under the same conditions to generate comparable results. As a matter of a wide range of different methods [27] to characterize the interaction with water (water binding, holding, and swelling) as well as a strong influence of the rehydration conditions, it is impossible to compare literature data and values of company brochures. Due to the different

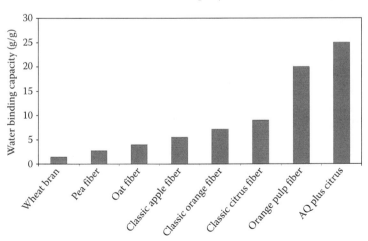

Figure 28.1 Water binding of commercial dietary fibers using a centrifugation method: 1 g dietary fibers is dispersed in 60 g water at 20°C, soaked for 24 h and centrifuged at 3000 × g for 10 min. The bound water is determined by weight measurement after discarding the supernatant.

ultra structure, the water-binding properties of fruit fiber are higher than cereal-based fiber. By-products like cereal bran or husks are composed of a rigid cellulose coat [28] to protect the germ and should not bind water at all, a biological need. Therefore, chemical activation is necessary to increase the water-binding properties as is done to produce, for example, CMC, MC, or HPMC.

The natural high functionality is a big benefit of fruit fiber compared to modified starches or modified celluloses. They are derived from succulent and attractive-to-eat plant material, which has always been a normal part of human nutrition, and help to fulfill consumer wishes for clean label ingredients.

28.2 Application of Fruit Fibers

"Fiber is of interest to product designers for not only its nutritional value but for its versatility as a functional ingredient" [29]. Indeed, the old conceptions, especially that insoluble fiber has been related with a rough mouthfeel, have disappeared and are replaced by multiple technological benefits [3,30,31]. In the past, the use of insoluble fruit fiber was limited to semidry applications such as bread or bars [32–35]. Nowadays, fruit fiber types are available with improved rehydration properties, and, with this better water uptake, the fibrous material is becoming softer and can be applied even for oil/water emulsion or ice cream without the formation of a sandy or grainy character [31,36–38]. This milestone in fiber technology enables new application possibilities for fibers as food ingredients, which are used because of a positive health effect but simultaneously offer technological and sensorial advantages. The use of citrus fiber in low-fat mayonnaise to mimic the characteristic of fat [39] is one of the best examples of what became possible with fruit fiber.

As in fruits or fruit-based products, the cell wall matrix is the principal structural component [22,40] and is responsible for moisture control; vice versa, fruit fiber can be added to food to create texture and to control moisture.

Without a doubt, the key property of fruit fiber is the hydration. Hydration summarizes the ability to swell, to bind water, to enhance the viscosity, or to prevent syneresis (see Table 28.2). Especially fruit fibers that are produced carefully without collapse of the cell wall architecture [21] are able to swell in a very short time and form a sponge like network. This matrix is able to immobilize water to a high degree. Scanning electron micrographs (see Figure 28.2) visualize the mechanism responsible for the superior water binding. It is mainly the cell architecture and to a smaller extent the chemical composition with the relative high content of pectin substances.

The high water binding is a technological as well as a physiological benefit [40,41].

However, dietary fibers with a high functionality (in respect to water binding) are typically used at a relatively low usage level to perform a specific function and then, only consequentially, add fiber at a low level. Nevertheless, they are advantageous to be used in low-fat or low-calorie products [42,43]. Some applications of fruit fiber to food products are shown in Table 28.2. The use in baked products has a long history, especially for apple fibers [44–46]. But why use fruit fibers in sausages, sauces, and dressings or in ice cream? The answer is simple: water has to be bound, and the leaner a product is, the more water needs to be structured.

Table 28.2 Applications and Benefits of Fruit Fibers with High Water Binding to Calorie-Reduced Food

---

Low fat o/w emulsions (mayonnaise-like)
Replacement of modified starch
Creamy, fat-like consistency even below 10% fat
Pseudoelastic flow behavior

Spreads
Stabilization of fat-reduced margarines
Replacement of nuts or beans
Replacement of starch or milk powders

Liver sausage and pâté
Mimic fat
Improved succulence
Improved consistency
Replacement of cereal-based binders

Frankfurter sausage
Improved succulence
Enhanced shelf life (less syneresis)
Improved bite

Sponge cake and muffins
Improved succulence
Replacement of flour and/or fat
Stabilization of shape

On the whole, meat products are far from being regarded as sources of dietary fiber. However, the high functionality and sensory improvement of some fruit fibers opened the doors to this new field [47–50]. Especially in boiled sausages, the addition of 3% dietary fiber in low-fat products is easy to achieve with a fiber blend of a soluble fiber such as inulin and a fruit fiber with high water-binding capacity. A 30% fat-reduced product just by using lean meat is very dry and firm due to the high meat protein content. Better results are achieved by keeping the protein level lower and adding a dispersion of fiber in water to substitute the fat.

A similar principle is applied to produce low-fat varieties of baked products such as brownies, which originally have a high fat content [25,33,51,52,54].

It is also possible to produce low-fat dressings, low-fat fresh cheese, or even ice cream without reduction of creaminess or mouthfeel. A prerequisite for such application is that the fiber can be rehydrated in a way that the grainy structure completely disappears (which is a result of cell wall collapse during production [21]). In some products, the fruit fibers should be rehydrated by using intensive stirring or shear treatment [25,53,54] to achieve the best results. Figure 28.3 shows the rheological behavior of a low-fat o/w

	"Starch"	"Starch + Citrus fiber"
Ingredients	[%]	[%]
Water	68	71.0
Vegetable oil	9	9
Modified waxy maize	6	1.8
Citrus fiber (Herbacel AQ Plus)	0	1.2
Vinegar (5% acid)	6	6
Egg yolk	3	3
Sugar	3	3
Mustard	2	2
Salt	1.5	1.5
Lemon juice	1	1
Spices	0.5	0.5

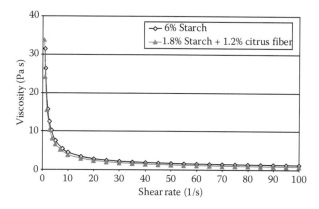

Figure 28.2 Flow behavior of fat-reduced Mayonnaise on basis of starch versus starch and citrus fiber.

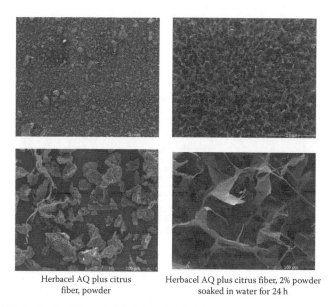

Herbacel AQ plus citrus fiber, powder

Herbacel AQ plus citrus fiber, 2% powder soaked in water for 24 h

Figure 28.3 Scanning electron micrographs of citrus fiber in powdered form and after swelling in distilled water at 20°C for 20 h. (From Herbafood 2006.)

emulsion. Citrus fiber, dispersed in water, created a very high yield point and can be used after this treatment similar to the known starchy slurry. The pseudoplastic properties allow the use in products with typical shear thinning such as mayonnaise or salad dressing.

28.3 Physiological Benefits of Fruit Fibers

As listed in Table 28.1, fruits consist mainly of water and are very low in fat. Many studies reveal that fruits (and vegetables) are a very important part of a healthy diet [55–57] as fruits are rich in vitamins, minerals, secondary plant substances such as flavonoids, and dietary fiber. The last is definitely the difference (or what is lacking) between juice and whole fruit. A high fruit and vegetable consumption is important in the prevention of two leading causes of death, cardiovascular disease and cancer. Convincing evidence exists on the positive effect of dietary fiber and energy-diluted food, such as fruits and vegetables, on obesity [58], an important risk factor.

According to a WHO report [55], "benefits of fruits and vegetables cannot be ascribed to a single mix of nutrients and bioactive substances," but as a food group, they contribute to cardiovascular health. The daily intake of 400–500 g fruits and vegetables is recommended to reduce the risk of coronary heart disease, stroke, and high blood pressure through the variety of phytonutrients, potassium, and fiber they contain. These recommendations [56–58] are broadly known as five-a-day (eat five or more portions of fruits or vegetables per day), and the concept is used as a strong marketing tool.

In regard to cancer prevention, fruit consumption is strongly linked to three of the eight recommendations given by the experts of World Cancer Research Fund [59]:

- Be as lean as possible within the normal range of body weight.
- Limit consumption of energy-dense foods.
- Eat mostly foods of plant origin.

In the United States, two health claims (101.76: might reduce the risk of some types of cancer and 101.77: might reduce the risk of heart disease) reflect the importance of a diet rich in fruit, vegetable, and grain that contain fiber in combination with low in saturated fat and cholesterol. However, there is no scientific agreement whether a particular soluble fiber is beneficial; the observed protective effects are due to other components or other fiber components or displacement of saturated fat and cholesterol [60].

Besides these general aspects on the benefit of fruit consumption, some reports focus more on subcategories of fruits such as citrus [61].

Although much work has been done to point out the advantages of fruits, which finally ended in nutrition guidelines [59,62], studies focusing on fruit fibers (in the sense of complex cell matrix and not isolated fraction like pectin) are rare.

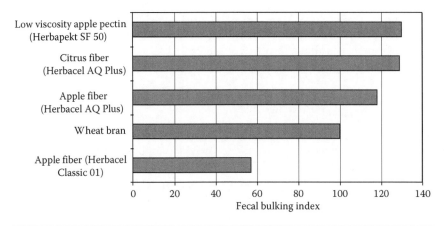

Figure 28.4 Fecal bulking index (FBI) (according to [69]) reflects non-digested food matter, hindgut bacterial biomass and the water-holding capacity of the whole. Reference was 12.5% wheat bran (100) to the normal diet (bases = 0).

Some work has been done on the bulking of fruit fibers [63,64]. This effect can be considered as beneficial to prevent constipation, a major health problem mainly for elderly women. Furthermore, bulking and transit time is an important risk factor for colon cancer.

Responsible for a high bulking effect is the good water binding of fruit fiber that is stable during the passage through the intestine. In addition, the relative filigree morphological structure allows good growth of the bacteria. Figure 28.4 shows results of a comparative study of different commercial fruit fibers. Additionally, some integral parts of fruit fibers are metabolized by desirable bacteria and, with that, have a prebiotic nature.

A few studies have been published concerning the link between the general health benefit of fruits and their dietary fiber content. An Italian study [65] supports the hypothesis that dietary fiber in fruits (and vegetable but not cereal) is one of the beneficial components that protects against laryngeal cancer risk. A Harvard research group [66] analyzed whether the source of dietary fiber has an influence on the reduction of heart disease risk by pooling results of studies on more than 91,000 men and 245,000 women. In this study, the strongest protective effect against coronary heart disease–caused deaths is a reduction in risk of 30% with fruit fiber and 25% with cereal fiber for each 10 g per day.

In a human intervention study with healthy volunteers, the effect of isolated soybean, lupin, and citrus fiber has been studied [67]. The supplementation with 25 g/day of the fibers resulted in significant increased fecal mass, reduction of secondary bile salt concentration, and enhancement of the short-chain fatty acid concentration. All three insoluble fibers positively influence the putative risk factors for colon cancer, thus being beneficial for colon health.

A recent intervention study with hypercholesterolemic subjects showed the positive effect of a high-fiber diet on the basis of food enriched with either citrus or lupin fiber against low-fiber food (placebo). In this single-blind, randomized crossover study, every subject had to consume three times over 4 weeks a pattern of experimental food that offered additional 25 g dietary fiber/day in case of both fibers with a 2 week break (baseline). After each block, the effect on blood lipids was studied. The study showed that citrus fiber could lower the LDL level of mild to clinical hypercholesterolemic persons to 6% compared to baseline [68].

From all data, it is obvious that fruit fibers offer beneficial effects to health and are able to prevent death. Even if generally the intake is recommended to be via a high consumption of whole fruits, it is evident that isolated fruit fiber can add a benefit to food or a diet. This happens either directly by the fiber itself or indirectly by energy dilution of food due to high water binding. Naturally, fruit fiber–free products such as dairy dessert and sausages of baked products can be enriched to improve the health benefit of these food categories. For the future, we like to see more studies on specific effect of different isolated fibers in food. The present fiber claims in most countries do not consider the difference in physiological effect of, for example, 1 g of fiber coming from inulin, wheat fiber, or apple fiber. This is a prerequisite of the food industry to develop functional food without being driven by price.

References

1. Hipsley, E.H., Dietary "fiber" and pregnancy toxaemia, *Brit. Med. J.*, 2, 420, 1953.
2. Trowell, H., Burkitt, D., and Heaton, K., *Dietary Fiber—Fiber Depleted Foods and Diseases*. Academic Press, London, U.K., 1985.
3. Meuser, F., Technological aspects of dietary fiber, in *Advanced Dietary Fiber Technology*, McCleary and Prosky, Eds., Blackwell Science, Oxford, U.K., 2001, Chapter 23.
4. Selvendran, R.R., Steven, B.J.H., and DuPont, M.S., Dietary fiber: Chemistry, analysis and properties, *Adv. Food Res.*, 31, 117, 1987.
5. Waldron, K.W., Parker, M.L., and Smith, A.C., Plant cell walls and food quality, *Comp. Rev. Food Sci. Food Safety*, 2, 128–146, 2003.
6. MacDougall, A.J. and Selvendran, R.R., Chemistry, architecture, and composition of dietary fiber from plant cell walls, *Handbook of Dietary Fiber*, Cho and Dreher, Eds., Marcel Dekker, New York, 2001, Chapter 19.
7. Pena, M.J., Vergara, C.E., and Carpita, N.C., The structure and architecture of plant cell walls define dietary fiber composition and the texture of foods, in *Advanced Dietary Fiber Technology*, McCleary and Prosky, Eds., Blackwell Science, Oxford, U.K., 2001, Chapter 5.
8. Selvendran, R.R., Dietary fiber in foods: Amount and type, physico-chemical properties of dietary fiber and effect of processing on micronutrient availability, *Proceeding of a Workshop, COST 92*, Amado, Barry, and Frolich, Eds., Commission of the European Communities, Luxemburg, IA, 1993.
9. Thomas, M. et al., Characterisation of dietary fiber and cell-wall polysaccharides from different tissue zones and entire fruit of *Chaenomeles japonica*, Poster at First *International Conference on Dietary Fiber*, Dublin, Ireland, 2000.
10. Martin-Cabrejas, M.A. et al., By-products of food industries as source of dietary fiber, physico-chemical properties of dietary fiber and effect of processing on micronutrient availability, *Proceeding of a Workshop, COST 92*, Amado, Barry, and Frolich, Eds., Commission of the European Communities, Luxemburg, IA, 1993.

11. Licandro, G. and Odio, C.E., Citrus by-products, in *Citrus*, Dugo and DiGiacomo, Eds., Taylor & Francis, London, U.K., 2002, Chapter 11.

12. Larrauri, J.A., New approaches in the preparation of high dietary fiber powders from fruit by-products, *Trends Food Sci. Technol.*, 10, 3, 1999.

13. Martin-Cabrejas, M.A. et al., Dietary fiber content of Pear and Kiwi pomace, *J. Food Chem.*, 43, 662, 1995.

14. Valiente, C. et al., Grape pomace as a potential food fiber, *J. Food Sci.*, 60, 818, 1995.

15. Walter, R.H. et al., Edible fiber from Apple pomace, *J. Food Sci.*, 50, 747, 1985.

16. Arrigoni, E. et al., Chemical composition and physical properties of modified dietary fiber sources, *Food Hydrocolloids*, 1, 57, 1986.

17. Braddock, R.J. and Graumlich, T.R., Composition of fiber from citrus peel, membranes, juice vesicles and seeds, *Lebensm. Wiss. Technol.*, 14, 229, 1980.

18. Dongowski, G. and Bock, W., Rohstoffressourcen für die Herstellung von pektinhaltigen Ballaststoffen und Ballaststoffpräparate, in *Aktuelle Aspekte der Ballaststofforschung*, Schulze and Bock, Eds., Behr's Verlag, Hamburg, Germany, 1993, Chapter 4.

19. Bock, W. and Ohm, G., Einfluss der gewachsenen Struktur auf die Wasserbindungskapazität ausgewählter Obst und Gemüsepräparate, *Food/Nahrung*, 27, 205, 1983.

20. Kunzek, H. and Dongowski, G., Der Einfluß des mechanolytischen Abbaus von Obst- und Gemüsetrockenpräparaten auf die Bestimmung des Wasserbindevermögens unter Verwendung verschiedener Methoden, *Lebensm. Ind.*, 38, 77, 1991.

21. Kunzek, H., Krabbert, R., and Gloyna, D., Aspects of material science in food processing: Changes in plant cell walls of fruits and vegetables, *Z. Lebensm. Unters. Forsch. A*, 208, 233, 1999.

22. Krabbert, R., Herrmuth, K., and Kunzek, H., Wasserbindekapazität und Makrostruktur von Apfelgewebepartikeln, *Z. Lebensm. Unters. Forsch.*, 197, 219, 1993.

23. Müller, S. and Kunzek, H., Material properties of processed fruits and vegetables, *Z. Lebensm. Unters. Forsch. A*, 206, 264, 1998.

24. Kunzek, H. et al., Einsatz der Druckhomogenisierung zur Herstellung von zellstrukturiertem Apfelmaterial, *Z. Lebensm. Unters. Forsch.*, 198, 239, 1994.

25. Fischer, J., Functional properties of Herbacel AQ Plus fruit fibers, *Poster at First International Conference on Dietary Fiber*, Dublin, Ireland, 2000.

26. Vetter, S., Kunzek, H., and Senge, B., The influence of the pre-treatment of apple cell wall samples on their functional properties, *Eur. Food Res. Technol.*, 212, 630, 2001.

27. Chen, J.V., Piva, M., and Labuza, T.P., Evaluation of water binding capacity (WBC) of food fiber sources, *J. Food Sci.*, 49, 59, 1984.

28. Canadian Harvest, Fiber Facts, Company brochure, Cambridge, MN, USA.

29. Bahr, P., New ways to apply fiber; Food Product Design, October, foodproductdesign. com/archive/1996/1096DE.html

30. Amado, R., Physico-chemical properties related to type of dietary fiber, *Physico-Chemical Properties of Dietary Fiber and Effect of Processing on Micronutrient Availability*, Amado, Barry, and Frolich, Eds., Commission of the European Communities, Luxembourg, IA, 1993.

31. Endress, H.U. and Fischer, J., Fibers and fiber blends for individual needs: A physiological and technological approach, in *Advanced Dietary Fiber Technology*, McCleary and Prosky, Eds., Blackwell Science, Oxford, U.K., 2001, Chapter 26.

32. Miller, E., Lassbeck, A., and Bender, M., Apple—The fruit for more than one application, *Food Tech. Europe*, March/April, 88, 1995.

33. Fischer, J., Dietary fibers-ingredients for sweet and bakery goods, *Zucker und Suesswarenwirtschaft*, 10, 20, 2001.

34. Bender, M., Citrusfaser, *Food Tech. M,* October, 22, 1996.

35. Duxbury, D.D., Apple fiber powder yields higher pectin, moisture retention, *Food Processing*, November, 82, 1987.
36. Fischer, J., Improved fruit fibers for modern food processing, *Food Ingredients Anal.*, May/June 29, 2001.
37. Figuerola, F. et al., Fiber concentrates from apple pomace and citrus peels as potential fiber source for food enrichment, *Food Chem.*, 91, 395, 2005.
38. Fischer, J., Fibers in ice cream, *Inter-Ice 2000, International Symposium*, Solingen, Germany, May 2000.
39. Meijer, E., Powerful technologies for differentiating vitality innovation, *SVP Food R&D* presented at Unilever Inventor Seminar, March 2007.
40. Schneeman, B.O., Dietary fiber and gastrointestinal function, in *Advanced Dietary Fiber Technology*, McCleary and Prosky, Eds., Blackwell Science, Oxford, U.K., 2001, Chapter 14.
41. Viuda-Martor, M., Role of fiber in cardiovascular diseases: A review, *Comp. Rev. Food Sci. Food Safety*, 9, 240–258, 2010.
42. Sandrou, D.K. and Arvanitoyannis, I.S., Low-fat/calorie foods: Current state and perspective, *Crit. Rev. Food Sci. Nutr.*, 40(5), 427, 2000.
43. Fischer, J., Dietary fibers, no.1 ingredients for calorie reduction, *Wellness Foods Europe*, April/May, 4, 2004.
44. Bollinger, H., Ballaststoffe—Eigenschaften und ihre Anwendungsmöglichkeiten, *Suesswaren*, 7–8, 384, 1990.
45. Bollinger, H., Calorie-reduced snacks, *Food Market. Technol.*, April, 18, 1993.
46. Hanneforth, U. and Brack, G., Apfelballaststoffe: Eigenschaften und Eignung für die Verarbeitung in Feinen Backwaren, *Brot und Backwaren*, 3, 80, 1991.
47. Perez-Alvarez, J.A. et al., Effect of citrus fiber (albedo) incorporation in cooked pork sausages, *IFT Annual Meeting*, New Orleans, 2001.
48. Fischer, J., Leichter ballast, *Lebensmitteltechnik*, 6, 48, 2001.
49. Garcia, M.L. et al., Utilisation of cereal and fruit fibers in low fat dry fermented sausages, *Meat Sci.*, 60(3), 227, 2002.
50. Garcia, M.l., Caeres, E., and Selgas, M.D., Utilisation of fruit fibers in conventional and reduced-fat cooked sausages, *J. Sci. Food Agric.*, 87(3), 624, 2007.
51. Köz, P., Boyacioglu, D., Özcelik, B., Development of a functional Turkish dessert: Dietetic and diabetic baklava, *IFT Annual Meeting*, Las Vegas, NV, 2004.
52. Hughes, K., Reduced fat with pulp fiber, *Prepared Food*, January 2007.
53. Fischer, J., Fruit fibers to count down the calories, *Innov. Food Technol.*, November, 20, 2005.
54. Auffret, A. et al., Effect of grinding and experimental conditions on the measurement of hydration properties of dietary fibers, *Lebensmittel-Wissenschaft und Technologie*, 27(2), 166, 1994.
55. WHO/FAO, Expert consultation on diet, nutrition and the prevention of chronic diseases, WHO Technical Report Series 916, Geneva, Switzerland, 2003.
56. US Department of Health and Human Service, Healthy people 2000, National health promotion and disease prevention objectives, DHHS Publ. 91-50212, Washington, DC, 1991.
57. Bazzano, L.A., Dietary intake of fruit and vegetables and risk of diabetes mellitus and cardiovascular diseases, *Background Paper for the Joint FAO/WHO Workshop on Fruit and Vegetables for Health*, September 1–3, 2004, WHO, Kobe, Japan, 2005.
58. Ludwig, D.S. et al., Dietary fiber, weight gain, and cardiovascular disease risk factors in young adults, *JAMA*, 282(16), 1999.
59. World Cancer Research Fund international/American Institute for Cancer Research, *Food, Nutrition, Physical Activity and the Prevention of Cancer: A Global Perspective*. AICR, Washington, DC, 2007, Chapter 12.

60. U.S. Food and Drug Administration, Health claims 21 CFR 101.76, 21 CFR 101.77 and 21 CFR 101.78, www.cfsan.fda.gov, 2004.
61. Baghurst, K., The health benefits of citrus fruits, CSIRO Health Science and Nutrition, Report to Horticulture Australia Ltd, Project No. CT01037, June 2003.
62. Deutsche Gesellschaft für Ernährung, Kohlenhydratzufuhr und Prävention ausgewählter ernährungsbedingter Krankheiten, Version 2011, DGE, Bonn, Germany, 2011.
63. Bravo, L., Saura-Calixto, F., and Goni, I., Effects of dietary fiber and tannins from apple pulp on the composition of faeces in rats, *Brit. J. Nutr.*, 67(3), 463, 1992.
64. Bird, A.R. and Topping, D.L., CSIRO Human Nutrition PTI/FITA report, June 1999.
65. Pelucchi, C. et al., Fiber intake and laryngeal cancer risk, *Ann. Oncol.*, 14, 162, 2003.
66. Pereira, M.A. et al., Dietary fiber and risk of coronary heart disease: A pooled analysis of cohort studies, *Arch. Int. Med.*, 164(4), 370, 2004.
67. Fechner, A. et al., Influence of legume kernel fibers on risk factors for colon cancer, *Poster at Fourth International Conference on Dietary Fiber*, Vienna, Austria, July 2009.
68. Jahreis, G., Intervention with lupin kernel fiber in hypercholesterolemic subjects, www.clinicaltrials.gov/ct2/show/record/NCT01035086, December 2009.
69. Monro, J., Faecal bulking index and wheat bran equivalents for dietary management of distal colonic bulk, *Poster at First International Conference on Dietary Fiber*, Dublin, Ireland, 2000.

29

Fig Fruit By-Products (*Ficus carica*) as a Source of Dietary Fiber

ELENA SÁNCHEZ-ZAPATA, EVANGÉLICA FUENTES-ZARAGOZA, MANUEL VIUDA-MARTOS, ANA MARTIN-SÁNCHEZ, JUANA FERNÁNDEZ-LÓPEZ, ESTHER SENDRA, ESTRELLA SAYAS-BARBERÁ, CASILDA NAVARRO, and JOSÉ A. PÉREZ-ÁLVAREZ

Contents

29.1 Fig Fruit

Figs (*Ficus carica*) are one of the earliest fruits cultivated.[1] Figs are dried and stored for later consumption. There was a fig tree in the Garden of Eden, and the fig is the most mentioned fruit in the Bible.[2] The fig tree (*Ficus carica* L.) is one of the unique *Ficus* species widely spread in tropical and subtropical countries, which has edible fruits with high commercial value. Commercial fig production is either located around the Mediterranean Sea or is realized in countries possessing Mediterranean climate as in the case of California, Australia, or South America. In Turkey, the major fig producer, around 65% of fig trees are in the western Aegean region especially in small and big Meander valleys. The major variety grown in this region is Sarilop, which is commercially sun dried.[3]

Although considered a fruit, the fig is actually a flower inverted into itself. The seeds are the real fruit in figs. They are the only fruit to ripen fully and semidry on the tree. Native to areas from Asiatic Turkey to northern India, figs spread to all the countries around the Mediterranean. Today, the United States, Turkey, Greece, and Spain are the primary producers of dried figs. The Spaniards brought figs to the Americas in the early sixteenth century.[4]

29.1.1 Fig Production

The total fig production in the world is more than 1,000,000 ton; Turkey is the highest fig producer, followed by Iran and other Mediterranean countries, like Spain. Today, Turkey, Iran, Algeria, and Spain are the primary producers of dried figs.[5] In Spain, the fig consumption is reduced, and the production is formed for common varieties with low commercial qualities, and so a lot of figs are lost along the production chain.

29.1.1.1 Fig Fruit Composition   Preservation of fruits by solar drying has been practiced for centuries. It is limited to climates with a hot sun and a dry atmosphere and to certain fruits, such as figs.[6] Figs are one of the highest plant sources of calcium and fiber. Dried figs are richest in carbohydrates, fiber, copper, manganese, magnesium, potassium, calcium, and vitamin K, relative to human needs.[1,7] They have smaller amounts of many other nutrients. The composition of dry figs is presented in Table 29.1. Figs have a laxative effect and contain many antioxidants. They are good source of flavonoids and polyphenols; a 40 g portion of dried figs (two medium size figs) produced a significant increase in plasma antioxidant capacity.[8]

29.1.1.2 Fig Industrialization and Its By-Products   Food processing by-products may still contain many valuable substances, such as dietary fiber, pigments, organic acids, flavors, and antibacterial or antifungal substances.[9–12] Some of these products have been recognized by several organizations (FDA and EFSA) to possess proved health benefits. Public institutions are supporting the food industry to implement new technologies to recover value-added ingredients from by-products. Depending on the availability of an adequate technology, these by-products can be converted into commercial products as raw materials for secondary processes (intermediate food ingredients), as operating supplies, or as ingredients of new products. Numerous valuable substances in food

Table 29.1 Dry Fig Composition

Component	g/100 g
Carbohydrate	66.16
TDF	12.21
Insoluble dietary fiber	8.74
Soluble dietary fiber	3.47
Protein	3.14
Fat	0.52
Potassium	609 mg
Sodium	12.26 mg
Vitamin A	9.76 IU
Vitamin C	0.68 mg
Calcium	133 mg
Iron	3.07 mg

Source: Vinson, J.A., *Cereal Food World*, 44(2), 82, 1999.

production are suitable for separation and recycling at the end of their life cycle, even though the available separation and recycling technologies are not necessarily cost efficient.[13]

Fig (*Ficus carica* L.) is one of the favorite dried fruits in the world. It is widely used in confectionery, snack foods, and pastry industries. The fig industrialization produces a lot of by-products.[14] This by-product is generally discarded or used in animal feeding. The nonuse of this by-product constitutes a real economic loss since it is rich in nutrients and bioactive compounds, which can be extracted and used as value-added materials. The aims of this study were (i) to develop a process to obtain a stable paste from these by-products and (ii) to characterize this fig paste in view of its possible incorporation in food.

29.1.2 Materials and Methods

29.1.2.1 Raw Material   Fig by-products from fresh fig processing were homogenized and triturated with the aim of obtaining a stable paste (Figure 29.1). This paste was packed in vacuum pouches made of polyethylene and polyamide laminate of water vapor permeability 1.1 g/m²/24h at 23°C, nitrogen permeability 10 cm³/m²/24h at 23°C, carbon dioxide permeability 140 cm³/m²/24h at 23°C, and oxygen permeability 30 cm³/m²/24h at 23°C (Fibran, Girona, Spain). The pouches were evacuated and heat sealed. The vacuum-packed paste was immediately frozen at −30°C until use.

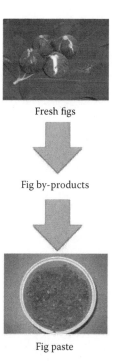

Fresh figs

Fig by-products

Fig paste

Figure 29.1 Fig paste obtention.

29.1.2.2 Chemical Analysis   Moisture, ash, protein, fat, and dietary fiber content were determined by AOAC methods.[15] Moisture (g water/100 g sample) was determined by drying a 3 g sample at 105°C to constant weight. Ashing was performed on a 2–3 g sample after combustion in a muffle furnace at 550°C for 8 h (g ash/100 g sample). Protein (g protein/100 g sample) was analyzed according to the Kjeldahl method, using a factor of 6.25 for the conversion of nitrogen to crude protein. Fat (g fat/100 g sample) was calculated by weight loss by extraction for 8 h with petroleum ether in a Sohxlet apparatus. Total dietary fiber (TDF) was determined by AOAC 985.29 method.

29.1.2.3 Physicochemical Analysis   The pH was measured in a suspension resulting from blending a 10 g sample with 10 mL deionized water for 2 min using a pH-meter (Mod. pH/Ion 510, Eutech Instruments Pte Ltd., Singapore). Water activity (A_w) was determined in a Novasina Thermoconstanter Sprint TH-500 (Pfäffikon, Switzerland). Color was studied in the CIELAB color space using a Minolta CM-2600d (Minolta Camera Co., Osaka, Japan), with D_{65} as illuminant and an observer angle of 10°. Low reflectance glass (Minolta CR-A51/1829-752) was placed between the samples and the equipment. The CIELAB coordinates studied were lightness (L*), coordinate red/green (a*), and coordinate yellow/blue (b*).

29.1.2.4 Technological Properties   Water-holding capacity (WHC) and oil-holding capacity (OHC) were determined according to Robertson et al.[16] WHC was expressed as g of water held per g of sample, and OHC was expressed as g of oil held per g of sample. Water adsorption capacity (WA_dC) and water absorption capacity (WA_bC) were determined according to Vázquez-Ovando et al.[17] WA_dC was expressed as g of water adsorbed per g of sample, and WA_bC was expressed as g of water absorbed per g of sample. Emulsion capacity (EC) and emulsion stability (ES) were evaluated according to Chau et al.,[18] with slight modifications. One hundred milliliter of 2% (w/v) sample suspension in water was homogenized at 11,000 rpm for 30 s using a homogenizer IKA T-25. One hundred milliliter of sunflower oil was then added and homogenized for another 1 min. The emulsions were centrifuged in 10 mL graduated centrifuged tubes at 1200 g for 5 min, and the volume of the emulsion left was measured. EA was calculated as volume of emulsified layer/volume of whole layer in centrifuge tube. To determine the ES, emulsions prepared by the procedures mentioned earlier were heated at 80°C for 30 min, cooled to room temperature, and centrifuged at 1200 g for 5 min. ES was calculated as volume of remaining emulsified layer/original emulsion volume.

29.1.2.5 Total Phenol Content   Total phenolics were determined colorimetrically using Folin–Ciocalteau reagent as described by Al-Farsi et al.[19] using a UV-1601 spectrophotometer (Shimazu, Kyoto, Japan). The concentrations are expressed as milligrams of gallic acid equivalents (GAE) per 100 g of fresh weight.

29.1.2.6 Antioxidant Properties The antioxidant activity of fig paste was measured using three complementary test systems, namely, diphenyl-1-picrylhydrazyl (DPPH) radical scavenging capacity assay, ferric reducing antioxidant power (FRAP), and ferrous ion chelating (FIC) assay.

29.1.2.6.1 DPPH Assay The antioxidant activity of fig paste was measured in terms of hydrogen-donating or radical-scavenging ability, using the stable radical DPPH.[20] A volume of 50 μL of a methanolic fig paste solution was put into a cuvette, and 2 mL 6 × 10–5 M methanolic solution of DPPH was added. Ascorbic acid and butylated hydroxytoluene (BHT; in the same concentration) were used as references. The mixtures were well shaken in a vortex (2500 rpm) for 1 min and then placed in a dark room. The decrease in absorbance at 517 nm was determined using an HP 8451 spectrophotometer (Hewlett-Packard) after 1 h for all samples. Methanol was used to zero the spectrophotometer. Absorbance of the radical without antioxidant (control) was measured daily. Inhibition (%) was plotted against the sample concentration in the reaction system. The percentage inhibition of the DPPH radical was calculated according to the formula of Yen and Duh[21]:

$$\%I = [(A_B - A_S)/A_B] \times 100$$

where
  I is the DPPH inhibition (%)
  A_B is the absorbance of control sample (t = 0 h)
  A_S is the absorbance of a tested sample at the end of the reaction (t = 1 h)

29.1.2.6.2 Ferric Reducing Antioxidant Power The reducing power of the fig paste was determined according to the method of Oyaizu.[22] Briefly, various concentrations of DW were mixed with 2.5 mL of 200 mmol/L sodium phosphate buffer (pH 6.6) and 2.5 mL of 1% potassium ferricyanide. The mixture was incubated in a water bath at 50°C for 20 min. Afterward, 2.5 mL of 10% trichloroacetic acid (w/v) was added; the mixture was centrifuged at 650 rpm for 10 min. The upper layer (2.5 mL) was mixed with 2.5 mL deionized water and 0.5 mL of 0.1% of ferric chloride (w/v), and the absorbance was measured at 700 nm (higher absorbance indicates higher reducing power). Trolox was used as standard. The assays were carried out in triplicate, and the results are expressed as mean values ± standard deviations.

29.1.2.6.3 Ferrous Ion Chelating Ability Assay The FIC assay was carried out according to the method of Singh and Rajini[23] with some modifications. Solutions of 2 mM $FeCl_2 \cdot 4H_2O$ and 5 mM ferrozine were diluted 20 times. Briefly, an aliquot (1 mL) of fig paste extract was mixed with 1 mL $FeCl_2 \cdot 4H_2O$. After 5 min incubation, the reaction was initiated by the addition of ferrozine (1 mL). The mixture was shaken vigorously, and, after a further 10 min incubation period, the absorbance of the solution was measured spectrophotometrically at 562 nm. The percentage inhibition of ferrozine–Fe + 2 complex formation was calculated by using the formula:

$$\text{Chelating effect } (\%) = [(1 - A_S)/A_B] \times 100$$

where

A_B is the absorbance of control sample (the control contains $FeCl_2$ and ferrozine, complex formation molecules)

A_S is the absorbance of a tested sample

29.1.3 Results and Discussion

29.1.3.1 Chemical Composition   The chemical composition of the fig paste (by-products) analyzed is presented in Table 29.2. The chemical composition of fig paste was 17.41%, sugars 53.40%, TDF 16.53%, fats 5.11%, proteins 3.36%, and ash 0.77%. Thus, fig paste provides a good source of rapid energy (sugars) and a good nutritional value, based on their dietary fiber contents. The main sugars found were glucose and fructose, in order of concentration.

29.1.3.2 Physicochemical Properties   The physicochemical properties of fig paste are shown in Table 29.3. The low water activity and pH of the fig paste, both parameters highly related to product deterioration, indicate that the risk of deterioration (by microorganism, enzymes, or nonenzymatic reactions) is minimal. The results on color measurements of fig paste in terms of CIEL*a*b* color coordinate values were lightness (L*) 31.73, redness (a*) 8.79, and yellowness (b*) 13.67. CIELAB a* and b* values represent red and yellow color of paste, respectively, and, therefore, fig paste showed an attractive color.

Table 29.2 Fig Paste Composition

Component	g/100 g
Carbohydrate	53.40
Protein	3.36
TDF	16.53
Moisture	17.41
Fat	5.11
Ash	0.77

Table 29.3 Physicochemical Properties of Fig Paste

Parameter	Value
pH	3.91
Water activity	0.686
Lightness (L*)	31.73
Redness (a*)	8.79
Yellowness (b*)	13.67

Table 29.4 Technological Properties of Fig By-Product Paste

Property	
Water holding capacity	1 g water/g fig paste
Oil holding capacity	0.36 g oil/g fig paste
Water adsorption capacity	0.12 g water/g fig paste
Water absorption capacity	0.27 g water/g fig paste
Emulsion capacity	45.50 mL/100 mL of emulsion
Emulsion stability	100 mL/100 mL of emulsion

29.1.3.3 Technological Properties The technological properties of fig paste are presented in Table 29.4. WHC is related to the chemical and physical structure of the plant polysaccharides. Dietary fiber has an important effect on this technological property because it holds water by adsorption (water adsorption capacity: 0.12 g/g fig paste) and absorption (water absorption capacity: 0.27 g/g fig paste) phenomena. Some water is also retained outside the fiber matrix (free water; 0.60 g/g fig paste). Fig paste exhibited a WHC 1.00 times its own weight (Table 29.4). These hydration properties of fig paste determine their optimal usage levels in foods as they provide desirable texture properties. The OHC is also a technological property related to the chemical structure of the plant polysaccharides and depends on their chemical and physical structure.[24] Fig paste exhibited an OHC 0.36 times its own weight (Table 29.4). OHC is important to flavor retention and product yield especially for cooked meat products, which normally lose fat during cooking.[25]

29.1.3.4 Total Phenol Content The total phenolic compound (TPC) content of the investigated fig paste is presented in Table 29.5. It showed a high content of total phenols (5.72 mg/g GAE), although this content is half of the content present in the fresh fig fruit.[1] This reduction in the TPC could be due to the processing conditions applied to obtain the fig paste. In spite of this reduction, the TPC of fig paste was similar to or higher than the TPC in other fresh fruits as blueberries, blackberries, strawberry, and grapes.[1,26]

Table 29.5 Total Phenol Content in the Fig Paste Extract

Total Phenol Content	**mg GAE/g**
Fig paste (by-product)	**5.72**
Fig (whole fruit)	10.90
Blueberries	5.56
Blackberries	4.87
Strawberry	2.18
Grape	4.90

The results of fig paste (by-products) analyzed is present in bold.

The phenolic compound content could be used as an important indicator of the antioxidant capacity, which may be used as a preliminarily screen for fig paste when intended as natural sources of antioxidants in functional foods.[20] Many authors have described the potential antioxidant properties of polyphenols. These compounds act as antioxidants by donating of a hydrogen atom, as an acceptor of free radicals, by interrupting chain oxidation reactions, or by chelating metals.

29.1.3.5 Antioxidant Properties

29.1.3.5.1 DPPH Assay The DPPH free radical does not require any special preparation and is considered a simple and very fast method for determining antioxidant activity. In contrast, DPPH can only be dissolved in organic media, especially in ethanol, which is an important limitation when interpreting the role of hydrophilic antioxidants.

The radical-scavenging capacity of the fig paste was tested using the "stable" free radical, DPPH. Table 29.6 shows the effective concentrations of fig paste compared with some essential oil, studied for our group, required to scavenge DPPH radical and the scavenging values as inhibition percentage. It can be seen that the methanolic fig solution at 100 g/L exhibited scavenging capacity, lower than Clove essential oil, ascorbic acid, or BHT, but higher than rosemary EO methanolic solutions at 5 g/L.[20]

The DPPH assay measures the ability of the extract to donate hydrogen to the DPPH radical, resulting in bleaching of the DPPH solution, and a linear correlation between the TPC content and antioxidant capacity has been demonstrated.[21]

29.1.3.5.2 Ferric Reducing Antioxidant Power The FRAP method is a simple, very rapid, inexpensive, and reproducible method, which can be applied to the assay of antioxidants in plasma or botanicals.[20] Table 29.7 shows the ferric reducing capacity obtained using the FRAP assay.

Methanolic solutions of fig paste showed lower ferric reducing capacity in terms of trolox concentrations than fig fruit and cherry, but similar to apple and higher than banana.[26]

Table 29.6 Radical-Scavenging Capacity of the Fig Paste Extract

DPPH	% Inhibition
Fig paste (100 g/L)	**90.39**
Clove essential oil (5 g/L)	97.85
Rosemary essential oil (5 g/L)	47.54
Ascorbic acid (5 g/L)	96.61
BHT (5 g/L)	95.93

The results of fig paste (by-products) analyzed is present in bold.

Table 29.7 Ferric Reducing Antioxidant Power
of Fig Paste Extract

FRAP	TEAC (mM Trolox/g)
Fig paste (by-product)	**1.68**
Fig (whole fruit)	3.54
Apple	1.6
Cherry	2.7
Banana	0.6

The results of fig paste (by-products) analyzed is
    present in bold.

29.1.3.5.3 Ferrous Ion Chelating Ability Assay   One of the possible mechanisms of the antioxidant action is the chelation of transition metals. Transition metal ions can stimulate lipid peroxidation in two ways:[20]

1. Participating in the generation of initiating species
2. Accelerating peroxidation, decomposing lipid hydroperoxides into other components that are able to abstract hydrogen, and perpetuating the chain of reaction of lipid peroxidation

Analysis of metal ion-chelating properties showed that fig paste from fig by-products (Table 29.8) was capable of chelating iron.

When the FIC values of fig paste were compared with the values obtained for different spice essential oils and other antioxidant products, rosemary essential oils showed the highest values.[20] The concentration of fig paste used for this assay was half of the other compounds, so, at the same concentration, fig paste will show a similar ferrous chelation activity than ascorbic acid. Therefore, it can be said that the fig paste, at this concentration, showed mild chelating activity, which is of great significance because the chelation of transition metals is of great potential interest in the food industry, where transition metal ions, by catalyzing the interaction and decomposition of hydroperoxides, contribute to lipid oxidation, which is the main source of degradation of food products.[23]

Table 29.8 Ferrous Ion-Chelating Ability of Fig Paste Extract

FIC Assay	% Chelating Effect
Fig paste (by-product) (100 g/L)	**63.22**
Clove essential oil (50 g/L)	60.04
Rosemary essential oil (50 g/L)	76.06
Ascorbic acid (50 g/L)	36.07
BHT (50 g/L)	44.67

The results of fig paste (by-products) analyzed is present
    in bold.

29.1.4 Conclusion

- Fig fruit by-products can be used to produce stable fig paste, which is a potential ingredient in food products, increasing their content of TDF. Due to its sugar content, the fig paste could be specially suitable for dry-cured meat products since they would be a source of carbon for the microbiota present in this kind of products.
- The results obtained using different methods to evaluate the antioxidant activity (DPPH, FRAP, and FIC) showed that fig paste, obtained from fig by-products, can be considered a good source of natural compounds with significant antioxidant activity, which can be attributed to the high percentage of the main constituents (phenols) or to synergy among the different fig constituents.

References

1. Vinson, J.A., The functional food properties of figs, *Cereal Food World*, 44(2), 82, 1999.
2. Goor, A., The history of the fig in the Holy Land from ancient times to the present day, *Econ. Bot.*, 19, 124, 1965.
3. Irget, M.E. et al., Effect of calcium based fertilization on dried fig (*Ficus carica* L. cv. Sarılop) yield and quality, *Sci. Hort.*, 118, 308, 2008.
4. Statistical Review of the California Fig Industry, Report, California Fig Advisory Board, Fresno, California, 1998, www.californiafigs.com (accessed April 6, 2010).
5. Amanlou, Y. and Zomorodian, A., Evaluation of air flow resistance across a green fig bed for selecting an appropriate pressure drop prediction equation, *Food Bioprod. Process.*, 89(2), 157, 2011.
6. Isman, B. and Biyik, H., The aflatoxin contamination of fig fruits in Aydin City (Turkey), *J. Food Safety*, 29, 318, 2009.
7. Waheed, S. and Siddique, N., Evaluation of dietary status with respect to trace element intake from dry fruits consumed in Pakistan: A study using instrumental neutron activation analysis, *Int. J. Food Sci. Nutr.*, 60(4), 333, 2009.
8. Lansky, E.P. et al., *Ficus* spp. (fig): Ethnobotany and potential as anticancer and anti-inflammatory agents, *J. Ethnopharm.*, 119, 195, 2008.
9. Fernández-López, J. et al., Physico-chemical and microbiological profiles of "salchichón" (Spanish dry-fermented sausage) enriched with orange fiber, *Meat Sci.*, 80, 410, 2008.
10. Mckee, L.H. and Latner, T.A., Underutilized sources of dietary fibre: A review, *Plant Food Hum. Nutr.*, 55, 285, 2000.
11. Lario, Y. et al., Preparation of high dietary fibre extract from lemon juice by-products, *Innov. Food Sci. Emerg. Technol.*, 5, 113, 2004.
12. Ku, C.S. and Mun, S.P., Optimization of the extraction of anthocyanin from Bokbunja (*Rubus coreanus* Miq.) marc produced during traditional wine processing and characterization of the extracts, *Bioresource Technol.*, 99, 8325, 2008.
13. Sánchez-Zapata, E. et al., Preparation of dietary fibre extract from tiger nut (*Cyperus esculentus*) milk ("Horchata") by-products and its physicochemical properties, *J. Agric. Food Chem.*, 57, 7719, 2009.
14. Doymaz, I., Sun drying of figs: An experimental study. *J. Food Eng.*, 71, 403, 2005.
15. AOAC., *Official Methods of Analysis of AOAC International*, 16th edn., Association of Official Analytical Chemists: Washington, DC, 1997.

16. Robertson, J.A. et al., Hydration properties of dietary fibre and resistant starch: A European collaborative study, *LWT Food Sci. Technol.*, 33, 72, 2000.
17. Vázquez-Ovando, A. et al., Physicochemical properties of a fibrous fraction from chia *(Salvia hispanica* L.), *Food Sci. Technol.*, 42, 168, 2009.
18. Chau, C., Cheung, K., and Wong, Y., Functional properties of protein concentrate from three Chinese indigenous legume seeds, *J. Agric. Food Chem.*, 45, 2500, 1997.
19. Al-Farsi, M. et al., Comparison of antioxidant activity, anthocyanins, carotenoids, and phenolics of three native fresh and sun-dried date (*Phoenix dactylifera* L.) varieties growth in Oman, *J. Agr. Food Chem.*, 53, 7592, 2005.
20. Viuda-Martos, M. et al., Antioxidant activity of essential oils of five Spice plants widely used in a Mediterranean diet, *Flavour Fragr. J.*, 25, 13, 2010.
21. Yen, G.C. and Duh, P.D., Scavenging effect of methanolic extracts of peanut hulls on free radical and active oxygen species, *J. Agr. Food Chem.*, 42, 629, 1994.
22. Oyaizu, M., Studies on products of browning reactions: Antioxidative activities of products of browning reaction prepared from glucosamine, *Jpn. J. Nutr.*, 44, 307, 1986.
23. Singh, N. and Rajini, P.S., Free radical scavenging activity of an aqueous extract of potato peel, *Food Chem.* 85, 611, 2004.
24. Fernández-López, J. et al., Storage stability of a high dietary fiber powder from orange by-products, *Int. J. Food Sci. Tech.*, 44, 748, 2009.
25. Thebaudin, J.Y. et al., Dietary fibers: Nutritional and technological interest, *Trends Food Sci. Tech.*, 8, 41, 1997.
26. Pande, G. and Akoh, C.C. 2010. Organic acids, antioxidant capacity, phenolic content and lipid characterization of Georgia-grown underutilized fruit crops, *Food Chem.*, 120, 1067, 2010.

30

Tiger Nut Fiber and Its Technological Applications in Meat Products

ELENA SÁNCHEZ-ZAPATA, EVANGÉLICA FUENTES-ZARAGOZA,
MANUEL VIUDA-MARTOS, ANA MARTIN-SÁNCHEZ, JUANA
FERNÁNDEZ-LÓPEZ, ESTHER SENDRA, ESTRELLA SAYAS-
BARBERÁ, CASILDA NAVARRO, and JOSÉ A. PÉREZ-ÁLVAREZ

Contents

30.1 Tiger Nut Fiber

Tiger nuts or "chufas" (*Cyperus esculentus* L. var. *sativus* Boeck.) are tubers mainly used to produce "horchata de chufa" (tiger nut milk), yielding high quantity of by-products. The development of optimized systems for the recovery of valuable compounds will assist in the reduction of wastes. However, as a previous step, these by-products should be characterized in order to optimize the recovery processing techniques. The presence of valuable compounds in "horchata de chufa" (protected designation of origin [PDO] "Chufa de Valencia") is not well documented; although "horchata" has been used in traditional medicine for its antihepatotoxic, choleretic, diuretic, hypocholesterolemic, and antilipidemic properties, none of these properties have been attributed to specific compounds.[1]

Spain is one of the main producers of "horchata de chufa." The annual value of tiger nut production is close to 5 million euros.[1] In the recent years, the popularity of "horchata" has been extended to other countries, as the United Kingdom. However, PDO horchata de chufa must be distinguished from different types of "horchata" based on rice and vanilla, which are from Central and South America. Chufa (or tiger nut) is also used to obtain other nonalcoholic beverages in African countries, such as Mali, where it is known as "kunnu."

Horchata by-products can form up to 60% of the harvested plant material, the management of which represents an additional problem for the industry.[1] Until now, the most common disposal method of "horchata" by-products (solid and liquid) has been its use as organic mass for combustion, composting, and animal feed. The term "by-product," which is common in industry, suggests that these wastes might be in fact usable and have their own market value. Food by-products can be used for the production of food ingredients, for example, polyphenols, protein isolates, and dietary fibers.[2] Fibers extracted from some grains and seeds exhibit physiological and functional properties that make them promising ingredients for the food industry and for health applications. Food researchers are looking for novel raw materials that meet these needs, with a particular focus on the by-products or other components from raw materials such as legumes.[3] There is a parallel interest in new sources of dietary fiber with a similar profile to those of cereal and legume by-products such as wheat, rice and oat bran, lupine, etc.[4] Fiber source research has focused on tubers, cereals, seeds, vegetables, fruits, and algae, all of which are characterized by their high dietary fiber content with low digestibility and low caloric content.[5-19] By-products from tiger nut (*Cyperus esculentus*) milk production have similar characteristics.[20]

The objective of this chapter was to develop a process to obtain a stable product from the by-products generated during the production of "horchata" from tiger nuts, which could be used as functional ingredient in food processing. The chemical, technological, and physicochemical properties of this product were also evaluated.

30.1.1 Tiger Nut Fiber Obtention

The raw material (Figure 30.1) was obtained from a local "horchata" producer, member of the "Asociación de Horchateros Artesanos de la Comunidad Valenciana." This association oversees the production of "horchata" from tiger nut PDO "Chufa de Valencia." By-products were taken during summer and transported to the pilot plant facilities of the IPOA Research Group, at the Universidad Miguel Hernández (Orihuela, Alicante, Spain) in refrigerated conditions (4°C). The whole waste was pressed in order to drain liquid waste and keep the solid residue for further analysis. All tests were carried out in triplicate ($4 \times 3 = 12$ samples). Results are expressed as means ± standard deviations (SPSS 16.0 for Windows, SPSS Inc., Chicago, Illinois).

30.1.1.1 Composition and Properties of Tiger Nut Fiber

30.1.1.1.1 Chemical Analysis Proximate composition analysis of solid "tiger nut by-product" (TNBP) is shown in Table 30.1. The total dietary fiber (TDF) content of the TNBP was 59.71 g/100 g ± 0.03, mainly insoluble dietary fiber (IDF) (59.610 g/100 g ± 0.08; 99.82% from TDF) and little soluble dietary fiber (SDF) (0.105 g/100 g; 0.17% from TDF). TNBP had more TDF than oat bran, rice bran, or orange peel,[5,9,21] but less TDF than cauliflower, pineapple, or date wastes.[5,19,22]

The high IDF content of TNBP points to a promising application in food products. IDF ingestion causes sensation of satiety, since it absorbs water and increases bolus size. It also increases the volume and weight of the fecal bolus, promoting

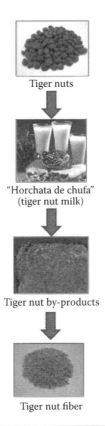

Tiger nuts

"Horchata de chufa"
(tiger nut milk)

Tiger nut by-products

Tiger nut fiber

Figure 30.1 Tiger nut fiber obtention.

Table 30.1 Proximate Composition of Solid "TNBP" (Mean Values ± SD) (g/100 g Fresh Weight)

Component	TNBP
Moisture	61.23 ± 4.12
Protein	1.75 ± 0.12
Fat	8.85 ± 1.11
Ash	0.99 ± 0.24
TDF	59.71 ± 0.03
IDF	59.61 ± 0.08
SDF	0.105 g ± 0.08

improved functioning of the digestive system and preventing disorders such as constipation and colon cancer.[6] Dietary fiber from several sources (vegetable, fruit, cereal, etc.) can increase the nutritional value of different foods like bread, cookies, muffins, cake,[23] meat products,[21] fish products,[24] and milk products;[25] thus, TNBP can be considered a potential ingredient for these types of food.

Table 30.2 WHC and OHC of "TNBP" (Mean Values ± SD)

Property	g/g of TNBP
WHC	8.01 ± 0.19
OHC	6.92 ± 0.26

30.1.1.1.2 Technological Properties (WHC and OHC) Table 30.2 shows the technological properties of tiger nut fiber. The water-holding capacity (WHC) is the ability of a moist material to retain water when subjected to an external centrifugal gravity force or compression. It consists of the sum of bound water, hydrodynamic water, and, mainly, physically trapped water.[6] Dietary fiber holds water by adsorption and absorption phenomena. Some water is also retained outside the fiber matrix (free water). Particle size, chemical composition, and structure of dietary fiber influence the WHC. The hydration properties of dietary fibers determine their optimal usage levels in foods as they provide desirable texture properties.[26] The WHC of TNBP is presented in Table 30.2. Tiger nuts exhibited a WHC 8.01 times its own weight (Figure 30.3). This is higher than that reported for fibrous residues from soybean,[27] sugarcane,[28] pear,[5] and coconut fiber,[29] but lower than the fibrous residues of some fruits with a higher SDF content, such as citrus by-products.[2,30] WHC depends on fiber processing and also on its chemical and physical structure, and it is also related to the SDF content.[2] TNBP had the lowest SDF content (Table 30.1). This proves that even though the SDF content of TNBP was relatively low, it still had a high WHC, due to the high proportion of hemicellulose and lignin (both have certain WHC) in the TNBP that may have increased its WHC. Fiber structure may also increase WHC.[9] Some vegetable fibers with high WHC have been added to meat and fish products.[21,32] TNBP has potential applications in products requiring hydration, viscosity development, and freshness preservation, such as baked foods or cooked meat products.

TNBP had an oil-holding capacity (OHC) of 6.92 g oil/g product (Table 30.2). This is similar to the OHC of pea fibrous residues.[5] It is higher than most of the vegetable processing wastes found in the literature, but lower than the OHC of asparagus[8] and date fiber.[30] OHC is also a functional property related to the chemical structure of the plant polysaccharides and depends on the chemical and physical structure;[9] it is also related with the IDF content.[26] When IDF is added to any formulation, it can absorb the oil present; the extent of this absorption is being measured as fat absorption capacity.[29] OHC is important to flavor retention and product yield especially for cooked meat products, which normally lose fat during cooking.[26] WHC and OHC had close values (Table 30.2). It has been shown that other fruit fibers with similar WHC and OHC values are useful as emulsifiers for meat products and as thickening or bulking agents.[31] Fiber particle size may influence OHC; smaller particles have relatively wider surface area and therefore would theoretically be able to hold more oil than higher particles.[6] In this sense, TNBP particles may be small enough to provide a high OHC. Due to its high OHC, TNBP is a potential ingredient for cooked meat products, but not for fried products since it would provide a greasy sensation.

30.2 Tiger Nut Fiber Application in Meat Products

Many efforts have been made to improve the quality and stability of meat products (fresh and cooked) because consumer demand for fast food has been increasing rapidly in the recent years. Most of the products used in fast food are rich in fats and sugar, but deficient in complex carbohydrates. Epidemiological research has demonstrated a relationship between this type of diet and the increase of a number of chronic diseases, including colon cancer, obesity, cardiovascular diseases, and several other disorders; therefore, an increase in the level of dietary fiber (and complex carbohydrates) in the daily diet has been recommended.[2,32] For these reasons, there is an interest in increasing the consumption of all foods that can supply fiber to daily food intake. Fiber addition to food products would help to overcome the current fiber deficit.

Fiber is one of the most common functional ingredients in food products and has been used as fat replacer, fat reducing agent during frying, volume enhancer, binder, bulking agent, and stabilizer.[32] The source of fiber is important because the differences on the structure and constitution of plant cells can affect fiber properties. Some dietary fiber ingredients could be desirable not only for their nutritional properties but also for their functional and technological properties. Some fiber applications had been successful in improving cooking yield, reducing formulation costs, and enhancing texture in food products.[32] Its technological effects on foods differ according to the quantity and nature of dietary fiber. No reports have been published on the properties of burgers or bologna sausages containing different levels of tiger nut fiber.

The objective of this chapter was to study the viability to use TNBP (at different concentrations) as functional ingredient in two meat products: burger (fresh meat product) and bologna (cooked meat product). The effect of this functional ingredient on the nutritional, technological, and physicochemical properties of these two meat products was also evaluated.

30.2.1 Pork Burgers

30.2.1.1 Burger Manufacture Three independent replicates of each batch were prepared at the IPOA Meat Research Group Pilot Plant of the Miguel Hernández University (Figure 30.2). A simple traditional formulation was used to obtain a base batter as follows (percentages of nonmeat ingredients are related to meat): 55% lean pork meat, 45% pork back fat, 18% (w/w) water (ice), 1.5% (w/w) sodium chloride, and 0.2% white pepper. This mixture was divided into batches with different tiger nut fiber concentration (0%, 5%, 10%, and 15%).

To obtain the base mixture, pork trimmings were ground through a 5 mm plate in a mincer attached to a mixer (Mod EM20, Crypto Peerless, Birmingham, U.K.),

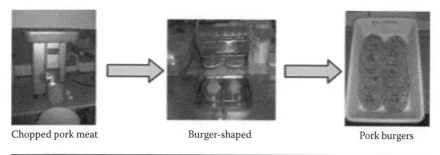

Chopped pork meat   Burger-shaped   Pork burgers

Figure 30.2 Pork burgers manufacture.

and then water, salt, and pepper were added into the bowl and mixed with the spiral dough hook at medium speed (80 rpm) during 5 min. For each treatment, the corresponding proportions of tiger nut fiber were added and then mixed again for 5 min. This mixture was shaped using a commercial burger maker (9 cm internal diam) to obtain patties of approximately 70 g and 1 cm thickness. Plastic packaging film was used to help maintain the shape of the patties prior to freezing at −30°C in a commercial plate freezer (Mod. LR 30QFADT, Foster Refrigerator U.K., Ltd., King's Lynn, Norfolk) for 15 min, packed into PVC-lined hermetic boxes, and stored at 4°C. Chemical composition and pH determinations were made immediately after elaboration, and the rest of tests were made on samples after cooking.

30.2.1.2 Pork Burgers with Tiger Nut Fiber Addition A significant decrease of water activity in burgers was observed due to the different addition of TNBP. No differences were observed in pH, moisture, and fat content among the different burger formulations. However, the burgers formulated with 10% TNBP and control had significantly higher ash and protein content than burgers with 5% and 15% TNBP added.

Exudation during the cooking process is a very important transformation in meat products with high moisture content (around 75% or more) and represents economic loses, alterations of the nutritional value of the product due to the release of soluble vitamins and amino acids, and some negative effects on texture and juiciness.[33,34] The cooking process led to water evaporation and lipid migration in the pork burgers, and the intensity of these changes is important to product acceptance. Moisture and fat retention are related to the ability of the protein matrix to retain water and bind fat. Results showed that formulation with 15% TNBP added had the highest cooking yield, fat retention, and moisture retention. These findings indicate that TNBP addition causes desirable changes in the cooking characteristics of pork burgers, suggesting that texture and juiciness of products were possibly improved. Results of cooking yield and moisture retention were similar to those reported for beef burgers added with lemon albedo, while fat retention was somewhat higher.[32]

The addition of 10% TNBP in burger formulations resulted in brighter samples with L* (lightness) values higher than those of control, 5% and 15% TNBP formulations ($P < 0.05$). The TNBP addition increased the coordinate a*, except in the samples with 10% TNBP addition. A significant increase of yellowness (b*), chroma (saturation), and hue angle values was observed with the addition of TNBP in the pork burger formulations. These results may be due to the higher amount of yellow components from tiger nut remaining in the by-products from "horchata" production.[33]

30.2.2 Bologna Sausages

30.2.2.1 Bologna Manufacture Bolognas were manufactured according to a traditional formula (Figure 30.3) (only the meat percentages add up to 100%, while the percentage of the other ingredients are related to meat): 50% lean pork meat and 50% pork back fat, 15% water (ice, w/w), 3% potato starch (w/w), 2.5% sodium chloride (w/w), 300 mg/kg sodium tripolyphosphate, 500 mg/kg sodium ascorbate, 150 mg/kg sodium nitrite, and spices (0.01% black pepper, 0.005% nutmeg, and 0.2% garlic powder). This original mixture was used as control sample, and, for the other sausages, TNBP was added in different proportions: 5%, 10%, and 15%.

The products were prepared in a pilot plant and followed industrial processing techniques. Frozen raw material of animal origin, except pork back fat, was transferred to the cutter (Tecator 1094 Homogenizer, Tekator, Höganäs, Sweden) with the sodium chloride to extract salt-soluble proteins; after comminution, the other ingredients and additives were added. Then, pork back fat, previously divided into cubes 10 × 10 × 10 cm, was added. After homogenization, the mixture was stuffed into artificial casing Fibran-Pack (Fibran, Girona, Spain) 100 × 150 mm long, clipped at both ends (Polyclip system/Niedecker, Germany), and cooked in a water bath. The sausages were kept in the bath until the coldest point reached 72°C (geometric center of bologna, which corresponds to the thickest part of the product). A thermocouple probe (Omega Engineering, Inc., Stamford, CT, United States) positioned in the geometric center of the bologna was used to monitor product temperature. When the endpoint temperature was achieved, the sausages were immediately chilled in ice. After reaching chilling temperature, the product was transferred to the lab in insulated boxes containing ice.

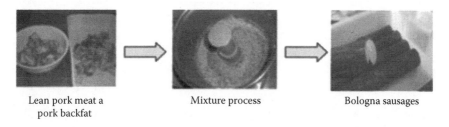

Lean pork meat a   Mixture process   Bologna sausages
pork backfat

Figure 30.3 Bologna sausages manufacture.

30.2.2.2 Bologna Characteristics   When the effect of the addition of TNBP in bologna sausages was analyzed, an increase in moisture and ash content and a decrease in protein and fat content, with respect to the sample control, were observed. These results indicate that TNBP retains water and increases the mineral content on the product. Similar behavior was reported by Alesón-Carbonell et al. [32] in English breakfast sausages added with different amount of functional ingredients (albedo, oat fiber, wheat flour rusk, and its combinations).

All color parameters were significantly ($P < 0.05$) affected by the TNBP content. The results showed that the addition of TNBP, at different concentrations, caused a decrease in L* (lightness coordinate) and b* (yellow-blue coordinate) values. However, there was a slight increase in a* values (red-green coordinate) as the concentration was increased.

Although color changes have been reported as being induced by the presence of functional ingredients of various origins in various meat products,[32,35–37] in other cases, no such effect was observed.[38]

pH levels did not differ ($P > 0.05$) between control and varying concentration of TNBP. This indicates that TNBP did not have any positive or negative effects on pH changes for bolognas. It is not surprising because the pH of TNBP was very similar to control sausage.

Water activity did not differ ($P > 0.05$) between control and varying concentration of TNBP. All bolognas had water activity values in the range of the values reported by Fennema and Carpenter[39] for bologna-type sausages (0.93–0.98). As in the case of meat and meat products, water activity and pH values are considered good predictors for food stability[39]; the values of both parameters in all bolognas (control, 5%, 10%, and 15% TNBP) determined that the product must be classified as highly perishable, and so to increase its shelf-life, it must be stored under refrigerated conditions (<5°C).

30.3 Conclusions

The results presented here suggest that by-products from "horchata" production from tiger nuts can be successfully used to obtain a "functional ingredient," which is a potential source of valuable nutrients (high proportion of TDF composed mainly of IDF). The technological properties of this "functional ingredient" (high WHC and OHC in comparison with other dietary fiber sources from vegetal origin) suggested that it could be used in food industries as an important and inexpensive source of dietary fiber that has nutritional and technological values.

This tiger nut fiber by-product has been successfully added (until 15%) to a fresh meat product (burger) and to a cooked meat product (type bologna). The addition of tiger nut fiber by-product to burgers and bolognas improves its nutritional value (decreases its fat content and increases TDF content) without relevant modifications in their physicochemical characteristics.

The beneficial results obtained for fiber enrichment of these two meat products suggest other potential applications for this type of by-products and the need for further research such as the nutritional enrichment of other meat products and applications in dairy and bakery products.

Acknowledgment

This work was supported by a predoctoral grant from Caja Mediterráneo (CAM).

References

1. CRDO, Consejo Regulador de la Denominación de Origen Chufa de Valencia, 2010, Available on line: www.chufadevalencia.org (accessed November 12, 2010).
2. Lario, Y. et al., Preparation of high dietary fiber powder from lemon juice by-products, *Innov. Food Sci. Emerg.*, 5, 113, 2004.
3. Betancur-Ancona, D. et al., Physicochemical characterization of Lima bean (*Phaseolus lunatus*) and Jack bean (*Canavalia ensiformis*) fibrous residues, *Food Chem.*, 84, 287, 2004.
4. Vázquez-Ovando, A. et al., Physicochemical properties of a fibrous fraction from chia (*Salvia hispanica* L.), *Food Sci. Technol.*, 42, 168, 2009.
5. Mckee, L.H. and Latner, T.A., Underutilized sources of dietary fiber: A review, *Plant Food Hum. Nutr.*, 55, 285, 2000.
6. Ku, C.S. and Mun, S.P., Optimization of the extraction of anthocyanin from Bokbunja (*Rubus coreanus* Miq.) marc produced during traditional wine processing and characterization of the extracts, *Bioresour. Technol.*, 99, 8325, 2008.
7. Dalgetty, D. and Baik, B., Isolation and characterization of cotyledon fibers from peas, lentils, and chikpeas, *Cereal Chem.*, 80(3), 310, 2003.
8. Fuentes-Alventosa, J.M. et al., Effect of extraction method on chemical composition and functional characteristics of high dietary fiber powders obtained from asparagus by-products, *Food Chem.*, 113, 665, 2009.
9. Fernández-López, J. et al., Storage stability of a high dietary fiber powder from orange by-products, *Int. J. Food Sci. Technol.*, 44, 748, 2009.
10. Jongaroontaprangsee, S. et al., Effects of drying temperature and particle size on hydration properties of dietary fiber powder from lime and cabbage by-products, *Int. J. Food Prop.*, 10, 887, 2007.
11. Jiménez-Escrig, A. et al., Guava fruit (*Psidium guajava* L.) as a new source of antioxidant dietary fiber, *J. Agric. Food Chem.*, 49, 5489, 2001.
12. Rincón, A.M., Vázquez, A.M., and Padilla, F.C., Composición química y compuestos bioactivos de las harinas de cáscaras de naranja (*Citrus sinensis*) mandarina (*Citrus reticulata*) y toronja (*Citrus paradisi*) cultivadas en Venezuela, *Arch. Latinoam. Nutr.*, 55(3), 305, 2005.
13. Bravo, L., Propiedades y aplicaciones de la fibra de algarroba (*Prosopis pallida* L.), *Alimentaria*, March, 67, 1999.
14. Lecumberri, E. et al., Caracterización de la fibra de cacao y su efecto sobre la capacidad antioxidante en suero de animales de experimentación, *Nutr. Hosp.*, 21(5), 622, 2006.
15. Larrauri, J.A. et al., Seasonal changes in the composition and properties of a high dietary fiber powder from grapefruit peel, *J. Sci. Food Agric.*, 74, 308, 1997.
16. Espinosa-Martos, I. and Rupérez, P., Indigestible fraction of okara from soybean: Composition, physicochemical properties and in vitro fermentability by pure cultures of *Lactobacillus acidophilus* and *Bifidobacterium bifidum*, *Eur. Food Res. Technol.*, 228(5), 685, 2009.

17. Figuerola, F. et al., Fiber concentrates from apple pomace and citrus peel as potential fiber sources for food enrichment, *Food Chem.*, 91, 395, 2005.

18. Rodríguez-Ambriz, S.L. et al., Characterization of a fiber-rich powder prepared by liquefaction of unripe banana flour, *Food Chem.*, 107, 1515, 2008.

19. Larrauri, J.A., Rupérez, P., and Saura-Calixto, F., Pineapple shell as a source of dietary fiber with associated polyphenols, *J. Agric. Food Chem.*, 45, 4028, 1997.

20. Sánchez-Zapata, E. et al., Preparation of dietary fiber powder from tiger nuts (*Cyperus esculentus*) milk ("horchata") by-products and its physicochemical properties, *J. Agric. Food Chem.*, 57, 7719, 2009.

21. Fernández-López, J. et al., Physico-chemical and microbiological profiles of "salchichón" (Spanish dry-fermented sausage) enriched with orange fiber, *Meat Sci.*, 80, 410, 2008.

22. Elleuch, M. et al., Date flesh: Chemical composition and characteristics of the dietary fiber, *Food Chem.*, 111, 676, 2008.

23. Larrea, M.A., Chang, Y.K., and Martínez-Bustos, F., Some functional properties of extruded orange pulp and its effect on the quality cookies, *Food Sci. Technol.*, 38, 213, 2005.

24. Sánchez-Zapata, E. et al., Application of orange fiber for the control of oxidation in paté from yellowfin (*Thunnus albacares*) dark muscle ("sangacho"), *Alimentaria*, 400, 95, 2009.

25. Sendra, E. et al., Incorporation of citrus fibers in fermented milk containing probiotic bacteria, *Food Microbiol.*, 25, 13, 2008.

26. Thebaudin, J.Y. et al., Dietary fibers: Nutritional and technological interest, *Trends Food Sci. Technol.*, 8, 41, 1997.

27. Mongeau, R. and Brassard, M., Insoluble dietary fiber from breakfast cereals and brans bile salt and water holding capacity in relation to particle size, *Cereal Chem.*, 59, 413, 1982.

28. Sangnark, A. and Noomhorm, A., Effect of particle sizes on functional properties of dietary fiber prepared from sugarcane bagasse, *Food Chem.*, 80, 221, 2003.

29. Raghavendra, S.N. et al., Grinding characteristics and hydration properties of coconut residue: A source of dietary fiber, *J. Food Eng.*, 72, 281, 2006.

30. Larrauri, J.A. et al., High dietary fiber powders from orange and lime peels: Associated polyphenols and antioxidant capacity, *Food Res. Int.*, 29(8), 757, 1996.

31. Larrauri, J.A. et al., Mango peels as a new tropical fiber: Preparation and characterization, *Lebensm. Wiss. Technol.*, 29, 729, 1996.

32. Alesón-Carbonell, L. et al., Characteristics of beef burger as influenced by various types of lemon albedo, *Innov. Food Sci. Emerg. Technol.*, 6, 247, 2005.

33. Sánchez-Zapata, E. et al., Effect of tiger nut fibre on quality characteristics of pork burger, *Meat Sci.*, 85(1), 70, 2010.

34. Bochi, V.C. et al., Fish burgers with silver catfish (*Rhamdia quelen*) filleting residue, *Biores. Technol.*, 99, 8844, 2008.

35. Cofrades, S. et al., Plasma protein and soy fiber content effect on bologna sausage properties as influenced by fat level, *J. Food Sci.*, 65, 281, 2000.

36. Sánchez-Escalante, A. et al., Utilization of applesauce in a low-fat bologna-type product, *Food Sci. Technol. Int.*, 6, 379, 2000.

37. Fernández-Ginés, J.M. et al., Effects of storage conditions on quality characteristics of bologna sausages made with citrus fiber, *J. Food Sci.*, 68, 710, 2003.

38. Mansour, E.H. and Khalil, A.H., Characteristics of low-fat beefburgers as influenced by various types of wheat fibers, *J. Agr. Food Chem.*, 79, 493, 1999.

39. Fennema, O. and Carpenter, J., Water activity in muscle and related tissues, in 37th Reciprocal Meat Conference, American Meat Science Association, Chicago, IL, 1984, p. 19.

31

Technological Properties of Pomegranate (*Punica granatum* L.) Peel Extract Obtained as Coproduct of Juice Processing

MANUEL VIUDA-MARTOS, ELENA SÁNCHEZ-ZAPATA, ANA MARTIN-SÁNCHEZ, YOLANDA RUIZ-NAVAJAS, JUANA FERNÁNDEZ-LÓPEZ, ESTHER SENDRA, ESTRELLA SAYAS-BARBERÁ, CASILDA NAVARRO, and JOSÉ A. PÉREZ-ÁLVAREZ

Contents

31.1 Introduction

Sustainable food production and coproduct valorization have become important issues in the food industry. From an environmental perspective, it is vital that plant coproducts produced by the agrofood industry must be "reused." The industrial transformation of fruits generates large quantities of coproducts rich in bioactive compounds that may well be suitable for other purposes.[1] Some of these coproducts have been recognized by several organizations (FDA and EFSA) as possessing proven health benefits. Depending on the availability of an adequate technology, these coproducts can be converted into commercial products, either as raw materials for secondary processes (intermediate food ingredients) or as ingredients of new products.[2] The preparation of extracts rich in dietary fiber (DF), antioxidant fiber, and bioactive compounds (organic acid, polyphenols, and so on) from coproducts of the food industry could be used as a functional ingredient[3,4] since the fibers can interact physiologically to provide numerous health benefits that go far beyond supporting regularity. These benefits may include not only digestive health but also weight management, cardiovascular health, and general wellness.[5] From a functionality point of view, fiber can play a number of roles in the food industry such as (i) it may be used as a tool for improving texture, (ii) as a bulking agent in reduced-sugar applications, (iii) to manage moisture in the replacement of fat, (iv) to add color, and (v) as natural antioxidant.[6]

Pomegranate (*Punica granatum* L.), belonging to the *Punicacea* family, is one of the oldest edible fruits. Actually pomegranate is widely cultivated in Iran, India, Mediterranean countries (principally in Spain), Malaysia, the East Indies, tropical Africa, and, to some extent, in the United States (drier parts of California and Arizona), China, Japan, and Russia.[7] The fruit is consumed fresh, as juice, jam, wine or oil, and in extract supplements.[8] There is growing interest in this fruit because it is considered to be a functional product of great potential benefit in the human diet as it contains several groups of substances that are useful in disease risk reduction. In the process used to obtain juice from pomegranate fruit, several coproducts are obtained, among them the peel. Pomegranate peels have been used in traditional medicine. For example, in Yemen and other countries of the Arabian Peninsula, dried peels have been traditionally used for treating stomachache and for healing wounds.[9]

Pomegranate peel comprises about 50% of the total fruit weight and is an important source of minerals especially potassium, calcium, phosphorus, magnesium, and sodium; complex polysaccharides;[10] and high levels of a diverse range of bioactive compounds such as phenolics, flavonoids, proanthocyanidin compounds,[11] and ellagitannins, such as punicalagin and its isomers, as well as lesser amounts of punicalin, gallagic acid, ellagic acid, and ellagic acid glycosides (hexoside, pentoside, rhamnoside, etc.).[8,12]

The aim of this chapter was to determine the functional and physicochemical properties of pomegranate (*Punica granatum* L.) peel extract (PPE) coproduct as potential DF source for food enrichment.

31.2 Materials and Methods

31.2.1 Pomegranate Peel Extract Coproduct

The material (peel), obtained as a coproduct during pomegranate juice extraction, was transported to the pilot plant facilities of the IPOA Research Group at the Miguel Hernández University (Orihuela, Alicante, Spain) where it was triturated for 40 s in a vertical cutter (Tecator 1094 Homogeneizer, Tekator, Hoganas, Sweden) to obtain uniformly sized pieces and so increase the contact time during washing (1 L of water per kg of product).

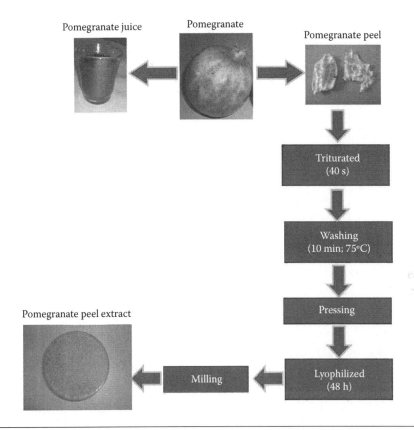

Figure 31.1 Flowchart of process to obtain an extract from pomegranate peel co-products.

The mixture was stirred constantly, and the water temperature was kept at 75°C during the 10 min that the washing process lasted. The whole coproduct was pressed to drain liquid waste and was then lyophilized in a Christ Alpha 2–4 lyophilizer (B. Braun Biotech, Melsungen, Germany) for 48 h to improve the product shelf-life without the addition of any chemical preservative. A grinder mill and sieves were used to obtain an extract particle size of less than 0.417 mm. Figure 31.1 describes the process used to obtain extract from pomegranate peel coproducts.

31.2.2 Chemical Analysis

Ash, protein, and fat contents were determined by AOAC methods.[13] Ash was performed at 550°C for 2 h (g ash/100 g sample). Protein (g protein/100 g sample) was analyzed according to the Kjeldahl method. Fat (g fat/100 g sample) was calculated by weight loss after a six-cycle extraction with petroleum ether in a Soxhlet apparatus. Total dietary fiber (TDF) and insoluble dietary fiber (IDF) were determined following 985.29 AOAC methods.[9] Soluble dietary fiber (SDF) was calculated by subtracting the IDF proportion from the TDF.

31.2.3 Physicochemical Analysis

The pH was measured in a suspension resulting from blending 10 g sample with 10 mL of deionized water for 2 min, using a pH meter (model pH/Ion 510, Eutech Instruments Pte Ltd., Singapore). The water activity (a_w) was determined in a Novasina Thermoconstanter Sprint TH-500 (Pfäffikon, Switzerland) at 25°C. The color was studied in the CIELAB color space using a Minolta CM-2600d (Minolta Camera Co., Osaka, Japan), with D_{65} as illuminant and an observer angle of 10°. Low reflectance glass (Minolta CR-A51/1829-752) was placed between the samples and the equipment. The CIELAB coordinates studied were lightness (L*), coordinate red/green (a*), and coordinate yellow/blue (b*).

31.2.4 Functional Properties

The water-holding capacity (WHC) and oil-holding capacity (OHC) were determined according to Robertson et al.[14] The WHC was expressed as g of water held per g of sample, and the OHC was expressed as g of oil held per g of sample. The water adsorption capacity (WA_dC) and water absorption capacity (WA_bC) were determined according to Vázquez-Ovando et al.[15] The WA_dC was expressed as g of water adsorbed per g of sample, and the WA_bC was expressed as g of water absorbed per g of sample.

Emulsifying activity (EA) and emulsion stability (ES) were evaluated according to Chau et al.[16] with some modifications. One hundred milliliters of 2% (w/v) sample suspension in water was homogenized at 11,000 rpm for 30 s using an IKA T-25 homogenizer. One hundred milliliters of sunflower oil was then added and homogenized for another 1 min. The emulsions were centrifuged in 10 mL graduated centrifuge tubes at 1200 g for 5 min, and the volume of the emulsion left was measured. The EA was calculated as the volume of emulsified layer/volume of whole layer in the centrifuge tube × 100. To determine the ES, emulsions prepared by the procedures mentioned earlier were heated at 80°C for 30 min, cooled to room temperature, and centrifuged at 1200 g for 5 min. The ES was calculated as the volume of remaining emulsified layer/original emulsion volume × 100.

31.2.5 Organic Acid and Sugar Content

One gram of PPE was homogenized in 20 mL of distilled water and shaken vigorously for 2 min and then left 1 h in a Selecta ultrasonic water bath (Selecta S.A. Barcelona, Spain) without temperature control. Extracts were centrifuged at 15,000 rpm for 15 min at 4°C. Two milliliters of the supernatant was filtered through a 0.45 μm Millipore filter (Millipore Corporation, Bedford, United States) and then 20 μL was injected into a Hewlett-Packard series 1100 HPLC according to the method described by Dougthy.[17] The elution system consisted of 0.1% phosphoric acid running isocratically with a flow rate of 0.5 mL min^{-1}. The organic acids were eluted through a Supelco column (Supelcogel C-610H, 30 cm 7.8 mm, Supelco Park, Bellefonte) and detected by absorbance at 210 nm. The standard curves of pure organic acids (L-ascorbic, malic, citric, oxalic, acetic, lactic, and succinic acids) purchased from Sigma (Poole, Dorset, United Kingdom) were used for quantification. For sugar concentrations, the same HPLC, elution system, flow rate, and column were used. The sugars were detected by refractive index detector (RID). The standard curves of pure sugars (glucose, fructose, and sucrose) purchased from Sigma were used for quantification.

31.3 Results and Discussion

31.3.1 Chemical Analysis

Table 31.1 shows the results obtained for the chemical analysis of the PPE coproduct. The proximate composition analysis of PPE showed lower protein and ash contents than other extracts from vegetable processing wastes such as peel from *Citrus sinensis* L. Cv. Liucheng or tiger nut by-products.[2,18] An important parameter in a fruit or vegetable powder extract is its lipid content. The PPE had a lipid content of 1.67 g/100 g (dry sample), which is lower than that reported in mango DF (2.3 g/100 g dry sample)[19] or grape skins (6.87–7.78 g/100 g dry sample).[20]

During the processing of fruit coproducts into fiber, the raw material undergoes two critical steps: scalding (which includes washing) and drying. In general terms, the ash, protein, and flavonoid contents decreased, while the fat content increased after these treatments.[21] Therefore, PPE might be considered a potential ingredient for the formulation of food products with a low caloric content.

The PPE was rich in TDF (72.68 g/100 g dry weight; being 42.53 g/100 dry weight IDF and 30.15 g/100 g dry weight SDF) and showed a moderate IDF/SDF ratio (1.41). The TDF content of PPE was found to be higher than that of some other fruit peels such as DF preparations from strawberry (20–22 g/100 g dry sample), mango DF (28.1 g/100 g dry sample), coconut fiber (60.9 g/100 g dry sample), apple (60.1 g/100 g dry sample), and cocoa fiber (60.54 g/100 g dry sample).[19,22–24] Extracts rich in DF obtained from fruits and vegetables are used as functional ingredients because they provide numerous health benefits such as their ability to decrease cholesterol levels, improve glucose tolerance and the insulin response, reduce hyperlipidemia and hypertension, contribute to gastrointestinal health, and prevent certain cancers such as colon cancer.[5]

DFs from cereals are more frequently used than those from fruits, even though fruit fibers, in general, have better nutritional qualities because of their higher levels of associated bioactive compounds (flavonoids, carotenoids, etc.) and more balanced composition (higher overall fiber content, greater IDF/SDF ratio, water- and fat-holding capacities, lower metabolic energy value, colonic fermentability, as well as lower phytic acid content).[25] Thus, DF from several sources

Table 31.1 Chemical Composition of PPE Coproduct (Mean Values ± SD)

Sample	Protein (g/100 g)	Fat (g/100 g)	Ash (g/100 g)	TDF (g/100 g)	IDF (g/100 g)	SDF (g/100 g)
PPP	1.84 ± 0.12	1.67 ± 0.13	0.69 ± 0.56	72.68 ± 0.26	42.53 ± 0.46	30.15 ± 0.31

TDF, total dietary fiber; IDF, insoluble dietary fiber; SDF, soluble dietary fiber.

Table 31.2 Physicochemical Properties: Water Activity, pH, and Color Coordinates of PPE Coproduct (Mean Values ± SD)

Sample	Water Activity	pH	Color L*	Color a*	Color b*
PPP	0.136 ± 0.00	4.31 ± 0.01	74.35 ± 1.23	1.87 ± 0.47	34.72 ± 0.47

(vegetable, fruit, cereal, etc.) can increase the nutritional value of different foods, including meat products,[26] breakfast cereals and bakery products,[19] and dairy products.[4] PPE can be considered a potential ingredient for these types of food.

31.3.2 Physicochemical Analysis

The physicochemical properties of PPE are given in Table 31.2. PPE showed a pH (4.36) very similar to that of other fruit fiber products such as orange DF (4.06) or lemon albedo (3.96),[27,28] while the water activity was 0.136. Due to its low pH and a_w, PPE is a highly stable product.

Color is one of the most important quality parameters in food products. Possible color changes caused by DFs would limit their potential application in food. Lightness (L*) in food is related with many factors, including the concentration and type of pigments present, the water content, and surface water availability. PPE presented a value for this coordinate of 74.35, similar to that other fiber product such as tiger nut by-product and higher than that of lemon by-product or sugarcane bagasse.[27,29]

As regards the red-green coordinate, redness, (a*), PPE showed a value of 1.87; this coordinate is affected by the structural integrity of the fiber and the pigment content and disposition (water or lipid soluble).[30] The yellow-blue coordinate, yellowness, (b*), presented a value of 34.72, which is higher than that of other fruit fibers. This high b* value could be due to the carotenoids present in the pomegranate peel fiber, which were not eliminated by washing.

31.3.3 Functional Properties

The functional properties of plant fiber depend on the IDF/SDF ratio, particle size, extraction condition, structure of the plant polysaccharides, and vegetable source.[31] The functional properties of PPE are given in Table 31.3.

Table 31.3 Functional Properties of PPE Coproduct (Mean Values ± SD)

Sample	WHC (g Water/g Dry Sample)	OHC (g Oil/g Dry Sample)	WA$_d$C (g Water/g Dry Sample)	WA$_b$C (g Water/g Dry Sample)	EA (mL/100 mL)	ES (mL/100 mL)
PPP	5.03 ± 0.06	6.67 ± 0.12	0.29 ± 0.06	0.76 ± 0.01	20.33 ± 1.53	95.06 ± 0.36

WHC, water-holding capacity; OHC, oil-holding capacity; WA$_d$C, water adsorption capacity; WA$_b$C, water absorption capacity; EA, emulsifying activity; ES, emulsion stability.

WHC, a property that refers to the ability to retain water within the matrix, is an important property of DF from both physiological and technological points of view. DF holds water by adsorption and absorption phenomena, and some water is also retained outside the fiber matrix (free water).[2]

Fiber with strong hydration properties could increase stool weight and potentially slow the rate of nutrient absorption from the intestine.[32] The PPE coproduct exhibited a WHC 5.03 times its own weight, which is higher than that reported for other fibrous residues such as sugarcane (4.98 g water/g product) and pear (5 g water/g product)[29,33] but lower than other DF products such as asparagus fiber-rich extracts (11–20 g water/g product) or fiber extracts from Mexican lime peels (6.96–12.8 g water/g product).[34,35] WHC depends on (i) fiber processing (washing increases WHC probably due to the removal of sugars), (ii) particle size (typically, a reduction in the particle size of DFs has been associated with a lower ability to retain water and a lower oil-binding capacity,[29] although it has been speculated that in the absence of a matrix structure a reduction in the particle size might expose large surface areas, and at the same time more polar groups with water-binding sites, to the surrounding water[36]), and (iii) the chemical and physical structure (the WHC is related to the soluble DF content, and high levels of SDF produce a high WHC because soluble fibers, such as pectin and gums, possess a higher WHC than cellulosic fibers). PPE has potential applications in products requiring hydration, viscosity development, and freshness preservation, such as baked foods or cooked meat products.

The OHC is also an important property. This represents the capacity of a fiber to bind fat and depends on (i) porosity (the porosity of the fiber is more important than the molecular affinity to bind the fat),[37] (ii) particle size (the lower the particle size, the higher the OHC because smaller particles have relatively larger surface areas and therefore would theoretically be able to hold more oil than large particles), and (iii) drying (in general, dehydration promotes a general decrease in fiber OHC compared with the fresh fiber). PPE shows an OHC of 6.6 g oil/g dry fiber. This is similar to the OHC of lemon by-products (6.60 g oil/g fiber) or tiger nut by-product (6.90 g oil/g fiber).[2,27]

WA_bC and WA_dC: WA_bC is indicative of a structure's aptitude to spontaneously absorb water when placed in contact with a constantly moist surface or when immersed in water, while the WA_dC is the ability of a structure to spontaneously adsorb water when exposed to an atmosphere of constant relative humidity. The PPE had a WA_bC of 0.76 (g water/g dry sample), which is lower than other fruit fiber such as chia (11.73 water/g sample) or carrot (6.36 g water/g sample).[15,38] The PPE presents a WA_dC of 0.29 g water/g product, which is similar to that of tiger nut by-products (0.23 g water/g product).[2] The emulsifying capacity (EC) is a molecule's ability to act as an agent that facilitates solubilization or the dispersion of two immiscible liquids, and emulsifying stability (ES) is the ability to maintain the integrity of an emulsion. The EA of the PPE was 20.33 mL/100 mL, and its ES was 95 mL/100 mL. The low protein content of PPE (1.84 g/100 g dry weight) would explain its low EA and ES, since most proteins are strong emulsifying agents.

Table 31.4 Organic Acid and Sugar Contents of PPE Coproduct (Mean Values ± SD)

Sample	Oxalic Acid (mg/g Sample)	Glucose (mg/g Sample)	Fructose (mg/g Sample)
PPP	44.20 ± 2.73	73.86 ± 1.56	119.98 ± 2.79

31.3.4 Organic Acid and Sugar Content

Table 31.4 showed the organic acid and sugars present in the PPE. Oxalic acid was the one organic acid identified. No studies have been published on the organic acid content of the pomegranate peel coproduct resulting from pomegranate transformation, although several authors have studied this in pomegranate juice,[39,40] where citric and malic acid were the main acids found.

As regards sugars, the main ones found in PPE were fructose and glucose, in that order. The same sugars are the most prevalent in pomegranate pulp and, therefore, the juice and extracts obtained from it.[40] The fructose content depends on whether the fruit is acidic or not being lowest in acidic fruit and highest in nonacidic fruit.[41] The sugar content of PPE means that this coproduct shows a potential as ingredient in dry-cured meat products since they would be a source of carbon for the microbiota present in this kind of product.

31.4 Conclusions

The results of this study indicate that PPE coproducts may be considered a potential ingredient for its use in food products, increasing the content of TDF and improving the technological properties at the same time. The addition of fibers to food products is of great interest not only as a means of improving the functionality of food products but also as a means to create functional foods with health benefits.

To improve our knowledge of DF composition and structure, together with our understanding of its physiological effects on the human body, collaborative studies are needed involving the participation of researchers from different scientific areas: chemistry, biochemistry, biotechnology, biology, physiology, nutrition, and medicine.

References

1. Viuda-Martos, M. et al., Effect of adding citrus waste water, thyme and oregano essential oil on the chemical, physical and sensory characteristics of a bologna sausage, *Innov. Food Sci. Emerg. Technol.*, 10, 655, 2009.
2. Sánchez-Zapata, E. et al., Preparation of dietary fibre extract from tiger nut (*Cyperus esculentus*) milk ("Horchata") by-products and its physicochemical properties, *J. Agric. Food Chem.*, 57, 7719, 2009.
3. Fernández-López, J. et al., Orange fibre as potential functional ingredient for dry-cured sausage, *Eur. Food Res. Technol.*, 226(1–2), 1, 2007.
4. Sendra, E. et al., Incorporation of citrus fibers in fermented milk containing probiotic bacteria, *Food Microbiol.*, 25(1), 13, 2008.

5. Viuda-Martos, M. et al., Role of fibre in cardiovascular diseases: A review, *Comp. Rev. Food Sci. Food Safety,* 9, 240, 2010.
6. Viuda-Martos, M. et al., Citrus co-products as technological strategy to reduce residual nitrite content in meat products, *J. Food Sci.,* 74(8), 93, 2009.
7. Fadavi, A., Barzegar, M., and Azizi, H.M., Determination of fatty acids and total lipid content in oilseed of 25 pomegranates varieties grown in Iran, *J. Food Comp. Anal.,* 19, 676, 2006.
8. Gil, M.I. et al., Antioxidant activity of pomegranate juice and its relationship with phenolic composition and processing, *J. Agric. Food Chem.,* 48, 4581, 2000.
9. Al-Zoreky, N.S., Antimicrobial activity of pomegranate (*Punica granatum* L.) fruit peels, *Int. J. Food Microbiol.,* 134, 244, 2009.
10. Mirdehghan, S.H. and Rahemi, M., Seasonal changes of mineral nutrients and phenolics in pomegranate (*Punica granatum* L.) fruit, *Sci. Hort.,* 111(2), 120, 2007.
11. Li, Y. et al., Evaluation of antioxidant properties of pomegranate peel extract in comparison with pomegranate pulp extract, *Food Chem.,* 96(2), 254, 2006.
12. Devatkal, S.K., Narsaiah, K., and Borah, A., Anti-oxidant effect of extracts of kinnow rind, pomegranate rind and seed extracts in cooked goat meat patties, *Meat Sci.,* 85(1), 155, 2010.
13. AOAC., *Official Methods of Analysis of AOAC International,* 16th edn., Association of Official Analytical Chemists: Washington, DC, 1997.
14. Robertson, J.A. et al., Hydration properties of dietary fibre and resistant starch: A European collaborative study, *LWT Food Sci. Technol.,* 33, 72, 2000.
15. Vázquez-Ovando, A. et al., Physicochemical properties of a fibrous fraction from chia (*Salvia hispanica* L.), *Food Sci. Technol.,* 42, 168, 2009.
16. Chau, C., Cheung, K., and Wong, Y., Functional properties of protein concentrate from three Chinese indigenous legume seeds, *J. Agric. Food Chem.,* 45, 2500, 1997.
17. Dougthy, E., Separation of acids, carbohydrates in fermentation products by HPLC, *Lebensm. Biotech.,* 12(3), 100, 1995.
18. Chau, C.F. and Huang, Y.L., Comparison of the chemical composition and physicochemical properties of different fibres prepared from the peel of *Citrus sinensis* L. Cv. Liucheng, *J. Agric. Food Chem.,* 51, 2615, 2003.
19. Vergara-Valencia, N. et al., Fibre concentrate from mango fruit: Characterization, associated antioxidant capacity and application as a bakery product ingredient, *LWT Food Sci. Technol.,* 40, 722, 2007.
20. Bravo, L. and Saura-Calixto, F., Characterization of dietary fibre and the in vitro indigestible fraction of grape pomace, *Am. J. Enolo. Viticul.,* 49, 135, 1998.
21. Marín, F.R. et al., By-products from different citrus processes as a source of customized functional fibres, *Food Chem.,* 100, 736, 2007.
22. Torres, P. et al., Effects of industrial processing on content and properties of dietary fibre of strawberry wastes, In: *Total Food Sustainability of the Agri-Food Chain,* Waldron, K.W., Moates, G.K., Faulds, C.B., Eds., RSC Publishing: Cambridge, U.K., 2009, pp. 38–43.
23. Trinidad, T.P. et al., Dietary fibre from coconut flour: A functional food, *Innov. Food Sci. Emerg. Technol.,* 7(4), 302, 2006.
24. Lecumberri, E. et al., Dietary fibre composition, antioxidant capacity and physicochemical properties of a fibre-rich product from cocoa (*Theobroma cacao* L.), *Food Chem.,* 104(3), 948, 2007.
25. Figuerola, F. et al., Fibre concentrates from apple pomace and citrus peel as potential fibre sources for food enrichment, *Food Chem.,* 91, 395, 2005.
26. Viuda-Martos, M. et al., Effect of orange dietary fibre, oregano essential oil and packaging conditions on shelf-life of bologna sausages, *Food Control,* 21, 436, 2010.

27. Lario, Y. et al., Preparation of high dietary fibre extract from lemon juice by-products, *Innov. Food Sci. Emerg. Technol.*, 5, 113, 2004.
28. Garau, M.C. et al., Effect of air-drying temperature on physico-chemical properties of dietary fibre and antioxidant capacity of orange (*Citrus aurantium* v. Canoneta) by-products, *Food Chem.*, 104, 1014, 2007.
29. Sangnark, A. and Noomhorm, A., Effect of particle sizes on functional properties of dietary fibre prepared from sugarcane bagasse, *Food Chem.*, 80, 221, 2003.
30. Fernández-López, J. et al., Antioxidant and antibacterial activities of natural extracts: Application on cooked meat balls, *Meat Sci.*, 69, 371, 2005.
31. Jaime, L. et al., Structural carbohydrates differences and potential source of dietary fibre of onion (*Allium cepa* L.) tissues, *J. Agric. Food Chem.*, 50, 122, 2002.
32. Gallaher, D. and Schneeman, B.O., Dietary fibre, In: *Present Knowledge in Nutrition*, Bowman, B., Russel, R., Eds., 8th edn., ILSI: Washington, DC, 2001, p. 805.
33. Mckee, L.H. and Latner, T.A., Underutilized sources of dietary fibre: A review. *Plant Food Hum. Nutr.*, 55, 285, 2000.
34. Ubando-Rivera, J., Navarro-Ocaña, A., and Valdivia-López, M.A., Mexican lime peel: Comparative study on contents of dietary fibre and associated antioxidant activity, *Food Chem.*, 89(1), 57, 2005.
35. Fuentes-Alventosa, J.M. et al., Effect of extraction method on chemical composition and functional characteristics of high dietary fibre extracts obtained from asparagus by-products, *Food Chem.*, 113(2), 665, 2009.
36. Chau, C.F., Wen, Y.L., and Wang, Y.T., Improvement of the functionality of a potential fruit insoluble fibre by micron technology, *Int. J. Food Sci. Technol.*, 41, 1054, 2006.
37. Nelson, A.L., High-fibre ingredients, in: *High-Fibre Properties and Analyses*, American Association of Cereal Chemists: St. Paul, MN, 2001, pp. 29–44.
38. Zambrano, M., Meléndez, R., and Gallardo, Y., Propiedades funcionales y met-odología para su evaluación en fibra dietética, in: *Fibra Dietética en Iberoamérica. Tecnología y Salud*, Lajolo, F., Saura-Calixto, F., Witting, E., Wenzel de Menezes, E., Eds., Livraría LTDA: Brazil, 2001, pp. 195–209.
39. Özgen, M. et al., Chemical and antioxidant properties of pomegranate cultivars grown in Mediterranean region of Turkey, *Food Chem.*, 111, 703, 2008.
40. Tezcan, F. et al., Antioxidant activity and total phenolic, organic acid and sugar content in commercial pomegranate juices, *Food Chem.*, 115, 873, 2009.
41. Albertini, M.V. et al., Changes in organic acids and sugar during early stages of development of acidic and acidicless citrus fruit, *J. Agric. Food Chem.*, 54, 8335, 2006.

32

Mechanisms by Which Resistant Starch Produces Gut Hormones and Reduces Body Fat

MICHAEL J. KEENAN, JUNE ZHOU, ANNE M. RAGGIO,
KATHLEEN L. McCUTCHEON, RESHANI SENEVIRATHNE,
FELICIA GOLDSMITH, MARLENE JANES, RICHARD T. TULLEY,
LI SHEN, KIRK VIDRINE, CATHY WILLIAMS,
JASON A. CHARRIER, JIANPING YE, and ROY J. MARTIN

Contents

32.1 Introduction

Resistant starches (RS) are a type of nondigestible, fermentable fiber. Generally, RS is categorized into four categories [1]: RS1 is a result of the structured food matrix in unprocessed whole grains, seeds, or legumes; RS2 is generally high amylose, but is primarily the result of an organized granular structure tightly packed in a radial pattern as in high-amylose cornstarch products; RS3 is retrograded starch as in cooked then cooled potatoes; and RS4 is considered chemically modified starch with either constituent groups attached or linkages between starch molecules. RS potentially will have three major effects when included in the diet: (1) dilution of dietary metabolizable energy as the metabolizable energy of one type of RS2 is 2.8 kcal/g compared to the 3.6–4 kcal/g of typical starches [2], (2) a bulking effect similar to nonfermentable fiber, and (3) fermentation to short-chain fatty acids (SCFA) and an increase in expression of hormone genes in the gut and peptide hormones in plasma [3–6].

In our research group's studies using RS, we have mainly used an RS2 (Hi-Maize®260, National Starch and Food Innovation, Bridgewater, NJ). Hi-Maize®260 is a cornstarch product that is high in amylose (60%) compared to traditional starches that are around 80% amylopectin and 20% amylose. The product assays as 59% fiber with traditional fiber measures and 56% RS [7] according to National Starch and evaluations. Our focus with dietary RS has been predominantly on reduction of body fat.

In this chapter, we will review the following:

- Dietary RS and reduced body fat
- Strategy to reduce dietary dose of RS
- Focus on the large intestine
- Satiety or energy expenditure
- Role of gut-derived GLP-1 associated with fermentation of RS
- Knockout mice
- When RS is effective and not effective in reducing body fat
- Summary

32.2 Dietary Resistant Starch and Reduced Body Fat

The research of Jennifer Brand-Miller with low-glycemic-index diets in rodents [8] introduced us to RS as RS was used to lower the glycemic index of the diets. Our lab conducted several studies replacing traditional starch with Hi-Maize®260 that resulted in decreased abdominal fat in rodents fed RS in their diets without knowing the energy density value for the RS (Figure 32.1). Initially, the metabolizable energy density value specifically for Hi-maize®260 was unknown to us, although the literature had a range of energy density values for various fiber sources [2]. Therefore, we conducted a study using bomb calorimetry.

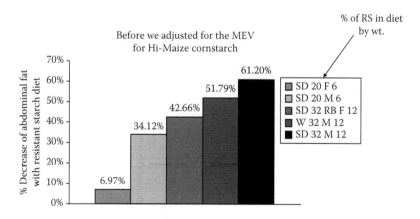

Figure 32.1 The percent decrease of abdominal body fat in rats fed a diet with resistant starch (RS) compared with rats fed a control diet. The control diets in the studies were not adjusted for the lower metabolizable energy of the Hi-maize®260 (determined after studies were completed) compared to the control starch. The legend in the figure gives the type of the rat (SD = Sprague Dawley or W = Wistar), the percent of RS in the diet by weight of diet (20 or 32%), the gender (F = female, M = male, RB = female retired breeder), and the number of rats in a treatment group (6 or 12).

National Starch and Food Innovation had also funded a study using a dietary energy titration method to also measure the metabolizable energy density of Hi-Maize®260. The two studies using different methods produced similar results with values of 2.8 and 2.7 kcal/g for the bomb calorimetry and the titration method, respectively, and were combined in publication [2]. This value is lower than the 3.6–4.0 kcal/g for the metabolizable energy density of traditional starches used in rodent diets. Thus, our early unpublished studies were not controlled for dietary energy density. We were interested in determining if there would be an effect of RS on abdominal body fat if the dietary energy density was controlled as any fiber, fermentable or nonfermentable, can dilute the energy density of the diet. Although the latter is still very important, determination of the metabolizable energy density allowed us to test if fermentation of RS in the large intestine had an effect on body fat.

Metabolizable energy density of the diet was controlled by adding purified cellulose to the base AIN-93 diet (G or M depending on the age of the rodents [9]), replacing traditional starch. Initially, our aim was to control diets for both energy density and total fiber, but this was not possible as purified cellulose is neither digested nor fermented in the rat gut, is 100% nonfermentable fiber, and has an energy density value of 0 kcal/g [10]. Hi-Maize®260, on the other hand, has an energy density value of 2.8 kcal/g, it assays as 59% fiber, and potentially the fiber is 100% fermentable. These various factors did not allow us to control for both energy density and total fiber in the diet. In addition, nonfermentable and fermentable fibers are very different entities, and one may not be a proper control for the other. The very practical solution was to use the energy density value of Hi-Maize®260 of 2.8 kcal and compare it to the energy density of ~4 kcal/g for traditional starch. This meant that ~1.2 kcal/g is neither digested nor fermented and is ~30% of the Hi-Maize®260. Using this value, we were able to estimate that both the diet with RS and the control diet had very similar amounts of fiber that was not fermented, and ~50% of the RS within the Hi-Maize®260 is not fermented. Thus, we were able to control for energy density of the diet with Hi-Maize®260 and for the nonfermentable fiber. In this way, we tested for the independent variable fermentable fiber. The reason for this level of RS not fermented was that we replace quite a bit of the high level of traditional starch in standard rodent diets with Hi-Maize®260 so that the level of RS in the diet is 25%–30% of the weight of the diet. This level of RS in the diet is effective in reducing rodent abdominal fat in 10–12 weeks of feeding when energy density of test and control diets is equal [3,4,11,12].

Our lab group has published three articles reporting reduced abdominal fat in rodents fed RS [3,4,11]. Our latest work demonstrated reduced abdominal fat in Goto-Kakizaki (GK) rats, a lean model of type 2 diabetes [12]. The reduced abdominal fat was associated with increased fermentation as indicated by decreased pH of the cecal contents and increased SCFA in the cecal contents [3,11]. Additionally, cecal cell gene expression [3,5] and plasma levels of the gut hormones PYY and GLP-1 [3,4,6,13] were increased in association with the reduced abdominal fat. It is possible that the fermentation of RS to SCFA leads to production of the gut hormones. In support of this hypothesis was increased gene expression for PYY and GLP-1 in primary cultures of cecal cells [5]. Also likely is the role of PYY and GLP-1 in the mechanism for the reduced body fat. PYY [5,14–16] and GLP-1 [17–19] are both reported to be involved in energy metabolism.

Thus, it appears from rodent studies that replacing the standard large amount of traditional starch with HiMaize®260 so that the diet has 25%–30% RS results in reduced body fat. This level of RS in the rodent diet appears to not be a problem with rodents as they eat the same or more diet than control rodents. However, this dietary level of RS would likely be too uncomfortable for humans because of the level of fermentation. It may be argued that similar effects of RS may occur in humans at lower doses based on the difference in metabolic body size of rodents versus humans. This is because rodents are more metabolically active than a human based on larger surface area to body size ratio. An alternative approach for lowering the dietary dose of RS is to combine RS with other dietary bioactive compounds that have similar effects in reducing body fat.

32.3 Strategy to Reduce Dietary Dose of RS

Currently there are strategies being tested or planned to use combinations or cocktails of drugs in the fight against obesity [20–22]. This type of strategy appears to be more effective because it overcomes redundancies of controls of body weight and prevents side effects of drugs because the strategy allows for lower doses of the drugs. Our lab has begun to investigate a similar strategy by using the combination of dietary RS and dietary sodium butyrate [23].

Butyrate is a histone deacetylase (HDAC) inhibitor and has been shown to dramatically reduce fat and increase fatty acid oxidation in rodents without altering food intake [24]. Because of the odor of sodium butyrate, the goal was to lower the dietary dose, and so we used a metabolic body size calculation to reduce this dietary dose of sodium butyrate for mice of 5%–3.2% of the weight of the diet for rats. A study was conducted using a 2 × 2 factorial arrangement of treatments with two levels of one independent variable, dietary sodium butyrate, with 0% and 3.2% of weight of diet and two levels of the other independent variable, dietary RS, with 0% and 28% of weight of the diet. There were significant decreases in abdominal fat and percent abdominal fat to body weight for both dietary sodium butyrate and dietary RS. However, there was not a significant interaction indicating that the effects on body fat for the two variables in combination were not additive. Individual *t*-tests comparing the combination group to the individual dietary sodium butyrate group or the dietary RS group indicated that the combination significantly lowered abdominal fat compared to either individual group.

Our lab also determined that the initial mechanism of action for dietary sodium butyrate and dietary RS appears to be different. Dietary sodium butyrate, as expected, appeared to be absorbed in the upper gut as there was no significant effect for dietary sodium butyrate on butyrate levels in the cecal contents. However, there was a significant effect for dietary RS for increased butyrate levels in the cecal contents as a result of fermentation of RS. As in previous research, dietary RS significantly increased plasma levels of PYY and GLP-1, but dietary sodium butyrate had no effect on these hormones. It was theoretically possible that dietary sodium butyrate might increase plasma levels of PYY and GLP-1. Plasma levels of GLP-1 can be increased by either an indirect or a direct stimulation mechanism of ʟ-endocrine cells [25]. The indirect mechanism would occur when nutrients in the small intestine stimulate κ cells to release glucose-dependent insulinotropic peptide (GIP), which then stimulates vagal efferent fibers resulting in a neural loop involving the central nervous system (CNS) that stimulates ʟ-endocrine cells. Nutrients that escape the proximal portions of the small intestine and reach the distal small intestine and large intestine directly stimulate ʟ-endocrine cells located in the distal gut. Dietary sodium butyrate could also be absorbed into the portal blood, enter the systemic blood, and then theoretically circulate to ʟ-endocrine cells. None of these possible mechanisms occurred for dietary sodium butyrate (Figure 32.2).

Interestingly, the group that had both dietary sodium butyrate and dietary RS had lower plasma levels of PYY and GLP-1 than the group with only dietary RS so that there were significant interactions indicating that dietary sodium butyrate

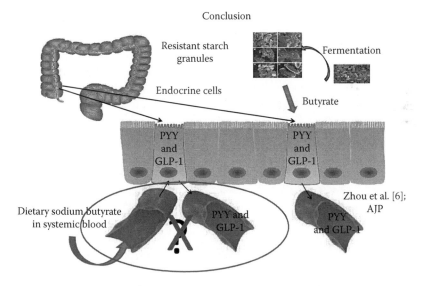

Figure 32.2 Possible mechanisms for the actions of resistant starch (RS) and dietary sodium butyrate in increasing production of the serum hormones produced by the gut, PYY and GLP-1. Fermentation of RS to butyrate and other short chain fatty acids in the lumen of the large intestine is associated with increased serum PYY and GLP-1. However, dietary sodium butyrate does not reach the large intestine and is absorbed in the upper gut. Theoretically this butyrate in the systemic blood could increase production of PYY and GLP-1, but our unpublished data demonstrate that dietary sodium butyrate treatment is not associated with increased serum levels of PYY and GLP-1.

reduced the levels associated with dietary RS. It is proposed that there is a saturation of the effect with high doses of the combination of RS and dietary sodium butyrate used. If the two compounds share a convergent mechanism at the cellular level, there may be a signal that feeds back to limit the production of the hormones with the combination of butyrate and RS.

32.4 Focus on the Large Intestine

Our group's research has focused on fermentation of RS. This is because reduction of abdominal fat with dietary RS was associated with increased fermentation and increased plasma levels of PYY and GLP-1 [3]. In one study, gene expression along the GI tract was monitored with the feeding of RS [5]. Although gene expression for PYY and proglucagon (gene for GLP-1) was highest in the ileum, an increase in expression associated with feeding of RS was only observed in the cecum and large intestine. However, there is a recent report of a human study in which dietary RS increased postprandial satiety after a meal and before RS could reach the large intestine for fermentation [26]. This may indicate more than one mechanism for the effect of dietary RS on body fat and species differences, or it may reflect different dietary dosages between animal and human studies.

32.5 Satiety or Energy Expenditure

Food intake data from our studies demonstrate that the high levels of fermentation are tolerated by rodents as rats fed RS consume the same amount of food as rats fed control diets [3,4] and mice consume statistically significant more food [11]. As the metabolizable energy densities of the diet containing RS and the control diet are equal, energy intake follows the same pattern as food intake. These results were initially surprising as the hormones PYY and GLP-1 are considered satiety hormones. However, another research group used dietary RS at levels similar to dietary levels in our studies to lower the glycemic index and found that food intake did not differ between rats fed RS and control diets [27]. Additionally, Reidelberger et al. [28] gave repeated infusions of PYY to rats and found that initial infusions reduced food intake, but repeated infusions actually increased food intake. The researchers speculated a possible downregulation of PYY receptors and an increased tolerance to PYY. However, the rats that received repeated infusions of PYY had reduced body fat. With the feeding of RS to rodents at 25%–30% of the weight of the diet, the plasma levels of PYY and GLP-1 are consistently elevated over a 24 h period compared to control [6]. This likely reflects consistent fermentation over the day. Normal meal plasma level peaks of these satiety hormones appear to be absent. Thus, food intake is not affected with the dietary dosages our research group is using in rodent studies. On the other hand, we have observed increased fat oxidation with a lower respiratory exchange ratio or respiratory quotient for mice fed RS compared to control [11]. Additionally, oxygen consumption was higher in RS fed mice, and there was no difference in physical activity between mice fed RS and control mice. Thus, levels of RS used in the diet in our rodent studies give us data that indicate that there is not a satiety effect. The evidence demonstrates that dietary RS is associated with increasing the energy expenditure component of the energy equation rather than decreasing the energy intake component. PYY [11,14–16] and GLP-1 [18,19] are also reported to be associated with increased energy expenditure, and it appears that plasma levels of PYY and GLP-1 retain their effectiveness in inducing increased energy expenditure despite losing the effects of satiety. This was demonstrated by Reidelberger et al. [28] as continuing infusion doses of PYY initially reduced food intake, but later increased food intake. However, the infusions of PYY resulted in reduced body fat for rats. Thus, high serum levels of PYY and GLP-1 appear to increase energy expenditure and not reduce food intake.

Future studies need to address a range of intakes of dietary RS as lower dietary doses may have very different effects compared to higher dietary doses. At lower doses, satiety may be the dominant effect as less fermentation occurs in the large intestine and much lower levels of plasma PYY and GLP-1 are produced allowing peaks of these hormones after meals to be effective in reducing food intake. Support for the latter is evident in the recent study by Anderson et al. [26] demonstrating postprandial satiety before the RS could reach the large intestine for fermentation. Consistently high plasma levels of PYY and GLP-1 likely lead to tolerance of the hormones at least in regard to satiety effects as is reported for PYY [28].

32.6 Role of Gut-Derived GLP-1 Associated with Fermentation of RS

When proopiomelanocortin (POMC) neurons are stimulated, the result is improved energy balance in favor of reduced food intake and increased energy expenditure [29]. In one of our studies with dietary RS, POMC gene expression was increased in the arcuate nucleus of the hypothalamus in the brain of rats fed RS compared to control [4]. Thus, the sequence of events leading to reduced body fat for rodents fed RS appears to be (1) fermentation in the cecum of the large intestine resulting in SCFA [3], (2) butyrate or other SCFA stimulating PYY and GLP-1 production in L-endocrine cells [5], (3) plasma PYY and GLP-1 circulating to the brain and stimulating POMC neurons [4], and (4) increased stimulation of peripheral tissues to increase fat oxidation [4,11,30].

However, Burcelin et al. [31] argue that gut-derived GLP-1 is extremely short-lived due to the action of circulating dipeptidyl peptidase IV (DPP-IV) that converts active GLP-1 to an inactive form. They review evidence for the gut stimulation of production of GLP-1 in the brain and argue that this source of GLP-1 is responsible for the majority of effects of GLP-1. "Only 10–15% of the total GLP-1 reaches the systemic circulation in the active form," which may mean that the major effects of gut-derived GLP-1 may be in the liver. Ding et al. [32] report that exendin-4, an agonist for the GLP-1 receptor, upregulates genes for fatty acid oxidation when added to the culture medium of primary cultures of hepatocytes. These results support a direct effect of GLP-1 on peripheral tissues, or in the least, the liver. The POMC increase in the arcuate nucleus associated with dietary RS may be the result of brain-derived GLP-1 rather than gut-derived GLP-1.

Future dietary RS studies need to measure brain-derived GLP-1 and try to determine the signal from the gut that would elevate GLP-1 in the brain in response to ingestion of RS. Shen et al. [4] demonstrated that capsaicin-sensitive nonmyelinated vagal nerves were not required for the effects of RS in reducing body fat. However, myelinated efferent nerves may still be the source of signaling of the gut to the brain with dietary RS.

32.7 Knockout Mice

Our lab's unpublished data demonstrate that the GLP-1 receptor is required for reduction of body fat with dietary RS. We compared wild-type mice with GLP-1 receptor knockout (GLP-1RKO) mice. The wild-type mice demonstrated reduced abdominal fat when fed RS compared to control diet, but GLP-1RKO mice did not respond to dietary RS despite fermenting the RS and had the same levels of abdominal fat as GLP-1RKO mice fed the control diet. This requirement of an intact GLP-1 receptor for effects of GLP-1 is similar to that reported for the effects of fermentable fructans on improvement of diabetic signs in rodents [33]. Use of the GLP-1 receptor antagonist also eliminated the many beneficial effects of fructans that include improvements in "glucose tolerance, fasting blood glucose, glucose-stimulated insulin secretion, insulin-sensitive hepatic glucose production, and reduced body weight gain."

Research is lacking demonstrating the need for PYY actions for the beneficial effects of fermentable fibers. PYY knockout mice as well as PYY receptor knockout mice are available for these studies.

32.8 When RS is Effective and Not Effective in Reducing Body Fat

As stated earlier, our lab group has demonstrated that dietary RS is associated with reduced body fat in several published studies [3,4,11]. Additionally, we have observed the same effect in several other studies, either published only in abstracts [12,23,34] or unpublished. These studies included several types of rodents: C57BL/6J mice, Sprague Dawley rats, Wistar rats, Sprague Dawley ovariectomized rats, and GK diabetic rats. However, we have also observed several instances where dietary RS was not associated with decreased abdominal fat that are published [11], published only in abstracts [35–37], or unpublished. Several of these results are summarized in Table 32.1. The factors that appear to be associated with elimination of the effect of RS on reducing abdominal fat are a prior obesity either using obese models or high-fat diet-induced obesity. These results are somewhat disappointing as it appears that RS is effective in reducing body fat accretion, but not in reversing prior obesity. It is now known that diet and some forms of obesity can affect the types of microflora present in the GI tract [38–40]. This could negatively affect fermentation of fermentable fibers. Theoretically, high-fat diets and certain types of obesity can inhibit the growth of bacteria that ferment RS, or high-fat diets may slow the transit of RS through the small intestine, increasing transit time and allowing greater digestion of the RS. Previous research in ruminant animals has demonstrated that added fat reduced

Table 32.1 Examples of Successful Reduction of Abdominal Body Fat with Dietary Resistant Starch (RS) Compared with Studies When Abdominal Body Fat was not Reduced with RS

Reduced Abdominal Fat with RS[a]	**No Reduction in Abdominal Fat with RS[a]**
1. Keenan et al. [3]: Reduced abdominal fat in rats fed a low-fat diet	1. Zhou et al. [11]: No reduction of abdominal fat in two obese mouse models fed low- and medium-fat diets; mice appeared to not ferment the RS Changes in cecal bacteria in obese model?
2. Shen et al. [4]: Reduced abdominal fat in rats fed a low-fat diet	2. Goldsmith et al. [36]: Mice fed a high-fat diet-fermented fructans and combinations of Hi-Maize to some extent, but had no reduction in abdominal fat High-fat diet-induced obesity prior to feeding of RS
3. Zhou et al. [11]: Reduced abdominal fat in black six mice fed low- and medium-fat diets	3. Badkoobeh et al. [37]: No reduction in abdominal fat in mice initially fed a high fat diet to induce obesity and then fed low- and high-fat RS diets High-fat diet-induced obesity prior to feeding of RS
4. Vidrine et al. [23]: Reduced abdominal fat in rats fed a low-fat diet	Low fat: 7% wt, 18% energy
5. Reduced abdominal fat in black six mice fed a low-fat RS diet compared with GLP-1RKO mice[b]	Medium: 11% wt, 28% energy
6. Zhou et al.: Reduced abdominal fat in PYY-Y1RKO mice fed a low-fat RS diet[b]	High: 20% wt, 42% energy
7. Robert et al. [34]: Reduced abdominal fat in sham and OVX rats fed low-fat RS diet	
8. Shen et al. [12]: Reduced body fat in GK rats fed a low-fat diet	

[a] Compared to rodents fed control diet with equal energy density.
[b] Unpublished data.

fermentation of foodstuffs in the rumen [41–43], and one way to increase the transit time for digesta moving through the upper GI tract (stomach and small intestine) is to increase the fat content of the diet [44]. Our lab group has observed that with feeding of a high-fat diet to rodents, there is a reduction of bacteria in the cecum that ferment RS (Table 32.2).

Recently, our lab group completed a thorough study comparing effects of dietary RS with feeding of either a low- or high-fat diet [45]. The study began

Table 32.2 Total Culturable Lactic Acid Bacteria (Colony-Forming Units [CFU])

	Diets			
	EC		RS	
Population	High Fat	Low Fat	High Fat	Low Fat
Lactobacillus spp.	7.18 ± 0.10	7.65 ± 0.10	7.88 ± 0.10	8.42 ± 0.10

RS, $p < 0.001$; Fat, $p < 0.014$; interaction, NS.

with normal Sprague Dawley rats without prior inducement of obesity. There was a significant increase in fermentation for rats fed RS either in a low- (7% fat by weight or 18% fat by energy of diet) or high-fat (20% fat by weight or 42% fat by energy of diet) diet as demonstrated by statistically significant lower cecal content pH and increased cecal weights. There were also significantly higher levels of blood serum GLP-1 and PYY and lower abdominal body fat in rats fed RS. However, the rats fed RS with a high-fat diet had reduced effects as cecal weights and PYY serum levels were not as great as in rats fed RS with a low-fat diet. And, very importantly, the reduction in abdominal body fat was a 27% reduction in rats fed RS with the low-fat diet compared to control rats fed a low-fat diet, but rats fed RS with high-fat diet only had a 9% abdominal body fat reduction compared to control rats fed a high-fat diet.

Some of this reduced effect on body fat is likely due to the somewhat reduced fermentation for the reasons mentioned earlier. A second possible explanation for the lack of an equal reduction of abdominal body fat with RS in a high-fat diet compared to low-fat diet may be that the high-fat diet is having a negative effect distal from the gut, such as in the brain. It is known that high-fat diets blunt the effect of leptin in the brain [46]. Therefore, a decreased response to gut hormones may be affected similarly to leptin with feeding of a high-fat diet. It has been reported that GLP-1 receptor signaling in the CNS is blunted by high-fat, diet-induced obesity [47]. The researchers demonstrated that normally GLP-1 signaling in the CNS results in sympathetic nervous system signaling to white adipocytes resulting in reduced fat stores in nonobese mice. This signaling was reduced with a high-fat diet. Thus, high-fat diets and obesity may affect signaling distal to the gut.

Our lab group's recent results are encouraging to some extent because accretion of body fat was reduced with dietary RS in a high-fat diet. However, the lesser effect compared to the consumption of the low-fat diet may be a good argument for promotion of the recommendations for humans to consume low- to moderate-fat diets with fat content not greater than ~30% of the energy of the diet. This should maximize the effects of RS. Additionally, comparison of our results with rodents that were obese prior to the start of the study with our results of studies starting with nonobese rodents indicates that fermentable fibers may play a role in the prevention of obesity, but other methods may need to be applied to reduce obesity. These may include pharmaceutical drugs and gastric bypass surgery. Our studies of the mechanism of action for RS in reducing body fat may someday lead to the development of an effective pharmaceutical drug for treatment of obesity.

32.9 Summary

In summary, our lab group has reported reduced abdominal fat in rodents fed diets with 25%–30% of the weight of the diet as RS by replacing traditional high levels of starch in standard experimental rodent diets. We are currently investigating ways to reduce the dietary levels of RS by combination with dietary sodium butyrate, a compound that has also been shown to reduce body fat in rodents. The reduction of body fat with dietary RS is associated with increased fermentation in the cecum and increased gene expression and plasma levels of PYY and GLP-1. An initial study combining dietary RS and dietary sodium butyrate demonstrated that the combination reduced abdominal fat to an extent greater than either compound individually, but the effect was not additive. Dietary sodium butyrate did not increase butyrate in the cecum and did not increase plasma levels of PYY and GLP-1. A large amount of data points to fermentation of RS as important for reduction of body fat. In rodents, increased fat oxidation and energy expenditure rather than satiety appear to lead to reduced body fat. However, a human study with low dietary doses of RS indicates that postprandial satiety is evident before RS could reach the large intestine for fermentation. Dietary RS has been effective in reducing abdominal fat in rodents fed high-fat diets, as long as rodents were not obese before the start of the studies, either in obese rodent models or in diet-induced obesity. However, the effect of RS with a high-fat diet is not as great as with a low-fat diet. High-fat diets and obesity have been shown to affect the CNS GLP-1 signaling. Therefore, RS may be most effective in preventing obesity with a low-fat diet, and treatments such as pharmaceutical drugs and gastric bypass surgery may be necessary for treatment of existing obesity. The alternative is that prebiotics like RS and other fermentable carbohydrates that promote the growth of beneficial bacteria in the large intestine may not be adequate to reduce body fat and produce other healthy effects of prebiotics in obese individuals. Obese individuals may be called nonresponders because of a change in microflora, and treatment with probiotics, beneficial bacteria, may be necessary to observe the response of beneficial health effects with feeding of prebiotics.

References

1. Sajilata MG, Singhai RS, and Kulkarni PR. Resistant starch: A review. *Compr Rev Food Sci Food Safe* 2006;5:1–17.
2. Tulley RT, Appel MJ, Enos TG et al. Comparative methodologies for measuring metabolizable energy of various types of resistant high amylose corn starch. *J Agric Food Chem* 2009;57:8474–8479.
3. Keenan MJ, Zhou J, McCutcheon KL et al. Effects of resistant starch, a non-digestible fermentable fiber, on reducing body fat. *Obesity (Silver Spring)* 2006;14:1523–1534.
4. Shen L, Keenan MJ, Martin RJ et al. Dietary resistant starch increases hypothalamic POMC expression in rats. *Obesity (Silver Spring)* 2009;17:40–45.

5. Zhou J, Hegsted M, McCutcheon KL et al. Peptide YY and proglucagon mRNA expression patterns and regulation in the gut. *Obesity (Silver Spring)* 2006;14:683–689.

6. Zhou J, Martin RJ, Tulley RT et al. Dietary resistant starch upregulates total GLP-1 and PYY in a sustained day-long manner through fermentation in rodents. *Am J Physiol Endocrinol Metab* 2008;295:E1160–E1166.

7. Englyst H. Classification and measurement of nutritionally important starch fractions. *Eur J Clin Nutr* 1992;46(Suppl 2):S33–S50.

8. Pawlak DB, Bryson JM, Denyer GS, and Brand-Miller JC. High glycemic index starch promotes hypersecretion of insulin and higher body fat in rats without affecting insulin sensitivity. *J Nutr* 2001;131:99–104.

9. Reeves PG, Nielsen FH, and Fahey GC, Jr. AIN-93 purified diets for laboratory rodents: Final report of the American Institute of Nutrition ad hoc writing committee on the reformulation of the AIN-76A rodent diet. *J Nutr* 1993;123:1939–1951.

10. Campbell JM, Fahey GC Jr, and Wolf BW. Selected indigestible oligosaccharides affect large bowel mass, cecal and fecal short-chain fatty acids, pH and microflora in rats. *J Nutr* 1997;127:130–136.

11. Zhou J, Martin RJ, Tulley RT et al. Failure to ferment dietary resistant starch in specific mouse models of obesity results in no body fat loss. *J Agric Food Chem* 2009;57:8844–8851.

12. Shen L, Keenan MJ, Raggio A, Williams C, and Martin RJ. Dietary-resistant starch improves maternal glycemic control in Goto-Kakizaki rat. *Mol Nutr Food Res* 2011;55:1499–1508.

13. Woodall CE 3rd, Brock GN, Fan J et al. An evaluation of 2537 gastrointestinal stromal tumors for a proposed clinical staging system. *Arch Surg* 2009;144:670–678.

14. Adams SH, Lei C, Jodka CM et al. PYY[3–36] administration decreases the respiratory quotient and reduces adiposity in diet-induced obese mice. *J Nutr* 2006;136:195–201.

15. Batterham RL, Cowley MA, Small CJ et al. Gut hormone PYY(3-36) physiologically inhibits food intake. *Nature* 2002;418:650–654.

16. Boey D, Lin S, Enriquez RF et al. PYY transgenic mice are protected against diet-induced and genetic obesity. *Neuropeptides* 2008;42:19–30.

17. Brand-Miller JC and Colagiuri S. Evolutionary aspects of diet and insulin resistance. *World Rev Nutr Diet* 1999;84:74–105.

18. Osaka T, Endo M, Yamakawa M, and Inoue S. Energy expenditure by intravenous administration of glucagon-like peptide-1 mediated by the lower brainstem and sympathoadrenal system. *Peptides* 2005;26:1623–1631.

19. Pannacciulli N, Bunt JC, Koska J, Bogardus C, and Krakoff J. Higher fasting plasma concentrations of glucagon-like peptide 1 are associated with higher resting energy expenditure and fat oxidation rates in humans. *Am J Clin Nutr* 2006;84:556–560.

20. Chan JL, Roth JD, and Weyer C. It takes two to tango: Combined amylin/leptin agonism as a potential approach to obesity drug development. *J Investig Med* 2009;57:777–783.

21. Neary NM, Small CJ, Druce MR et al. Peptide YY3-36 and glucagon-like peptide-17–36 inhibit food intake additively. *Endocrinology* 2005;146:5120–5127.

22. Roth JD, Roland BL, Cole RL et al. Leptin responsiveness restored by amylin agonism in diet-induced obesity: Evidence from nonclinical and clinical studies. *Proc Natl Acad Sci USA* 2008;105:7257–7262.

23. Vidrine K Keenan MJ, Martin RJ, Gao Z, Finley J, McCutcheon KL, Raggio AM, Tulley RT, Geenway F, Zhou J, and Ye J. Combining resistant starch and sodium butyrate for reducing body fat in rats. *FASEB J* 2010;24:95.5.

24. Gao Z, Yin J, Zhang J et al. Butyrate improves insulin sensitivity and increases energy expenditure in mice. *Diabetes* 2009;58:1509–1517.

25. Brubaker PL and Anini Y. Direct and indirect mechanisms regulating secretion of glucagon-like peptide-1 and glucagon-like peptide-2. *Can J Physiol Pharmacol* 2003;81:1005–1012.

26. Anderson GH, Cho CE, Akhavan T, Mollard RC, Luhovyy BL, and Finocchiaro ET. Relation between estimates of cornstarch digestibility by the Englyst in vitro method and glycemic response, subjective appetite, and short-term food intake in young men. *Am J Clin Nutr* 2010;91:932–939.

27. Scribner KB, Pawlak DB, Aubin CM, Majzoub JA, and Ludwig DS. Long-term effects of dietary glycemic index on adiposity, energy metabolism, and physical activity in mice. *Am J Physiol Endocrinol Metab* 2008;295:E1126–E1131.

28. Reidelberger RD, Haver AC, Chelikani PK, and Buescher JL. Effects of different intermittent peptide YY (3-36) dosing strategies on food intake, body weight, and adiposity in diet-induced obese rats. *Am J Physiol Regul Integr Comp Physiol* 2008;295:R449–R458.

29. Xu AW and Barsh GS. MC4R neurons weigh in differently. *Nat Neurosci* 2006;9:15–16.

30. Zigman JM and Elmquist JK. Minireview: From anorexia to obesity—The yin and yang of body weight control. *Endocrinology* 2003;144:3749–3756.

31. Burcelin R, Cani PD, and Knauf C. Glucagon-like peptide-1 and energy homeostasis. *J Nutr* 2007;137:2534S–2538S.

32. Ding X, Saxena NK, Lin S, Gupta NA, and Anania FA. Exendin-4, a glucagon-like protein-1 (GLP-1) receptor agonist, reverses hepatic steatosis in ob/ob mice. *Hepatology* 2006;43:173–181.

33. Delzenne NM, Cani PD, and Neyrinck AM. Modulation of glucagon-like peptide 1 and energy metabolism by inulin and oligofructose: Experimental data. *J Nutr* 2007;137:2547S–2551S.

34. Robert JA, Zhou J, Raggio AM, Tulley RT, McCutcheon KL, Martin RJ, and Keenan MJ. Resistant starch is effective in lowering body fat in a rat model of human endocrine obesity. *FASEB J* 2008;22:702.14.

35. Tripathy S, Loebig SL, Raggio AM, Zhou J, McCutcheon KL, Hegsted M, Tulley RT, Martin RJ, and Keenan MJ. Resistant starch in a high fat diet produces signaling from the gut, but not reduced body fat. *FASEB J* 2007;21:550.25.

36. Goldsmith F, Martin RJ, Raggio AM, McCutcheon KL, Vidrine V, Goita M, Zhou J, and Keenan MJ. A high fat diet attenuates fermentation effects of resistant starch and fructans. *FASEB J* 2010;24:102.6.

37. Badkoobeh D, Tulley R, Martin RJ, Raggio AM, McCutcheon KL, Goldsmith F, Zhou J, and Keenan MJ. Effects of dietary fat on resistant starch fermentation in mice. *FASEB J* 2010;24:926.2.

38. Backhed F, Ding H, Wang T et al. The gut microbiota as an environmental factor that regulates fat storage. *Proc Natl Acad Sci USA* 2004;101:15718–15723.

39. Cani PD and Delzenne NM. Gut microflora as a target for energy and metabolic homeostasis. *Curr Opin Clin Nutr Metab Care* 2007;10:729–734.

40. DiBaise JK, Zhang H, Crowell MD, Krajmalnik-Brown R, Decker GA, and Rittmann BE. Gut microbiota and its possible relationship with obesity. *Mayo Clin Proc* 2008;83:460–469.

41. Ferguson JD, Sklan D, Chalupa WV, and Kronfeld DS. Effects of hard fats on in vitro and in vivo rumen fermentation, milk production and reproduction in dairy cows. *J Dairy Sci* 1990;73:2864–2879.

42. Harvatine KJ and Allen MS. Effects of fatty acid supplements on ruminal and total tract nutrient digestion in lactating dairy cows. *J Dairy Sci* 2006;89:1092–1103.

43. Jenkins TC. Lipid metabolism in the rumen. *J Dairy Sci* 1993;76:3851–3863.

44. Saunders DR and Sillery JK. Absorption of triglyceride by human small intestine: Dose-response relationships. *Am J Clin Nutr* 1988;48:988–991.

45. Charrier JA, Martin RJ, Brown IL, McCutcheon KL, Raggio AM, Zhou J, Shen L, Goldsmith FR, Goita M, Lammi-Keefe C, and Keenan MJ. Resistant starch in the diet of rodents promotes an increase in fermentation and a reduction in body fat, which is not lost in a high fat diet. *FASEB J* 2011;25:438.6.

46. Lin S, Thomas TC, Storlien LH, and Huang XF. Development of high fat diet-induced obesity and leptin resistance in C57Bl/6J mice. *Int J Obes Relat Metab Disord* 2000;24:639–646.

47. Nogueiras R, Perez-Tilve D, Veyrat-Durebex C et al. Direct control of peripheral lipid deposition by CNS GLP-1 receptor signaling is mediated by the sympathetic nervous system and blunted in diet-induced obesity. *J Neurosci* 2009;29:5916–5925.

Resistant Starch Content of Brown Rice Increases after Refrigeration in Selected Varieties

MARIA STEWART and YU-TING CHIU

Contents

33.1 Introduction

Definitions of dietary fiber range from including physiological effects to purely analytical. Many substances recognized by one dietary fiber definition are not included in other definitions. For example, in the United States, the FDA defines dietary fiber as end products of the AOAC dietary fiber analysis methods 985.29 and 991.43 (DeVries, 2004). Unfortunately, these methods exclude some types of resistant starch (RS) and all oligofructans. RS is considered to be the fraction of starch that resists digestion to human alimentary enzymes and acts as dietary fiber in the large intestine. RS is present in every food containing starch, but the quantity of RS depends on the type and amount of starch, food processing techniques, storage, and ingestion (as cited by reference [Brown, 2004]). The only formal definition of RS by a government-related agency is the definition put forth by EURSETA (European Flair Concerted Action on Resistant Starch), backed by the European Union, defining RS as "the total amount of starch and the products of starch degradation that resists digestion in the small intestine of healthy people." The AACC definition of dietary fiber includes some types of RS, classified as indigestible starches (DeVries, 2004). The IOM definition of fiber would classify RS based on source and physiological effects (Food Nutrition Board, Institute of Medicine, 2001). In the context of the IOM's definitions of fiber, RS that is found in its native food source, such as potatoes or green bananas, is categorized as *dietary fiber*. When the starch is isolated and/or modified to confer resistance to digestion, it is classified as *functional fiber* as long as it confers beneficial physiological effects in humans.

Total dietary fiber content often does not agree with RS content of both prepared foods and isolated RS sources (Sanz et al., 2010). Englyst and other were the first to recognize RS, when performing a nonstarch polysaccharide determination in raw potatoes, cooked and cooled potatoes (containing retrograded RS, RS3), and cooked, warm potatoes (Englyst et al., 1982). In 2002, the AOAC adopted method 2002.02 as its official RS measure (McCleary et al., 2002). This method was validated against in vivo data from ileostomy patients. Measurement of RS is dependent on methods used (Walter et al., 2005). The methods of Siljestrom and Asp (direct RS measurement) and AOAC 996.11 (indirect RS measurement) resulted in substantial differences when white and parboiled rice were analyzed. Compared with the AOAC total dietary fiber analysis method, AOAC 985.29, not all RS analyzes as dietary fiber (Brown, 2004). Altering enzymatic incubation time, pH, or mixing method (shaking or stirring) results in variable amounts of RS in a given sample (McCleary and Rossiter, 2004).

RS intake in the United States averages 4.9 g/day, with breads, cooked cereals and pasta, and vegetables making to greatest contributions to total RS intake (Murphy et al., 2008).

Starchy foods, such as rice, are the primary source of RS in the diet. Rice is a staple carbohydrate in many parts of the world. In the United States, 17.4%–18.2% of adults (ages 20 years and older) consume 1/4 c or more of rice per day, based on NHANES (2001–2002) and CSFII (1994–1996) data (Batres-Marquez et al., 2009). However, in specific regions of the United States, rice intake is much higher. The state of Hawaii is located in the central Pacific Ocean, and local diet patterns are strongly influenced by Japanese, Thai, Korean, Filipino, and Chinese customs. Rice is a staple food in Hawaii. Depending on ethnic group, rice contributes 16.9%–51.1% of daily carbohydrate intake (Takata et al., 2004).

RS content of rice is influenced by rice variety, cooking method, and as described earlier, analytical method. Additionally, some studies report RS content of raw rice, not prepared rice (Walter et al., 2005). The relevance of these RS content is raw rice is questionable, as RS content can be altered by cooking and/or cooling. Most studies report the content or RS in white (milled) rice. Rashmi and Urooj reported that cooking method (pressure cooker, boiling, straining, and steaming) influenced RS content. Within one variety of rice (parboiled white rice), RS content ranged from 0.6 g/100 g cooked to 16.5 g/100 g cooked, depending on cooking method. This suggests that RS content may not be uniform within a single food, depending on cooking method. We previously reported no significant difference in RS content based on cooking method (Abstract # 7478, FASEB meeting 2010). Brown (unmilled) rice is gaining popularity due to its higher dietary fiber and naturally occurring vitamin and mineral content, compared with white rice. Although the starchy endosperm in brown rice contains the same amount of carbohydrate as white rice, the presence of bran and other nondigestible components may decrease the carbohydrate digestibility. Murphy et al. reported that brown rice contains an average of 1.7 g RS per 100 g cooked rice, with a range of 0–3.7 g. The studies cited in this report employ a variety of analytical methods, namely, the Englyst method. Since analytical method impacts RS determination, the present study aimed to build the body of knowledge by determining RS content of five brown rice samples using AOAC method 2002.02 of analysis.

33.2 Methods

33.2.1 Rice Selection and Cooking Method

A survey of available rice varieties was conducted in four major supermarkets in Honolulu, Hawaii. Five rice varieties were chosen for the study: short grain (Tamanishiki®), medium grain (Hinode®), medium grain (Family®), long grain (Hinode®), and quick cooking (Nishiki®). All varieties of rice were cooked in household rice cooker (Aroma brand).

33.2.2 Resistant Starch Analysis

A commercially available RS analysis kit (Megazyme International Ireland Limited) was used for determination of RS found in rice samples. Six replicates of each rice sample (variety x refrigeration) were analyzed. Approximately 0.5 g of fresh rice sample was inserted into glass screw cap tube. Four milliliters of pancreatic α-amylase containing amyloglucosidase (AMG, 3 U/mL) was added, tube vortexed, and incubated in a shaking water bath at 37°C with continuous shaking for 16 h. Tubes were removed from water bath and treated with 4 mL of 99% ethanol with stirring on a vortex mixer. Tubes were centrifuged at 2000 g for 10 min noncapped. Supernatants were decanted, and pellets were resuspended in 2 mL of 50% ethanol again with stirring on vortex. Six milliliters of 50% ethanol was added, tubes were mixed and centrifuged again at 2000 g for 10 min. Supernatants were decanted, suspension and centrifugation step repeated again, and supernatants were decanted once more.

A magnetic bar and 2 mL of 2 M KOH were added to each tube. Pellets were resuspended by stirring for 20 min in an ice/water bath over magnetic stirrer. Eight milliliters of 1.2 M sodium acetate buffer and 0.1 mL of AMG (3300 U/mL) were added, mixed, and placed in water bath at 50°C. Tubes were incubated for 30 min with intermittent mixing on vortex.

For samples containing >10% RS content, tube contents were transferred to a 100 mL volumetric flask. Stirrer bars were taken out with external magnets. Tubes were washed twice by distilled water and pour the residue into the volumetric flask. Solution was adjusted to 100 mL with distilled water, mixed well, and centrifuged at 2000 g for 10 min.

For samples containing <10% RS content, tubes were centrifuged at 2000 g for 10 min with no dilution. In duplicate of supernatants, 0.1 mL of aliquots were transferred into glass test tubes. GOPOD reagent of 3.0 mL was added, and tubes were incubated for 20 min. Absorbance was measured at 510 nm against reagent blank by spectrophotometer. Laboratory data were analyzed using analysis of variance (ANOVA) using SAS statistical software (v. 9.1.3).

33.3 Results and Discussion

Data from this study indicate that RS content of brown rice varies with grain length and significantly increases after refrigeration in medium grain rice (Table 33.1). Rosin et al. reported similar results: a 108% increase in RS content after brown rice was frozen (Rosin et al., 2002). RS content of brown rice was reported to be 2.63 g/100 g dry weight (cooked) and 5.48 g/100 g dry weight (frozen). Percent moisture in our brown rice samples ranged from 42% (long grain) to 73% (short grain). The adjusted RS content per 100 g dry weight ranged 0.55–1.05 g RS/100 g dwb for fresh rice and 0.86–1.20 g RS/100 g dry weight for refrigerated brown rice, which is much lower than the values reported by Rosin et al. (2002). The method used by Rosin et al. was similar to AOAC 2002.02 but had minor modifications that may have altered RS recovery. Additionally, Rosin et al. oven dried the samples at 60°C for 18 h. It is unclear how oven drying affects RS content, if at all.

Other studies measured RS content of brown rice indirectly. Indirect measurement is based on difference of starch fractions (RS = total starch − [rapidly digested starch + slowly digested starch]) via Englyst method. RS content of two varieties of short-grain brown rice were 11.2 and 16.3 g/100 g dry weight, using indirect measurement (Ortuno et al., 1996). These values are 3–4 times greater than the values presented by Rosin et al. and in this study. A report by Englyst et al., also employing indirect measurement of RS, reported that long-grain RS has 0 g RS/100 g as eaten (Englyst et al., 1996).

Brown rice should not be considered as a single food, but rather variety, grain length (long, medium, and short), and cooking methods need to be considered when discussing the availability of carbohydrate. RS content ranged from 0.204 g/100 g cooked rice to 0.883 g/100 g cooked rice. RS content increased significantly after refrigeration for the two medium grain rice samples, but not for quick-cook, long-grain or short-grain brown rice. We expected long-grain rice to have the greatest RS content, both fresh and refrigerated due to its expected amylose content. Six samples of each rice variety were analyzed for RS content. Greater sample size would increase the power to detect significant differences

Table 33.1 Amount of RS per 100 g in Varied Brown Rice

Brand	Fresh Rice	Refrigerated Rice
Tamanishiki (short grain)	0.256 ± 0.061[a]	0.351 ± 0.132[a]
Nishiki (quick cooking)	0.204 ± 0.026[a]	0.368 ± 0.112[a]
Hinode (medium grain)	0.320 ± 0.066[ab*]	0.393 ± 0.047[ab*]
Family (medium grain)	0.465 ± 0.063[bc*]	0.885 ± 0.177[c*]
Hinode (long grain)	0.609 ± 0.163[c]	0.697 ± 0.112[bc]

Values are mean ± standard deviation. Different letters within the same column are statistical differences, $P < 0.05$.

* Indicates that RS within the same row is significantly different between fresh and refrigerated samples.

and more rice samples. However, statistical differences in nutrient content do not necessarily translate to physiological differences in the human body.

A number of physiological effects have been credited to RS, including improved glycemic responses, bowel health, blood lipid profile, increased satiety and reduced energy intake, and increased micronutrient absorption (Nugent, 2005). RS also has considerable benefits to human colonic health. Its fermentation in the large intestine results in the production of short-chain fatty acids. Short-chain fatty acids are the preferred respiratory fuel of colonocytes, increase colonic blood flow, lower luminal pH, and help prevent the development of abnormal colonic cells (Topping and Clifton, 2001). It also appears to impact hunger and food consumption over several hours, corresponding with its fermentation in the large intestine (Bodinham et al., 2010). RS can also confer benefits to heart health, impacting both lipid and glucose metabolism.

RS content in brown rice may be influenced by the bran fraction—inhibiting enzymatic degradation of starch. However, previous studies do not necessarily support this (Englyst et al., 1996). Compared with other foods such as white beans (4.2 g/100 g food as eaten) and bananas (4.0 g/100 g food as eaten), RS content of brown rice is relatively low (Murphy et al., 2008). As a single food, brown rice is not likely to alter chronic disease risk. However, it can make a contribution toward total dietary fiber intake as part of a balanced diet.

Acknowledgments

Funding for this project was provided by the College of Tropical Agriculture and Human Resources at the University of Hawaii at Manoa and USDA Hatch project # HAW00262H.

References

Batres-Marquez S.P., Jensen H.H., and Upton J. Rice consumption in the United States: Recent evidence from food consumption surveys. *J Am Diet Assoc.* 109, 1719, 2009.

Bodinham C.L., Frost G.S., and Robertson M.D. Acute ingestion of resistant starch reduces food intake in healthy adults. *Br J Nutr.* 103, 917, 2010.

Brown I.L. Applications and uses of resistant starch. *J AOAC Int.* 87, 727, 2004.

DeVries J.W. Dietary fiber: The influence of definition on analysis and regulation. *J AOAC Int.* 87, 682, 2004.

Englyst H.N., Veenstra J., and Hudson G.J. Measurement of rapidly available glucose (RAG) in plant foods: A potential in vitro predictor of the glycaemic response. *Br J Nutr.* 75, 327, 1996.

Englyst H.N., Wiggins H.S., and Cummings J.S. Determination of the non-starch polysaccharides in plant foods by gas-liquid chromatography of constituent sugars as alditol acetates. *Analyst.* 107, 307, 1982.

Food Nutrition Board, Institute of Medicine. *Dietary Reference Intakes: Proposed Definition of Dietary Fiber.* Washington, DC: National Academy Press, 2001.

McCleary B.V. and Rossiter P. Measurement of novel dietary fiber. *J AOAC Int.* 87, 707, 2004.

McCleary B.V., McNally M., and Rossiter P. Measurement of resistant starch by enzymatic digestion in starch and selected plant materials: Collaborative study. *J AOAC Int.* 85, 1103, 2002.

Murphy M.M., Douglass J.S., and Birkett A. Resistant starch intakes in the united states. *J Am Diet Assoc.* 108, 67, 2008.

Nugent A.P. Health properties of resistant starch. *Nutr Bull.* 30, 27, 2005.

Ortuno J. et al. Cooking water update and starch digestible values of selected spanish rices. *J Food Qual.* 19, 79, 1996.

Rosin P.M., Lajolo F.M., and Menezes E.W. Measurement and characterization of dietary starches. *J Food Comp Anal.* 15, 367, 2002.

Sanz T. et al. Resistant starch content and glucose release of different resistant starch commercial ingredients: Effect of cooking conditions. *Euro Food Res Tech.* 231, 655, 2010.

Takata Y. et al. A comparison of dietary habits among women in Japan and Hawaii. *Public Health Nutr.* 7, 319, 2004.

Topping D.L. and Clifton P.M. Short-chain fatty acids and human colonic function: Roles of resistant starch and nonstarch polysaccharides. *Physiol Rev.* 81, 1031, 2001.

Walter M., Picolli da Silva L., and Denardin C.C. Rice and resistant starch: Different content depending on methodology. *J Food Comp Anal.* 18, 279, 2005.

34
Acacia Gum

SEBASTIEN BARAY

Contents

34.1 Characteristics

34.1.1 Definition

Acacia gum (also known as gum arabic) is an all-natural sap that exudes from stems and branches of acacia trees (Leguminosae), which grow in the Sahel zone of Africa. The Codex Alimentarius Commission's Committee on Food Additives and Contaminants (CCFAC) determined in 1999 that the only two botanical species allowed for food applications are *Acacia senegal* and *Acacia seyal*. This position is reflected in the Joint FAO/WHO Expert Committee on Food Additives (JECFA) monograph for acacia gum (FAO Food and Nutrition Paper 52 Add 7, 1999).

Over 80% of this natural polysaccharide is made up of sugars (L-arabinose, D-galactose, L-rhamnose, and D-glucuronic acid and its 4-O-methyl derivative), the remaining part consisting of protein (1%–2% depending on the specie),

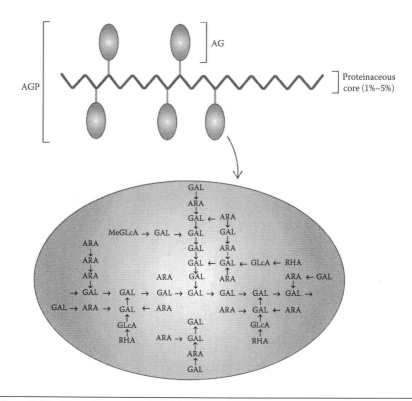

Figure 34.1 Schematic representation of Acacia Gum molecule (Fincher et al., 1983).

polyphenols (catechins, epicatechins, etc.), and minerals (magnesium, potassium, calcium, and sodium). It has a very complex highly branched structure with an average molecular weight varying from 300 to 800 kDa.

The "wattle blossom" model represents the highly branched and compact structure of acacia gum (see Figure 34.1): arabinogalactans are linked with a protein skeleton. The polysaccharidic fraction is made up of a linear chain of galactose β1,3 linked. This chain is branched in position 1,6 with chains of galactose and arabinose. Rhamnose, glucuronic acid, or methyl glucuronic acid units are found at the end of chains.

34.1.2 Safety

Acacia gum has been used in the food industry for decades as a food additive or ingredient. The JECFA recognizes acacia gum as a food additive (INS 414) that can be used with no specified ADI (acceptable daily intake). In February 2005, FDA has issued memoranda specifically on the lack of cancer potential [1] and allergenicity [2,3] for acacia gum. In the United States, acacia gum is recognized as a GRAS (generally recognized as safe) ingredient (CFR 184.1330). In Europe, acacia gum is permitted both as a food additive (E 414) and as a food ingredient under the "quantum satis" principle.

34.2 Nutritional Aspects

34.2.1 Metabolism

Acacia gum generally contains more than 80% soluble dietary fiber on a dry weight basis by the internationally recognized and official AOAC 985.29 method.

Fibregum™ (a range of branded acacia gum products from Nexira) has a soluble dietary fiber content of more than 90% on a dry weight basis.

Acacia gum is not metabolized in the upper digestive tract due to a lack of proper depolymerizing enzymes such as galactanases or arabinases. It will only be fermented by lactic acid bacteria in the large bowel. Upon arrival in the colon, acacia gum represents an extra carbon source providing fuel for microbial fermentation. After a few days of adaptation, no acacia gum is found in rat [4] or human [5] feces, meaning that acacia gum is totally degraded by colonic flora and then fermented. For that reason, slightly less than half of the actual bond energy (as measured by calorimetry) is available under physiological conditions. Research done in 2008 by G. Livesey and Nexira has established the acacia gum caloric value at approximately 1.7 kcal/g. As a result, this value has been recognized by FDA as acceptable on labels. In Europe, Commission Directive 2008/100/EC recommends the use of an energy conversion factor of 2 kcal/g for any fiber, including acacia gum. Caloric value of acacia gum is 1.8 and 1 kcal/g in, respectively, Australia and Japan.

Acacia gum's mechanical roles, such as increasing satiety rate or transit time in the upper intestinal tract, are minimal, as compared with viscous soluble fibers and with insoluble fibers having a high water retention capacity. However, the influence of acacia gum on gastric emptying time, for instance, could be an indirect influence through its colonic fermentation metabolites such as the short-chain fatty acids (SCFAs).

34.2.2 Intestinal Tolerance

The fermentation of soluble fibers may produce abdominal discomfort, abdominal cramps, or diarrhea in some persons. Cherbut et al. studied the intestinal tolerance of Fibregum as compared to sucrose (placebo) and fructooligosaccharides (FOS) in 20 healthy subjects [6]. The results showed that acacia gum does not exhibit laxative side effects at dosages up to 50 g/day (see Figure 34.2) and that flatus, bloating, and borborygmi occurred at lower doses with FOS. The greater tolerance of Fibregum compared to FOS was attributed to its much higher molecular weight and slower colonic fermentation pattern [6].

34.2.3 Prebiotic Effect

Fermentation of acacia gum in the large bowel stimulates the growth of lactic acid bacteria (lactobacilli and bifidobacteria), which is beneficial to human health and wellness. The prebiotic effect of acacia gum has been extensively studied.

First in vitro studies showed that among different genus of bacteria from human feces, bifidobacteria strains [7], more specifically from the *B. longum* and

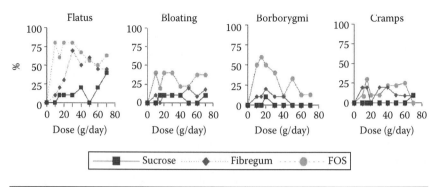

Figure 34.2 Tolerance of Acacia Gum vs. FOS in human.

B. adolescentis [8] species, were able to use acacia gum for their growth. In an in vitro system batch, May et al. [9] were able to demonstrate an increase in the total anaerobe quantity with acacia gum. With a continuous system, Michel et al. [10] showed that the lactobacilli count was increased by 6.75 times and the Clostridium count was decreased by 1.8 log with acacia gum compared to a control, and the decrease was even better compared to FOS. In rats, 10% of acacia gum added to the diet allowed to increase the diaminopimelic acid index in the cecum and feces, measured as an indicator of the total bacterial mass, compared to control and wheat bran [11].

In a case study with a 32 year old female volunteer consuming 10 g/day of acacia gum during 18 days, the proportion of bacteria able to ferment acacia gum rose from 6.5% at the beginning of the study to 53.6% at the end of the treatment, indicating an adaptation of the microflora [12]. After cessation of the consumption, this proportion decreased slightly to come back to initial value after 45 days.

In a single blind controlled study performed on 10 healthy volunteers consuming either Fibregum or sucrose as control at the dose of 10 g/day during 10 days, concentrations of bifidobacteria, lactobacilli, and total lactic acid bacteria groups were significantly increased by, respectively, 0.62 log, 0.48 log, and 0.77 log with Fibregum compared to control without affecting neutral groups such as bacteroides [6]. The bifidogenic effect was even more pronounced (+1 log) in subjects having low initial bifidobacteria count (<9.5 log).

In a randomized double blind controlled trial with six parallel test groups involving 54 healthy volunteers, Calame et al. [13] demonstrated that consumption of 10 g/day of acacia gum for 4 weeks yielded an increase in counts of bifidobacteria and lactobacilli (respectively 40-fold and 6-fold) as compared to water (negative control). Numbers of bifidobacteria, lactobacilli, and bacteroides were found to be significantly higher with the intake of 10 g/day of acacia gum than with the same dose of inulin.

In a randomized double blind controlled study involving 96 healthy volunteers [14], an intake of 6 g/day of Fibregum induced a 0.7 log increase of fecal bifidobacteria after 1 week of consumption. Moreover, this effect was greater compared to FOS that induced a 0.3 log increase at the same dosage. A mix of 3 g of Fibregum plus 3 g of FOS had a synergetic bifidogenic effect (+1.38 log increase).

Acacia gum is widely fermented and results in greater production of total SCFAs when compared to other sources of oligo- or polysaccharides, including pectin, psyllium, xylooligosaccharides, FOS, and others, as seen in the in vitro model [9,10,15–19] using either fecal bacteria from human or pig origin.

Increased total pool and concentration of SCFAs were also demonstrated in cecum, feces, cecum blood flow, and hepatic portal venous plasma of rats [4,11,20–25]. Acacia gum is considered one of the most soluble and most fermentable polysaccharides. However, because SCFAs are progressively absorbed in the colon, it is rather difficult to detect a variation in their concentration in human feces. McLean Ross et al. [5] and Rochat et al. [14] were not able to demonstrate an SCFA fecal concentration increase after a daily intake of, respectively, 25 and 6 g of acacia gum.

The shift from acetate to higher proportions of propionate and butyrate with acacia gum compared with control period and with other sources of fiber (e.g., pectin) has been described in vitro [9,10,17–19], in rats [4,20–25] as well as in humans [5]. This shift probably partly explains the health benefits on the gut epithelium (e.g., stimulation of intestinal mobility, reduction of inflammation and colorectal cancer risk) but also the possible effects on lipid metabolism.

34.3 Potential Health Benefits of Acacia Gum

34.3.1 Reduction of Diarrhea and Constipation

Benefits of acacia gum on water/electrolyte absorption and on recovery from diarrhea have been well detailed in studies on malnourished rats or animals with diarrhea induced by use of cathartics [26–28]. In rat intestine exposed to cholera toxin, acacia gum reduced chloride secretion and normalized sodium transport [29].

The mechanisms of action of acacia gum have not been fully elucidated. Evidence suggests that acacia gum may be an indirect regulator of nitric oxide (NO) metabolism, scavenging some of the NO diffused from the enterocyte into the lumen and thereby promoting fluid absorption [30]. Alternatively, acacia gum may modify bulk transport by enhancing diffusive mechanisms but had no effect on sodium-dependent carriers [31].

The efficacy of acacia gum might derive, at least in part, from regulation of NO-dependent gating of the basolateral membrane potassium channel [32]. However, considering that acacia gum is not absorbed at all in the upper gastrointestinal tract, the possible linkage might be exerted via a purely physical mechanism, such as NO gas adsorption or scavenging.

Additional studies indicate that acacia gum, in addition to its ability to remove NO diffused into the intestinal lumen, may also partially inhibit intestinal NO synthase and thus modulate intestinal absorption through these mechanisms [33,34].

More recently, Wapnir et al. showed in animal models with intestinal dysfunction induced by cathartics that the addition of 10 or 20 g/L acacia gum could reduce the expression of the nuclear factor kappa B (NF-κB), which is associated with an inflammatory response in the small intestinal mucosa [35]. In addition, a tendency to normalize several genes expressed in the small intestinal mucosa, upregulated by the cathartics, was observed according to evidence obtained with microarray chips (Affymetrix rat specific).

Several human studies clearly showed that supplementation with acacia gum reduces fecal incontinence and improves stool consistency [36–38]. In addition, acacia gum, from the dose of 15 g/day, allows increasing stool wet weight and stool humidity in healthy adults [12]. More than a drug, acacia gum is interesting because it behaves as a regulator: it is able to reduce diarrhea and, alternatively, reduce constipation risk.

34.3.2 Improvement of Nitrogen Excretion

In a prospective single blind crossover study, a greater nitrogen excretion in stools and lower serum urea nitrogen have been measured in 16 patients (male and female) with chronic renal failure when 50 g/day of acacia gum was added to a low-protein diet during 4 weeks [39]. Significant decrease of plasma urea (-11%, $p < 0.05$) was also observed in patients with slowly progressive uremia with 30 g acacia gum daily [40]. This could be dependent on an increase in bacterial growth and activity in the gut. More recent studies, in rat models of acute renal failure, suggest that acacia gum may also improve renal function independently of its action on fecal bacterial ammonia metabolism [41,42]. Acacia gum may act by reducing the amount of urea nitrogen excreted in urine and by increasing urea disposal in the large intestine, where it is degraded. It has been also reported that acacia gum can decrease urea nitrogen excretion, urea production, and urea cycling in rats [43,44] without having a net effect on nitrogen balance.

Latest data support the hypothesis that dietary supplementation with acacia gum may have a potential beneficial effect in renal disease by increasing systemic levels of butyrate and thus suppressing the profibrotic cytokine TGF-β1 activity [45].

The regular intake of acacia gum in addition to a low-protein/high-calorie diet can contribute to the postponement of the need for hemodialysis or peritoneal dialysis in children with end-stage renal disease [46]. More recently, the use of acacia gum in adult patients with symptomatic uremia has been investigated in 11 patients [47]. Assimilation of acacia gum was associated with amelioration of the uremic symptoms and improvement of general well-being as long as patients were compliant with the therapeutic protocol. The most significant finding in this study is the achievement of hemodialysis freedom in two patients, both of whom had a previous vascular access [48].

These effects enable lowering of the kidneys' workload with the objective of decreasing adverse clinical symptoms such as nausea, anorexia, and fatigue associated with renal failure. Acacia gum could also be used to prevent renal damage that could be associated with a high-protein diet.

Moreover, acacia gum can help normalize parameters such as increase in urine volume, in serum creatinine, or in urea induced by nephrotoxicity [49]. Acacia gum has notably been shown to protect the kidneys from gentamicin-induced nephrotoxicity in rats [50]. Its administration lessened the negative effects of this nephrotoxicity possibly by inhibiting free radical–mediated process and prevents histological changes in renal tissues. Acacia gum can thus help the body to detoxify or eliminate deleterious components and thus prevent tissue damages.

34.3.3 Reduction of Cholesterol

Physiological effects of acacia gum from human studies include the lowering of serum triglyceride and cholesterol levels [51,52]. A study in five healthy human volunteers taking 25 g/day of acacia gum shows a significant reduction of total serum cholesterol concentrations [5,53]. Another study in seven nonobese hypercholesterolemic men consuming 15 g acacia gum twice a day along with their main meals for 30 days indicates that acacia gum causes a significant decrease in serum total cholesterol levels, especially LDL and VLDL fractions [54], which confirms previous results obtained in rats [55]. But other studies come to different conclusions either in normal [56] or in hypercholesterolemic subjects [57]. In the same way, some studies in rats exhibit contradictory conclusions on the ability of acacia gum to reduce plasma cholesterol levels. Those variations among studies are possibly due to the variability of acacia gum used or the dose and the duration of consumption.

The potential ability of acacia gum to decrease serum cholesterol may be linked to its globular structure and its emulsifying and film-forming properties [58]. The production of SCFAs (especially propionate) and also possible binding with cholesterol and bile acids in the small intestine may be responsible for this outcome.

34.3.4 Hypoglycemic Effect

Acacia gum not only has a negligible impact on blood glycemia but also has been proven to reduce the glycemic index (GI) of food products. Glucose tolerance test was conducted in 12 healthy subjects. The addition of 20 g acacia gum to 100 g load of glucose resulted in a significant reduction of plasma glucose response (−18.6%) and serum insulin (−12.4%) [59].

Twelve healthy Japanese males consumed consecutively in a random order a sucrose loading (100 g) plus 0, 5, or 10 g of acacia gum dissolved in 300 mL of water [60]. Blood samples were taken from each subject before examination and at intervals of 30 min during 150 min after supplementation. Blood glucose level was determined by glucose oxidase method using Glutest Ace. Blood glucose concentration reached peak level 30 min after the supplementation with sucrose and acacia gum. Compared to the peak glucose level after taking the placebo (171.1 ± 7.65 mg/dL), the level was significantly lowered after taking 5 or 10 g acacia gum (153.5 ± 7.5 and 146.0 ± 9.8 mg/dL, respectively). Similarly, the glucose concentration at 60 min after supplementation was significantly decreased in test groups compared to placebo group. Additionally, a dose-response relationship was observed in the blood glucose lowering effect of acacia gum.

Fourteen overweight or obese women suffering from type 2 diabetes consumed 50 g of available carbohydrate from white bread (100 g) as reference food and, 7 days later, the same reference product plus 15 g of Fibregum, dissolved in 180 mL of water [61]. Addition of Fibregum to the diet allowed a significant GI reduction (−18.6%).

Glycemic and insulin index of three crisp breads proportionally decreased in a group of 12 healthy people when increasing quantities of Fibregum (0%, 6%, and 11% by weight) were added to the breads [62]: GI of crisp bread decreased from 78 for the standard product to 69 when 6% Fibregum was added and 65 with 11% Fibregum.

Torres y Torres et al. showed that soy beverages with low concentration of carbohydrate (maltodextrine) and added soluble fiber (Fibregum) may be recommended in obese and diabetic patients thanks to their low GI and the low level of insulin secreted after ingestion [63].

34.4 Applications of Acacia Gum in Food Products

Acacia gum is available in the form of a highly soluble and pure powder that is tasteless and odorless. Acacia gum requires no heating or shearing for activation, but it is resilient to high shear and also temperature or pH extremes.

Due to its low viscosity and high solubility, it is very easy to add a significant amount of acacia gum into many food products without altering their original characteristics. The acacia gum can simply be added to an existing formulation with no negative interaction or unwanted increase in viscosity (see Figure 34.3).

In the human mouth, acacia gum resists hydrolysis by salivary enzymes and local flora, which allows it to be classified as noncariogenic and makes it safe for teeth [64]. Acacia gum can be used in dietetic products and can safely be used in sugar-free formulations.

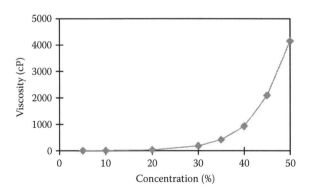

Figure 34.3 Influence of concentration on viscosity of Acacia Gum (at 25°C).

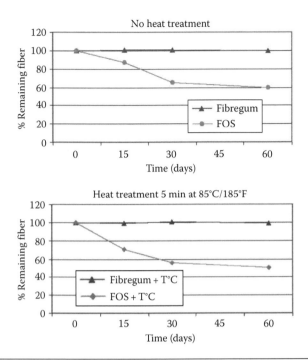

Figure 34.4 Fiber stability of Acacia gum vs. FOS at low pH (3.8) and high temperature.

Due to its highly branched structure, acacia gum is extremely resistant to heat treatments, acidic conditions, and yeast fermentation; it remains stable against the most severe temperatures, even at very low pH for several months (see Figure 34.4).

Acacia gum not only brings nutritional benefits but it also provides many technical functionalities to food applications such as beverages (fruit juice blends, smoothies, etc.), dairy products (milk, yogurt, etc.), baked goods (breads, muffins, cookies, wraps, etc.), confectionery, extruded snacks, cereals, sauces and dressings, nutrition bars (cereal, high protein, etc.), meal replacement shakes and powders, or nutraceutical tablets.

34.4.1 Beverages

Acacia gum is being widely used in reduced-sugar or low-juice beverages because the roundness and mouthfeel it provides perfectly matches the texture brought by sucrose or fruit juice. Studies on rats clearly showed that water, glucose, and mineral absorption were significantly enhanced when acacia gum was added into oral rehydration solutions or sports drinks [26–29].

34.4.2 Bakery Products

Due to its moisture regulation and film-forming properties, acacia gum brings many benefits to baked goods in terms of processing, texture, and shelf life. Addition of acacia gum to bakery products has been proved to enhance their texture (smoothness and fullness), especially in freeze/thaw or freeze/bake applications. Those benefits lead to a reduced staling effect and a shelf-life extension. For instance, studies carried out by The Food Development Group in Toronto, Canada, clearly showed that the texture of bakery products such as soft cookies or muffins was improved at increased acacia gum levels (0%–3% by weight). In the meantime, superior eating qualities over the standard cookie without acacia gum were noted during the entire duration of the shelf life. The softness brought by the addition of acacia gum is perceived by the consumer as freshness.

34.4.3 Cereal Bars

Acacia gum develops unique binding and sticking properties that enable a partial or total replacement of sugar, glucose syrup, and high-fructose corn syrup (HFCS) in the binding solution. Addition of 4%–8% acacia gum is usually required to effectively bind the dry components of the formula (fruits, cereals). Its high moisture stabilization properties and its film-forming ability favor extending the shelf life and delaying the hardening of the bar.

34.4.4 Extruded Snacks and Breakfast Cereals

Acacia gum acts as a lubricant during the extrusion process, which leads to a more consistent shape and texture of the snacks. During extrusion, the addition of acacia gum into the snack dough has been reported to help decrease the mechanical energy while increasing both efficiency and output of the extruder. Such benefits have been obtained with addition of 2%–5% acacia gum, and optimum reduction of electrical intensity, engine torque, and heat buildup have been observed with 3.5% acacia gum. Acacia gum's high moisture control properties help increase the crispiness and reduce the staling effect during storage.

34.4.5 Confectionery

Acacia gum is not considered a thickening hydrocolloid when dissolved in water at low concentration (up to 30%). Meanwhile, when used in sucrose or sugarless system (polyols and artificial sweeteners) at high level of dry substances, acacia gum provides a unique texture to European-type molded confectionery products such as jujubes or gum pastilles. In coated sweet goods, acacia gum is used for its film-forming ability in order to improve the physical and mechanical properties of the centers and make the hard and soft coating layers more effective. The addition of a low level (1%–3%) of acacia gum in a sugarless hard candy based on sorbitol, maltitol, or mannitol slightly increases the amount of residual water (1%–3%) after cooking and therefore decreases the cooking temperature from 40°F to 60°F. Hygroscopicity of the candy is reduced, recrystallization of polyols is avoided, and wrapped sweets are not sticky.

Acacia gum is used as a binder for tableting by direct compression or wet granulation in food and pharmaceutical products. For the direct compression, purified and agglomerated acacia gum is mixed with the other powders (having the same mesh size) before filling the die. In the wet granulation, acacia gum in solution is added to the powders to make a slurry, which is dried and sieved to produce a free-flowing material that is then compressed.

34.4.6 Encapsulation of Active Components

Acacia gum exhibits colloidal film-forming properties that are widely used to protect sensitive nutritional components against oxygen, acidity, moisture, temperature, and light by spray-drying encapsulation.

Examples of active ingredients that can be protected with acacia gum–based carrier are as follows: essential oils, polyunsaturated fatty acid, probiotics such as *Lactobacillus paracasei* NFBC 338 [65], minerals, polyphenols, liposoluble vitamins (A, E, D, and K), ascorbic acid [66], or fruit juices such as acerola or camu-camu juices [67] rich in vitamin C.

References

1. Ekelman K. Gum arabic, *Memorandum of Conference, Cancer Assessment Committee Meeting*, Washington, DC, January 6, 1998.
2. Griffiths J, FDA's Additives Evaluation Branch, Memorandum to Coker C, FDA's Case and Advisory Branch, Gum arabic and immunogenicity; updated literature survey, March 8, 1998.
3. Griffiths J, FDA's Additives Evaluation Branch, Memorandum to Flamm E, FDA's Direct Additives Branch, Gum arabic and immunogenicity; literature from Dr. D.M.W. Anderson, November 9, 1998.
4. McLean Ross AH, Eastwood MA, Brydon WG, Busuttil A, McKay LF. A study of the effects of dietary gum arabic in the rat. *Br. J. Nutr.* 1984; 51:47–56.
5. McLean Ross AH, Eastwood MA, Brydon WG, Anderson JR, Anderson DM. A study of the effects of dietary gum arabic in humans. *Am. J. Clin. Nutr.* 1983; 37:368–375.
6. Cherbut C, Michel C, Raison V, Kravtchenko TP, Meance S. Acacia gum is a bifidogenic dietary fiber with high digestive tolerance in healthy humans. *Microbial Ecol. Health Dis.* 2003; 15:43–50.
7. Salyers AA, Palmer JK, Wilkins TD. Degradation of polysaccharides by intestinal bacterial enzymes. *Am. J. Clin. Nutr.* 1978; 31:S128–S130.
8. Crociani F, Alessandrini A, Mucci MM, Biavati B. Degradation of complex carbohydrates by Bifidobacterium spp. *Int. J. Food Microbiol.* 1994; 24:199–210.
9. May T, Mackie RI, Fahey GC, Jr., Cremin JC, Garleb KA. Effect of fiber source on short-chain fatty acid production and on the growth and toxin production by *Clostridium difficile*. *Scand. J. Gastroenterol.* 1994; 29:916–922.
10. Michel C, Kravtchenko T, David A, Gueneau S, Kozlowski F, Cherbut C. In vitro prebiotic effects of Acacia gums onto the human intestinal microbiota depend on both botanical origin and environmental pH. *Anaerobe* 1998; 4:257–266.
11. Walter DJ, Eastwood MA, Brydon WG, Elton RA. Fermentation of wheat bran and gum arabic in rats fed on an elemental diet. *Br. J. Nutr.* 1988; 60:225–232.
12. Wyatt GM, Bayliss CE, Holcroft JD. A change in human faecal flora in response to inclusion of gum arabic in the diet. *Br. J. Nutr.* 1986; 55:261–266.
13. Calame W, Weseler AR, Viebke C, Flynn C, Siemensma AD. Gum arabic establishes prebiotic functionality in healthy human volunteers in a dose-dependent manner. *Br. J. Nutr.* 2008 Dec; 100(6):1269–75. Epub 2008 May 9. Erratum in: *Br. J. Nutr.* 2009 Aug; 102(4):642.
14. Rochat F, Baumgartner M, Jann A, Rochat C, Nielsen G, Reuteler G, Ballèvre O. Synergistic effect of prebiotics on human intestinal microflora. Personal Communication, 2001.

15. Tomlin J. Which fibre is best for the colon? *Scand. J. Gastroenterol.* 1987; 129(Suppl):100–104.

16. Adiotomre J, Eastwood MA, Edwards CA, Brydon WG. Dietary fiber: In vitro methods that anticipate nutrition and metabolic activity in humans. *Am. J. Clin. Nutr.* 1990; 52:128–134.

17. Mortensen PB, Hove H, Clausen MR, Holtug K. Fermentation to short-chain fatty acids and lactate in human faecal batch cultures. Intra- and inter-individual variations versus variations caused by changes in fermented saccharides. *Scand. J. Gastroenterol.* 1991; 26:1285–1294.

18. Titgemeyer EC, Bourquin LD, Fahey GC, Jr., Garleb KA. Fermentability of various fiber sources by human fecal bacteria in vitro. *Am. J. Clin. Nutr.* 1991; 53:1418–1424.

19. Bourquin LD, Titgemeyer EC, Fahey GC, Jr., Garleb KA. Fermentation of dietary fibre by human colonic bacteria: Disappearance of, short-chain fatty acid production from, and potential water-holding capacity of, various substrates. *Scand. J. Gastroenterol.* 1993; 28:249–255.

20. Storer GB, Illman RJ, Trimble RP, Snoswell AM, Topping DL. Plasma and caecal volatile fatty acids in male and female rats: Effects of dietary gum arabic and cellulose. *Nutr. Res.* 1984; 4:701–707.

21. Topping DL, Mock S, Trimble RP, Storer GB, Illman RJ. Effects of varying the content and proportions of gum arabic and cellulose on caecal volatile fatty acid concentrations in the rat. *Nutr. Res.* 1988; 8:1013–1020.

22. Topping DL, Illman RJ, Trimble RP. Volatile fatty acid concentrations in rats fed diets containing gum arabic and cellulose separately and as a mixture. *Nutr. Rep.* 1985; 32:809–814.

23. Tulung B, Remesy C, Demigne C. Specific effect of guar gum or gum arabic on adaptation of cecal digestion to high fiber diets in the rat. *J. Nutr.* 1987; 117:1556–1561.

24. Walter DJ, Eastwood MA, Brydon WG, Elton RA. An experimental design to study colonic fibre fermentation in the rat: The duration of feeding. *Br. J. Nutr.* 1986; 55:465–479.

25. Annison G, Trimble RP, Topping DL. Feeding Australian Acacia gums and gum arabic leads to non-starch polysaccharide accumulation in the cecum of rats. *J. Nutr.* 1995; 125:283–292.

26. Wapnir RA, Teichberg S, Go JT, Wingertzahn MA, Harper RG. Oral rehydration solutions: Enhanced sodium absorption with gum arabic. *J. Am. Coll. Nutr.* 1996; 15:377–382.

27. Wapnir RA, Wingertzahn MA, Moyse J, Teichberg S. Gum arabic promotes rat jejunal sodium and water absorption from oral rehydration solutions in two models of diarrhea. *Gastroenterology* 1997; 112:1979–1985.

28. Teichberg S, Wingertzahn MA, Moyse J, Wapnir RA. Effect of gum arabic in an oral rehydration solution on recovery from diarrhea in rats. *J. Pediatr. Gastroenterol. Nutr.* 1999; 29:411–417.

29. Turvill JL, Wapnir RA, Wingertzahn MA, Teichberg S, Farthing MJ. Cholera toxin-induced secretion in rats is reduced by a soluble fiber, gum arabic. *Dig. Dis. Sci.* 2000; 45:946–951.

30. Wingertzahn MA, Teichberg S, Wapnir RA. Jejunal nitric oxide (NO) levels are reduced by gum arabic (GA). *J. Am. Coll. Nutr.* 1998; Abstract 52:509.

31. Wingertzahn MA, Teichberg S, Wapnir RA. Stimulation of non-sodium-dependent water, electrolyte, and glucose transport in rat small intestine by gum arabic. *Dig. Dis. Sci.* 2001; 46:1105–1112.

32. Rehman KU, Wingertzahn MA, Harper RG, Wapnir RA. Proabsorptive action of gum arabic: Regulation of nitric oxide metabolism in the basolateral potassium channel of the small intestine. *J. Pediatr. Gastroenterol. Nutr.* 2001; 32:529–533.

33. Rehman KU, Codipilly CN, Wapnir RA. Modulation of small intestinal nitric oxide synthase by gum arabic. *Exp. Biol. Med. (Maywood.)* 2004; 229:895–901.
34. Rehman KU, Wingertzahn MA, Teichberg S, Harper RG, Wapnir RA. Gum arabic (GA) modifies paracellular water and electrolyte transport in the small intestine. *Dig. Dis. Sci.* 2003; 48:755–760.
35. Wapnir RA, Sherry B, Codipilly CN, Goodwin LO, Vancurova I. Modulation of rat intestinal nuclear factor NF-κB by gum arabic. *Dig. Dis. Sci.* 2008; 53:80–87.
36. Bliss DZ, Jung HJ, Savik K et al. Supplementation with dietary fiber improves fecal incontinence. *Nurs. Res.* 2001; 50:203–213.
37. Korula J. Dietary fiber supplementation with psyllium or gum arabic reduced fecal incontinence in community-living adults. *ACP J. Club.* 2002; 136:23.
38. Campbell S. Dietary fibre supplementation with psyllium or gum arabic reduced incontinent stools and improved stool consistency in community living adults. *Evid. Based. Nurs.* 2002; 5:56.
39. Bliss DZ, Stein TP, Schleifer CR, Settle RG. Supplementation with gum arabic fiber increases fecal nitrogen excretion and lowers serum urea nitrogen concentration in chronic renal failure patients consuming a low-protein diet. *Am. J. Clin. Nutr.* 1996; 63:392–398.
40. Rampton DS, Cohen SL, Crammond VD et al. Treatment of chronic renal failure with dietary fiber. *Clin. Nephrol.* 1984; 21:159–163.
41. Ali BH, Al Qarawi AA, Haroun EM, Mousa HM. The effect of treatment with gum Arabic on gentamicin nephrotoxicity in rats: A preliminary study. *Ren. Fail.* 2003; 25:15–20.
42. Ali BH, Alqarawi AA, Ahmed IH. Does treatment with gum Arabic affect experimental chronic renal failure in rats? *Fundam. Clin. Pharmacol.* 2004; 18:327–329.
43. Assimon SA, Stein TP. Digestible fiber (gum arabic), nitrogen excretion and urea recycling in rats. *Nutrition* 1994; 10:544–550.
44. Younes H, Garleb K, Behr S, Remesy C, Demigne C. Fermentable fibers or oligosaccharides reduce urinary nitrogen excretion by increasing urea disposal in the rat cecum. *J. Nutr.* 1995; 125:1010–1016.
45. Matsumoto N, Riley S, Fraser D et al. Butyrate modulates TGF-beta1 generation and function: Potential renal benefit for Acacia(sen) SUPERGUM (gum arabic)? *Kidney Int.* 2006; 69:257–265.
46. Al Mosawi AJ. Acacia gum supplementation of a low-protein diet in children with end-stage renal disease. *Pediatr. Nephrol.* 2004; 19:1156–1159.
47. Al-Mosawi AJ. Continuous renal replacement in the developing world: Is there any alternative? *Therapy* 2006; 3:265–272.
48. Al-Mosawi AJ. Acacia gum therapeutic potential: Possible role in the management of uremia—A new potential medicine (8 articles). *Therapy* 2006; 3:301–321.
49. Al-Mosawi AJ. The challenge of chronic renal failure in the developing world: Possible use of acacia gum. *Pediatr. Nephrol.* 2002; 17:390–391.
50. Al-Majed AA, Mostafa AM, Al Rikabi AC, Al Shabanah OA. Protective effects of oral Arabic gum administration on gentamicin-induced nephrotoxicity in rats. *Pharmacol. Res.* 2002; 46:445–451.
51. Meyer D, Tungland B. Non-digestible oligosaccharides and polysaccharides: Their physiological effects and health implications. In: McCleary BV, Prosky L, eds. *Advanced Dietary Fibre Technology*, Blackwell Science Ltd, Oxford, UK, 2006. p. 464.
52. Schneeman BO, Lefevre M. Effects of fiber on plasma lipoprotein composition. In: Vahouny GV, Kritchevsky D, eds. *Dietary Fiber: Basic Clinical Aspects*, Plenum Press, New York, 1984. p. 309–321.
53. McLean Ross AH, Eastwood MA, Brydon WG, McKay LF, Anderson DM, Anderson JR. Gum arabic metabolism in man. *Proc. Nutr. Soc.* 1982; 41:64A.

54. Sharma RD. Hypocholesterolemic effect of gum acacia in men. *Nutr. Res.* 1985; 5:1321–1326.
55. Sharma RD. Hypocholesterolemic activity of some Indian gums. *Nutr. Res.* 1984; 4:381–389.
56. Haskell WL, Spiller GA, Jensen CD, Ellis BK, Gates JE. Role of water-soluble dietary fiber in the management of elevated plasma cholesterol in healthy subjects. *Am. J. Cardiol.* 1992; 69:433–439.
57. Jensen CD, Spiller GA, Gates JE, Miller AF, Whittam JH. The effect of acacia gum and a water-soluble dietary fiber mixture on blood lipids in humans. *J. Am. Coll. Nutr.* 1993; 12:147–154.
58. Eastwood MA, Brydon WG, Anderson DM. The effect of the polysaccharide composition and structure of dietary fibers on cecal fermentation and fecal excretion. *Am. J. Clin. Nutr.* 1986; 44:51–55.
59. Sharma RD. Hypoglycemic effect of gum acacia in healthy human subjects. *Nutr. Res.* 1985; 5:1437–1441.
60. Castellani F. Fibregum (acacia gum) helps reduce the glycemic index of food products. *Agro Food Industry Hi-tech.* 2006; 16:24–26.
61. Meance S, Mescheriakova VA, Charaphétdinov CC, Plotnikova OA. Glycemic index with a supplementation of acacia gum or a viscous acacia gum mix in type 2 diabetic women. Personal Communication, 2004.
62. Fremont G. Glycemic index and insulin index values of Fibregum enriched crispbreads. Personal Communication, 2006.
63. Torres y Torres N, Palacios-González B, Noriega-López L, Tovar-Palacio A. Glycemic, insulinemic index, glycemic load of soy beverage with low and high content of carbohydrates. *Rev. Invest. Clin.* 2006; 58(5):487–497.
64. Imfeld T, Meance S. Evaluation of the safe for teeth of the acacia gum Fibregum at different concentrations in humans. Personal Communication, 2003.
65. Desmond C, Ross RP, O'Callaghan E, Fitzgerald G, Stanton C. Improved survival of *Lactobacillus paracasei* NFBC 338 in spray-dried powders containing gum Acacia. *J. Appl. Microbiol.* 2002; 93:1003–1011.
66. Trindade MA, Grosso CR. The stability of ascorbic acid microencapsulated in granules of rice starch and in gum arabic. *J. Microencapsul.* 2000; 17:169–176.
67. Dib Taxi CM, de Menezes HC, Santos AB, Grosso CR. Study of the microencapsulation of camu-camu (*Myrciaria dubia*) juice. *J. Microencapsul.* 2003; 20:443–448.

35

Nondigestible Saccharide Enhances Transcellular Transport of Myricetin Glycosides in the Small Intestine of Rats
A Newly Defined Mechanism of Flavonoid Absorption

NORIKO MATSUKAWA, MEGUMI MATSUMOTO, and HIROSHI HARA

Contents

35.1 Introduction

Quercetin and myricetin are flavonols, a class of flavonoid, and are abundant in plant as secondary metabolites. Quercetin and quercetin glycosides are known to have many beneficial effects on health [1,2]. Myricetin, which has an additional hydroxyl group at 5′ position of B-ring in quercetin, is also known to be abundantly present in tea, wine, and grapes [3] and is known to have some physiological effects, such as the improvement of glucose intolerance [4,5] and cancer prevention [6,7]. Intestinal absorption of quercetin and quercetin-3-O-glucoside has been well-studied in animals and humans [8–10], and it has been reported that quercetin-3-O-glucoside is hydrolyzed into aglycone in the small intestinal lumen by lactase-phloridine hydrolase, then transported into the intestinal epithelial cells, where it is conjugated as quercetin glucuronides or sulfides, before release into the mesenteric blood [11,12]. Another reported mechanism suggests that quercetin-3-O-glucoside is absorbed as a glycoside via the sodium-dependent glucose transporter 1 (SGLT1) [13]. However, there

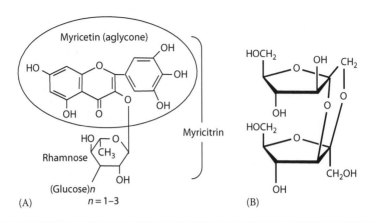

Figure 35.1 Chemical structure of a water-soluble flavonoid, glucosylated myricitrin (A) and DFAIII (B).

is little information on intestinal absorption of myricetin and myricetin glycosides. One report describes the transport of myricitrin (myricetin 3-O-α-L-rhamnoside) via the paracellular pathway in Caco-2 monolayer, a model of the intestinal epithelium [14].

We have recently found that a nondigestible saccharide, difructose anhydride III (DFAIII) (Figure 35.1A), promotes the absorption and bioavailability of αG-rutin and quercetin-3-O-glucoside [15–17]. Absorption of the water-soluble glycoside, αG-rutin, was increased via the paracellular transport pathway through the tight junction of the small intestinal epithelium [18], a result supported by the fact that portal absorption of intact αG-rutin was largely enhanced by DFAIII after duodenal injection of αG-rutin in portal and duodenal cannulated conscious rats [15].

The aims of the present study were to examine effects of DFAIII on a water-soluble myricetin glycoside, glucosylated myricitrin, and to define the absorptive mechanism of the flavonoid glycoside through the intestinal epithelium using small intestinal loops in anesthetized rats. We found that this myricetin glycoside was absorbed into the intestinal epithelial cells as glycosides, not as aglycone, and released into the mesenteric blood as glucuronide or sulfide.

35.2 Materials and Methods

35.2.1 Chemicals

A glucosylated myricitrin mixture (G-Myr, Figure 35.1A) composed of 73.5 mol% myricitrin (myricetin 3-O-α-L-rhamnoside), 13.4 mol% myricetin 3-O-D-glucosy [1–3] α-L-rhamnoside (monoglucose adduct of myricitrin), 12.1 mol% α-1, 4 diglucose adduct of myricitrin, and 7.2 mol% α-1, 4 triglucose adduct of myricitrin (Figure 35.1A) was kindly donated by San-Ei Gen F.F.I., Inc. (Osaka, Japan). Standard compounds of myricetin and myricitrin were also provided by San-Ei Gen F.F.I., Inc. All other reagents and chemicals were of the highest grade commercially available. DFAIII (Figure 35.1B, DFAIII; di-D-fructofuranosyl 1, 2′: 2, 3′ dianhydride), a disaccharide comprising two fructose residues with two glycoside linkages, was provided by Fancl Co. (Yokohama, Japan).

35.2.2 Animals

Male Wistar/ST rats (6 weeks old; Japan Clea, Tokyo, Japan), weighing about 150 g, were housed in individual stainless-steel cages. The cages were placed in a room with controlled temperature (22°C–24°C), relative humidity (40%–60%), and lighting (lights on 09:00–21:00 h). The rats had free access to water and a flavonoid-free semipurified diet based on the AIN93G formulation for an acclimation period of 7 days. This study was approved by the Hokkaido University Animal Committee, and the animals were maintained in accordance with the Hokkaido University guideline for the care and use of laboratory animals.

35.2.3 Absorption by Ligated Jejunum and Ileum of Anesthetized Rats

Sixteen acclimated rats were divided into two groups and placed on a warm plate under ketamine-xylazine anesthesia after fasting for 18 h. Ligated 15 cm jejunal (at 3 cm distal from the ligament of Treitz) and an ileal (at 3 cm proximal to the ileocecal junction) segments were prepared through an abdominal midline incision (3–4 cm) in each rat. The ligated intestinal segment was washed out with warmed saline, and then 1.5 mL of G-Myr solution (100 mmol/mL as aglycone in sum of myricetin glycosides) was instilled with or without DFAIII 100 mmol/mL. To adjust osmotic pressure between the two groups, 50 mmol/mL NaCl was added to the DFAIII-free solution. Blood was collected from the mesenteric vein in the ligated jejunal and ileal segments and from the aorta using heparinized syringes at 60 min after instillation. The rats were killed by withdrawal of aortic blood, and both the jejunal and ileal segments were removed together with their contents and stored at −40°C until subsequent analyses. The luminal contents of the segments were collected together with the mucosa after thawing [19].

35.2.4 Sample Treatment for Measurement of Quercetin Derivatives

Plasma (100 μL) from the mesenteric and aortic blood was acidified (to pH 4.9) with 10 μL of acetic acid (0.58 mol/L) and treated with (total flavonoids) or without (nonconjugated flavonoids) 10 μL of Helix pomatia extract (Sigma G0876, 5, 106 U/L, β-glucuronidase and 2.5, 105 U/L sulfatase) for 30 min at 37°C. To extract myricetin derivatives, the reaction mixture was added to 100 μL of methanol, heated at 100°C for 1 min, and centrifuged (9000 × g, 5 min). This procedure was repeated three times. The combined supernatant was then applied to a C18 cartridge (Oasis HLB, Waters Co. Ltd., Milford, MA). After washing with 1 mL of water, the eluent with methanol was dried and dissolved in a 100 μL of 50% methanol (sample solution). The appropriately diluted solution of homogenized luminal contents including the mucosa (100 μL, Exp. 3) was treated in the same manner as the plasma. We confirmed that conjugates were not degraded by the extraction procedure.

35.2.5 Quantification of Myricetin Derivatives by Liquid Chromatography/Mass Spectrometry

Myricetin and its metabolites were identified and quantified using a liquid chromatography/mass spectrometry (LC/MS) system with an electric spray ionization (ESI) interface (Acquity UPLC, Waters Co. Ltd., Milford, MA). The capillary heater and the vaporization heater were maintained at 100°C and 300°C, respectively. The flow rate of the sheath gas (nitrogen) was 70 arb. The UPLC system was fitted with a 1.7 μm C18 column (ACQUITY UPLC BEH, 2.1 × 100 mm, Waters Co. Ltd.) set at 40°C. Solvents A (water:methanol:trifluoroacetic acid, 70:30:0.1) and B (methanol:trifluoroacetic acid, 100:0.1) were run at a flow rate of 0.2 mL/min using a linear gradient from 10% up to 20% solvent B for 20 min then returning to 10% solvent B for 5 min. The injection volume was 20 μL.

LC/ESI-MS was carried out in scan mode from (m/z) +50 to 2000 and in selected ion monitoring (SIM) mode at m/z: +319, +465, +627, +789, and +951 for myricetin, myricitrin, and mono-, di-, and triglucosylated myricitrin, respectively. We also identified m/z +545, +641, +707, and +803 as myricitrin sulfate, myricitrin glucuronide, monoglucosylated sulfate, and monoglucosylated glucuronide, respectively. Concentrations of myricetin, myricitrin, and mono-, di-, and triglucosylated myricitrin were calculated from the peak area of each mass spectrum and calibration curves of each standard compound. The concentrations of conjugated derivatives (sulfates and glucuronides) in the blood plasma were estimated as myricitrin or monoglucosylated myricitrin concentrations after enzymatic treatment.

35.2.6 Statistics

Statistical analyses were performed using STATCEL2 (OMS, Saitama, Japan). The differences between the means of the groups with and without DFAIII were determined by Student's t-test. Statistical analyses were also performed by two-way ANOVA for DFAIII treatment and intestinal segment (jejunum and ileum, Table 35.1). Differences were considered significant at $P < 0.05$.

35.3 Results

Figure 35.2 shows representative chromatograms of myricetin derivatives detected in the mesenteric blood before and after deconjugation by glucuronidase and sulfatase, as described in Section 35.2. In the sample before deconjugation (hydrolysis), we found only glucuronides and sulfides of myricitrin and monoglucosylated myricitrin and did not detect any peaks for nonconjugated forms of the myricitrin derivatives. After the enzyme treatment, all four peaks corresponding to the conjugated forms of myricitrin derivatives disappeared, and only two peaks were observed: those for myricitrin and monoglucosylated myricitrin. Unexpectedly, we did not detect a myricetin (aglycone) peak after deconjugation, or peaks for the conjugated and nonconjugated forms of myricetin before enzyme treatment. These results reveal that myricetin glycosides,

Table 35.1 Remaining Myricetin Glycosides in the Closed Segments of the Jejunum and Ileum 60 min after an Instillation of Glucosylated Myricetin Mixture (G-Myr)

	Remaining Glycosides		Rate of Absorption	
	Jejunum	Ileum	Jejunum	Ileum
	mol		%	
NaCl	143.9 ± 2.0^a	142.2 ± 1.2	4.1 ± 1.3^b	5.2 ± 0.8
DFAIII	136.0 ± 1.6^b	139.9 ± 1.6	9.3 ± 1.1^a	6.7 ± 1.1
Student's *t*-test *P*-values				
	0.012	0.280	0.012	0.286
Two-way ANOVA %-values				
Saccharide		0.005	0.005	
Intestine		0.497	0.505	
Saccharide × intestine		0.099	0.099	

The values are mean ± SEM.
[a,b] Significant differences between means of NaCl and DFAIII groups ($P < 0.05$).

Before hydrolysis of conjugates

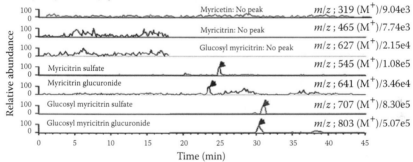

After hydrolysis of conjugates

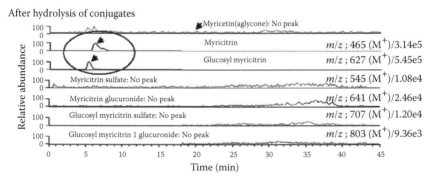

Figure 35.2 Representative LC/MS chromatograms of myricetin derivatives in the intestinal mesenteric blood before and after treatment by glucuronidase and sulfatase. Peaks appearing after hydrolysis corresponded to myricitrin and monoglucosyl myricitrin, and no peak for aglycone.

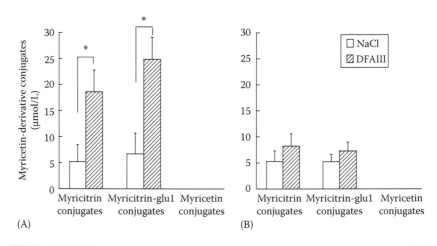

Figure 35.3 DFAIII markedly increased the release of myricetin glycoside into the mesenteric blood of the jejunum, but not of the ileum, 60 min after instillation of glucosyl myricitrins (G-Myr) into the jejunal and ileal segments. No myricetin conjugates or nonconjugated forms of myricetin derivatives were detected. Values are mean ± SEM (*n* = 6). Myricitrin-glu1: monoglucosyl myricitrin. (A) Jejunal mesenteric blood and (B) ileal mesenteric blood. * Shows significant differences between 2 groups (*P* < 0.05).

myricitrin, and   monoglucosylated myricitrin, but not aglycone, are absorbed into the mesenteric blood as conjugated forms of the glycosides.

The mesenteric blood concentrations of myricetin derivatives 60 min after administration of G-Myr solution with or without DFAIII into the jejunal and ileal lumen in the anesthetized rats are shown in Figure 35.3. As mentioned earlier, only conjugated forms of myricitrin and monoglucosylated myricitrin were detected, and these concentrations markedly higher in the jejunal mesenteric blood, but not in the ileal mesenteric blood, in the DFAIII group than in the control group. The values for the two myricetin derivatives in the ileal blood were very similar to those of the jejunal blood in the control group; however, these flavonoid concentrations were not enhanced in the ileal blood by coadministration of DFAIII. The sum of these myricetin glycoside conjugates in the jejunal mesenteric blood was 2.5-fold higher in the DFAIII group than in the control group (Figure 35.4). The levels of these conjugates were much lower in the aortic blood (inflow into the intestine) than in the mesenteric blood (outflow from the intestine) with or without DFAIII, which indicates that the conjugated flavonoids released into the mesenteric blood were produced in the intestinal mucosa.

The myricetin glycosides found to be remaining 60 min after instillation of the G-Myr solution in both the jejunal and ileal lumen consisted of myricitrin and monoglycosylated myricitrin, and sum of these glycosides was significantly lower in the jejunal loops, but not in the ileal loops, in the DFAIII group than in the control group (Table 35.1). Absorptive rates (%), which were calculated from the instilled and remaining amounts of myricetin glycosides in the intestinal loops, were doubled by coadministration with DFAIII in the G-Myr solution.

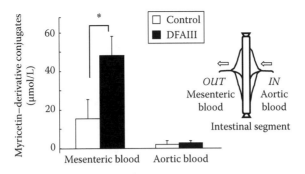

Figure 35.4 Sum of myricetin glycosides (conjugated forms) in the jejunal mesenteric and abdominal aortic blood 60 min after instillation of glucosyl myricitrins (G-Myr) into the jejunal segment. Values are mean ± SEM ($n = 6$). * Shows significant difference between 2 groups ($P < 0.05$).

35.4 Discussion

First, in this study, we found that myricitrin and glucosyl myricitrin, which are glycoside forms of myricitrin, are absorbed via transcellular pathway in the small intestinal epithelium. The second finding is that a nondigestible disaccharide, DFAIII, markedly enhanced jejunal absorption of these myricetin glycosides. Both are novel findings—that intestinal epithelial cells could take up flavonoids with one or two sugar moieties and that DFAIII could promote not only the paracellular transport, as our previous finding [15], but also the transcellular transport of flavonoids.

The DFAIII-mediated increase in myricetin glycosides absorption seen in situ closed intestinal loops is supported by the results regarding the remaining myricetin glycosides in the intestinal loops. Table 35.1 clearly shows that absorption rates for 60 min were doubled by addition of DFAIII to the osmotic pressure-adjusted intestinal fluid. The absorption intensity of myricetin glycoside shown by increased mesenteric blood concentration was only promoted in the jejunal loops and not in the ileal loops by the addition of DFAIII. The absorption intensities of the control fluid without DFAIII were comparable between the jejunum and ileum. The reason for the different response to DFAIII in the jejunum and ileum is still unknown. It is possible that the sensitivity to DFAIII is lower in the ileum than in the jejunum. However, the in vivo contribution of the ileum to flavonoid absorption may be higher than that of the jejunum because of the longer transit time. To clarify this, it is necessary to observe the effects of DFAIII on myricetin glycoside absorption in an in vivo study.

We provide evidence that myricetin glycosides are absorbed via transcellular transport through the intestinal epithelium because myricetin derivatives appearing in the mesenteric blood of the intestinal loops were all conjugated forms. The levels of these conjugated myricetin glycosides in the mesenteric were much higher than those in the aortic blood. These results clearly indicate that the conjugation of myricetin glycoside occurs in the intestine, not in the liver, and that the conjugation, via glucuronidation and sulfation, only takes place within the epithelial cells, not outside of the cells. Taken together, the aforementioned results indicate that myricitrin (myricetin rhamnoside) and glucosylated myricitrin are incorporated into the epithelial cells, where they are conjugated and then released as the only existing forms of myricetin derivatives into the mesenteric blood. DFAIII promotes some steps of these transcellular transport processes. The conjugation of quercetin glycosides has not been clarified, but it has been reported that anthocyanidine glycosides are absorbed as glycoside forms [20]. This is the first observation that a nondigestible saccharide enhances the transcellular transport of flavonoids in the small intestine.

As mentioned earlier, we have previously demonstrated that DFAIII enhances the absorption of a water-soluble quercetin glycoside via the paracellular transport pathway. The disaccharide has also been shown to increase calcium absorption via the paracellular pathway through the tight junction [21,22]. The present study provides evidence that myricetin glycosides are absorbed by transcellular transport, though there have been no previous observations of the promotion of transcellular transport by any nondigestible saccharides. We proposed possible mechanisms for this finding: first, that myricetin glycosides are taken up into the epithelial cells through a glucose transporter, GLUT2, which is known to interact with flavonoids [23] and also known to translocate to the apical membrane in the epithelial cells during the postprandial state [24], and second, that flavonoid glycosides are incorporated into the cells by endocytosis. There have been no previous reports that nondigestible saccharides influence

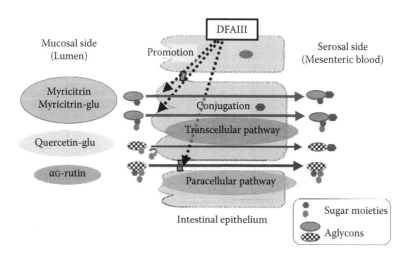

Figure 35.5 Myricitrin (myricetin rhamnoside) and monoglucosyl myricitrin (myricitrin-glu) are incorporated into the intestinal epithelial cells as glycosides, conjugated within the cells, and then released into the mesenteric blood as conjugated forms of myricetin glycosides. In contrast, quercetin glucoside (quercetin-glu) is incorporated into the epithelial cells after removal of a sugar moiety, conjugated, and released into the blood as conjugated forms of aglycone. Both absorption processes are enhanced by nondigestible disaccharide, DFAIII.

endocytosis process. However, we cannot rule out this possibility as many compounds, including minerals, are known to be incorporated into the intestinal cells by endocytosis [25–27].

In conclusion, we found that myricetin glycosides are absorbed by a different mechanism from that of quercetin glycosides and that DFAIII strongly promotes this process in the proximal small intestine. The increase in the bioavailability of myricitrin glycosides by this nondigestible saccharide may enhance many beneficial effects on health attributed to this flavonoid. We summarized the transport mechanisms for myricitrin glycoside and quercetin glycoside in Figure 35.5.

References

1. Bischoff, S.C., Quercetin: Potentials in the prevention and therapy of disease. *Curr. Opin. Clin. Nutr. Metab. Care*, 11, 733, 2008.
2. Hertog, M.G., Kromhout, D., Aravanis, C. et al., Flavonoid intake and long-term risk of coronary heart disease and cancer in the seven countries study. *Arch. Intern. Med.*, 155, 381, 1995.
3. Manach, C., Williamson, G., Morand, C. et al., Bioavailability and bioefficacy of polyphenols in humans. I. Review of 97 bioavailability studies. *Am. J. Clin. Nutr.*, 81, 230S, 2005.
4. Ong, K.C. and Khoo, H.E., Effects of myricetin on glycemia and glycogen metabolism in diabetic rats. *Life Sci.*, 67, 1695, 2000.
5. Liu, I.M., Tzeng, T.F., Liou, S.S. et al., Myricetin, a naturally occurring flavonol, ameliorates insulin resistance induced by a high-fructose diet in rats. *Life Sci.*, 81, 1479, 2007.
6. Kumamoto, T., Fujii, M., and Hou, D.X., Myricetin directly targets JAK1 to inhibit cell transformation. *Cancer Lett.*, 275, 17, 2009.
7. Kumamoto, T., Fujii, M., and Hou, D.X., Akt is a direct target for myricetin to inhibit cell transformation. *Mol. Cell Biochem.*, 332, 33, 2009.
8. Morand, C., Manach, C., Crespy, V. et al., Quercetin 3-O-beta-glucoside is better absorbed than other quercetin forms and is not present in rat plasma. *Free Radic. Res.*, 33, 667, 2000.
9. Hollman, P.C., Bijsman, M.N., van Gameren, Y. et al., The sugar moiety is a major determinant of the absorption of dietary flavonoid glycosides in man. *Free Radic. Res.*, 31, 569, 1999.
10. Hollman, P.C., van Trijp, J.M., Buysman, M.N. et al., Relative bioavailability of the antioxidant flavonoid quercetin from various foods in man. *FEBS Lett.*, 418, 152, 1997.
11. Day, A.J., Gee, J.M., DuPont, M.S. et al., Absorption of quercetin-3-glucoside and quercetin-4′-glucoside in the rat small intestine: The role of lactase phlorizin hydrolase and the sodium-dependent glucose transporter. *Biochem. Pharmacol.*, 65, 1199, 2003.
12. Sesink, A.L., Arts, I.C., Faassen-Peters, M. et al., Intestinal uptake of quercetin-3-glucoside in rats involves hydrolysis by lactase phlorizin hydrolase. *J. Nutr.*, 133, 773, 2003.
13. Wolffram, S., Block, M., and Ader, P., Quercetin-3-glucoside is transported by the glucose carrier SGLT1 across the brush border membrane of rat small intestine. *J. Nutr.*, 132, 630, 2002.
14. Yokomizo, A. and Moriwaki, M., Transepithelial permeability of myricitrin and its degradation by simulated digestion in human intestinal Caco-2 cell monolayer. *Biosci. Biotechnol. Biochem.*, 69, 1774, 2005.

15. Matsumoto, M., Matsukawa, N., Chiji, H. et al., Difructose anhydride III promotes absorption of the soluble flavonoid alphaG-rutin in rats. *J. Agric. Food Chem.*, 55, 4202, 2007.

16. Matsukawa, N., Matsumoto, M., Chiji, H. et al., Oligosaccharide promotes bioavailability of a water-soluble flavonoid glycoside, alpha G-rutin, in rats. *J. Agric. Food Chem.*, 57, 1498, 2009.

17. Matsukawa, N., Matsumoto, M., Shinoki, A. et al., Nondigestible saccharides suppress the bacterial degradation of quercetin aglycone in the large intestine and enhance the bioavailability of quercetin glucoside in rats. *J. Agric. Food Chem.*, 57, 9462, 2009.

18. Matsumoto, M., Chiji, H., and Hara, H., Intestinal absorption and metabolism of a soluble flavonoid, alphaG-rutin, in portal cannulated rats. *Free Radic. Res.*, 39, 1139, 2005.

19. Kasai, T., Tanaka, T., Kiriyama, S. et al., Facile preparation of rat intestinal mucosa for assay of mucosal enzyme activity. *J. Nutr. Sci. Vitaminol. (Tokyo)*, 39, 399, 1993.

20. Matsumoto, H., Inaba, H., Kishi, M. et al., Orally administered delphinidin 3-rutinoside and cyanidin 3-rutinoside are directly absorbed in rats and humans and appear in the blood as the intact forms. *J. Agric. Food Chem.*, 49, 1546, 2001.

21. Mineo, H., Hara, H., Shigematsu, N. et al., Melibiose, difructose anhydride III and difructose anhydride IV enhance net calcium absorption in rat small and large intestinal epithelium by increasing the passage of tight junctions in vitro. *J. Nutr.*, 132, 3394, 2002.

22. Suzuki, T. and Hara, H., Various nondigestible saccharides open a paracellular calcium transport pathway with the induction of intracellular calcium signaling in human intestinal Caco-2 cells. *J. Nutr.*, 134, 1935, 2004.

23. Kwon, O., Eck, P., Chen, S. et al., Inhibition of the intestinal glucose transporter GLUT2 by flavonoids. *FASB J.*, 21, 366, 2007.

24. Kellett, G.L., Brot-Laroche, E., Mace, O.J. et al., Sugar absorption in the intestine: The role of GLUT2. *Annu. Rev. Nutr.*, 28, 35, 2008.

25. Nemere, I. and Norman, A.W., 1,25-Dihydroxyvitamin D3-mediated vesicular transport of calcium in intestine: Time-course studies. *Endocrinology*, 122, 2962, 1988.

26. Gnoth, M.J., Rudloff, S., Kunz, C. et al., Investigations of the in vitro transport of human milk oligosaccharides by a Caco-2 monolayer using a novel high performance liquid chromatography-mass spectrometry technique. *J. Biol. Chem.*, 276, 34363, 2001.

27. Moriya, M. and Linder, M.C., Vesicular transport and apotransferrin in intestinal iron absorption, as shown in the Caco-2 cell model. *Am. J. Physiol. Gastrointest. Liver Physiol.*, 290, G301, 2006.

36

Efficacy and Safety of Xylooligosaccharides

ALICE FU, ALBERT W. LEE, STEPHANIE NISHI,
IRIS L. CASE, and SUSAN S. CHO

Contents

36.1 Introduction

Xylooligosaccharide (XOS) is a nondigestible oligosaccharide (NDO) composed of two to seven xylose molecules bonded with β (1–4) glycosidic bonds. Molecular formula of XOS is $C5^{n}H^{8n+2} O^{4n+1}$, where n = 2–7. XOS is naturally present in fruits, vegetables, bamboo, honey, and milk. It can be produced on an industrial scale by enzymatic hydrolysis of xylan-rich food ingredients, such as corncob or wheat bran. Xylan is the major component of plant hemicelluloses that are composed of xylose and arabinose backbones with side chains of galactose, glucose, and/or mannose (Southgate, 1979).

    XOS has a sweet taste and is stable in acidic conditions (Courtin et al., 2009). Thus, it is used as an alternative sweetener in variety of foods, including juice-based beverages and dairy foods. It functions as a prebiotic by stimulating the growth of healthy microflora, such as bifidobacteria, in the gut (FAO, 2007; Grootaert et al., 2007; Kabel et al., 2002; Moure et al., 2006; Vázquez et al., 2000). NOs are completely or partially fermented in the large intestine. XSO has acceptable organoleptic properties and does not exhibit toxicity or negative effects on human health (Vázquez et al., 2000).

Most of XOS is made from corncob, which contains approximately 35% xylan (Aachary and Prapulla, 2009; Moure et al., 2006; Oliveira et al., 2010) and is an important by-product of the corn industry. Corncob is used to produce XOS, xylose, and xylitol (Aachary and Prapulla, 2009). A partial hydrolysis of xylan (polysaccharides) results in XOS, while a complete hydrolysis produces xylose, a monosaccharide.

D-xylose (monosaccharide) is a hydrolysis product of XOS and xylan that is found as a component of the polysaccharide xylan in fruit juices, such as those from apples and peaches (Hardinge et al., 1965).

XOS is stable after heating to 100°C under acid conditions (pH = 2.5–8), which covers the pH value of the vast majority of food systems (Courtin et al., 2009; Vázquez et al., 2000). In food processing, XOS shows advantages over inulin in terms of resistance to both acids and heat, allowing their utilization in low-pH juices and carbonated drinks (Vázquez et al., 2000).

XOS is produced from xylan-rich corncob by chemical methods, autohydrolysis, direct enzymatic hydrolysis of a susceptible substrate, or a combination of chemical and enzymatic treatments (Vázquez et al., 2000). However, enzymatic production of XOS is preferred in the food industry (Ai et al., 2005; Jiang et al., 2005, 2006).

36.2 Regulatory Status of XOS

FDA has no questions on the NDI notice of XOS and the GRAS notice of a mixture of XOS and AXOS derived from wheat bran (GRN 343; wheat bran extract composed of primarily xylo- and arabinoxylooligosaccharides). The 2007 FAO Technical Meeting Report on Prebiotics classified XOS as a prebiotic, defined as a food component that confers a health benefit on the host associated with modulation of the microbiota (FAO, 2007). XOS is commercially used as a food ingredient in Japan. The FOSHU (Food for Specified Health Use) has been used in Japan since 1991 (Vázquez et al., 2000). FOSHU foods are expected to have a specific effect on health due to the relevant constituent(s) of the foods.

Other NDOs, such as FOS (FDA, GRN 44), GOS (FDA, GRN 236, 285, and 286), and IMO (FDA, GRN 246), already are listed as GRAS substances. Also, xylose and xylitol (xylose-based sugar alcohol) are listed as GRAS substances and are included in the *"Everything" Added to Food in the United States* (EAFUS) list. The EAFUS list of substances contains ingredients added directly to food that FDA has either approved as food additives or listed or affirmed as GRAS. Many dietary fiber ingredients containing xylose backbones (i.e., xylans or arabinoxylans), such as psyllium, corn bran, rice bran, and wheat bran, are considered as GRAS ingredients by the U.S. FDA (21 CFR, Part 184.1890, 182.8890, and 182.8892) when used in accordance with good manufacturing practice. FDA has approved a health claim for psyllium fiber and heart disease risk reduction.

In addition, XOS is a component of dietary fiber that is considered as an essential nutrient low in the American diet. The Institute of Medicine (IOM, 2002) has recommended increased consumption of dietary fiber for Americans of all ages.

In Japan, D-xylose is widely used as a natural food additive in the fishery products and baking industries (JETRO, 2010; MHLW, 1996a,b).

36.3 Metabolic Fate and Health Benefits of XOS

Like other NDOs, including FOS and GOS, XOS is fermented to short-chain fatty acids (SCFA) in the lower gastrointestinal tract (Alles et al., 1996, 1999; Campbell et al., 1997; Fleming et al., 1983; Fleming and Lee, 1983; Fleming and Rodriguez, 1983) and promotes the growth of bifidobacteria (Bouhnik et al., 1997, 2004; Crittenden et al., 2002; Fujikawa et al., 1991; van Loo et al., 1999; Moura et al., 2008; Park et al., 1992; Ryu et al., 2002; Van Laere et al., 2000; Yazawa et al., 1978). The 2007 FAO Technical Meeting Report on Prebiotics classified XOS, FOS, GOS, soya oligosaccharides, and isomaltooligosaccharides (IMO) as prebiotics. These are defined as food components that confer a health benefit on the host via modulation of the microbiota (FAO, 2007).

Clinical trials report advantages of XOS with no adverse effects. Research shows that in healthy men and elderly subjects, XOS is strongly bifidogenic (Chung et al., 1973; Kajihara et al., 2000; Na and Kim, 2007; Okazaki et al., 1990). The lowest dose for XOS prebiotic efficacy was 1.4 g/day (Na and Kim, 2007). Like other fiber ingredients, XOS maintains fecal water content within the normal range and relieves constipation as well as diarrhea without side effects. No adverse effects have been reported at intakes of 0.4–10 g/day (Chung et al., 1973; Iino et al., 1997; Kobayashi et al., 1991; Okazaki et al., 1990).

36.4 Human Tolerance Test (Kobayashi et al., 1991)

Ten male volunteers aged 30–60 years consumed XOS at the dose of 2, 5, or 10 g/day for 5 days. Diarrhea is defined as a ratio of six score or watery defecation. The incidence of diarrhea was 7.7% before XOS intake and was reduced to 2.1%, 5.0%, or 6.7% after consumption of 2, 5, or 10 g XOS for 5 days. However, on day 1, increased incidence of diarrhea (18%) was associated with consumption of XOS. However, this symptom was transient: The incidence of diarrhea started to decrease, and the average diarrhea incidence during the 5 days was reduced to 6.7% from initial 8%. The frequency of fecal evacuation was 1.4 times/day before intake, 1.1 times/day after 2 g XOS intake ($p < 0.05$), 1.2 times/day after 5 g XOS intake, and 1.3 times/day after 10 g XOS intake. In this trial, the maximum frequency of defecation was 4 times/day. The hardness of stool before XOS intake was 4.1 points; the feces was slightly soft. After the intake of 2, 5, or 10 g, the scores were decreased to 3.4 ($p < 0.01$), 3.7 ($p < 0.05$), or 3.9 points, respectively. These scores were close to the normal score (three points). The results indicate that the best fecal state was observed at the dose of 2 g XOS. With the intake of 10 g, the fecal characteristics were close to those found during the no-intake period, and stools tended to be soft.

36.5 Preclinical Safety Studies of XOS

Published studies indicate that XOS is of low toxicity to animals. The acute toxicity of XOS has been reported to be 10 g/kg BW in the rat (Park et al., 1999) and >20 g/kg BW in mice (Gao et al., 2012). Table 36.1 summarizes the toxicity studies on XOS. A subacute toxicity of XOS in young rats demonstrated that the NOAEL of XOS was 3000 mg/kg BW (Park et al., 2000) and 4% in the diet in chicks (Graham et al., 2004). Gao et al. (2012) confirmed the previous findings; NOAEL was found to be 8000 mg/kg BW. Other animal studies measuring various endpoints reported no adverse effects of XOS (Gobinath et al., 2010; Howard et al., 1995; Hsu et al., 2004). In addition, various studies showed no mutagenic, teratogenic, or genotoxic effects of XOS (Oh et al., 1999). Related compounds such as xylose, xylan, and fibers containing a xylose backbone were found to be safe (Fleming and Lee, 1983; Imazawa et al., 1999; Kuroiwa et al., 2005).

Table 36.1 Acute, Subacute, and Subchronic Toxicity Studies of XOS

Species	Length of the Study	Measurement Endpoints	Results	Reference
Rat	Single dose, observed 14 days	Acute toxicity	LD_{50} = 10 g/kg BW	Park et al. (1999)
Mouse	Single dose, observed 14 days	Acute toxicity	LD_{50} >20 g/kg BW	Gao et al. (2012)
Dog	Single dose, observed 14 days	Acute toxicity	LD_{50} >14 g/kg BW	Gao et al. (2012)
Rat	13 weeks	Subacute toxicity	NOAEL—3000 mg/kg BW/day; the highest dose administered	Park et al. (2000)
Rat	30 days	Subacute toxicity	NOAEL—4000 mg/kg BW/day; the highest dose administered	Gao et al. (2012)
Chick	21 days	Subacute toxicity	4% in the diet in chicks; the highest dose administered	Graham et al. (2004)
Dog	6 months	Subchronic toxicity	NOAEL—4000 mg/kg BW/day; the highest dose administered	Gao et al. (2012)

36.5.1 Acute Toxicity Test in Rats and Mice (Park et al., 1999)

Park et al. (1999) demonstrated that XOS had no toxic effects in Sprague Dawley® (SD) rats and that the LD_{50} value of XOS was above 10 g/kg BW. In another study by Park et al. (2000), 20 mice (10 males and 10 females) weighing 18–22 g were infused with 20 g/kg BW of XOS twice daily and observed for 14 days. The researchers found no obvious toxicity in any mice, and no animals died at 14 days (Table 36.1). Thus, the LD_{50} value of XOS in both male and female mice exceeded 20 g/kg BW.

36.5.2 Acute Toxicity in Beagle Dogs (Gao et al., 2012)

Four beagle dogs weighing 7.9–8.2 kg were infused with XOS at the dosage of 4, 6, 9, and 14 g/kg BW (single dose; 1 animal/group) and were observed at 14 days. There were no obvious toxicity symptoms and no death of animals at 14 days (Table 36.1). The only side effects noted in the high-dose groups (6, 9, or 14 g/kg BW) were vomiting and diarrhea, which disappear in 48 h. Thus, it was concluded that the LD_{50} value of XOS in both male and female mice was greater than 14 g/kg BW.

36.5.3 Subacute Toxicity in Rats (Tables 36.2 through 36.8; Park et al., 2000)

Park et al. (2000) evaluated subacute toxicity of XOS in SD rats. Groups of 60 male and 60 female rats were orally administered 0, 333, 1000, or 3000 mg/kg for 13 weeks. Administration of XOS did not influence body weight gain and feed consumption (Tables 36.2 and 36.3). No deaths or toxic effects were observed during the test periods. Statistically significant changes were seen in several criteria, but these had no direct relationship to dosage. Gross necropsy and histopathology found no XOS in target organs of treated mice. No XOS-related changes in BW were noted during the treatment period. Except for transient changes noted on day 1 in males, daily food intake in the XOS-treated groups did not differ significantly from that of the controls. The NOAEL of XOS was estimated at over 3000 mg/kg.

36.5.3.1 Hematological Values (Tables 36.4 through 36.6) Hematological values and histopathological findings were investigated at the end of 13 and 17 weeks. No XOS-related changes in hematological values (white blood cell [WBC], red blood cell [RBC], hematocrit [HCT], mean corpuscular hemoglobin ([MCH], mean corpuscular hemoglobin concentration [MCHC], and lymphocyte values) were noted during the treatment period. A significant decrease in MCH values (19.8 ± 0.5 vs. 19.2 ± 0.4 pg; $p < 0.05$) was observed in males in the 3000 mg/kg group at 4 weeks of recovery compared with controls. However, all hematological values were within physiologically normal ranges.

36.5.3.2 Serum Biochemistry (Tables 36.7 and 36.8) Serum analysis showed no XOS-related changes in concentrations of aspartate aminotransferase (AST or SGOT), alanine aminotransferase (ALT or SGPT), alkaline phosphatase (ALP), blood urea nitrogen (BUN), creatine (CREA), glucose, total cholesterol (T-C), total

Table 36.2 Subacute Toxicity of XOS in Rats: Body Weights (g) in Male and Female Rats Treated Orally with XOS

Gender	Male				Female			
Dose, mg/kg	0	333	1000	3000	0	333	1000	3000
0 day	132.7 ± 9.2	133.2 ± 9.2	135.4 ± 10.1	134.5 ± 8.8	110.7 ± 6.4	112.1 ± 8.1	111.4 ± 7.0	111.6 ± 7.0
28 days	353.2 ± 29.2	355.3 ± 21.9	350.4 ± 17.9	351.0 ± 22.0	217.1 ± 18.7	211.7 ± 18.4	211.9 ± 17.4	215.6 ± 17.3
56 days	456.8 ± 44.2	453.2 ± 29.3	460.1 ± 30.8	451.0 ± 29.3	262.0 ± 19.3	252.7 ± 26.5	253.1 ± 19.8	257.6 ± 22.4
89 days	511.9 ± 49.7	502.6 ± 36.8	508.3 ± 46.1	510.1 ± 35.3	287.5 ± 22.8	277.1 ± 26.6	276.6 ± 17.3	279.6 ± 21.0
118 days	531.3 ± 56.4	NM	NM	550.7 ± 52.3	292.4 ± 9.6	NM	NM	294.7 ± 16.9

Source: Park, Y.J. et al., *J. Food Hyg. Saf.*, 15, 151, 2000.
NM = not measured.

Table 36.3 Subacute Toxicity of XOS in Rats: Food Consumption by Male and Female Rats Treated Orally with XOS

Gender	Male				Female			
Dose, mg/kg	0	333	1000	3000	0	333	1000	3000
1 day	26.0 ± 1.0	25.1 ± 0.8	24.6 ± 1.2[a]	24.7 ± 1.0[a]	19.8 ± 2.3	19.6 ± 1.5	21.6 ± 1.9	20.0 ± 1.6
29 days	34.1 ± 3.3	33.1 ± 2.8	31.5 ± 1.1	32.9 ± 2.0	22.6 ± 2.6	21.0 ± 2.4	22.4 ± 1.6	21.5 ± 2.0
57 days	32.1 ± 3.3	32.0 ± 1.9	31.9 ± 1.5	31.0 ± 2.2	22.3 ± 1.7	21.3 ± 1.5	22.7 ± 0.8	22.2 ± 1.9
90 days	31.9 ± 2.6	32.5 ± 2.6	31.9 ± 2.8	30.7 ± 3.1	21.6 ± 2.3	20.5 ± 1.5	20.5 ± 5.5	18.6 ± 3.2
119 days	30.8 ± 2.4	NM	NM	31.9 ± 1.9	20.9 ± 1.4	NM	NM	20.7 ± 1.7

Source: Park, Y.J. et al., *J. Food Hyg. Saf.*, 15, 151, 2000.

NM = not measured.

[a] Significantly different from control ($p < 0.01$).

Table 36.4 Subacute Toxicity of XOS in Rats: Hematological Values in Male Rats Treated Orally with XOS at 13 Weeks

	Dose, mg/kg			
Item	0	333	1000	3000
WBC, 10^3/μL	13.73 ± 2.8	11.56 ± 4.2	13.31 ± 4.4	12.31 ± 2.6
RBC, 10^6/μL	8.22 ± 0.3	8.33 ± 0.3	8.25 ± 0.5	8.22 ± 0.3
HGB, 10^3/μL	15.6 ± 0.4	15.8 ± 0.3	15.5 ± 0.7	15.6 ± 0.6
HCT, %	45.2 ± 1.5	45.7 ± 1.4	45.2 ± 2.0	45.3 ± 1.8
MCV, fl	55.0 ± 1.5	54.9 ± 1.1	54.9 ± 1.9	55.0 ± 1.3
MCH, pg	18.9 ± 0.7	18.9 ± 0.4	18.8 ± 0.7	19.0 ± 0.4
MCHC, g/μL	34.4 ± 0.5	34.5 ± 0.4	34.3 ± 0.4	34.5 ± 0.4
PLT, 10^3/μL	1034 ± 84.0	959 ± 55.4	1004 ± 100.1	1014 ± 55.2
Neutrophil, 10^3/μL	1.73 ± 0.8	1.46 ± 0.6	2.35 ± 1.9	1.44 ± 0.6
Eosinophil, 10^3/μL	0.11 ± 0.11	0.13 ± 0.1	0.1 ± 0.1	0.09 ± 0.1
Basophil, 10^3/μL	0.0 ± 0.0	0.0 ± 0.0	0.0 ± 0.0	0.0 ± 0.0
Lymphocyte, 10^3/μL	11.85 ± 2.9	9.94 ± 4.0	10.84 ± 4.2	10.74 ± 2.6
Monocyte, 10^3/μL	0.05 ± 0.1	0.03 ± 0.1	0.03 ± 0.1	0.04 ± 0.1

Source: Park, Y.J. et al., *J. Food Hyg. Saf.*, 15, 151, 2000.
HGB, hemoglobin; MCV, mean corpuscular volume; PLT, platelets.
The values in various treatment groups are not significantly different.

Table 36.5 Subacute Toxicity of XOS in Rats: Hematological Values in Female Rats Treated Orally with XOS at 13 Weeks

	Dose, mg/kg			
Item	0	333	1000	3000
WBC, 10^3/μL	7.71 ± 2.4	7.76 ± 3.0	6.52 ± 1.7	6.5 ± 1.3
RBC, 10^6/μL	7.38 ± 0.6	7.61 ± 0.4	7.81 ± 0.3	7.59 ± 0.3
HGB, 10^3/μL	14.6 ± 1.1	14.6 ± 0.6	15.1 ± 0.5	15.1 ± 0.5
HCT, %	42.5 ± 2.9	42.7 ± 2.0	44.3 ± 1.8	43.6 ± 1.5
MCV, fl	57.6 ± 1.8	56.1 ± 1.0	56.8 ± 1.4	57.5 ± 1.5
MCH, pg	19.8 ± 0.5	19.2 ± 0.4	19.4 ± 0.5	19.8 ± 0.5
MCHC, g/μL	34.3 ± 0.5	34.2 ± 0.3	34.2 ± 0.4	34.5 ± 0.2
PLT, 10^3/μL	9641 ± 84.4	9461 ± 15.3	942 ± 71.3	930 ± 79.7
Neutrophil, 10^3/μL	0.98 ± 0.4	1.15 ± 0.6	0.66 ± 0.3	0.75 ± 0.2
Eosinophil, 10^3/μL	0.04 ± 0.1	0.06 ± 0.1	0.05 ± 0.1	0.04 ± 0.1
Basophil, 10^3/μL	0.0 ± 0.0	0.0 ± 0.0	0.0 ± 0.0	0.0 ± 0.0
Lymphocyte, 10^3/μL	6.67 ± 2.2	6.55 ± 2.5	5.81 ± 1.8	5.69 ± 1.3
Monocyte, 10^3/μL	0.01 ± 0.0	0.01 ± 0.0	0.0 ± 0.0	0.01 ± 0.0

Source: Park, Y.J. et al., *J. Food Hyg. Saf.*, 15, 151, 2000.
HGB, hemoglobin; MCV, mean corpuscular volume; PLT, platelets.

Table 36.6 Subacute Toxicity of XOS in Rats: Hematological Values in Male and Female Rats Treated Orally with XOS at 4 Weeks of Recovery

	Dose, mg/kg			
	Males		Females	
Item	0	3000	0	3000
WBC, $10^3/\mu L$	12.27 ± 2.7	9.22 ± 2.4^a	7.6 ± 1.4	8.11 ± 2.3
RBC, $10^6/\mu L$	8.45 ± 0.4	8.01 ± 0.3^a	7.74 ± 0.3	7.84 ± 0.3
HGB, $10^3/\mu L$	15.4 ± 0.7	14.9 ± 0.7	15.1 ± 0.6	15.4 ± 0.5
HCT, %	45.5 ± 2.0	43.6 ± 1.7^a	44.0 ± 1.6	44.8 ± 1.2
MCV, fl	53.9 ± 1.2	54.5 ± 1.4	56.9 ± 1.5	57.2 ± 0.6
MCH, pg	18.2 ± 0.5	18.6 ± 0.6	19.5 ± 0.6	19.6 ± 0.4
MCHC, $g/\mu L$	33.8 ± 0.2	34.2 ± 0.4^b	34.2 ± 0.3	34.4 ± 0.4
PLT, $10^3/\mu L$	984 ± 65.6	1028 ± 87.5	893 ± 71.4	913 ± 68.6
Neutrophil, $10^3/\mu L$	1.64 ± 1.1	1.19 ± 0.4	0.77 ± 0.5	0.75 ± 0.3
Eosinophil, $10^3/\mu L$	0.14 ± 0.1	0.1 ± 0.1	0.09 ± 0.1	0.10 ± 0.1
Basophil, $10^3/\mu L$	0.0 ± 0.0	0.0 ± 0.0	0.0 ± 0.0	0.0 ± 0.0
Lymphocyte, $10^3/\mu L$	10.49 ± 2.7	7.92 ± 2.6^a	6.7 ± 1.4	7.27 ± 2.2
Monocyte, $10^3/\mu L$	0.0	0.01 ± 0.0	0.0 ± 0.0	0.0 ± 0.0

Source: Park, Y.J. et al., *J. Food Hyg. Saf.*, 15, 151, 2000.

HGB, hemoglobin; MCV, mean corpuscular volume; PLT, platelets.

[a] Significantly different from control ($p < 0.05$).

[b] Significantly different from control ($p < 0.01$).

bilirubin (T-BIL), total protein (TP), albumin (ALB), the ratio of ALB to globulin (A/G ratio), creatine phosphokinase (CPK), triglyceride (TG), calcium (Ca), inorganic phosphorus (IP), Na, K, and Cl. The only exception was an increased phospholipid (PL-E) concentration (148.6 ± 28.1 vs. 123.8 ± 3.2 mg/dL; $p < 0.05$) in the 1000 mg/kg males at 13 weeks. However, the effect was not treatment related.

36.5.3.3 Gross and Histopathological Findings in Male and Female Rats Treated Orally with XOS (Tables 36.9 through 36.11)   Oral treatment with XOS in male and female rats has produced no abnormalities in the brain, hypophysis, adrenal gland, liver, spleen, kidney, heart, testis, ovary, prostate/uterus, lung, thymus, thyroid gland, salivary gland, urinary bladder, seminal vesicle, epididymis, preputial gland, pancreas, skin, stomach, duodenum, jejunum, ileum, cecum, colon, rectum, artery, cervical spinal cord, lumbar spinal cord, tongue, trachea, esophagus, sciatic nerve, muscle, femur, sternum, eyes, harderian gland, mesenteric lymph node, submandibular lymph node, or abdominal cavity.

36.5.3.4 Urine Analysis   Urine analysis showed no XOS-related changes in concentrations of glucose, bilirubin, ketone, protein, urobilinogen, nitrite, or specific gravity, pH, occult blood, or color during the treatment period.

Table 36.7 Subacute Toxicity of XOS in Rats: Serum Metabolite Concentrations in Male and Female Rats Treated Orally with XOS[a] at 16 Weeks

| | Dose, mg/kg | | | | | | | |
| | Male | | | | Female | | | |
Item	0	333	1000	3000	0	333	1000	3000
AST, IU/L	120.7 ± 28.3	110.7 ± 24.4	120.1 ± 38.0	113.0 ± 22.6	125.5 ± 17.3	117.2 ± 29.1	100.6 ± 21.7	100.0 ± 17.7
ALT, IU/L	42.0 ± 6.5	47.2 ± 6.7	45.0 ± 7.5	48.0 ± 7.5	39.8 ± 9.6	41.6 ± 17.1	29.8 ± 2.8	32.6 ± 7.0
ALP, IU/L	173.5 ± 35.1	195.8 ± 13.6	169.8 ± 29.1	185.8 ± 41.1	82.6 ± 18.1	96.1 ± 19.7	87.4 ± 20.4	107.2 ± 26.5
BUN, mg/dL	15.1 ± 0.9	16.2 ± 1.7	15.4 ± 2.5	15.4 ± 1.7	17.8 ± 3.0	18.2 ± 3.7	16.2 ± 2.9	17.2 ± 2.1
CREA, mg/dL	0.51 ± 0.1	0.55 ± 0.1	0.50 ± 0.1	0.48 ± 0.1	0.53 ± 0.1	0.50 ± 0.1	0.5 ± 0.1	0.54 ± 0.1
GLU, mg/dL	122.2 ± 12.8	129.6 ± 13.8	124.8 ± 18.4	141.1 ± 24.8	117.6 ± 12.9	110.5 ± 14.6	113.4 ± 20.5	118.0 ± 6.7
T-C, mg/dL	94.3 ± 23.5	94.3 ± 16.3	78.1 ± 14.1	88.0 ± 16.7	89.2 ± 10.5	78.7 ± 18.4	71.0 ± 16.0	81.1 ± 11.1
T-BIL, mg/dL	0.10 ± 0.0	0.09 ± 0.0	0.09 ± 0.0	0.09 ± 0.0	0.11 ± 0.0	0.1 ± 0.4	0.11 ± 0.0	0.12 ± 0.0
TP, g/dL	6.27 ± 0.3	6.43 ± 0.3	6.12 ± 0.6	6.39 ± 0.3	6.29 ± 0.5	6.10 ± 0.4	5.84 ± 0.7	6.12 ± 0.3
ALB, g/dL	4.34 ± 0.2	4.42 ± 0.2	4.24 ± 0.3	4.44 ± 0.1	4.65 ± 0.3	4.54 ± 0.3	4.44 ± 0.5	4.56 ± 0.1
A/G ratio	2.26 ± 0.2	2.22 ± 0.2	2.33 ± 0.4	2.32 ± 0.3	2.96 ± 0.6	2.97 ± 0.5	3.27 ± 0.5	2.95 ± 0.3
CPK, IU/L	334.8 ± 170.8	240.4 ± 134.4	301.1 ± 197.8	245.7 ± 92.6	340.4 ± 106.0	262.0 ± 110.6	237.9 ± 103.4	222.7 ± 88.6
TG, mg/dL	115.8 ± 48.1	100.4 ± 19.6	82.6 ± 25.0	100.0 ± 34.5	54.9 ± 20.8	47.2 ± 27.8	44.5 ± 27.7	52.0 ± 14.9
CA, mg/dL	10.18 ± 0.5	10.33 ± 0.4	10.21 ± 1.1	10.54 ± 0.5	10.33 ± 0.8	10.11 ± 0.7	9.72 ± 1.5	10.38 ± 0.7
IP, mg/dL	7.14 ± 0.8	7.08 ± 0.8	7.14 ± 1.1	7.36 ± 1.0	6.42 ± 1.3	6.5 ± 1.1	6.31 ± 1.4	6.42 ± 1.6
PL-E, mg/dL	148.6 ± 28.1	145.8 ± 19.5	123.8 ± 13.2[a]	139.4 ± 16.2	174.7 ± 13.1	156.4 ± 32.1	145.0 ± 27.5	163.2 ± 16.4
Na, mmol/L	144.4 ± 0.8	144.4 ± 1.2	143.8 ± 2.8	143.1 ± 2.1	148.1 ± 10.5	144.2 ± 2.2	147.6 ± 7.5	143.6 ± 4.8
K, mmol/L	4.95 ± 0.3	4.79 ± 0.3	5.49 ± 1.21	5.49 ± 1.2	5.03 ± 0.7	4.67 ± 0.3	5.23 ± 1.1	4.51 ± 0.5
Cl, mmol/L	107.6 ± 0.8	108.0 ± 1.2	108.1 ± 2.4	107.0 ± 2.3	112.3 ± 9.8	109.8 ± 3.29	112.2 ± 6.2	108.7 ± 4.7

Source: Park, Y.J. et al., *J. Food Hyg. Saf.*, 15, 151, 2000.

[a] Significantly different from control ($p < 0.05$).

Table 36.8 Subacute Toxicity of XOS in Rats: Serum Metabolite Concentrations in Male and Female Rats Treated Orally with XOS at 4 Weeks of Recovery

	Dose, mg/kg			
	Male		Female	
Item	0	3000	0	3000
AST, IU/L	116.9 ± 19.5	129.3 ± 30.5	122.9 ± 37.3	126.2 ± 21.8
ALT, IU/L	47.9 ± 7.7	48.5 ± 6.6	35.5 ± 5.3	39.8 ± 12.3
ALP, IU/L	170.2 ± 35.3	159.1 ± 17.5	74.4 ± 16.0	80.7 ± 18.1
BUN, mg/dL	16.2 ± 1.5	17.6 ± 2.0	21.0 ± 3.5	20.2 ± 2.5
CREA, mg/dL	0.60 ± 0.1	0.56 ± 0.1	0.68 ± 0.0	0.66 ± 0.1
GLU, mg/dL	127.4 ± 10.8	134.6 ± 11.5	150.2 ± 26.9	138.4 ± 19.3
T-CHO, mg/dL	88.2 ± 13.2	95.5 ± 13.9	98.2 ± 15.0	89.3 ± 19.1
T-BIL, mg/dL	0.10 ± 0.0	0.1 ± 0.0	0.12 ± 0.0	0.12 ± 0.0
TP, g/dL	6.37 ± 0.3	6.34 ± 0.4	6.81 ± 0.3	6.63 ± 0.5
ALB, g/dL	4.25 ± 0.1	4.19 ± 0.2	4.80 ± 0.2	4.76 ± 0.3
A/G ratio	2.03 ± 0.2	1.96 ± 0.2	2.40 ± 0.2	2.56 ± 0.2
CPK, IU/L	267.4 ± 138.2	340.8 ± 172.1	309.5 ± 176.5	313.1 ± 133.7
TG, mg/dL	96.53 ± 0.4	125.1 ± 49.3	53.6 ± 24.6	52.0 ± 21.3
CA, mg/dL	10.60 ± 0.3	10.63 ± 0.4	11.24 ± 0.5	11.37 ± 0.8
IP, mg/dL	6.78 ± 0.7	6.60 ± 0.6	6.97 ± 0.9	7.31 ± 1.1
PL-E, mg/dL	133.3 ± 15.5	143.2 ± 21.1	180.8 ± 23.3	167.3 ± 25.2
Na, mmol/L	143.6 ± 2.6	144.0 ± 1.4	143.8 ± 1.3	144.1 ± 2.0
K, mmol/L	5.44 ± 1.6	5.42 ± 1.1	4.84 ± 0.9	5.27 ± 1.0
Cl, mmol/L	107.2 ± 1.6	107.5 ± 1.9	106.6 ± 1.5	106.9 ± 1.1

Source: Park, Y.J. et al., *J. Food Hyg. Saf.*, 15, 151, 2000.
HGB, hemoglobin; MCV, mean corpuscular volume; PLT, platelets.
The values in various treatment groups are not significantly different.

36.5.4 Subacute Toxicity Study in Chicks (Table 36.1; Graham et al., 2004)

Day-old chicks were fed diets with 0, 0.4, 4,000, or 40,000 mg/kg XOS to 21 days (18 chicks/diet). XOS did not influence growth, liver weight, gut length, or ileal digesta dry matter. However, XOS decreased ileal lactic acid concentration and increased cecal butyric acid and SCFA. XOS was rapidly fermented in the ceca and elevated plasma xylose levels. It decreased overall cecal bacterial numbers but had little influence on the overall bacterial community profile. No adverse effects were noted in any test group. The NOAEL was 4% of the diet.

36.5.5 30 Day Feeding Study in Rats (Table 36.1; Gao et al., 2012)

This study supported the NOAEL of 4000 mg/kg BW/day in rats. Eighty weaning rats, weighing 50–60 g, were randomly assigned to four groups: control, 1000,

Table 36.9 Subacute Toxicity of XOS in Rats: Absolute and Relative Organ Weights in Male Rats Treated Orally with XOS at 13 Weeks

Dose, mg/kg	0	333	1000	3000
Brain, g	2.076 ± 0.066	2.068 ± 0.141	2.014 ± 0.062	2.010 ± 0.066
Rel.wt., %[b]	427 ± 0.045	0.435 ± 0.034	0.424 ± 0.034	0.425 ± 0.026
Hypophysis, g	0.013 ± 0.003	0.014 ± 0.003	0.013 ± 0.002	0.013 ± 0.002
Rel.wt., %	0.003 ± 0.001	0.003 ± 0.001	0.003 ± 0.001	0.003 ± 0.001
Adrenal gland—left, g	0.033 ± 0.007	0.030 ± 0.004	0.030 ± 0.004	0.029 ± 0.007
Rel.wt., %	0.007 ± 0.002	0.006 ± 0.001	0.006 ± 0.001	0.006 ± 0.001
Adrenal gland—right, g	0.030 ± 0.003	0.029 ± 0.003	0.029 ± 0.005	0.032 ± 0.007
Rel.wt., %	0.006 ± 0.000	0.006 ± 0.001	0.006 ± 0.001	0.007 ± 0.001
Adrenal gland—total, g	0.063 ± 0.008	0.059 ± 0.006	0.059 ± 0.007	0.061 ± 0.007
Rel.wt., %	0.013 ± 0.002	0.013 ± 0.001	0.012 ± 0.002	0.013 ± 0.001
Liver, g	13.158 ± 1.492	12.322 ± 1.207	12.429 ± 1.786	12.135 ± 0.814
Rel.wt., %	2.678 ± 0.110	2.584 ± 0.154	2.590 ± 0.176	2.562 ± 0.112
Spleen, g	0.758 ± 0.073	0.709 ± 0.070	0.750 ± 0.129	0.674 ± 0.126
Rel.wt., %	0.155 ± 0.010	0.150 ± 0.018	0.158 ± 0.027	0.142 ± 0.024
Kidney—left, g	1.485 ± 0.190	1.422 ± 0.150	1.447 ± 0.167	1.466 ± 0.159
Rel.wt., %	0.303 ± 0.033	0.298 ± 0.018	0.302 ± 0.018	0.309 ± 0.028
Kidney—right, g	1.498 ± 0.153	1.449 ± 0.153	1.451 ± 0.166	1.426 ± 0.127
Rel.wt., %	0.306 ± 0.029	0.304 ± 0.018	0.303 ± 0.015	0.301 ± 0.020
Kidney—total, g	2.984 ± 0.338	2.871 ± 0.297	2.897 ± 0.329	2.892 ± 0.282
Rel.wt., %	0.609 ± 0.061	0.602 ± 0.034	0.605 ± 0.032	0.610 ± 0.047
Heart, g	1.487 ± 0.120	1.371 ± 0.115	1.403 ± 0.149	1.426 ± 0.116
Rel.wt., %	0.304 ± 0.029	0.288 ± 0.023	0.294 ± 0.027	0.301 ± 0.014
Testis/ovary—left, g	1.715 ± 0.307	1.777 ± 0.112	1.814 ± 0.150	1.773 ± 0.169
Rel.wt., %	0.351 ± 0.070	0.374 ± 0.021	0.382 ± 0.045	0.375 ± 0.038
Testis/ovary—right, g	1.713 ± 0.354	1.765 ± 0.124	1.814 ± 0.119	1.724 ± 0.179
Rel.wt., %	0.350 ± 0.077	0.371 ± 0.027	0.382 ± 0.039	0.365 ± 0.041
Testis/ovary—total, g	3.427 ± 0.650	3.542 ± 0.232	3.628 + 0.267	3.497 ± 0.345
Rel.wt., %	0.702 ± 0.145	0.745 ± 0.048	0.764 ± 0.084	0.740 ± 0.079
Prostate/uterus, g	0.650 ± 0.136	0.740 ± 0.131	0.720 ± 0.109	0.705 ± 0.147
Rel.wt., %	0.135 ± 0.038	0.156 ± 0.030	0.151 ± 0.019	0.148 ± 0.027
Lung, g	1.626 ± 0.132	1.588 ± 0.139	1.597 ± 0.130	1.644 ± 0.191
Rel.wt., %	0.332 ± 0.013	0.334 ± 0.025	0.335 ± 0.018	0.347 ± 0.033
Thymus, g	0.446 ± 0.144	0.311 ± 0.089	0.303 ± 0.069	0.331 ± 0.095
Rel.wt., %	0.091 ± 0.027	0.065 ± 0.018	0.064 ± 0.015	0.070 ± 0.018

Table 36.9 (continued) Subacute Toxicity of XOS in Rats: Absolute and Relative Organ Weights in Male Rats Treated Orally with XOS at 13 Weeks

Dose, mg/kg	0	333	1000	3000
Thyroid gland—left, g	0.011 ± 0.003	0.013 ± 0.003	0.010 ± 0.002	0.010 ± 0.003
Rel.wt., %	0.002 ± 0.001	0.003 ± 0.001	0.002 ± 0.001	0.002 ± 0.001
Thyroid gland—right, g	0.011 ± 0.003	0.012 ± 0.003	0.012 ± 0.003	0.012 ± 0.003
Rel.wt., %	0.002 ± 0.001	0.002 ± 0.001	0.002 ± 0.001	0.002 ± 0.001
Salivary gland, g	0.762 ± 0.111	0.758 ± 0.058	0.734 ± 0.082	0.746 ± 0.062
Rel.wt., %	0.155 ± 0.017	0.160 ± 0.013	0.154 ± 0.015	0.158 ± 0.010

Source: Park, Y.J. et al., *J. Food Hyg. Saf.*, 15, 151, 2000.
HGB, hemoglobin; MCV, mean corpuscular volume; PLT, platelets.
The values in various treatment groups are not significantly different.

2000, or 4000 mg/kg BW/day (10 male and 10 female rats per group). All animals showed normal growth activity. There were no significant differences in BW, food intake, or food availability between test groups and controls.

Hematological and serum chemistry values (e.g., hemoglobin, RBC count, WBC count, aminotransferase, BUN, creatine, cholesterone, nitroglycerin, blood sugar, TP, and ALB) were in the normal range, with no significant differences between the treatment and control groups. General inspection showed no abnormalities of urine bladder and liver duct stone and organ coefficient. In test groups, there were no significant microscopic pathological changes in liver, spleen, kidney, gastric, duodenum, testis, or ovaries compared with controls.

36.5.6 *Subchronic (6 Months) Toxicity Study in Beagle Dogs (Table 36.4; Gao et al., 2012)*

From this study, the NOAEL was determined to be 5000 mg/kg BW/day. In this study, 32 beagle dogs (7–8 months old, 7.9–9.8 kg) were randomly assigned to four groups (8 dogs/group): control, 1250, 2500, or 5000 mg/kg BW/day for 6 months. All animals showed normal growth activity. There were no significant differences in BW, food intake, or food availability between any test group and the control group. Hematological values and serum chemistry values, such as hemoglobin, RBC count, WBCs, ALT, AST, ALP, TP, glucose, and lipid profiles, BUN, and mineral concentrations, were in the normal range, and there were no significant differences among treatment groups and control groups. Also, there were no significant microscopic pathological changes in liver, spleen, kidney, stomach, duodenum, testis, or ovary in any treatment group compared with the control group. Detailed data are presented in the appendix.

36.5.7 *Other Animal Studies Showing No Adverse Effects of XOS*

Other animal studies also reported no adverse effects of XOS. Even a diet with 6%–10% XOS produced no adverse effects in rats.

Table 36.10 Subacute Toxicity of XOS in Rats: Absolute and Relative Organ Weights in Female Rats Treated Orally with XOS at 13 Weeks

Dose, mg/kg	0	333	1000	3000
Brain, g	1.807 ± 0.253	1.882 ± 0.081	1.823 ± 0.166	1.899 ± 0.111
Rel.wt., %[b]	0.667 ± 0.110	0.729 ± 0.059	0.702 ± 0.078	0.732 ± 0.044
Hypophysis, g	0.014 ± 0.004	0.013 ± 0.002	0.014 ± 0.003	0.014 ± 0.002
Rel.wt., %	0.005 ± 0.001	0.005 ± 0.001	0.005 ± 0.001	0.005 ± 0.001
Adrenal gland—left, g	0.044 ± 0.008	0.038 ± 0.005	0.040 ± 0.005	0.036 ± 0.006[a]
Rel.wt., %	0.016 ± 0.002	0.015 ± 0.002	0.015 ± 0.002	0.014 ± 0.003
Adrenal gland—right, g	0.038 ± 0.004	0.033 ± 0.006[a]	0.038 ± 0.004	0.034 ± 0.004
Rel.wt., %	0.014 ± 0.001	0.013 ± 0.003	0.015 ± 0.002	0.013 ± 0.002
Adrenal gland—total, g	0.083 ± 0.012	0.071 ± 0.010[a]	0.077 ± 0.008	0.070 ± 0.009[a]
Rel.wt., %	0.030 ± 0.003	0.027 ± 0.005	0.030 ± 0.004	0.027 ± 0.004
Liver, g	7.017 ± 0.857	6.241 ± 0.644[a]	6.457 ± 0.426	6.164 ± 0.397[b]
Rel.wt., %	2.565 ± 0.148	2.404 ± 0.099	2.482 ± 0.164	2.379 ± 0.1093[a]
Spleen, g	0.488 ± 0.055	0.458 ± 0.067	0.420 ± 0.047	0.423 ± 0.071
Rel.wt., %	0.179 ± 0.018	0.178 ± 0.032	0.161 ± 0.015	0.163 ± 0.022
Kidney—left, g	0.879 ± 0.153	0.824 ± 0.063	0.826 ± 0.095	0.811 ± 0.056
Rel.wt., %	0.320 ± 0.033	0.318 ± 0.016	0.318 ± 0.038	0.312 ± 0.013
Kidney—right, g	0.920 ± 0.206	0.829 ± 0.060	0.857 ± 0.048	0.833 ± 0.085
Rel.wt., %	0.335 ± 0.057	0.320 ± 0.015	0.330 ± 0.020	0.321 ± 0.025
Kidney—total, g	1.799 ± 0.355	1.653 ± 0.116	1.683 ± 0.132	1.644 ± 0.135
Rel.wt., %	0.655 ± 0.090	0.638 ± 0.027	0.647 ± 0.054	0.633 ± 0.035
Heart, g	0.962 ± 0.106	0.882 ± 0.065	0.931 ± 0.075	0.948 ± 0.091
Rel.wt., %	0.353 ± 0.029	0.342 ± 0.035	0.358 ± 0.033	0.365 ± 0.027
Testis/ovary—left, g	0.046 ± 0.013	0.045 ± 0.010	0.047 ± 0.008	0.047 ± 0.007
Rel.wt., %	0.017 ± 0.004	0.017 ± 0.003	0.018 ± 0.003	0.018 ± 0.003
Testis/ovary—right, g	0.048 ± 0.010	0.048 ± 0.009	0.053 ± 0.010	0.048 ± 0.007
Rel.wt., %	0.018 ± 0.003	0.019 ± 0.004	0.020 ± 0.005	0.018 ± 0.003
Testis/ovary—total, g	0.094 ± 0.021	0.094 ± 0.015	0.100 ± 0.014	0.095 + 0.011
Rel.wt., %	0.035 ± 0.007	0.036 ± 0.006	0.038 ± 0.007	0.037 ± 0.005
Prostate/uterus, g	0.549 ± 0.183	0.558 ± 0.213	0.466 ± 0.084	0.540 ± 0.179
Rel.wt., %	0.201 ± 0.065	0.213 ± 0.066	0.180 ± 0.041	0.207 ± 0.062
Lung, g	1.249 ± 0.138	1.118 ± 0.100	1.171 ± 0.104	1.201 ± 0.135
Rel.wt., %	0.458 ± 0.046	0.434 ± 0.049	0.450 ± 0.041	0.461 ± 0.033
Thymus, g	0.285 ± 0.062	0.267 ± 0.044	0.234 ± 0.028	0.252 ± 0.043
Rel.wt., %	0.104 ± 0.018	0.103 ± 0.015	0.090 ± 0.009	0.097 ± 0.015

Table 36.10 (continued) Subacute Toxicity of XOS in Rats: Absolute and Relative Organ Weights in Female Rats Treated Orally with XOS at 13 Weeks

Dose, mg/kg	0	333	1000	3000
Thyroid gland—left, g	0.009 ± 0.004	0.007 ± 0.003	0.008 ± 0.002	0.010 ± 0.002
Rel.wt., %	0.003 ± 0.001	0.003 ± 0.001	0.003 ± 0.001	0.004 ± 0.001
Thyroid gland—right, g	0.009 ± 0.003	0.009 ± 0.002	0.007 ± 0.002	0.009 ± 0.002
Rel.wt., %	0.003 ± 0.001	0.003 ± 0.001	0.003 ± 0.001	0.003 ± 0.001

Source: Park, Y.J. et al., *J. Food Hyg. Saf.,* 15, 151, 2000.
[a] Significantly different from control ($p < 0.05$).
[b] Significantly different from control ($p < 0.01$).

36.5.7.1 Colonic Health Study in Mice Howard et al. (1995) added soluble fiber (XOS, FOS, or gum arabic) to a semielemental diet to assess the impact on colonic epithelial cell proliferation and microflora. Consumption of XOS increased cecal crypt depth (175.8 vs. control, 168.5 µm; $p < 0.05$) and labeling index (0.21 vs. control, 0.17; $p < 0.05$) compared to the other two treatments. Consumption of XOS and the control diet resulted in comparable cell density (number of cells in a vertical half of the crypt), crypt depth, cell proliferation zone, and labeling index of cecum and distal colon. No adverse effects of XOS were reported.

36.5.7.2 Bifidogenic Effect of XOS in Streptozotocin-Induced Diabetic Wistar Rats XOS from alkali-pretreated corncob was supplemented at 10% (w/w) in the basal diet of streptozotocin-induced diabetic Wistar rats while controls were fed a basal diet for a period of 6 weeks (Gobinath et al., 2010). XOS supplementation significantly improved respective body weight gain (XOS, −19.9 ± 10.2 vs. control, −37.3 ± 6.1 g; $p < 0.05$) and reduced both hyperglycemia and plasma cholesterol (XOS, 12146 ± 101 vs. control, 2295 ± 175 mg/L; $p < 0.05$). It increased the activity of antioxidant enzymes (catalase and glutathione reductase) in the blood of diabetic rats. XOS and FOS supplementation also led to a significant increase in bifidobacteria ($\log_{10}$ CFU/g wet contents; XOS, 10.2 ± 0.12 vs. control, 8.89 ± 0.21; $p < 0.05$) and lactobacilli ($\log_{10}$ CFU/g wet contents; XOS, 7.81 ± 0.23 vs. control, 7.45 ± 0.16; $p < 0.05$) in the cecum of normal rats. No adverse effects were reported.

36.5.8 Carcinogenicity Test

From a study of 1,2-dimethylhydrazine (DMH, 15 mg/kg BW/week for 2 weeks) treatment in rats, Hsu et al. (2004) found that both XOS and FOS markedly decreased the cecal pH (XOS, 6.08 ± 0.11 vs. FOS, 6.16 ± 0.07 vs. DMH control, 6.53 ± 0.12; $p < 0.05$). It also increased the total cecal weight (XOS, 18.5 ± 0.8 vs. FOS, 19.0 ± 0.1 vs. DMH control, 14.6 ± 0.9 g; $p < 0.05$) and bifidobacteria population ($\log_{10}$ CFU/g wet contents; XOS, 10.93 ± 0.07 vs. FOS, 10.09 ± 0.12 vs. DMH control, 8.95 ± 0.26; $p < 0.05$). XOS had a greater effect on the bacterial

Table 36.11 Subacute Toxicity of XOS in Rats: Absolute and Relative Organ Weights in Male and Female Rats Treated Orally with XOS[a] at 4 Weeks of Recovery[a]

Dose, mg/kg	0	3000	0	3000
Brain, g	2.115 ± 0.067	2.090 ± 0.058	1.908 ± 0.070	1.915 ± 0.070
Rel.wt., %[b]	0.428 ± 0.047	0.406 ± 0.040	0.698 ± 0.032	0.698 ± 0.043
Hypophysis, g	0.013 ± 0.002	0.014 ± 0.002	0.014 ± 0.003	0.014 ± 0.003
Rel.wt., %	0.003 ± 0.001	0.003 ± 0.001	0.005 ± 0.001	0.005 ± 0.001
Adrenal gland—left, g	0.033 ± 0.007	0.030 ± 0.003	0.033 ± 0.005	0.039 ± 0.007
Rel.wt., %	0.007 ± 0.001	0.006 ± 0.001	0.012 ± 0.002	0.015 ± 0.003
Adrenal gland—right, g	0.028 ± 0.007	0.026 ± 0.003	0.035 ± 0.004	0.038 ± 0.006
Rel.wt., %	0.006 ± 0.001	0.005 ± 0.001	0.013 ± 0.001	0.014 ± 0.002
Adrenal gland—total, g	0.061 ± 0.012	0.057 ± 0.006	0.068 ± 0.006	0.077 ± 0.012
Rel.wt., %	0.012 ± 0.002	0.011 ± 0.002	0.025 ± 0.003	0.028 ± 0.005
Liver, g	13.128 ± 1.902	13.699 ± 1.742	6.781 ± 0.228	6.934 ± 0.642
Rel.wt., %	2.644 ± 0.127	2.634 ± 0.133	2.478 ± 0.075	2.520 ± 0.170
Spleen, g	0.769 ± 0.116	0.739 ± 0.105	0.446 ± 0.048	0.452 ± 0.041
Rel.wt., %	0.155 ± 0.017	0.143 ± 0.018	0.163 ± 0.016	0.165 ± 0.019
Kidney—left, g	1.575 ± 0.170	1.501 ± 0.132	0.825 ± 0.034	0.884 ± 0.092
Rel.wt., %	0.316 ± 0.019	0.290 ± 0.024	0.302 ± 0.018	0.322 ± 0.032
Kidney—right, g	1.572 ± 0.183	1.525 ± 0.146	0.846 ± 0.046	0.929 ± 0.095
Rel.wt., %	0.316 ± 0.023	0.295 ± 0.029	0.309 ± 0.018	0.339 ± 0.038
Kidney—total, g	3.146 ± 0.349	3.026 ± 0.265	1.672 ± 0.072	1.813 ± 0.179
Rel.wt., %	0.632 ± 0.041	0.5854 ± 0.050	0.612 ± 0.034	0.660 ± 0.068
Heart, g	1.526 ± 0.184	1.500 ± 0.161	0.961 ± 0.085	0.927 ± 0.068
Rel.wt., %	0.306 ± 0.020	0.290 ± 0.025	0.352 ± 0.035	0.338 ± 0.31
Testis/ovary—left, g	1.834 ± 0.170	1.814 ± 0.123	0.041 ± 0.006	0.047 ± 0.009
Rel.wt., %	0.371 ± 0.048	0.351 ± 0.027	0.015 ± 0.002	0.017 ± 0.004
Testis/ovary—right, g	1.808 ± 0.135	1.817 ± 0.108	0.041 ± 0.007	0.048 ± 0.008
Rel.wt., %	0.366 ± 0.047	0.352 ± 0.023	0.015 ± 0.002	0.018 ± 0.004
Testis/ovary—total, g	3.642 ± 0.301	3.630 ± 0.228	0.082 ± 0.011	0.095 ± 0.016
Rel.wt., %	0.737 ± 0.094	0.702 ± 0.050	0.030 ± 0.003	0.035 ± 0.007
Prostate/uterus, g	0.5959 ± 0.150	0.602 ± 0.184	0.549 ± 0.121	0.506 ± 0.125
Rel.wt., %	0.119 ± 0.028	0.116 ± 0.035	0.201 ± 0.048	0.185 ± 0.048
Lung, g	1.663 ± 0.146	1.590 ± 0.150	1.174 ± 0.090	1.238 ± 0.120
Rel.wt., %	0.336 ± 0.033	0.308 ± 0.038	0.429 ± 0.031	0.450 ± 0.039
Thymus, g	0.294 ± 0.086	0.275 ± 0.093	0.252 ± 0.049	0.200 ± 0.044
Rel.wt., %	0.060 ± 0.019	0.053 ± 0.018	0.092 ± 0.016	0.073 ± 0.015

Table 36.11 (continued) Subacute Toxicity of XOS in Rats: Absolute and Relative Organ Weights in Male and Female Rats Treated Orally with XOS[a] at 4 Weeks of Recovery[a]

Dose, mg/kg	0	3000	0	3000
Thyroid gland—left, g	0.013 ± 0.004	0.010 ± 0.002	0.008 ± 0.002	0.008 ± 0.002
Rel.wt., %	0.003 ± 0.001	0.002 ± 0.001	0.003 ± 0.001	0.003 ± 0.001
Thyroid gland—right, g	0.013 ± 0.004	0.011 ± 0.002	0.009 ± 0.003	0.007 ± 0.001
Rel.wt., %	0.003 ± 0.001	0.002 ± 0.001	0.003 ± 0.001	0.003 ± 0.001
Salivary gland, g	0.748 ± 0.097	0.732 ± 0.084	0.477 ± 0.044	0.447 ± 0.057
Rel.wt., %	0.151 ± 0.018	0.142 ± 0.020	0.174 ± 0.018	0.163 ± 0.017

Source: Park, Y.J. et al., *J. Food Hyg. Saf.*, 15, 151, 2000.

[a] Values are expressed as means ± SD.

[b] Relative organ weights were expressed as the percentage of organ weights to BWs.

population than FOS did. Moreover, both XOS and FOS markedly reduced the number of aberrant crypt foci in the colon of DMH-treated rats (number of 2 crypts/focus; XOS, 1.20 ± 0.33 vs. FOS, 3.10 ± 0.69 vs. DMH control, 4.80 ± 1.00; $p < 0.05$: number of >4 crypts/focus; XOS, 0.30 ± 0.15 vs. FOS, 0.60 ± 0.27 vs. DMH control, 2.80 ± 1.04; $p < 0.05$). The authors concluded that dietary supplementation with such NDOs as XOS and FOS may improve gastrointestinal health and that XOS is more effective than FOS. No adverse effects of XOS were reported.

36.5.9 Mutagenicity and Genotoxicity Tests of XOS

Table 36.12 shows that there were no adverse effects from XOS in mice after the Ames test, the polychromatophilic normocyte micronucleus test of bone marrow (BM), and sperm abnormality and testis chromosome aberration tests.

36.5.9.1 Bacterial Reverse Mutation Assay of XOS (Table 36.12; Oh et al., 1999) From the in vitro Ames test using *Salmonella typhimurium* (TA98, TA100, TA1535, and TA1537) and *Escherichia coli* (WP2 uvrA) with and without rat liver microsomal enzyme (S-9 fraction), Oh et al. (1999) showed that XOS at a concentration up to 5000 ug/plate did not cause bacterial reverse mutation.

Table 36.12 Summary of Mutagenicity and Genotoxicity Studies Showing No Adverse Effects of XOS

Test	Dosage of XOS	References
Ames test	5000 ug/plate	Oh et al. (1999)
Ames test	5000 ug/plate	Gao et al. (2012)
Polychromatophilic normocyte micronucleus test of BM in mice, 5 days	10.0 g/kg BW	Gao et al. (2012)

36.5.9.2 Ames Test (Table 36.12; Gao et al., 2012)   In two experiments, another Ames test with four strains of *Salmonella typhimurium* (TA97, TA98, TA100, and TA102) with or without S-9 found no mutagenicity with XOS at five concentrations (250, 500, 1000, 2500, or 5000 μg/plate). The number of revertant colonies did not exceed two times that of spontaneous revertant colonies in all dosage groups (Table 36.10). No dose-response relationship was observed. The data indicate those four strains of *Salmonella typhimurium* with or without S-9 had no inherent toxicity.

36.5.9.3 Polychromatophilic Normocyte Micronucleus Test in Mice (Table 36.12; Gao et al., 2012)   A polychromatophilic normocyte micronucleus test in 50 mice (25–30 g of BW) with XOS doses of 2.5, 5.0, and 10.0 g/kg BW showed no significant difference in micronucleus rate between test and control groups. This indicated that the sample did not cause micronucleus change of polychromatophilic normocyte of BM in mice. In this study, distilled water was given by gastric perfusion two times within 24 h to the negative control group; the positive control group received cyclophosphamide (CTX, 40 mg/kg BW) in the same fashion.

36.6 Summary and Conclusions

The nutritional benefits and safety of the prebiotic ingredient XOS are well established in animal models and human clinical trials. The literature showed no significant adverse effects related to XOS consumption.

References

Aachary AA and Prapulla SG. Value addition to corncob: Production and characterization of xylooligosaccharides from alkali pretreated lignin-saccharide complex using *Aspergillus oryzae* MTCC 5154. *Bioresour Technol* 2009;100:991–995.

Ai Z, Jiang Z, Li L, Deng W, Kusakabe I, and Li H. Immobilization of *Streptomyces olivaceoviridis* E-86 xylanase on Eudragit S-100 for xylo-oligosaccharide production. *Process Biochem* 2005;40:2707–2714.

Alles MS, Hartemink R, Meyboom S, Harryvan JL, Van Laere KMJ, Nagengast FM, and Hautvast JGAJ. Effect of transgalactooligosaccharides on the composition of the human intestinal microflora and on putative risk markers for colon cancer. *Am J Clin Nutr* 1999;69:980–991.

Alles MS, Hautvast JGAJ, Nagengast FM, Hartemink R, Van Laere KMJ, and Jansen JBMJ. Fate of fructo-oligosaccharides in the human intestine. *Br J Nutr* 1996;76:211–221.

Bouhnik Y, Flourie B, D'Agay-Abensour L, Pochart P, Gramet G, Durand M, and Rambaud JC. Administration of transgalacto-oligosaccharides increases fecal bifidobacteria and modifies colonic fermentation metabolism in healthy humans. *J Nutr* 1997;127:444–448.

Bouhnik Y, Raskine L, Simoneau G, Vicaut E, Neut C, Flourie B, Brouns F, and Bornet FR. The capacity of nondigestible carbohydrates to stimulate fecal bifidobacteria in healthy humans: A double-blind, randomized, placebo-controlled, parallel-group, dose response relation study. *Am J Clin Nutr* 2004;80:1658–1664.

Campbell JM, Fahey GC Jr, and Wolf BW. Selected indigestible oligosaccharides affect large bowel mass, cecal and fecal short-chain fatty acids, pH and microflora in rats. *J Nutr* 1997;127:130–136.

Chung M, Chien C, Huang P, and Tung T. Effects of prolonged feeding of D-xylose on rats. *J Formosan Med Assoc* 1973;72:467–471.

Courtin CM, Swennen K, Verjans P, and Delcour JA. Heat and pH stability of prebiotic arabinoxylooligosaccharides, xylooligosaccharides and fructooligosaccharides. *Food Chem* 2009;112:831–837.

Crittenden R, Karppinen S, Ojanen S, Tenkanen M, Fagerstrom R, Matto J, Saarela M, Mattila-Sandholm T, and Poutanen K. In vitro fermentation of cereal dietary fibre carbohydrates by probiotic and intestinal bacteria. *J Sci Food Agric* 2002;82:781–789.

Fleming SE and Lee B. Growth performance and intestinal transit time of rats fed purified and natural dietary fibers. *J Nutr* 1983;113:592–601.

Fleming SE, Marthinsen D, and Kuhnlein H. Colonic function and fermentation in men consuming high fiber diets. *J Nutr* 1983;113:2535–2544.

Fleming SE and Rodriguez MA. Influence of dietary fiber on fecal excretion of volatile fatty acids by human adults. *J Nutr* 1983;113:1613–1625.

Food and Agriculture Organization of the United Nations (FAO). Technical meeting report on prebiotics. Rome, Italy, September 15–16, 2007.

Food and Drug Administration (FDA). GRN 44. Fructooligosaccharides, filed by GTC nutrition, 2000.

Food and Drug Administration (FDA). GRN 236. Galacto-oligosaccharides, filed by Friesland foods domo, Friesland, the Netherlands, 2008.

Food and Drug Administration (FDA). GRN 246. Isomalto-oligosaccharide mixture (IMOM), filed by BioNeutra Inc., Alberta, Canada.

Food and Drug Administration (FDA). GRN 285. Galacto-oligosaccharides, filed by GTC nutrition, 2009.

Food and Drug Administration (FDA). GRN 286. Galacto-oligosaccharides, filed by GTC nutrition, 2009.

Food and Drug Administration (FDA). GRN 343. Wheat bran extract composed primarily of xylo- and arabinoxylo-oligosaccharides, filed by Fugeia NV, 2010.

Fujikawa S, Okazaki M, and Matsumoto N. Effect of xylooligosaccharide on growth of intestinal bacteria and putrefaction products'. *J Jpn Soc Nutr Food Sci* 1991;44:37–40.

Gao et al. 2012. Safety of xylooligosaccharides. Manuscript in preparation.

Gibson GR and Roberfroid MB. Dietary modulation of the human colonic microbiota. Introducing the concept of prebiotics. *J Nutr* 1995;125:1401–1412.

Gobinath D, Madhu AN, Prashant G, Srinivasan K, and Prapulla SG. Beneficial effect of xylo-oligosaccharides and fructo-oligosaccharides in streptozotocin-induced diabetic rats. *Br J Nutr* 2010;104:40–47.

Graham H, Apajalahti J, and Peuranen S. Xylo-oligosaccharides alter metabolism of gut microbes and blood xylose levels in chicks. In *Dietary Fibre; Bioactive Carbohydrates for Food and Feed*. Van de Kamp et al. (Ed.). Wagningen Academic Publishers, Wagningen, the Netherlands. 2004, pp. 329–333.

Grootaert C, Delcour JA, Courtin CM, Broekaert WF, Verstraete W, and Van de Wiele T. Microbial metabolism and prebiotic potency of arabinoxylan oligosaccharides in the human intestine. *Trends Food Sci Technol* 2007;18:64–71.

Hardinge MG, Swarner JB, and Grooks H. Carbohydrates in foods. *J Am Diet Assoc* 1965;46,197–204.

Howard MD, Gordon DT, Garleb KA, and Kerley MS. Dietary fructooligosaccharide, xylo-oligosaccharide and gum arabic have variable effects on cecal and colonic microbiota and epithelial cell proliferation in mice and rats. *J Nutr* 1995;125:2604–2609.

Hsu CK, Liao JW, Chung YC, Hsieh CP, and Chan YC. Xylooligosaccharides and fructooligosaccharides affect the intestinal microbiota and precancerous colonic lesion development in rats. *J Nutr* 2004;134:1523–1528.

Iino T, Nishijima Y, Sawada S, Sasaki H, Harada H, Suwa Y, and Kiso Y. Improvement of constipation by a small amount of xylooligosaccharides ingestion in adult women. *J Jpn Assoc Dietary Fiber Res* 1997;1:19–24.

Imazawa T, Nishikawa A, Furukawa F, Ikeda T, Nakamura H, Miyauchi M, and Hirose M. A 13-week subchronic toxicity study of D-xylose in F344 rats. *Bull Natl Inst Health Sci* 1999;117:115–118 (in Japanese).

Institute of Medicine (IOM). *Dietary Reference Intakes for Energy, Carbohydrates, Fiber, Fat, Fatty Acids, Cholesterol, Protein, and Amino Acids.* National Academy Press, Washington, DC. 2002.

Jeong KJ, Park IY, Kim MS, and Kim SC. High-level expression of an endoxylanase gene from Bacillus sp. in *Bacillus subtilis* DB104 for the production of xylobiose from xylan. *Appl Microbiol Biotechnol* 1998;50:113–118.

JETRO (Japan External Trade Organization), Specifications and Standards for Foods, Food Additives, etc. Under the Food Sanitation Act, 2010. Available from http://www.jetro.go.jp/se/e/standards_regulation/foodadd2004apr-e.pdf (accessed January 2, 2011).

Jiang ZQ, Deng W, Li XT, Ai ZL, Li LT, and Kusakabe I. Characterization of a novel, ultra-large xylanolytic complex (xylanosome) from *Streptomyces olivaceoviridis* E-86. *Enz Microbial Technol* 2005;36:923–929.

Jiang Z, Deng W, Yan Q, Zhai Q, Li L, and Kusakabe I. Subunit composition of a large xylanolytic complex (xylanosome) from *Streptomyces olivaceoviridis* E-86. *J Biotechnol* 2006;126:304–312.

Joo GJ, Rhee IK, Kim SO, and Rhee SJ. Effect of dietary xylooligosaccharide on indigestion and retarding effect of bile acid movement across a dialysis membrane. *Han'guk Sikp'um Yongyang Kwahak Hoechi* 1998;27:705–711.

Kabel MA, Kortenoeven L, Schols HA, and Voragen AG. In vitro fermentability of differently substituted xylo-oligosaccharides. *J Agric Food Chem* 2002;50:6205–6010.

Kajihara M, Kato S, Konishi M, Yamagishi Y, Horie Y, and Ishii H. Xylooligosaccharide decreases blood ammonia levels in patients with liver cirrhosis. *Am J Gastroenterol* 2000;95: 2514.

Kobayashi T, Okazaki M, Fujikawa S, and Koga K. Effect of xylooligosaccharides on feces of men. *J Jpn Soc Biosci Biotech Agrochem* 1991;65:1651–1653.

Kuroiwa Y, Nishikawa A, Imazawa T, Kitamura Y, Kanki K, Umemura T, and Hirose M. Lack of carcinogenicity of D-xylose given in the diet to F344 rats for two years. *Food Chem Toxicol* 2005;43:1399–1404.

van Loo J, Cummings J, Delzenne N, Englyst H, Franck A, Hopkins M, Kok N, Macfarlane G, Newton D, Quigley M, Roberfroid M, van Vliet T, and van den Heuvel E. Functional food properties of non-digestible oligosaccharides: A consensus report from the ENDO project (DGXII AIRII-CT94–1095). *Br J Nutr* 1999;81:121–132.

MHLW (Ministry of Health, Labor and Welfare of Japan). List of existing food additives, Notification No. 120 of the Ministry of Health and Welfare, Tokyo, Japan. 1996a.

MHLW (Ministry of Health, Labor and Welfare of Japan). Guidelines for designation of food additives, and for revision of standard for use of food additives, Article No. 29 of the life and sanitation bureau. Ministry of Health, Labor and Welfare, Tokyo, Japan. 1996b.

Moura P, Cabanas S, Lourenço P, Gírio F, Maria C, Loureiro-Dias M, and Esteves P. In vitro fermentation of selected xylo-oligosaccharides by piglet intestinal microbiota. *Food Sci Technol* 2008;41:1952–1961.

Moure A, Gullón P, Domínguez H, and Parajó JC. Advances in the manufacture, purification and applications of xylo-oligosaccharides as food additives and nutraceuticals. *Process Biochem* 2006;41:1913–1923.

Na MH and Kim WK. Effects of xylooligosaccharide intake on fecal Bifidobacteria, lactic acid and lipid metabolism in Korean young women. *Korean J Nutr* 2007;40:154–161.

Oh HG, Park YJ, Lee UT, Lee JW, Lee CS, Rhew BK, Yang CK, Yoon SW, and Kang BH. Bacterial reverse mutation assay of xylooligosaccharide. *J Food Hyg Saf* 1999;14:259–264.

Okazaki M, Fujikawa S, and Matumoto N. Effect of xylooligosaccharide on the growth of bifidobacteria. *Bifidobacteria Microflora* 1990;9:77–86.

Okazaki M, Koda H, Izumi R, Fujikawa S, and Matsumoto N. In vitro digestibility and in vivo utilization of xylobiose. *Nippon Eiyo Shokuryo Gakkaishi* 1991;44:41–44.

Oliveira EE, Silva AE, Júnior TN, Gomes MC, Aguiar LM, Marcelino HR, Araújo IB, Bayer MP, Ricardo NM, Oliveira AG, and Egito ES. Xylan from corn cobs, a promising polymer for drug delivery: Production and characterization. *Bioresour Technol* 2010;101:5402–5406.

Park YJ, Lee UT, Lee JW, Lee CS, Rhew BK, Yang CK, Yoon SW, and Kang BH. Subacute toxicity of xylooligosaccharide in rats. *J Food Hyg Saf* 2000;15:151–166.

Park YJ, Oh HG, Lee UT, Lee JW, Lee CS, Rhew BK, Yang CK, Yoon SW, and Kang BH. Acute oral toxicity of xylooligosaccharide in rats. *J Food Hyg Saf* 1999;14:255–258.

Park JH, Yoo JY, Shin OH, Shin HK, Lee SJ, and Park KH. Growth effect of branched oligosaccharides on principal intestinal bacteria. *Kor J Appl Microbiol Biotechnol* 1992;20:237–242.

Ryu BG, Lee JW, Lee CS, Hyeon SI, Park YJ, An JB, and Yang CG. Effects of xylooligosaccharides on the growth of intestinal microflora. *Korean J Microbiol Biotechnol* 2002;30:380–386.

Southgate DAT. The definition, analysis and properties of dietary fiber. In: *Dietary Fiber: Current Developments of Importance to Health*. Heaton, K.W. (Ed.). J. Libbey & Co., London, U.K. 1979, pp. 9–19.

Van Laere KMJ, Hartemink R, Bosveld M, Schols HA, and Voragen AGJ. Fermentation of plant cell wall derived polysaccharides and their corresponding oligosaccharides by intestinal bacteria. *J Agric Food Chem* 2000;48:1644–1652.

Vázquez MJ, Alonso JL, Domínguez H, and Parajó JC. Xylooligosaccharides: Manufacture and applications. *Trends Food Sci Technol* 2000;11:387–393.

Yazawa K, Imai K, and Tamura Z. Oligosaccharides and polysaccharides specifically utilizable by bifidobacteria. *Chem Pharm Bull* 1978;26:3306–3311.

Appendix: Global Suppliers of Fiber Ingredients

SUSAN S. CHO

Alpha cyclodextrin
Wacker Chemical
www.wacker.com; info.finechemicals@wacker.com

CAVAMAX® W6 Alpha Cyclodextrin: Wacker Chemicals is the global leader in cyclodextrin products. All CAVAMAX® cyclodextrins are FDA-notified GRAS. CAVAMAX® W6 is a colorless natural dietary fiber. It is heat stable even under acidic conditions and stable in carbonated beverages. With a viscosity like sucrose, a neutral taste, and no browning effect, it can be used even in complex food systems. CAVAMAX W6 also lowers the glycemic index of starch-containing food.

3301 Sutton Road, Adrian, MI 49221-9397, USA
Phone l: +1-517-264-8671; Fax: +1-517-264-8795

Microcrystalline cellulose (MCC), microcrystalline cellulose gel (MCG), methyl cellulose (MC), hydroxypropylmethyl cellulose (HPMC)
J. Rettenmaier USA LP
www.jrsusa.com; www.jrs.de; info@jrsusa.com

Vivapur® microcrystalline cellulose (MCC), methyl cellulose (MC), and hydroxypropylmethyl cellulose (HPMC): Vitacel® modified cellulose products are available in a variety of types that are suitable for use in pharmaceutical (tableting) and stabilizing food systems (increased viscosity, suspension, adhesion, and/or shelf life).

Contact for United States and Canada
J. Rettenmaier USA LP
16369 US Highway 131, Schoolcraft, MI 49087
Phone: +1-269-679-2340; Toll-free: +1-877-895-4099; Fax: +1-269-679-2364

Contact outside United States and Canada
J. Rettenmaier & Söhne GmbH + Co. KG
Holzmühle 1, D-73494 Rosenberg (Germany)
Phone: +49-(0)7967-152-0; Fax: +49-(0)7967-152-222

Cellulose and hydroxymethylpropyl cellulose (HMPC)
Dow Chemical
www.fortefiber.com; fortefiber@dow.com
FORTEFIBER™ soluble dietary fiber from cellulose

FORTEFIBER™ HB Plus (medium viscosity)
FORTEFIBER™ HB Ultra (high viscosity): The products have been shown to help maintain healthy levels of cholesterol, blood glucose, and insulin.

North America
1650 N. Swede Rd, Larkin 100, Midland, MI 48674, USA
Phone: 1-800-488-5430; Fax 1-989-638-9836

Europe, India, Africa, and the Middle East
Toll-free: +800-3-694-6367; Toll-free for Italy: +800-783-82
Phone: +32-3-450-2240; Fax: +32-3-450-2815

Latin America
Phone: +55 11 5188 9222; Fax +55-11-5188-9749

The Pacific
Toll-free call: 800-7776-7776; Toll-free fax: 800-7779-7779
Phone: +60-3-7958-3392; Fax: +60-3-7958-5598

Cellulose
International Fiber Corporation
www.ifcfiber.com; info@ifcfiber.com

Alpha-cel, Keycel, and QualFlo
International Fiber Corporation
50 Bridge Street, North Tonawanda, New York 14120
Phone: 1-888-698-1936 or +1-716-693-4040; Fax: +1-716-693-3528

Fruit fiber
Herbafood Ingredients GmbH
www.herbafood.dep; info@herbafood.de; www.herbafood.com; usa@herbstreith-fox.com

Herbacel® Classic: insoluble fruit fiber with the typical flavor and taste and a moderate water binding. Fiber content is about 60%, available from apples, lemon, or orange in different grain sizes.
Herbacel® Classic Plus: insoluble fruit fiber with a fiber content of about 80% and a moderate water binding, available from apples.
Herbacel® AQ Plus: insoluble fruit fiber with a fiber content of about 90% and a high water binding, available from citrus fruits and apples.
Herbapekt® LV: soluble fruit fiber with a fiber content (pectin with low viscosity) of about 80%, available from citrus fruits and apples.

Herbafood Ingredients GmbH
Phöbener Chaussee 12, D-14542 Werder/Havel, Germany
Phone: +49-3327-785-202; Fax: +49-3327-785-201

Herbstreith & Fox Inc.
570 Taxter Road, Elmsford, New York 10523, USA
Phone: +1-914-345-9501; Fax: +1-914-345-0919

Gum arabic (acacia gum)
Colloïdes Naturels International
www.cniworld.com; information@cniworld.com

Fibregum™ and its organic-certified versions, (Fibregum™ Bio and Fibregum™ Bio L), are all-natural soluble dietary fibers (guaranteed 90% minimum level) from acacia gum.

129 Chemin de Croisset—BP 4151-76723 Rouen cedex 3, France
Phone: +33-0-232-83-1818; Fax: +33-0-232-83-1919

1140 US Highway 22 East, Center Point IV, Suite 102
Bridgewater, NJ 08807, USA
Ph: +1-908-707-9400; Fax: +1-908-707-9405

Inulin/fructooligosaccharides
GTC Nutrition

Orafti
www.orafti.com or www@beneo.com; afi@orafti.com

BENEO™ L60/L85/L95/P95 (oligofructose)
BENEO™ ST/GR/ST-Gel (inulin)
BENEO™ HP/HP-Gel/HPX (long-chain inulin)
BENEO™ HSI (high-soluble inulin)
BENEO™ Synergy1 (oligofructose-enriched inulin): The products are prebiotic dietary fibers and have been shown to contribute to gut health, better calcium absorption, and immunity.

Orafti Active Food Ingredients
Aandorenstraat, 1, 3300 Tienen, Belgium
Phone: +32-16-801-301; Fax: +32-16-801-308

2740 Route 10 West, Suite 205, Morris Plains, NJ 07950, USA
Phone: +1-973-867-2140; Fax: +1-973-867-2141

Sensus
www.sensus.us. Email: contact@sensus.us
Frutafit® and Frutalose® inulin and oligofructose from the chicory root
Frutafit® HD (highly dispersable)
Frutafit® IQ (instant quality)
Frutafit® TEX! (texturizing)
Frutafit® CLR (highly soluble)
Frutalose® L90 (sweet liquid fiber)

Head Office: Sensus Operations C.V
PO Box 1308, 4700 BH Roosendaal, the Netherlands
Phone: +31-165-582-578; Fax: +31-165-567-796
Email: info.sensus@sensus.nl; www.sensus.nl

North American Office: Sensus America, Inc.
1 Deer Park Dr., Suite J, Monmouth Junction, NJ 08852
Phone: 1-646-452-6150; 1-866-456-8872; Fax: 1-646-452-6150
www.sensus.us. Email: contact@sensus.us

Asian office: Sensus Asia
Off. Mid Valley City, Lingkaran Syed Putra, 59200 Kuala Lumpur, Malaysia
Phone: 603-2140-2462; Fax: 603-2140-2463

Cargill
www.cargill.com; www.hft@cargill.com

Oliggo-Fiber™ Instant (native)
Oliggo-Fiber™ XL (fat mimetic properties)
Oliggo-Fiber™ F97 (high solubility)

Oat beta-glucan, concentrated
Garuda International
bfaress@garudaint.com

Garuda International's B-CAN™ oat beta-glucan is an unique oat (*Avena sativa*) derived, free-flowing powder that contains high concentration of oat beta-glucan. In addition to 70% oat beta-glucan, which is currently one of the highest concentrations of beta-glucan on the market today, Garuda International also offers a 55% and 20% oat beta-glucan ingredient.

Garuda's B-CAN™ 70% oat beta-glucan is water soluble and has a neutral taste/smell profile and, along with its stability to heat, allows for a wide variety of formulations in food, beverage, nutraceutical, and cosmeceutical industries. Garuda International's B-CAN™ oat beta-glucan products are certified Kosher and Halal, and an organically certified product is also currently offered. There is extensive research linking the consumption of oat beta-glucan (combined with a low-fat diet) to supporting healthy LDL cholesterol levels, cardiovascular health, and glycemic control. The U.S. FDA and, more recently, the European EFSA may allow a "heart healthy" claim for some foods containing beta-glucan soluble fiber.

Contact for United States and Canada
PO Box 159, Exeter, CA 93221, USA
Phone: +1-559-594-4380

Oat hull fiber

Vitacel® oat fibers: Vitacel® oat fibers are available in a variety of grades suitable for use in meat, bakery, cereal, and beverage applications for fiber fortification, calorie reduction, and structural enhancement.

United States and Canada
J. Rettenmaier USA LP
16369 US Highway 131, Schoolcraft, MI 49087, USA
Phone: (269)-679-2340; Toll-free: (877)-895-4099; Fax: (269)-679-2364

Outside United States and Canada
J. Rettenmaier & Söhne GmbH + Co. KG
Holzmühle 1, D-73494 Rosenberg (Germany)
Phone: +49-0-7967-152-0
Fax: +49-0-79 67-1522 22

SunOpta Ingredients Group
www.sunopta.com/ingredients; ingredients@sunopta.com

Canadian Harvest® oat fibers: SunOpta Ingredients Group offers a family of quality fibers and the experience to help you select the right fiber for your product whether your goal is to enhance texture, increase yield, extend shelf-life, improve strength and flexibility, or increase the level of total dietary fiber.

100 Apollo Drive, Chelmsford MA 01824
Toll-free: +1-800-353-6782
Phone: +1-781-276-5100

Partially hydrolyzed guar gum (PHGG)

Taiyo International, Inc.
www.taiyointernational.com and www.sunfiber.com; email: sales@taiyoint.com; scott@taiyoint.com

Sunfiber® soluble dietary fiber
Sunfiber® R (regular)
Sunfiber® AG (agglomerated): Sunfiber® has been clinically shown to maintain digestive health and microflora balance, lower glycemic index, improve mineral absorption, inhibit gas production, and control symptoms of IBS.

North America: Taiyo International, Inc.
5960 Golden Hills Drive, Minneapolis, MN 55416, USA
Phone: +1-763-398-3003; Fax: +1-763-398-3007

Europe
Phone: +49-711-779-8291; Fax +49-711-779-8292

Japan
Phone: +81-593-47-5427; Fax +81-593-47-5438

Call from Latin America
Phone: +1-763-398-3003; Fax: +1-763-398-3007

Pea fiber

SunOpta Ingredients Group
www.sunopta.com/ingredients; ingredients@sunopta.com

Pectin

Herbstreith & Fox KG
www.herbstreith-fox.de
info@herbstreith-fox.de

H&F Classic Pectin: pectins from apples or citrus fruits ranging from high ester and medium ester to low ester products.
H&F Instant Pectin: pectins with improved solubility due to an agglomeration process; especially suitable for nutritional supplements or instant drinks.
H&F Amid Pectin: low and high ester pectins from apples or citrus fruits, partially amidated.

Herbstreith & Fox KG
Pektin-Fabriken, Turnstr. 37
D-75305 Neuenburg, Germany
Phone: +49-7082-79130; Fax: +49-7082-20281

Herbstreith & Fox Inc
570 Taxter Road, Elmsford, New York 10523, USA
www.herbstreith-fox.com
usa@herbstreith-fox.com
Phone: +1-914-345-9501; Fax: +1-914-345-0919

Polydextrose

Danisco
Tate and Lyle

Resistant maltodextrin: Fibersol®-2

Matsutani Chemical
webmaster@matsutani.com

Fibersol®-2 (dietary fiber ≥90%)
Fibersol®-2H (hydrogenated Fibersol®-2, available in Asia-Pacific region)
Fibersol®-2 is a soluble dietary fiber that helps promote intestinal regularity and healthy levels of blood glucose, insulin, and triglyceride

Website address: www.matsutani.com
Physical address: Matsutani Chemical Industry Co., Ltd.
5-3 Kita-itami, Itami, Hyogo 664-8508
Phone: +81-72-771-2013; Fax: +81-72-771-7447

Resistant maltodextrin: Nutriose
NUTRIOSE® FM06—Resistant dextrin made from cornstarch with 85% soluble fiber
NUTRIOSE® FM10—Resistant dextrin made from cornstarch with 70% soluble fiber
NUTRIOSE® FB06—Resistant dextrin made from wheat starch with 85% soluble fiber
NUTRIOSE® FB10—Resistant dextrin made from wheat starch with 70% soluble fiber

Roquette Frères
Corporate headquarters
62080 Lestrem, France
Phone: +33-32163-3600; Fax: +33-32163-3850

Roquette America, Inc.
1417 Exchange Street, PO Box 6647, Keokuk. IA 52632-6647, USA
Phone: +1 319-524-5757; Fax: + 1-319-526-2345

National Starch—Distribution in North America:
www.foodinnovation.com
10 Finderne Avenue, Bridgewater, New Jersey 07830, USA

Resistant starch
National Starch
www.foodinnovation.com

Hi-maize 5 in 1 fiber: Benefits range from weight management, glycemic (blood sugar) management, energy management, and digestive health. More than 40 human studies using natural Hi-maize and Novelose provide a high level of confidence that the benefits are reliable and real.
Hi-maize® 220 Resistant Starch—High-amylose corn with 20% insoluble dietary fiber
Hi-maize® 260 Resistant Starch—High-amylose corn with 60% insoluble dietary fiber
Hi-maize® Flour 120—Natural corn flour, resistant starch with 20% fiber
Hi-maize® Flour 150—Natural corn flour, resistant starch with 50% fiber
Hi-maize® Meal 130—Natural corn meal, resistant starch with 30% fiber
Hi-maize® Meal 150—Natural corn meal, resistant starch with 50% fiber
Hi-maize® Whole Grain Corn Flour—Resistant starch with 25% fiber
NOVELOSE® 330—Source of RS3 resistant starch with 30% dietary fiber

Rice bran fiber
CJ Cheiljedang and CJ America
http://cjamerica.com
foodingredients@cj.net; jenniferjang@cj.net; jinhpark@cj.net636

Riber®, rice fiber, prepared from defatted rice bran, is an excellent source of insoluble hypoallergenic and gluten-free fiber. It can be applied to various foods to enhance texture, increase yield, extend shelf life, or increase the level of total dietary fiber.

CJ Cheiljedang
600 5-Ga Namdaemun-Ro Jung-Gu, Seoul, Korea
Phone: +82-2-2629-5394; Fax: +82-2-2629-5560

CJ America
3500 Lacey Road # 230
Downers Grove, IL 60515-5423, USA
+1-630-241-0112

Rice Fiber 300
Rice hull fiber has >91% total fiber, of which >97% is insoluble dietary fiber. The rice hull fiber contains no sulfites, added flavors, components from an animal source, BHA, BHT, genetically altered plant material, or irradiated material.

Color: Cream to beige
Flavor: Bland to slightly sweet, no off flavors
Physical form: Fine powder (particle size; >40% retained on Mesh #325, >20% retained on Mesh #200, and less than 10% retained on Mesh #100)

Water holding capacity: >300% of fiber weight
Sun Opta Ingredient Group
ingredients@sunopta.com

Soy fiber
SunOpta Ingredients Group
www.sunopta.com/ingredients; ingredients@sunopta.com

The Solae Company
PO Box 88940, St. Louis, MO 63188, USA
Local: +1-314-659-3000; Phone: +1-800-325-7108

Solae Europe S.A.
2 chemin du Pavillon, CH-1218 Le Grand-Saconnex, Geneva, Switzerland
Phone: +41-22-717-6420; Fax: +41-22-717-6401

Sugar beet fiber
Danisco and IFC
Fibrex

Sugar cane fiber
JRS (J. Rettenmaier & Söhne)
www.jrsusa.com; www.jrs.de; info@jrsusa.com

Xylooligosaccharides
Shandong Longlive Bio-Technology Co., Ltd.
http://www.longlivegroup.com

A super prebiotic ingredient; XOS is effective in increasing the number of bifido-bacteria at a dose of 1.4 g/day.

No.91, Hanhuai St., Yucheng High-Tech Development Zone,
Shandong Province, 251200, China
Phone: +86-531-819-26176

Other fibers: wheat fiber, bamboo fiber, cottonseed fiber, potato fiber, pea fiber, apple fiber, orange fiber, psyllium
J. Rettenmaier
www.jrsusa.com, www.jrs.de
Email: info@jrsusa.com

Vitacel® fibers are available in a variety of grades suitable for use in bakery, cereal, bar, and beverage applications for fiber fortification, calorie reduction, fat reduction, and structural enhancement.

International Fiber Corporation: JustFiber® line including cottonseed fiber, white wheat fiber, and bamboo fiber
www.ifcfiber.com; industrialsales@ifcfiber.com

North Tonawanda, NY 14120, USA
Phone: +1-888-698-1936; Fax: +1-716-693-3528

Other carbohydrates behave like fiber
Tagatose
CJ Cheiljedang and CJ America
http://cjamerica.com
foodingredients@cj.net; jenniferjang@cj.net; jinhpark@cj.net636

- TagaSweet®, a naturally occurring epimer of D-fructose, is as sweet as sugar, yet it has only 1.5 kcal/g. Tagatose helps promote glycemic control and intestinal regularity. Tagatose has flavor-masking effects for stevia. Thus, tagatose can be used with or without stevia or high intensity sweeteners. TagaSweet can be used in beverages and ready-to-eat cereals.

Psicose

CJ Cheiljedang and CJ America

http://cjamerica.com

foodingredients@cj.net; jenniferjang@cj.net; jinhpark@cj.net636

Psicose is an ultralow-energy monosaccharide sugar with 0.2 kcal/g. Psicose helps promote glycemic control and intestinal regularity. It can be used as a sugar substitute in diet or low-calorie foods, such as soft and hard candy, desserts, bakery products, beverages, or table-top sugar.

Index